Experimental and Clinical Metastasis

Julia V. Burnier • Miguel N. Burnier, Jr.
Editors

Experimental and Clinical Metastasis

A Comprehensive Review

Springer

Editors
Julia V. Burnier
Centre for Genomic Regulation
Barcelona, Spain

Miguel N. Burnier, Jr.
Ophthalmology, Pathology, Oncology, Medicine
McGill University, Montreal, QC
Canada

ISBN 978-1-4614-3684-3 ISBN 978-1-4614-3685-0 (eBook)
DOI 10.1007/978-1-4614-3685-0
Springer New York Heidelberg Dordrecht London

Library of Congress Control Number: 2012954252

Printed on acid-free paper

Springer is part of Springer Science+Business Media (www.springer.com)

The student begins with the patient, continues with the patient, and ends his studies with the patient, using books and lectures as tools, as means to an end.

Sir William Osler

Preface

In the great majority of cases, cancer death is, in fact, "Death by Metastasis". Primary cancers, in and of themselves, are seldom fatal, and it is only the distal colonization of vital organs by metastatic cells that results in the demise of the patient.

Metastatic disease is a late event in the evolution of a cancer, and requires the development of a subset of cells in the tumour that can survive the successful cellular odyssey required for metastatic disease to occur. Amongst the biological properties that such cells must acquire include those of self-sufficiency, the capacity to withstand anti-growth signals, resistance to factors inducing apoptosis, and the limitless capacity for reproductive potential. In addition, the metastatic cellular invaders must be able to establish sustained angiogenesis for metastatic lesions to become entrenched and grow. The events resulting in secondary tumours is a remarkably orchestrated change in both the genetic and proteomic expression of the malignant cells. This is a magnificent biological process, but unfortunately it almost invariably results in a terrible outcome for the patient.

The individual steps that allow the relatively fragile metastatic cells to detach from the mother lode of the primary cancer and then interact with what must be considered the hostile microenvironment of the host continue to be unravelled. Indeed, the tumour microenvironment plays a critical role in both primary and metastatic tumour development. This interstitium consists of both a blood and lymphatic vasculature with endothelial linings, as well as a variety of cells (fibroblasts, adipocytes, and host inflammatory cells) secreting extracellular matrix proteins, with all of which the primary and metastatic cells must interact successfully, to survive and grow.

After accomplishing the journey through either the blood or lymphatic vasculature, the metastatic cells must find an appropriate tissue in which to establish secondary tumour sites. Here, the 'seed and soil' hypothesis requires that the micrometastases find what has been referred to as "fertile soil" in which to come to rest, often referred to as site-specific metastasis, or 'homing'. Just exactly what "fertile soil" implies, has not really been clearly defined. The possibility that breast cancer metastases, having developed in a calcium rich environment, seek bone with a comparable microenvironment, is an interesting concept. However, breast cancer cells will also make their way to the liver and the lung. Regardless of the secondary target organ selected, there can be little doubt that the establishment of a secondary tumour site again requires successful interaction with the unique microenvironment of the target organ.

It is well established that the vast majority of metastatic cells never go on to develop secondary lesions. Whether this is due to apoptotic cancer cell death, through host-generated immune reactions, by inhibition of angiogenesis, or by factors yet to be determined, is under intense investigation. Metastatic dormancy certainly occurs in many tumours, the prototype of which may well be uveal melanoma. Micrometastatic uveal melanoma cells are clearly demonstrable in the circulation both before and after tumour excision or radiation, yet it is not at all uncommon for the initial clinically manifestations of liver metastases from a uveal melanoma to occur only a decade later. Have the metastatic cells taken up initial residence in the liver and simply 'waited' for the appropriate opportunity in order to multiply, or have they been resident elsewhere, and only latterly moved into the liver, with immediate growth?

With the foregoing factors in mind, the co-editors of this splendid volume, Miguel and Julia Burnier, father and daughter, have compiled a remarkable text with contributions from outstanding experts in every aspect of the metastatic process. Many of the cellular and molecular factors in metastatic disease that have been noted above, and many others, are addressed in the various comprehensive chapters of the book, each written by an expert in the field. The problems of metastatic cell survival, the route around metastatic suppressor factors, the role of growth factor systems and angiogenesis are clearly defined, and the problems yet to be solved are discussed. Our knowledge about the ever- increasing importance of the role of the microenvironment in tumour progression is expertly defined, and such parameters as metastatic cell dormancy as it occurs in such tumours as uvular melanoma, is considered.

Taken together, this is a volume that should find its way to the bookshelves of virtually all Oncologists and, indeed, all physicians and surgeons involved in the care and treatment of cancer patients.

Phil Gold CC, OQ, MD, PhD, FRSC, FRCP©
Douglas G. Cameron Professor of Medicine,
Professor of Physiology and Oncology,
McGill University
Executive Director Clinical Research Centre
McGill University Health Centre

Contents

Contributors

Murad Aljiffry Hepato Pancreato Biliary and Transplant, McGill University, Montreal, QC, Canada

Sarah Assadian Goodman Cancer Research Centre and Department of Biochemistry, McGill University, 1160 Pine Avenue, Montreal, QC H3A 1A3, Canada

Silvin Bakalian MD, PhD Henry C. Witelson Ocular Pathology Laboratory, McGill University, Montreal, QC, Canada
e-mail: sbakalian@hotmail.com

Nicholas R. Bertos Rosalind & Morris Goodman Cancer Research Centre, McGill University, 1160 Ave. des Pins O., Montreal, QC H3A 1A3, Canada
e-mail: nicholas.bertos@mcgill.ca

Department of Medicine, McGill University, Montreal, QC, Canada

Miguel N. Burnier, Jr. MD, PhD, FRCSC Ophthalmology, Pathology, Oncology, Medicine, McGill University, Montreal, QC, Canada
e-mail: miguel.burnier@mcgill.ca

Julia V. Burnier PhD Centre for Genomic Regulation, Barcelona, Spain
e-mail: julia.burnier@mail.mcgill.ca

Ann F. Chambers PhD Departments of Oncology, Medical Biophysics, and Pathology, University of Western Ontario, London, ON, Canada
e-mail: ann.chambers@Lhsc.on.ca

Prosanto Chaudhury Surgery and Oncology, King Saud University, Montreal, QC, Canada

Jonathan Cools-Lartigue MD Department of Surgery, McGill University, Montreal, QC, Canada
e-mail: jonathan.cools-lartigue@mail.mcgill.ca

Fabio Luis Cury Department of Radiation Oncology, McGill University, Montreal, QC, Canada

Jeremy Dupaul-Chicoine Department of Biochemistry, McGill University Health Centre, 687 Pine Ave. W., Montreal, QC H3G 1Y62, Canada

Wissal El-Assaad Goodman Cancer Research Centre, McGill University, 1160 Pine Avenue, Montreal, QC H3A 1A3, Canada

Dana Faingold MD, PhD Henry C. Witelson Ocular Pathology Laboratory, McGill University, Montreal, QC, Canada
e-mail: faingolddana@yahoo.com

Dominique Fausto de Souza MD Dermatologist from the Federal University of Rio de Janeiro, Rio de Janeiro, Brazil

Henry C Witelson Ocular Pathology Laboratory, McGill University, Montreal, QC, Canada

Bruno F. Fernandes MD, PhD Department of Ophthalmology & Pathology, Henry C. Witelson Ocular Pathology Laboratory McGill University, Montreal, Canada
e-mail: bruno.mtl@gmail.com

Mazen Hassanain MBBS, FRCS(C), PhD Prince Naif research institute, King Saud University, Riyadh, Saudi Arabi

Eli Kakiashvili Surgical Oncology, McGill University, Montreal, QC, Canada

Jennifer M. Kirstein Department of Medical Biophysics, University of Western Ontario, London, ON, Canada

Karen J. Lefebvre Goodman Cancer Research Centre and Department of Biochemistry, McGill University, 1160 Pine Avenue, Montreal, QC H3A 1A3, Canada
e-mail: jose.teodoro@mcgill.ca

Patrick T. Logan M.Sc McGill University, Montreal, QC, Canada
e-mail: patrick.logan@mail.mcgill.ca

Shawn C. Maloney Henry C. Witelson Ocular Pathology Laboratory, McGill University, Montreal, QC, Canada

Claudia Maria de Oliveira Martins MD, MSc Henry C. Witelson Ocular Pathology Laboratory, McGill University, Montreal, QC, Canada

Jean-Claude Marshall MSc., PhD. National Cancer Institute, 37 Convent Blvd, Building 37, Bethesda, MD, USA
e-mail: jeanclaude.marshall@gmail.com

Ari-Nareg Meguerditchian MD, MSc, FRCS Department of Surgery, Faculty of Medicine, McGill University, Montreal, QC, Canada

McGill University Health Centre, Montreal, QC, Canada

Sarkis H. Meterissian MD, MSc, FRCS, FACS McGill University, Montreal, QC, Canada

Peter Metrakos FRCS(C), FACS Multi-Organ Transplant Program, MUHC, McGill University, Montreal, QC, Canada

Hepatic, Pancreatic and Biliary Surgery, McGill University, Montreal, QC, Canada

Catalin Mihalcioiu MD, FRCPC Medicine & Oncology, Royal Victoria Hospital, McGill University, Montreal, QC, Canada

Dr. Mohib Morcos MD Faculty of Medicine, Laval University, Quebec, QC, Canada

William J. Muller PhD, FRSC Department of Biochemistry and Medicine, McGill University, Montreal, QC, Canada
e-mail: william.muller@mcgill.ca

Alexandre Nakao Odashiro MD, PhD Département de Pathologie & Cytologie du Centre Hospitalier Affilié universitaire de Québec (CHA), Hôpital l'Enfant-Jésus, local 1210 1401, 18e rue, Québec, QC G1J 1Z4, Canada

Morag Park Rosalind & Morris Goodman Cancer Research Centre, McGill University, 1160 Ave. des Pins O., Montreal, QC H3A 1A3, Canada

Department of Medicine, McGill University, Montreal, QC, Canada

Departments of Oncology and Biochemistry, McGill University, Montreal, QC, Canada

Department of Medicine, McGill University Health Centre, Montreal, QC, Canada

Patricia Rusa Pereira MD, PhD Henry C. Witelson Ocular Pathology Laboratory, McGill University, Montreal, Canada
e-mail: bruno.mtl@gmail.com

Marissa Grace Ponzo MD, PhD McGill University, Montreal, QC, Canada

Abelardo A. Rodríguez-Reys MD Asociación Para Evitar la Ceguera en México, Hospital "Dr. Luis Sánchez Bulnes", Faculty of Medicine, Universidad Nacional Autónoma de Mexico (UNAM), Ciudad de México, México
e-mail: bruno.mtl@gmail.com

Dawn Russell-Hermanns MD McGill University, Montreal, QC, Canada

Maya Saleh Department of Biochemistry, McGill University Health Centre, 687 Pine Ave. W., Montreal, QC H3G 1Y62, Canada

Department of Medicine, McGill University, Montreal, QC H3G 1Y62, Canada

Department of Microbiology and Immunology, McGill University, Montreal, QC H3A 2B4, Canada
e-mail: maya.saleh@mcgill.ca

George Shenouda MBBCh, PhD, FRCP(C) Radiation Oncology, McGill University Health Centre, McGill University, Montreal, QC, Canada

Jonathan Spicer MD Department of Surgery, McGill University, Montreal, QC, Canada

Ian Swanson M.Sc., MD Department of Biochemistry and Medicine, McGill University, Montreal, QC, Canada

Jose G. Teodoro Goodman Cancer Research Centre and Department of Biochemistry, McGill University, 1160 Pine Avenue, Montreal, QC H3A 1A3, Canada
e-mail: jose.teodoro@mcgill.ca

Part I
Introduction to Metastatic Diseases

Editors:
Julia V. Burnier and Miguel N. Burnier, Jr.

Chapter 1
Introduction

Julia V. Burnier and Miguel N. Burnier, Jr.

Metastatic disease is the most lethal aspect of human malignancies, making the understanding and continued research into the process of metastasis a crucial step in treating cancer. The lethality of malignant neoplasms is attributable directly to the development of secondary growths in organs often at a distance from the primary tumor mass (Fidler et al. 1978). While most primary tumors are treatable and manageable by local resection or irradiation, disseminated cancer cells are often immune to our methods of treatment. Few therapeutic options for patients have demonstrated potential in curing metastatic disease. The molecular mechanisms underlying site-specific metastasis and the factors mediating tumor cell homing remain largely unknown. In this introductory chapter, the metastatic cascade will be reviewed, with emphasis on the individual steps of the metastatic process and the routes of cell dissemination. In addition, the molecular mechanisms driving site-specific metastasis and tumor cell homing to specific sites will be discussed.

1.1 Metastatic Cascade

Tumor metastasis is a complex multi-step process that involves many cell and organ-mediated steps culminating in the establishment of metastatic tumors in distant organ sites (Steeg 2006). As metastatic cells detach from the primary tumor, migrate and invade through tissue barriers, enter the circulation, arrest and interact with endothelial cells of the vascular network, extravasate and grow in the target organ, they must communicate with their rapidly changing microenvironments through cell-cell and cell-ECM contacts and the release of soluble mediators (reviewed in Steeg 2006;

J. V. Burnier (✉)
Centre for Genomic Regulation, Barcelona, Spain
e-mail: julia.burnier@mail.mcgill.ca

M. N. Burnier, Jr.
Ophthalmology, Pathology, Oncology, Medicine, McGill University, Montreal, QC, Canada
e-mail: miguel.burnier@mcgill.ca

J. V. Burnier, M. N. Burnier, Jr. (eds.), *Experimental and Clinical Metastasis*,
DOI 10.1007/978-1-4614-3685-0_1, © Springer Science+Business Media New York 2013

Chambers et al. 2002; Langley and Fidler 2007). These cells must acquire the genetic and epigenetic changes necessary to survive all of these steps. The expression of a distinct set of genes involved in cell-cell and cell-ECM interactions as well as migration, growth, angiogenic and inflammatory factors plays a major role in permitting or restricting metastasis (Nguyen and Massague 2007; Hanahan and Weinberg 2000; Baylin and Ohm 2006). For metastasis to successfully develop, all steps of the cascade need to be completed; i.e. all steps are rate-limiting. Mouse models using transformed cells show us that oncogenic transformation is not always sufficient to cause tumors and that a stimuli can lead to tumors in a specific organ. Moreover, not all patients with circulating malignant cells, i.e. cells with metastatic potential, will go on to suffer from metastatic disease. Indeed it is evident that metastasis is a series of steps that culminate to metastatic tumors in a highly specific manner. Although a great deal of research has focused on all of the metastatic steps, and the biology of the cascade has been extensively studied, there has been little progress in effectively preventing or treating metastatic disease.

1.1.1 Change in Phenotype

The metastatic process is a highly inefficient process with a higher tendency of cells to die than to metastasize (Luzzi et al. 1998). First, cell populations of the primary tumor acquire mutations resulting in a change of phenotype. In fact, metastatic cells are characterized by genetic changes causing them to be more invasive and motile. Tumor cells are more prone to mutation that their normal counterparts (Cifone and Fidler 1981; Eccles and Welch 2007) and this genetic instability results in the accumulation of genetic changes enabling a more aggressive phenotype. Experimentally transformed cells are also characterized by genetic and phenotypic flux (Cifone and Fidler 1981). In addition, the proliferation and progression of certain cell populations are mediated through a selection pressure based on the tumor environment, immune system, and host factors. Cell subpopulations, even in large metastatic tumors, can have a wide variety of gene expression profiles and display distinct behavior in vitro (Eccles and Welch 2007; Welch and Goldberg 1997). A variety of transient and permanent genetic changes are required for cells to survive the metastatic cascade, including changes in the expression of integrins, chemokines, proteases, angiogenic factors, and adhesion molecules. To date, most of the gene profiling performed on metastatic cells compare end point lesions to benign or primary tumors. These studies do not account or provide data on the many transitory cell population characteristics not seen in the primary tumor or in established metastasis. To compliment these end-point assays, new studies have emerged which involve real-time analyses of gene changes in tumor cells over the course of the metastatic cascade (Luzzi et al. 1998; Cameron et al. 2000).

One major occurrence that initiates metastasis is the change in cell adhesion markers on the tumor cell surface, enabling the cell to detach from the primary tumor. It has been well documented that integrins, the cell surface receptors for the extracellular matrix, are altered in metastatic cell populations (Hood and Cheresh 2002;

Felding-Habermann 2003). In addition, secretion of ECM and proteolytic enzymes leads to the degradation of the basement membrane, allowing the cells to invade. Evidence suggests that many of these changes are stimulated by growth factors in the tumor milieu. Proteolytic degradation of the ECM can also release sequestered growth factors that further promote the invasive phenotype (Saad et al. 2002).

Many of these changes can occur by a process of dedifferentiation, referred to as the epithelial to mesenchymal transition (EMT) (Thompson et al. 2005). Neoplastic cells can dedifferentiate to a more motile mesenchymal phenotype during the process of metastasis, which is often also accompanied by a resistance to apoptosis (Robson et al. 2006). This can be induced by TGF signaling as well as other oncogenic signaling pathways (Siegel et al. 2003). Once in the metastatic site, there can be a reversion back to the differentiated epithelial phenotype as the cells no longer require motility or invasiveness.

1.1.2 Survival in the Bloodstream

Tumors are unable to grow beyond 0.4 mm in diameter without a vascular system to support the proliferating tumor cells (Bergers and Benjamin 2003; Gimbrone et al. 1972). A leaky network of neovessels not only provides oxygen and nutrients for the primary tumor, but can also act as a route through which malignant cells can enter the bloodstream (Wyckoff et al. 2000). It has been documented that tumors with high metastatic potential are more angiogenic than non-metastatic tumors (Folkman 1996). As millions of cells are shed from the primary tumor and enter the bloodstream, they encounter a harsh environment where less than 0.01 % of circulating malignant cells go on to successfully form metastasis (Luzzi et al. 1998). The shear stress and velocity-associated pressure of the bloodstream, as well as the presence of immune cells, can result in tumor cell death of the greater proportion of circulating cancer cells. In addition, whereas in the primary tumor, cells are attached to the substratum of the host organ and to the network of cancer cells within the tumor; once they detach and migrate they must survive in an anchorage-independent manner. Anoikis is a term used to describe apoptosis in the absence of cellular attachment. In experimental models, anchorage requirement is lost upon oncogenic transformation. Metastatic cells often have mechanisms to evade anoikis, such as over expression of RTKs, which may contribute this may contribute to tumor cell survival in the circulation. Indeed, malignant cells possess signaling mechanisms that protect them from anoikis (Grossmann 2002). Furthermore, as more is known about the mechanisms contributing to anoikis, it has become evident that anchorage-independent growth as an anti-anoikis process is a major characteristic contributing to malignancy.

1.1.3 Attachment and Extravasation

During circulation, malignant cells that survive the bloodstream, must arrest and extravasate into the target organ. In order to enter the target organ, malignant cells must adhere to capillary beds and interact with endothelial cells. Two different types of cell arrest have been demonstrated. Nonspecific arrest due to coagulation factors and capillary diameter results in cells lodging (Weiss et al. 1986). This means that tumor cells enter capillaries and are unable to pass through due to their size. Once lodged, they can extravasate between endothelial cells of the organ lining. Specific interactions can also occur and are mediated through tumor cell expression of vascular adhesion factors specific to the organ (such as selectins and tumor necrosis factor-alpha) and by secretion of factors by the vascular microenvironment (Steeg 2006). In fact, endothelial cells from different organs capillary beds possess different vascular markers and this can add to the site-specificity of tumor cell infiltration (Trepel et al. 2002). The changes, or re-expression of adhesion molecules likely occur through post-translational modification of cell surface receptors. Due to the short time frame for this process to occur, it is unlikely that cancer cells alter their gene expression during circulation (Eccles and Welch 2007; Christofori 2003). It is possible that, both specific and non-specific arrest occurs during metastasis, and successful colonization depends on the affinity of tumor cells to their new environment.

1.1.4 Colonization and Proliferation

Once cells have extravasated into the parenchyma of the target site, they must form metastatic foci. The time gap between infiltration of metastatic cells and the occurrence of colonization represents the latency of the disease (Nguyen et al. 2009). Colonization of the organ is the most extensively in vivo studied step of the metastatic cascade because of the use of experimental metastasis animal models. Successful metastatic colonization involves reciprocal interactions between infiltrating tumor cells and a foreign microenvironment. Organ microenvironments vary from site to site and the requirements for tumor cell growth in the microenvironment of the secondary site is therefore distinct from that at the primary tumor site. The extracellular matrix as well as cells such as fibroblasts, endothelial cells and inflammatory cells secrete growth factors, chemokines, cytokines, and proteases that can act as signals for the promotion or deterrent of metastatic growth. For example, the insulin growth factor 1 - receptor has been found to be a regulator of liver metastasis and this is at least in part due to the abundance of the receptor's ligand, IGF-I secreted by hepatocytes (Long et al. 1994). Infiltrating tumor cells, which express IGF-IR, will therefore receive a strong mitogenic signal from the liver, inducing metastatic growth. Moreover, the recent notion by Kaplan and colleagues that progenitor cells can migrate from the bone marrow to potential sites of metastasis, which they then condition as a 'pre-metastatic niche' by secretion of factors which facilitate or drive tumor cell homing to specific sites has further confounded our understanding of site-specific metastasis (Kaplan et al. 2006).

1.2 Routes of Cell Dissemination and Site-Specific Metastasis

The site, timing, and severity of metastasis vary among individuals and type of malignancy. The reasons for this remain mainly unknown. In 1988, Weiss et al showed that the primary site of metastasis occurs at the first capillary bed encountered (Weiss et al. 1988). This idea is centered upon different malignancies having distinct patterns of cancer spread, determined by the route of cell dissemination. It is increasingly apparent, however, that this is not the only factor mediating the development of metastatic disease. Weiss later showed, through a series of autopsy studies that only 66 % of tumors were predicted by blood flow patterns alone; other mechanisms must account for the remainder of the metastases (Weiss 1992).

Many routes of tumor cell dissemination are associated with metastatic occurrence. While many cancers spread via hematogenous dissemination, it is also common to see secondary tumors arise via the initial entry of cancer cells entry into lymphatics, ultimately draining to lymph nodes and the blood stream. The absence or presence of lymph node tumors can be a prognostic predictor (such as in the case of head and neck cancers) and is critical for prognosis (Wittekind 2000). The TNM prognostic grading system takes into account the extent of the primary tumor, lymph node positivity, and metastatic growth. In addition, local or proximity metastatic disease can occur by spreading across body cavities (such as in the case of ovarian tumors). In the absence of lymph node or metastatic positivity, patient blood is currently being assayed for the presence of disseminated tumor cells. Cytokeratins, for example, are being used as a marker for these cells (Wong and Hynes 2006). The significance of circulating malignant cells is still in debate, perhaps due to its overestimated value or inadequate techniques for detecting disseminated cells (Wong and Hynes 2006).

However, while we can explain some metastatic sites via anatomical dissemination, it remains unclear why some breast cancers metastasize to the liver and some to organs as distant as the bone, brain, and lungs. Uveal melanoma tumors, which grow in an immune-privileged site void of lymphatic association to the rest of the body, show site-predilection to the liver. Over 100 years ago, the surgeon Stephen Paget predicted that there are properties of both the cancer cell "seed", as well as factors in the microenvironment of the target organs "soil" that allow for metastatic growth (Paget 1889). However, the host and tumor-dependent factors that regulate the organ-selectivity of disseminating cancer cells and determine their ultimate destination remained until recently, largely unknown (Fidler 2003). Moreover, the relationship between these two entities and the pathways that synergize as a metastasis progresses, may be the central regulator of the site-specificity of metastasis. As previously mentioned, a "pre-metastatic" niche may be forming before tumor cells arrest in target organs, perhaps by stem-cell mediated organ conditioning for malignant growth, thereby mediating site-selectivity. Unknown factors influence stem cell recruitment to tissues, remodeling of the matrix, and modifications of the environment; these factors can precondition the growth of metastatic cells at that site (Kaplan et al. 2006).

1.3 Research in Metastatic Disease

While we appreciate the importance of clinical metastasis, little is known about what causes metastatic disease, what determines site of metastasis, and the biological mechanisms behind cancer spread. The difficulty in understanding metastatic disease lies in the wide variety of timing, distribution, and severity of secondary tumors. In humans, only the late stages of metastasis are generally clinically detected, such as a large enough tumor to be imaged. Extensive in vitro and in vivo work has been done to understand key steps of the metastatic cascade. Experimental metastasis models, in which tumor cells are injected directly into the blood stream of animals have facilitated research in this field. However, while this model presents advantages of ease, reproducibility, and time efficiency, it does not give insight into the metastatic process as an entity, but merely on the later steps of survival in the blood stream and colonization of the host organ. On the other hand, spontaneous metastasis models better mimic the disease occurrence and provide vital information as to early steps in metastatic occurrence. We have unfortunately learned however, that animal models of metastatic disease do not always adequately represent the disease progression in humans and valuable but limited knowledge can be learned from them.

Predicting tumor cell homing to specific sites has become a focus in cancer research. Recent advances in genomic and proteomic profiling of tumor cell populations have provided novel and powerful tools for identifying gene subsets that are preferentially expressed in tumor subpopulations with predilections for specific metastatic sites. High throughput micro array analysis technology capable of quickly and efficiently quantifying changes in the expression of thousands of genes has facilitated the study of genetic changes in cell and tissue models. These studies have begun to yield information on gene signatures that are associated with site-specific metastasis to organs such as the lung, bone, and brain (Fidler and Kripke 2003; Palmieri et al. 2006; Minn et al. 2005a, b). Since even the activation of a single gene can be sufficient to induce metastasis, and given that many gene changes show site-specificity (Pozzatti et al. 1986; Veer et al. 2002), determining distinct genetic profiles for metastatic cells is crucial to understanding tumor progression and spread. Moreover, prognosis and response to treatment have also been predicted (Sorlie et al. 2001; Vijver et al. 2002) as well as the involvement of angiogenic- and hypoxia-associated genes via the usage of gene expression profiling (Eynden et al. 2007). What is of crucial interest is two-fold: understanding why some cells metastasize and what determines preferential homing of cells to a specific site.

References

Baylin SB, Ohm JE (2006) Epigenetic gene silencing in cancer—a mechanism for early oncogenic pathway addiction? Nat Rev Cancer 6:107–116

Bergers G, Benjamin LE (2003) Tumorigenesis and the angiogenic switch. Nat Rev Cancer 3:401–410

Cameron MD et al (2000) Temporal progression of metastasis in lung: cell survival, dormancy, and location dependence of metastatic inefficiency. Cancer Res 60:2541–2546

Chambers AF, Groom AC, MacDonald IC (2002) Dissemination and growth of cancer cells in metastatic sites. Nat Rev Cancer 2:563–572

Christofori G (2003) Changing neighbours, changing behaviour: cell adhesion molecule-mediated signalling during tumour progression. EMBO J 22:2318–2323

Cifone MA, Fidler IJ (1981) Increasing metastatic potential is associated with increasing genetic instability of clones isolated from murine neoplasms. Proc Natl Acad Sci U S A 78:6949–6952

Eccles SA, Welch DR (2007) Metastasis: recent discoveries and novel treatment strategies. Lancet 369:1742–1757

Felding-Habermann B (2003) Integrin adhesion receptors in tumor metastasis. Clin Exp Metastasis 20:203–213

Fidler IJ (2003) The pathogenesis of cancer metastasis: the 'seed and soil' hypothesis revisited. Nat Rev Cancer 3:453–458

Fidler IJ, Kripke ML (2003) Genomic analysis of primary tumors does not address the prevalence of metastatic cells in the population. Nat Genet 34:23 (author reply 25)

Fidler IJ, Gersten DM, Hart IR (1978) The biology of cancer invasion and metastasis. Adv Cancer Res 28:149–250

Folkman J (1996) New perspectives in clinical oncology from angiogenesis research. Eur J Cancer 32A:2534–2539

Gimbrone MA Jr, Leapman SB, Cotran RS, Folkman J (1972) Tumor dormancy in vivo by prevention of neovascularization. J Exp Med 136:261–276

Grossmann J (2002) Molecular mechanisms of "detachment-induced apoptosis–Anoikis". Apoptosis 7:247–260

Hanahan D, Weinberg RA (2000) The hallmarks of cancer. Cell 100:57–70

Hood JD, Cheresh DA (2002) Role of integrins in cell invasion and migration. Nat Rev Cancer 2:91–100

Kaplan RN, Rafii S, Lyden D (2006) Preparing the "soil": the premetastatic niche. Cancer Res 66:11089–11093

Langley RR, Fidler IJ (2007) Tumor cell-organ microenvironment interactions in the pathogenesis of cancer metastasis. Endocr Rev 28:297–321

Long L, Nip J, Brodt P (1994) Paracrine growth stimulation by hepatocyte-derived insulin-like growth factor-1: a regulatory mechanism for carcinoma cells metastatic to the liver. Cancer Res 54:3732–3737

Luzzi KJ et al (1998) Multistep nature of metastatic inefficiency: dormancy of solitary cells after successful extravasation and limited survival of early micrometastases. Am J Pathol 153:865–873

Minn AJ et al (2005a) Genes that mediate breast cancer metastasis to lung. Nature 436:518–524

Minn AJ et al (2005b) Distinct organ-specific metastatic potential of individual breast cancer cells and primary tumors. J Clin Invest 115:44–55

Nguyen DX, Massague J (2007) Genetic determinants of cancer metastasis. Nat Rev Genet 8:341–352

Nguyen DX, Bos PD, Massague J (2009) Metastasis: from dissemination to organ-specific colonization. Nat Rev Cancer 9:274–284

Paget S (1889) The distribution of secondary growth in cancer of the breast. Lancet 1:3

Palmieri D et al (2006) Brain metastases of breast cancer. Breast Dis 26:139–147

Pozzatti R et al (1986) Primary rat embryo cells transformed by one or two oncogenes show different metastatic potentials. Science 232:223–227

Robson EJ, Khaled WT, Abell K, Watson CJ (2006) Epithelial-to-mesenchymal transition confers resistance to apoptosis in three murine mammary epithelial cell lines. Differentiation 74:254–264

Saad S, Gottlieb DJ, Bradstock KF, Overall CM, Bendall LJ (2002) Cancer cell-associated fibronectin induces release of matrix metalloproteinase-2 from normal fibroblasts. Cancer Res 62:283–289

Siegel PM, Shu W, Cardiff RD, Muller WJ, Massague J (2003) Transforming growth factor beta signaling impairs Neu-induced mammary tumorigenesis while promoting pulmonary metastasis. Proc Natl Acad Sci U S A 100:8430–8435

Sorlie T et al (2001) Gene expression patterns of breast carcinomas distinguish tumor subclasses with clinical implications. Proc Natl Acad Sci U S A 98:10869–10874

Steeg PS (2006) Tumor metastasis: mechanistic insights and clinical challenges. Nat Med 12:895–904

Thompson EW, Newgreen DF, Tarin D (2005) Carcinoma invasion and metastasis: a role for epithelial-mesenchymal transition? Cancer Res 65:5991–5995; discussion 5995

Trepel M, Arap W, Pasqualini R (2002) In vivo phage display and vascular heterogeneity: implications for targeted medicine. Curr Opin Chem Biol 6:399–404

van de Vijver MJ et al (2002) A gene-expression signature as a predictor of survival in breast cancer. N Engl J Med 347:1999–2009

Van den Eynden GG et al (2007) Differential expression of hypoxia and (lymph)angiogenesis-related genes at different metastatic sites in breast cancer. Clin Exp Metastasis 24:13–23

van 't Veer LJ et al (2002) Gene expression profiling predicts clinical outcome of breast cancer. Nature 415:530–536

Weiss L (1992) Comments on hematogenous metastatic patterns in humans as revealed by autopsy. Clin Exp Metastasis 10:191–199

Weiss L et al (1986) Haematogenous metastatic patterns in colonic carcinoma: an analysis of 1541 necropsies. J Pathol 150:195–203

Weiss L et al (1988) Metastatic patterns of renal carcinoma: an analysis of 687 necropsies. J Cancer Res Clin Oncol 114:605–612

Welch DR, Goldberg SF (1997) Molecular mechanisms controlling human melanoma progression and metastasis. Pathobiology 65:311–330

Wittekind C (2000) Diagnosis and staging of lymph node metastasis. Recent Results Cancer Res 157:20–28

Wong SY, Hynes RO (2006) Lymphatic or hematogenous dissemination: how does a metastatic tumor cell decide? Cell Cycle 5:812–817

Wyckoff JB, Jones JG, Condeelis JS, Segall JE (2000) A critical step in metastasis: in vivo analysis of intravasation at the primary tumor. Cancer Res 60:2504–2511

Chapter 2
Interactions of Normal Tissues and Systems with Metastatic Cells: Impact on Location, Survival and Growth

Jennifer M. Kirstein and Ann F. Chambers

2.1 Introduction

Tumor formation is not a cell autonomous phenomenon, but rather an evolution of disease within and responding to the host environment. In particular, metastatic spread from a primary tumor results from a complex interplay between tumor cells and the host. In order to form successful metastases, tumor cells must escape the primary tumor, enter the host vasculature, travel to and arrest in a distant tissue and survive and grow in that new organ (Chambers et al. 2002). Cells that progress through these stages must both escape and exploit host systems.

As tumor cells acquire a metastatic phenotype, they do so through interacting with and manipulating host responses (Brooks et al. 2010; Borsig 2008; Lorusso and Ruegg 2008). The tissue microenvironment is significantly altered by the presence of a primary tumor, with changes in stromal cell composition and activation and the presence of infiltrating immune cells. The individual components are specific to tumor type, but the net result is a cycle of mutual stimulation of host and tumor tissue, leading to increased tumor growth and aggressive behavior. For example, in melanoma, direct contact between keratinocytes and melanocytes is essential to maintain normal melanocyte growth characteristics. This contact is maintained by E-cadherin, which is often down-regulated as a first step toward melanoma tumorogenesis (Li et al. 2003). Interestingly, hepatocyte growth factor/scatter factor (HGF/SF) production by fibroblasts is capable of stimulating growth and reducing E-Cadherin expression in normal melanocytes resulting in decreased adhesion to keratinocytes. These normal melanocytes begin to express basic fibroblast growth factor (bFGF), platelet-derived growth factor (PDGF), vascular endothelial growth factor (VEGF) and transforming growth factor-β (TGFβ)—growth factor signals

A. F. Chambers (✉)
Departments of Oncology, Medical Biophysics, and Pathology, University of Western Ontario, London, ON, Canada
e-mail: ann.chambers@Lhsc.on.ca

J. M. Kirstein
Department of Medical Biophysics, University of Western Ontario, London, ON, Canada

J. V. Burnier, M. N. Burnier, Jr. (eds.), *Experimental and Clinical Metastasis*,
DOI 10.1007/978-1-4614-3685-0_2,

then expanded by neighboring fibroblasts which express insulin-like growth factor-1 (IGF-1), HGF/SF, bFGF and TGFβ in response, further stimulating the melanocytes. Therefore, the initial transformation of melanocytes does not necessarily involve major genetic changes, but is a result of losing contact and regulation from keratinocytes, leading to a cycle of mutual positive feedback between stromal cells and melanocytes (reviewed in (Li et al. 2003)). In breast cancer, a loss of tissue organization and polarity is also seen, with increasing disorganization and decreased cell-cell contact as tumor invasiveness increases (Weaver et al. 1997) (reviewed in (Takeichi 1993)).

After initial tumorigenesis, host systems and pathways are further co-opted by tumor cells. Herein we will focus on how particular tumor types are capable of exploiting host cells, growth factors, pathways and systems during each of the key steps in metastasis.

2.2 Tumor Cell Invasion and Intravasation

Excessive proliferation of neoplastic cells in a developing cancer leads to hypoxia and necrosis in the tumor microenvironment. Tumor and stromal cells react by secreting growth factors and cytokines such as colony stimulating factor (CSF)-1 and TGF-β, which are chemoattractants for immune cells (Robinson and Coussens 2005). Further host reaction to the developing neoplasm leads to recruitment of mesenchymal stem cells, activated fibroblasts, endothelial precursors, dendritic cells, macrophages, monocytes, lymphocytes, leukocytes and mast cells (Olumi et al. 1999; Le Bitoux and Stamenkovic 2008). Initially, it is likely that this recruitment is a host defense mechanism, but the tumor is able to capitalize on the pro-growth factors and counteract the growth-inhibitory capabilities of the recruited cells (Le Bitoux and Stamenkovic 2008). It would be expected that an abundance of immune cells would be beneficial for the host, yet it often correlates with poor clinical prognosis (Nonomura et al. 2007; Taskinen et al. 2008), a global indicator of a tumor's ability to subvert the host response.

A major effect of the inflammatory response to tumor development is an increase in tumor invasiveness. Breast cancer cells cultured in macrophage-conditioned media, or co-cultured with macrophages, show a significant increase in invasive behavior in vitro (Wu et al. 2009; Hagemann et al. 2005). This increase was found to be due to nuclear factor kappa B (NF-κB)-mediated stabilization of Snail, a major transcription factor for epithelial—mesenchymal transition (EMT) induction (Nieto 2002). Snail expression by tumor cells conferred metastatic ability to non-metastatic cell lines (MCF7 and T47D) and shRNA knockdown of Snail suppressed both innate and 'inflammation-enhanced' invasion and metastasis of MDA-MB-231 and MDA-MB-435 cells (Wu et al. 2009). Additionally, tumor necrosis factor-α (TNFα) produced by macrophages was found to induce expression of macrophage migration inhibiting factor (MIF) in tumor cells, which led to increased matrix metalloproteinase (MMP) production by macrophages, also through stimulation of NF-κB. This increase in MMP activity was found to aid tumor cell invasion (Hagemann et al. 2005). These

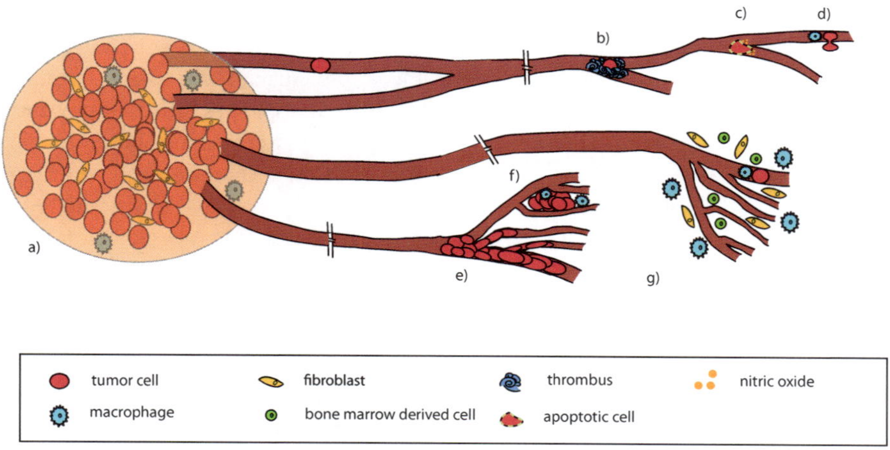

Fig. 2.1 Interaction between metastatic tumor cells and the host environment in early stages of metastasis. *a* A primary tumor is infiltrated with host-derived macrophages and fibroblasts that aid in tumor cell invasion and intravasation. Upon arrest in a secondary site, tumor cells often stimulate formation of a thrombus *b*, which provides adhesion contacts and protection from the host immune system. These arrested cells may undergo apoptosis due to release of nitric oxide from the vascular endothelium *c* or may extravasate, often with assistance from a host macrophage *d*. Not all metastatic cells extravasate prior to initiating growth in a secondary organ, and intravascular micrometastases are found *e*, especially in the lung. Extravascular micrometastatic growths *f* are also common, and often found to be associated with host macrophages. The site of metastatic growth is dependent on many factors, but formation of a pre-metastatic niche *g* is thought to direct and aid initial growth and survival of metastatic cells

results indicate that tumor cells can capitalize on the host immune response leading to increased invasiveness and subsequent metastasis.

Tumor-associated macrophages (TAMs) are often the most common immune cell in the tumor microenvironment and play an essential role in tumor metastasis. Using an in vivo model of mammary carcinoma, it was found that TAMs are most likely to be found at the margin of a primary tumor, with decreasing numbers upon imaging deeper into the tumor (Wyckoff et al. 2007). The few TAMs that were found in the tumor core were associated with blood vessels and were essential for tumor cell intravasation (Fig. 2.1a). There was a significant correlation between the number of perivascular TAMs and the number of circulating tumor cells in this rat model of mammary carcinoma. Additionally, time-lapse imaging was only able to detect tumor cell intravasation at the site of TAM association with the vasculature, and this intravasation was found to be dependent on epidermal growth factor (EGF)-CSF-1 signaling (Wyckoff et al. 2007; Wyckoff et al. 2004; Goswami et al. 2005). Further, deletion of CSF-1 in a murine model of mammary carcinogenesis showed limited tumor invasion coupled with decreased angiogenesis, resulting in abrogation of lung metastasis due to deficient macrophage recruitment to the tumor microenvironment (Lin and Pollard 2004). Analysis of murine and clinical samples found that TAMs may guide breast cancer cells toward blood vessels through EGF-CSF-1 signaling, as cancer cells were often found in contact with perivascular macrophages. The density of these interactions in clinical samples correlated with the histological grade of the tumor and positively associated with the risk of distant metastasis formation (Robinson et al. 2009). It has also been noted that macrophages are often present at the site of basement membrane breach and tumor cell dissemination (Pollard 2004).

Neutrophils, lymphocytes and TAMs all express and secrete MMPs, which collectively can degrade every extracellular matrix (ECM) protein. The association of these immune cells with the invasive border of a tumor leads to a degradation of the physical barrier that prevents tumor cell dissemination. This degradation releases and activates many growth factors (TGFβ, TNFα, Fas Ligand, heparin bound–epidermal growth factor and others) that are normally sequestered in the ECM (Ii et al. 2006; Hynes 2009). Additionally, the degradation products of many ECM proteins have their own activity. For example, degradation of laminin results in peptides that mimic epidermal growth factor receptor (EGFR) ligands and can result in increased cell migration and invasion in EGFR positive cells (Giannelli et al. 1997; Pirila 2003). It is understood that a tumor is not a uniformly organized mass—each tumor cell will have differential access to nutrients, oxygen and tumor stromal components depending on its individual location (Kedrin 2008). Direct imaging of murine mammary tumor growth using a mammary window was able to visualize individual cells longitudinally and evaluate differences in their behavior depending on their initial location. It was found that those cells in close proximity to blood vessels showed increased migration and invasion and were more likely to spread from the primary tumor to the lung than those cells that did not have immediate access to the vasculature (Kedrin 2008).

Immune cells are a key component of tumor stroma, but the most abundant stromal cell is the carcinoma associated fibroblast (CAF) (Orimo and Weinberg 2006) (Fig. 2.1a), which is also associated with an increase in tumor cell invasion. These fibroblasts have been recruited as normal fibroblasts and are activated to become myofibroblasts, or have been recruited as bone marrow derived cells (BMDCs) and differentiate into fibroblasts at the tumor site (Direkze et al. 2004). Using a 3D in vitro model of the epidermal/dermal microenvironment, it was found that invasion of squamous cell carcinoma (SCC) cells always followed a leading CAF (Gaggioli et al. 2007). This leading fibroblast was able to create a track in the matrigel matrix through both protease- and force-mediated remodeling that the SCC cells would follow. The track was found to be necessary and sufficient for SCC cell invasion as removal of the fibroblasts after track formation still allowed SCC cells to invade. These SCC cells have not undergone an epithelial—mesenchymal transition (EMT) and are non-invasive. It had been questioned how tumors that maintained an epithelial phenotype were able to intravasate; this work illustrates that those tumor cells that are not invasive are able to co-opt host cells in order to metastasize (Gaggioli et al. 2007).

During melanoma development, melanocytes lose expression of E-cadherin thereby losing regulatory contact with keratinocytes, and gain expression of N-cadherin and melanoma cell adhesion molecule (MCAM) which mediate adhesion between melanoma cells and fibroblasts, vascular endothelial cells and other melanoma cells (Hsu et al. 2002; Li et al. 2001). Signaling between melanoma cells, which produce PDGF, bFGF and TGFβ, and fibroblasts which produce IGF-1, HGF/SF, bFGF and TGFβ, results in increased melanoma tumor growth and invasiveness (Li et al. 2003; Hsu et al. 2002; Lee and Herlyn 2007). It has also been shown that TGFβ expression decreases E-cadherin expression, up-regulates β1 and β3 integrin expression and increases MMP-9 activity leading to increased migration (Janji et al. 1999) and enhanced adhesion of melanoma cells to the endothelium (Teti 1997). Re-expresion of E-cadherin in melanoma cells led to reduced invasion in vitro and tumorigenicitiy in vivo (Hsu et al. 2000). Additionally, during the transition of melanomas from the radial growth phase (RGP, flat, non-invasive tumor) to vertical growth phase (VGP, invasive growth), significant matrix remodeling is required; the majority of the enzymes and MMPs utilized are contributed by host fibroblasts and TAMs (Liotta and Kohn 2001).

Components of the host coagulation system are also involved in regulating tumor cell invasiveness. Tissue Factor (TF) is consistently upregulated in many human malignancies and is found to contribute to many facets of tumor aggressiveness (Rak et al. 2009). TF is expressed by tumor cells, often at high levels, but also by many host cells such as endothelial cells, TAMs and CAFs. The main function of TF is to activate thrombin which potentiates clot formation, but thrombin is also essential for activating protease activated receptor (PAR)-1 and -2. Activation of PAR-1 expressed by tumor cells leads to increased tumor invasion and metastasis through induction of proteases and cell adhesion molecules (Melnikova and Bar-Eli 2009).

2.3 Survival and Arrest in the Vasculature

The host coagulation system is known to play a significant role in tumor cell arrest and survival in the vasculature. Tumor cells activate or produce many components of the coagulation cascade such as thrombin, PAR-1, TF, fibrinogen, von Willebrand factor, and platelet-activating factor (PAF), leading to a 'platelet mimicry' phenotype (Timar et al. 2005). The hypoxic environment increases TF expression by endothelial cells, TAMs and CAFs leading to thrombin production within the primary tumor. This 'pre-treatment' with thrombin increases tumor cell adhesion to platelets and the vascular endothelium following tumor cell intravasation (Nierodzik and Karpatkin 2006).

Through expression of TF, tumor cells are able to exploit the host coagulation system to increase metastatic efficiency. In an elegant series of papers, Palumbo et al. (Palumbo et al. 2000; Palumbo et al. 2002; Palumbo et al. 2005; Palumbo et al. 2007; Palumbo et al. 2008) evaluated the interplay between metastatic cells and the individual components of coagulation. They found that loss of host fibrinogen significantly decreased lung metastasis formation, yet had no impact on the number of cells that originally arrested in the lung following experimental metastasis cell injection. However, fibrinogen was essential for sustained adherence of tumor cells in the lung vasculature (Palumbo et al. 2000). This role for fibrinogen also held true in a spontaneous model of metastasis, with reduced lung metastasis despite equivalent primary tumor formation in fibrinogen-null and wild type animals (Palumbo et al. 2002). Evaluation of metastasis in animals with activation-resistant platelets (platelets present in normal number, but not able to be activated by thrombin, adenosine diphosphate (ADP), or other coagulation stimulants) showed a significant decrease in experimental and spontaneous metastasis, again due to reduced survival or retention in the lung vasculature (Palumbo et al. 2005). Depletion of circulating natural killer (NK) immune cells prior to metastatic cell introduction resulted in equivalent metastasis number in platelet mutant, fibrinogen knock-out and wild type animals, indicating that platelet- and fibrinogen-mediated thrombus formation protects tumor cells from NK cell surveillance in the lung vasculature (Palumbo et al. 2005). The role of NK-mediated cell killing was strengthened through work on Factor XIII, which stabilizes fibrin and other ECM matricies through catalysis of crosslinkages. FXIII was found to be essential in preventing NK cell immunosurveillance of tumor cells (Palumbo et al. 2008).

To specifically evaluate the role of TF and TF signaling in metastasis, tumor cells were derived from TF knock-out animals and cell lines with and without TF, or TF lacking the cytoplasmic tail responsible for cell signaling. It was found that while TF expression was not essential for primary tumor formation, it was critical for lung metastasis but dependent on functional coagulation in the host. Interestingly, blockage of TF signaling had no effect on metastasis generation (Palumbo and Degen 2007).

The formation of a thrombus at the surface of an arrested tumor cell has also been linked to increased metastasis through maintenance of cell adherence in the pulmonary vasculature (Fig. 2.1b) (Borsig 2008; Kim et al. 1998; Im et al. 2004). Metastatic cells protected in a fibrin clot were able to change from a rounded morphology and spread along the inside of a vessel. Those cells that showed stable adherence to the lung vasculature were able to form significantly more lung metastases than those prevented from spreading through treatment with anticoagulant agents (Im et al. 2004). Treatment of animals with the clot-stabilizing drug aprotinin was found to increase metastasis of B16F10 melanoma cells through prolonging the interaction between tumor cells arrested in the pulmonary vasculature and cell surface thrombi (Kirstein et al. 2009). In accordance with this, prevention of thrombus formation with heparin (Kirstein et al. 2009) or hiruden (Esumi et al. 1991) is linked with reduced pulmonary metastasis due to decreased cell retention in the lung.

Stable adherence of tumor cells to the vasculature upon arrest appears to be a major determinant of metastatic efficiency. Comparison of metastatic and non-metastatic cells injected into the circulation showed no difference in the original number of cells that arrested in the lung, however only those cell lines that had a metastatic phenotype were able to persist and form micrometastases in the lung (Kim et al. 2004). Tumor cell arrest is also influenced by host expression of P-selectin. Platelets isolated from P-selectin knock-out mice were unable to bind to tumor cells in vitro, and experimental metastasis assays found that there was a decrease in the initial seeding of the lung tissue in P-selectin-null animals (Kim et al. 1998). Additionally, P-selectin was found to facilitate tumor cell tethering and rolling along the pulmonary vasculature, but further binding by $\alpha_{IIb}\beta_3$ was required to stabilize tumor cell adhesion (McCarty et al. 2000). Integrin $\alpha_3\beta_1$ is also involved in tumor cell adhesion to the vascular endothelium through sections of exposed basement membrane. Adhesion and migration of tumor cells was also stimulated by binding of TF on tumor cells to tissue factor pathway inhibitor -1 on tumor associated vessels which was a surprising consequence of receptor-inhibitor binding (Fischer et al. 1999).

Tumor cell-associated thrombus formation may also increase metastatic cell survival in the vasculature, as activation of PAR-1 by thrombin leads to transmission of survival signals and prevention of apoptosis (Shi et al. 2004). Additionally, many growth and survival factors are released from platelets upon activation and are therefore present within thrombi. Tumor cells are able to bind to the provisional matrix provided by a fibrin clot thereby increasing metastasis (Fig. 2.1b) (Palumbo et al. 2002; Reijerkerk et al. 2000; Dvorak et al. 1995). Further, plasmin-mediated clot dissolution may aid tumor cells with the next step in metastasis—extravasation from the host vasculature.

2.4 Extravasation and Growth Initiation in Secondary Tissue

Compared with the other steps in metastasis, relatively little is known about tumor cell extravasation at a secondary site. Using cell accounting techniques Luzzi, et al. (Luzzi et al. 1998) found that the majority of B16F1 murine melanoma cells had extravasated from the liver vasculature within 3 days of cell injection (Luzzi et al. 1998). Importantly, very few of these cells went on to form micrometastases (2 %) and even fewer were able to form macrometastases (0.02 %). Two weeks following tumor cell injection, over one-third of injected cells remained in the liver as solitary, extravasated cells and 95 % of those identifiable cells were not apoptotic or proliferating (as determined by histological staining for TUNEL and Ki67), indicating that in the liver, extravasation may not be an essential part of metastatic inefficiency. Additionally, using the chick chorioallantoic membrane (CAM) found that nearly all B16F1 cells were able to survive and extravasate following arrest. Tissue inhibitor of metalloproteinases-1 (TIMP-1) overexpressing B16F1 cells were poorly metastatic, and yet they were still able to successfully extravasate in the chick CAM model (Koop et al. 1995). Using *ras*-transformed and control fibroblasts, it was also found that extravasation was independent of metastatic ability (Koop et al. 1996). Nearly all *ras*-transformed fibroblasts and control fibroblasts (89 and 96 %, respectively) had extravasated from the chick CAM within 24 h of initial injection. Additionally, migration of both cell types within the mesenchymal layer was equivalent, despite having differential invasion capabilities in vitro (Koop et al. 1996).

Direct visualization of tumor cell extravasation was performed recently in a murine model of brain metastasis (Kienast et al. 2010). Using a cranial window, single cancer cells were visualized throughout arrest and extravasation. MDA-MD-435 cells were found to arrest in microvessel branch points and extravasate as single cells. These cells began to proliferate only after successful extravasation and only when extravasated cells maintained contact with an abluminal endothelial cell of a brain capillary (Kienast et al. 2010).

Study of metastasis to the lung vasculature shows a distinct difference from that seen in the liver and chick CAM, however. Using the 4T1 murine mammary carcinoma cell line it was found that these cells arrest in the lung as individuals attached to the vascular endothelium. The cells were able to form small colonies within three weeks, some entirely maintained within the vasculature. Following growth initiation, the colonies were able to extravasate as micro or macrometastases (Wong et al. 2002). Further to this, fewer than 2 % of HT1080 cells had extravasated from the lung vasculature within 24 h of tumor cell injection, and were found to form colonies within the lung vasculature within three days. These colonies showed tumor cells that projected outwards from the central focus as 'strings' following within the capillaries (Fig. 2.1e) (Al-Mehdi et al. 2000). Analysis of experimental metastasis of B16F10 melanoma cells in the mouse lung found that the majority of injected cells had extravasated, with no identifiable clusters or single cells within the pulmonary vasculature within 4 days of injection (Cameron et al. 2000). Using an orthotopic prostate cancer model, however, the majority of metastatic tumor cells and tumor cell clusters were found within the vasculature of both the liver and the lung (Zhang et al. 2010). Taken together, these data indicate that the role of extravasation in successful metastasis formation may be specific to the model, cell type and secondary organ of study.

Recent work has found a subset of macrophages ($CD11b^{+}Gr^{-}$) recruited to tumor cells arrested in the lung aids in tumor cell extravasation (Qian 2009). The timing of tumor cell extravasation was directly linked to macrophage recruitment, as depletion of macrophages at various times following tumor cell injection resulted in either reduced metastasis number and size, if macrophages were depleted prior to tumor cell injection, or equivalent number of metastases with reduced size, if macrophages were depleted after successful seeding of the lung with PyMT induced or MDA-MB-231 tumor cells. Ex vivo imaging of intact lung tissue at various times following tumor cell injection found that macrophages associated with tumor cells in the vasculature and increased extravasation (Fig. 2.1d). Five minutes after cell injection all tumor cells were retained in the lung vasculature. Within 24 h, there was a significant increase in macrophage association with arrested tumor cells, and ~75 % of tumor cells were outside of a vessel, and within 3 days no cells were found completely within a vessel. Some of the extravasated cells had begun to proliferate as several colonies were visualized, and these colonies showed extensive macrophage association (Fig. 2.1f). Macrophage depletion reduced tumor cell extravasation from 75–25 % within 24 h and within 48 h many fewer cells had survived in the lung. These studies found that macrophage recruitment to the lung promoted tumor cell extravasation and survival (Qian et al. 2009).

It is known that arrest of tumor cells is associated with the formation of a fibrin clot at the arrested cell site. These clots do not persist indefinitely—clot dissolution is mediated by the powerful protease plasmin (Reijerkerk et al. 2000). This clot breakdown may aid tumor cell extravasation through activation of MMPs and other proteinases. Tumor cells that express high amounts of urokinase type plasminogen activator (uPA) tend to be more aggressive and metastatic (reviewed in (Kramer et al. 1994)). Clinically, high levels of uPA, uPA receptor (uPAR), plasminogen activator inhibitor (PAI)-1 and PAI-2 is linked to poor prognosis and increased metastasis development (Duffy et al. 2008; Harbeck et al. 2004).

The site of metastatic cell arrest and growth has been debated for some time—from Stephen Paget's theory of 'seed and soil' whereby the tumor cell (seed) must arrest in a permissible secondary tissue (soil) in order to develop into a tumor (Chambers et al. 2002; Ribatti et al. 2006). This century-old theory still has merit as metastatic cells grow in different tissues depending on the tumor type they originated from. A type of hospitable 'soil' has been identified as a pre-metastatic niche. These regions of secondary tissue show recruitment of clusters of BMDCs prior to the arrival of tumor cells. It is thought that primary tumor and tumor stromal secretion of chemokines direct the migration of these cells, as in vivo injection of media conditioned by melanoma cells led to similar recruitment and pattern of metastasis as the presence of a melanoma primary tumor (Kaplan et al. 2005). The primary tumor stimulates pre-metastatic niche formation through secretion of VEGF and placental growth factor (PlGF), which recruit VEGF receptor 1 (VEGFR1)-positive cells. PlGF in particular increases the proliferation of fibroblast-like cells and stimulates their production of fibronectin (Ruzinova 2003).

BMDCs expressing VEGFR1 and $\alpha_4\beta_1$ arrest in regions of increased fibronectin synthesis by fibroblasts and fibroblast-like cells. These arrested BMDCs secrete MMP-9 which may degrade the basement membrane to allow extravasation of more BMDCs and/or metastatic cells. They are also found to express Id3, which is involved in proliferation and mobilization of hematopoietic progenitor cells (HPCs) from the bone marrow and maintains an activated state within the BMDC clusters. These clusters alter the local microenvironment and activate integrins and chemokines such as stromal derived factor –1 (SDF-1). This activation leads to further recruitment of BMDCs and increased attachment, survival, and growth of tumor cells (Fig. 2.1g) (Kaplan et al. 2005).

Pre-metastatic niche formation can also be directed by platelet aggregation (Massberg et al. 2006). At a site of endothelium disruption, platelet activation was essential for recruitment of BMDCs, which adhere to P-selectin and $\alpha_{IIb}\beta_3$ on the platelet surface, rather than to exposed ECM. Additionally, SDF-1 released from platelets leads to ongoing retention of BMDC and tumor cell arrest.

2.5 Angiogenesis and Sustained Growth

Sustained primary tumor and metastatic growth beyond $\sim 1\text{mm}^3$ requires the recruitment of a blood supply (Folkman 1995). Vascularization of tumors promotes growth by providing oxygen and nutrients and increases metastasis by providing an entry point into the circulation. Normal tissues undergo angiogenesis during development, wound healing and tissue regeneration, through a tightly regulated system leading to structured, hierarchical branching of vessels (Carmeliet 2005). Tumor vascularization is characterized by highly tortuous dysfunctional vessels due to improper regulation of angiogenesis (McDonald and Choyke 2003).

High levels of VEGF-A in the tumor microenvironment expressed by tumor cells, macrophages (Barbera-Guillem et al. 2002; Harmey et al. 1998; Evans 1992), neutrophils (McCourt et al. 1999), platelets (McCabe et al. 2006), fibroblasts (Hlatky et al. 1994) and endothelial cells (Nilsson et al. 2004) tips the balance of pro- and anti-angiogenic factors and leads to activation of angiogenesis. VEGF-A is elevated in response to hypoxia and inflammation, which are common in during tumor formation. Solid tumors tend to have a hypoxic core due to poorly functioning vasculature leading to constant stimulation of pro-angiogenic factors such as VEGF-A (Byrne et al. 2005).

The initial reaction to high levels of VEGF-A is destabilization of existing blood vessels. The number of endothelial cell interactions with stabilizing mural cells decreases, leading to leaky, dialated vessels (Carmeliet und Jain 2000; Bach et al. 2007). This destabilization is mediated by angiopoietin-2 (Ang-2) (Tait and Jones 2004; Maisonpierre et al. 1997), partly through up-regulation of MMP-1 and -9 (Etoh et al. 2001) and is found to increase tumor cell entry into the vasculature (Chung et al. 2006; Nakayama et al. 2005).

Following vessel destabilization, endothelial tip cells begin sprouting through tightly regulated signaling between Delta-like 4 (Dll4) and Notch (Suchting et al. 2007) which may be de-regulated in the tumor microenvironment resulting in incomplete vascular remodeling (Noguera-Troise 2006). Tip cells lead the migration of endothelial cells following chemotactic signals, especially VEGF-A. HPCs and endothelial progenitor cells (EPCs) are also recruited by VEGF-A signaling to further increase vessel growth (Hattori et al. 2001). In order for proper vascular function, vessel growth is followed by vasculature stabilization by pericytes due to PDGF and Ang-1 signaling (Abramsson et al. 2003; Milner et al. 2009). Ang-1 and PDGF can be overexpressed in the tumor microenvironment (Tait and Jones 2004; Nakamura 2008) yet tumor vessels are poorly stabilized, showing leakiness and poor pericyte coverage. This indicates that the balance of pro-angiogenic, destabilizing factors such as VEGF-A are present in higher functional concentration than Ang-1 and PDGF (Hall and Ran 2010). Recent work has also linked MMP-14 and TGFβ to vascular stability, as MMP inhibition was found to increase vascular leakiness due to reduced activation of TGFβ present in the ECM. TGFβ was found to signal through ALK5 to control leakage of small (10 kDa dextran) and large (70 kDa dextran) molecules in tumor and normal tissue though control of vasodilation and venular openings (Sounni et al. 2010). These data indicates that TGFβ in the ECM can modulate host response depending on its bioavailability, and its release by MMP activity in the tumor stroma may increase tumor cell extravasation through increased vascular leakiness.

Deregulated angiogenesis in a tumor is due to an imbalance between pro- and anti-angiogenic factors in the tumor microenvironment. The over-expression of pro-angiogenic factors VEGF-A, Ang-2, bFGF and TGFβ leads to constant stimulation of angiogenesis and a reduction in stabilized vessels. This leads to poor tissue perfusion, high vasculature permeability and chronic inflammation and an increase in metastasis due to ease of metastatic cell entry into the vasculature (Hall and Ran 2010).

The process of angiogenesis in the metastatic setting is thought to proceed through a similar path as seen in the primary tumor. Initial growth of a micrometastasis is halted without the recruitment of a blood supply, leading to a functionally dormant metastasis with balanced levels of proliferation and apoptosis (Naumov et al. 2008). Tumor cells and macrophages present at the metastatic site stimulate expression of VEGF-A leading to the same cascade of angiogenic events as seen in the primary tumor setting.

Blood clot formation at the metastatic site provides further angiogenic and growth signals as platelet activation results in the release of many growth and pro-angiogenic factors such as VEGF, PDGF, Ang-1, TGFβ, IGF-1, EGF, and platelet-derived epidermal growth factor (PD-EGF). Additionally, thrombin activity is linked to increased angiogenesis through up-regulation of cathepsin-D which increases endothelial cell growth, migration and tube formation in vitro (Hu et al. 2008). Thrombin may also play an important role in angiogenesis through induction of VEGF-A in tumor cells (Huang et al. 2002) and platelets (Mohle et al. 1997), as well as Ang-1 and -2 from platelets (Li et al. 2001) and endothelial cells (Huang et al. 2002) respectively.

2.6 Host-Mediated Inhibition of Metastasis

Successful metastasis formation results when tumor cells are able to exploit and avoid natural host defenses. Yet metastasis is an exceptionally inefficient process, (Chambers et al. 2002) indicating that the host is capable of preventing progression of the majority of metastatic cells. The mechanisms behind this prevention are largely unknown, yet several interesting examples of host triumph over tumor have been established.

Following tumor cell arrest in the liver vasculature, nitric oxide (NO) is released and induces apoptosis in B16F1 cells (Wang et al. 2000). B16F1 cell arrest in the pulmonary vasculature was also found to lead to an eNOS-dependent release of NO. NO may represent a natural host defense mechanism as it triggers apoptosis in melanoma cells and reduced the growth of metastatic tumors (Fig. 2.1c) (Qiu et al. 2003). Accordingly, comparison of metastatic (isolated from VGP tumor) and non-metastatic (isolated from RGP tumor) melanoma cells following arrest in the murine lung showed that non-metastatic cells were unable to survive in the pulmonary vasculature. Within 8 h of tumor cell injection, non-metastatic cells had apoptosed and were cleared from the lung, whereas metastatic cells persisted and were able to form metastatic colonies within 7 days (Kim et al. 2004).

Given the extensive interaction between tumors and the host, there is the potential to alter the microenvironment to create an anti-tumor rather than pro-tumor interface. It has been proposed that the large number of TAMs present in tumor stroma could be 're-educated' to target tumor cells (Hagemann et al. 2008). Using NF-κB signaling, tumor cells are able to keep TAMs in an immunosuppressive state. By introducing a dominant negative inhibitor of nuclear factor kappa B kinase β (IKKβ) into bone marrow derived macrophages, TAMs became tumoricidal through release of NO and through promotion of NK cell-mediated killing (Hagemann et al. 2008). The extensive interaction between TAMs and metastatic cells throughout invasion and extravasation as discussed earlier illustrates the great potential for manipulation of TAM activity to reduce tumor progression.

Normal tissue structure and function is maintained through proper ECM adhesion and tissue polarity. In breast and melanoma tumor development, dysregulation of cell adhesion represents an initiating step in tumor formation (Li et al. 2003; Takeichi 1993). Therefore the effect of re-establishing proper tissue architecture and adhesion in tumor tissues has been investigated (Bissell et al. 2002). It was found that restoration of proper integrin signaling within a 3D culture setting led to phenotypic reversion of breast cancer cells. Without alterations to tumor cell genotype, tumor cells were induced to form normal breast structures. Metastatic breast cancer cells could also be reverted to a non-malignant phenotype in 3D culture following treatment with anti-integrin antibodies (Wang et al. 2002). The global switch in cellular behavior as a direct result of modulation of environmental interaction indicates the powerful role that the tumor stroma and microenvironment has on tumor development and progression and illustrates that many treatment options are available beyond direct targeting of tumor tissue.

2.7 Summary

The study of tumor biology and metastasis has long been investigated from the perspective of the individual tumor cell. However, the importance of tumor cell interaction with host cells and systems has also been recognized. Tumor cells are unable to form metastases without interaction with many microenvironments—from the primary tumor stroma, through the host vasculature and host coagulation systems, to an entirely new environment in a secondary organ. The metastatic cell's ability to survive and proliferate in each of these new environments depends on the ability to influence and often exploit the host. Fundamental to this is the interaction of tumor cells with the host coagulation pathway and avoidance of the host immune system. These two major systems exist to maintain tissue homeostasis and health though elimination of non-normal cells, yet tumor cells are able to circumvent these host responses and turn them from anti-tumor to pro-metastatic. Full understanding of the interplay between tumor progression and host responses is essential for understanding metastatic disease and successful patient treatment.

Acknowledgments We would like to thank Kyle MacLean for his assistance with figure design. JMK is the recipient of a Translational Breast Cancer Studentship from the London Regional Cancer Program. AFC is a Cancer Research Chair in Oncology and receives salary support from the Canada Research Chairs Program.

References

Abramsson A, Lindblom P, Betsholtz C (2003) Endothelial and nonendothelial sources of PDGF-B regulate pericyte recruitment and influence vascular pattern formation in tumors. J Clin Invest 112:1142–1151

Al-Mehdi AB et al (2000) Intravascular origin of metastasis from the proliferation of endothelium-attached tumor cells: a new model for metastasis. Nat Med 6:100–102

Bach F, Uddin FJ, Burke D (2007) Angiopoietins in malignancy. Eur J Surg Oncol 33:7–15

Barbera-Guillem E, Nyhus JK, Wolford CC, Friece CR, Sampsel JW (2002) Vascular endothelial growth factor secretion by tumor-infiltrating macrophages essentially supports tumor angiogenesis, and IgG immune complexes potentiate the process. Cancer Res 62:7042–7049

Bissell MJ, Radisky DC, Rizki A, Weaver VM, Petersen OW (2002) The organizing principle: microenvironmental influences in the normal and malignant breast. Differentiation 70:537–546

Borsig L (2008) The role of platelet activation in tumor metastasis. Expert Rev Anticancer Ther 8:1247–1255

Brooks SA, Lomax-Browne HJ, Carter TM, Kinch CE, Hall DM (2010) Molecular interactions in cancer cell metastasis. Acta Histochem 112:3–25

Byrne AM, Bouchier-Hayes DJ, Harmey JH (2005) Angiogenic and cell survival functions of vascular endothelial growth factor (VEGF). J Cell Mol Med 9:777–794

Cameron MD et al (2000) Temporal progression of metastasis in lung: cell survival, dormancy, and location dependence of metastatic inefficiency. Cancer Res 60:2541–2546

Carmeliet P (2005) VEGF as a key mediator of angiogenesis in cancer. Oncology 69(Suppl 3):4–10

Carmeliet P, Jain RK (2000) Angiogenesis in cancer and other diseases. Nature 407:249–257

Chambers AF, Groom AC, MacDonald IC (2002) Dissemination and growth of cancer cells in metastatic sites. Nat Rev Cancer 2:563–572

Chung YC, Hou YC, Chang CN, Hseu TH (2006) Expression and prognostic significance of angiopoietin in colorectal carcinoma. J Surg Oncol 94:631–638

Direkze NC et al (2004) Bone marrow contribution to tumor-associated myofibroblasts and fibroblasts. Cancer Res 64:8492–8495

Duffy MJ, McGowan PM, Gallagher WM (2008) Cancer invasion and metastasis: changing views. J Pathol 214:283–293

Dvorak HF, Brown LF, Detmar M, Dvorak AM (1995) Vascular permeability factor/vascular endothelial growth factor, microvascular hyperpermeability, and angiogenesis. Am J Pathol 146:1029–1039

Esumi N, Fan D, Fidler IJ (1991) Inhibition of murine melanoma experimental metastasis by recombinant desulfatohirudin, a highly specific thrombin inhibitor. Cancer Res 51:4549–4556

Etoh T et al (2001) Angiopoietin-2 is related to tumor angiogenesis in gastric carcinoma: possible in vivo regulation via induction of proteases. Cancer Res 61:2145–2153

Evans R et al (1992) Tumor cell IL-6 gene expression is regulated by IL-1 alpha/beta and TNF alpha: proposed feedback mechanisms induced by the interaction of tumor cells and macrophages. J Leukoc Biol 52:463–468

Fischer EG et al (1999) Tumor cell adhesion and migration supported by interaction of a receptor-protease complex with its inhibitor. J Clin Invest 104:1213–1221

Folkman J (1995) Angiogenesis inhibitors generated by tumors. Mol Med 1:120–122

Gaggioli C et al (2007) Fibroblast-led collective invasion of carcinoma cells with differing roles for RhoGTPases in leading and following cells. Nat Cell Biol 9:1392–1400

Giannelli G, Falk-Marzillier J, Schiraldi O, Stetler-Stevenson WG, Quaranta V (1997) Induction of cell migration by matrix metalloprotease-2 cleavage of laminin-5. Science 277:225–228

Goswami S et al (2005) Macrophages promote the invasion of breast carcinoma cells via a colony-stimulating factor-1/epidermal growth factor paracrine loop. Cancer Res 65:5278–5283

Hagemann T et al (2005) Macrophages induce invasiveness of epithelial cancer cells via NF-kappa B and JNK. J Immunol 175:1197–1205

Hagemann T et al. (2008) "Re-educating" tumor-associated macrophages by targeting NF-kappaB. J Exp Med 205:1261–1268
Hall K, Ran S (2010) Regulation of tumor angiogenesis by the local environment. Front Biosci 15:195–212
Harbeck N et al (2004) Urokinase-type plasminogen activator (uPA) and its inhibitor PAI-I: novel tumor-derived factors with a high prognostic and predictive impact in breast cancer. Thromb Haemost 91:450–456
Harmey JH, Dimitriadis E, Kay E, Redmond HP, Bouchier-Hayes D (1998) Regulation of macrophage production of vascular endothelial growth factor (VEGF) by hypoxia and transforming growth factor beta-1. Ann Surg Oncol 5:271–278
Hattori K et al (2001) Vascular endothelial growth factor and angiopoietin-1 stimulate postnatal hematopoiesis by recruitment of vasculogenic and hematopoietic stem cells. J Exp Med 193:1005–1014
Hlatky L, Tsionou C, Hahnfeldt P, Coleman CN (1994) Mammary fibroblasts may influence breast tumor angiogenesis via hypoxia-induced vascular endothelial growth factor up-regulation and protein expression. Cancer Res 54:6083–6086
Hsu MY et al (2000) E-cadherin expression in melanoma cells restores keratinocyte-mediated growth control and down-regulates expression of invasion-related adhesion receptors. Am J Pathol 156:1515–1525
Hsu MY, Meier F, Herlyn M (2002) Melanoma development and progression: a conspiracy between tumor and host. Differentiation 70:522–536
Hu L, Roth JM, Brooks P, Luty J, Karpatkin S (2008) Thrombin up-regulates cathepsin D which enhances angiogenesis, growth, and metastasis. Cancer Res 68:4666–4673
Huang YQ, Li JJ, Hu L, Lee M, Karpatkin S (2002) Thrombin induces increased expression and secretion of angiopoietin-2 from human umbilical vein endothelial cells. Blood 99:1646–1650
Hynes RO (2009) The extracellular matrix: not just pretty fibrils. Science 326:1216–1219
Ii M, Yamamoto H, Adachi Y, Maruyama Y, Shinomura Y (2006) Role of matrix metalloproteinase-7 (matrilysin) in human cancer invasion, apoptosis, growth, and angiogenesis. Exp Biol Med (Maywood) 231:20–27
Im JH et al (2004) Coagulation facilitates tumor cell spreading in the pulmonary vasculature during early metastatic colony formation. Cancer Res 64:8613–8619
Janji B, Melchior C, Gouon V, Vallar L, Kieffer N (1999) Autocrine TGF-beta-regulated expression of adhesion receptors and integrin-linked kinase in HT-144 melanoma cells correlates with their metastatic phenotype. Int J Cancer 83:255–262
Kaplan RN et al (2005) VEGFR1-positive haematopoietic bone marrow progenitors initiate the pre-metastatic niche. Nature 438:820–827
Kedrin D et al (2008) Intravital imaging of metastatic behavior through a mammary imaging window. Nat Methods 5:1019–1021
Kienast Y et al (2010) Real-time imaging reveals the single steps of brain metastasis formation. Nat Med 16:116–122
Kim JW et al (2004) Rapid apoptosis in the pulmonary vasculature distinguishes non-metastatic from metastatic melanoma cells. Cancer Lett 213:203–212
Kim YJ, Borsig L, Varki NM, Varki A (1998) P-selectin deficiency attenuates tumor growth and metastasis. Proc Natl Acad Sci U S A 95:9325–9330
Kirstein JM et al (2009) Effect of anti-fibrinolytic therapy on experimental melanoma metastasis. Clin Exp Metastasis 26:121–131
Koop S et al (1995) Fate of melanoma cells entering the microcirculation: over 80 % survive and extravasate. Cancer Res 55:2520–2523
Koop S et al (1996) Independence of metastatic ability and extravasation: metastatic ras-transformed and control fibroblasts extravasate equally well. Proc Natl Acad Sci U S A 93:11080–11084
Kramer MD, Reinartz J, Brunner G, Schirrmacher V (1994) Plasmin in pericellular proteolysis and cellular invasion. Invasion Metastasis 14:210–222

Le Bitoux MA, Stamenkovic I (2008) Tumor-host interactions: the role of inflammation. Histochem Cell Biol 130:1079–1090

Lee JT, Herlyn M (2007) Microenvironmental influences in melanoma progression. J Cell Biochem 101:862–872

Li G. et al. (2003) Function and regulation of melanoma-stromal fibroblast interactions: when seeds meet soil. Oncogene 22:3162–3171

Li G, Satyamoorthy K, Herlyn M (2001a) N-cadherin-mediated intercellular interactions promote survival and migration of melanoma cells. Cancer Res 61:3819–3825

Li JJ, Huang YQ, Basch R, Karpatkin S (2001b) Thrombin induces the release of angiopoietin-1 from platelets. Thromb Haemost 85:204–206

Lin EY, Pollard JW (2004) Role of infiltrated leucocytes in tumour growth and spread. Br J Cancer 90:2053–2058

Liotta LA, Kohn EC (2001) The microenvironment of the tumour-host interface. Nature 411:375–379

Lorusso G, Ruegg C (2008) The tumor microenvironment and its contribution to tumor evolution toward metastasis. Histochem Cell Biol 130:1091–1103

Luzzi KJ et al (1998) Multistep nature of metastatic inefficiency: dormancy of solitary cells after successful extravasation and limited survival of early micrometastases. Am J Pathol 153:865–873

Maisonpierre PC et al (1997) Angiopoietin-2, a natural antagonist for Tie2 that disrupts in vivo angiogenesis. Science 277:55–60

Massberg S et al (2006) Platelets secrete stromal cell-derived factor 1alpha and recruit bone marrow-derived progenitor cells to arterial thrombi in vivo. J Exp Med 203:1221–1233

McCabe NP, Selman SH, Jankun J (2006) Vascular endothelial growth factor production in human prostate cancer cells is stimulated by overexpression of platelet 12-lipoxygenase. Prostate 66:779–787

McCarty OJ, Mousa SA, Bray PF, Konstantopoulos K (2000) Immobilized platelets support human colon carcinoma cell tethering, rolling, and firm adhesion under dynamic flow conditions. Blood 96:1789–1797

McCourt M, Wang JH, Sookhai S, Redmond HP (1999) Proinflammatory mediators stimulate neutrophil-directed angiogenesis. Arch Surg 134:1325–1331; (discussion 1331–2)

McDonald DM, Choyke PL (2003) Imaging of angiogenesis: from microscope to clinic. Nat Med 9:713–725

Melnikova VO, Bar-Eli M (2009) Inflammation and melanoma metastasis. Pigment Cell Melanoma Res 22:257–267

Milner CS, Hansen TM, Singh H, Brindle NP (2009) Roles of the receptor tyrosine kinases Tie1 and Tie2 in mediating the effects of angiopoietin-1 on endothelial permeability and apoptosis. Microvasc Res 77:187–191

Mohle R, Green D, Moore MA, Nachman RL, Rafii S (1997) Constitutive production and thrombin-induced release of vascular endothelial growth factor by human megakaryocytes and platelets. Proc Natl Acad Sci U S A 94:663–668

Nakamura Y et al (2008) PDGF-BB is a novel prognostic factor in colorectal cancer. Ann Surg Oncol 15:2129–2136

Nakayama T et al (2005) Expression and significance of Tie-1 and Tie-2 receptors, and angiopoietins-1, 2 and 4 in colorectal adenocarcinoma: Immunohistochemical analysis and correlation with clinicopathological factors. World J Gastroenterol 11:964–969

Naumov GN, Folkman J, Straume O, Akslen LA (2008) Tumor-vascular interactions and tumor dormancy. Apmis 116:569–585

Nierodzik ML, Karpatkin S (2006) Thrombin induces tumor growth, metastasis, and angiogenesis: Evidence for a thrombin-regulated dormant tumor phenotype. Cancer Cell 10:355–362

Nieto MA (2002) The snail superfamily of zinc-finger transcription factors. Nat Rev Mol Cell Biol 3:155–166

Nilsson I, Shibuya M, Wennstrom S (2004) Differential activation of vascular genes by hypoxia in primary endothelial cells. Exp Cell Res 299:476–485

Noguera-Troise I et al (2006) Blockade of Dll4 inhibits tumour growth by promoting non-productive angiogenesis. Nature 444 1032–1037
Nonomura N et al (2007) Decreased number of mast cells infiltrating into needle biopsy specimens leads to a better prognosis of prostate cancer. Br J Cancer 97:952–956
Olumi AF et al (1999) Carcinoma-associated fibroblasts direct tumor progression of initiated human prostatic epithelium. Cancer Res 59:5002–5011
Orimo A, Weinberg RA (2006) Stromal fibroblasts in cancer: a novel tumor-promoting cell type. Cell Cycle 5:1597–1601
Palumbo JS et al (2000) Fibrinogen is an important determinant of the metastatic potential of circulating tumor cells. Blood 96:3302–3309
Palumbo JS et al (2002) Spontaneous hematogenous and lymphatic metastasis, but not primary tumor growth or angiogenesis, is diminished in fibrinogen-deficient mice. Cancer Res 62: 6966–6972
Palumbo JS et al (2005) Platelets and fibrin(ogen) increase metastatic potential by impeding natural killer cell-mediated elimination of tumor cells. Blood 105:178–185
Palumbo JS et al (2007) Tumor cell-associated tissue factor and circulating hemostatic factors cooperate to increase metastatic potential through natural killer cell-dependent and-independent mechanisms. Blood 110:133–141
Palumbo JS et al (2008) Factor XIII transglutaminase supports hematogenous tumor cell metastasis through a mechanism dependent on natural killer cell function. J Thromb Haemost 6:812–819
Palumbo JS, Degen JL (2007) Mechanisms linking tumor cell-associated procoagulant function to tumor metastasis. Thromb Res 120(Suppl 2):S22–8
Pirila E et al (2003) Matrix metalloproteinases process the laminin-5 gamma 2-chain and regulate epithelial cell migration. Biochem Biophys Res Commun 303:1012–1017
Pollard JW (2004) Tumour-educated macrophages promote tumour progression and metastasis. Nat Rev Cancer 4:71–78
Qian B et al (2009) A distinct macrophage population mediates metastatic breast cancer cell extravasation, establishment and growth. PLoS One 4:e6562
Qiu H et al. (2003) Arrest of B16 melanoma cells in the mouse pulmonary microcirculation induces endothelial nitric oxide synthase-dependent nitric oxide release that is cytotoxic to the tumor cells. Am J Pathol 162:403–412
Rak J, Milsom C, Magnus N, Yu J (2009) Tissue factor in tumour progression. Best Pract Res Clin Haematol 22:71–83
Reijerkerk A, Voest EE, Gebbink MF (2000) No grip, no growth: the conceptual basis of excessive proteolysis in the treatment of cancer. Eur J Cancer 36:1695–1705
Ribatti D, Mangialardi G, Vacca A (2006) Stephen Paget and the 'seed and soil' theory of metastatic dissemination. Clin Exp Med 6:145–149
Robinson BD et al (2009) Tumor microenvironment of metastasis in human breast carcinoma: a potential prognostic marker linked to hematogenous dissemination. Clin Cancer Res 15: 2433–2441
Robinson SC, Coussens LM (2005) Soluble mediators of inflammation during tumor development. Adv Cancer Res 93:159–187
Ruzinova MB et al (2003) Effect of angiogenesis inhibition by Id loss and the contribution of bone-marrow-derived endothelial cells in spontaneous murine tumors. Cancer Cell 4:277–289
Shi X, Gangadharan B, Brass LF, Ruf W, Mueller BM (2004) Protease-activated receptors (PAR1 and PAR2) contribute to tumor cell motility and metastasis. Mol Cancer Res 2:395–402
Sounni NE et al (2010) Stromal regulation of vessel stability by MMP14 and TGFbeta. Dis Model Mech 3:317–332
Suchting S et al (2007) The Notch ligand Delta-like 4 negatively regulates endothelial tip cell formation and vessel branching. Proc Natl Acad Sci U S A 104:3225–3230
Tait CR, Jones PF (2004) Angiopoietins in tumours: the angiogenic switch. J Pathol 204:1–10
Takeichi M (1993) Cadherins in cancer: implications for invasion and metastasis. Curr Opin Cell Biol 5:806–811

Taskinen M, Karjalainen-Lindsberg ML, Leppa S (2008) Prognostic influence of tumor-infiltrating mast cells in patients with follicular lymphoma treated with rituximab and CHOP. Blood 111:4664–4667

Teti A et al (1997) Transforming growth factor-beta enhances adhesion of melanoma cells to the endothelium in vitro. Int J Cancer 72:1013–1020

Timar J et al (2005) Platelet-mimicry of cancer cells: epiphenomenon with clinical significance. Oncology 69:185–201

Wang F et al (2002) Phenotypic reversion or death of cancer cells by altering signaling pathways in three-dimensional contexts. J Natl Cancer Inst 94:1494–1503

Wang HH et al (2000) B16 melanoma cell arrest in the mouse liver induces nitric oxide release and sinusoidal cytotoxicity: a natural hepatic defense against metastasis. Cancer Res 60:5862–5869

Weaver VM et al. (1997) Reversion of the malignant phenotype of human breast cells in three-dimensional culture and in vivo by integrin blocking antibodies. J Cell Biol 137:231–245

Wong CW et al (2002) Intravascular location of breast cancer cells after spontaneous metastasis to the lung. Am J Pathol 161:749–753

Wu Y et al (2009) Stabilization of snail by NF-kappaB is required for inflammation-induced cell migration and invasion. Cancer Cell 15:416–428

Wyckoff J et al (2004) A paracrine loop between tumor cells and macrophages is required for tumor cell migration in mammary tumors. Cancer Res 64:7022–7029

Wyckoff JB et al (2007) Direct visualization of macrophage-assisted tumor cell intravasation in mammary tumors. Cancer Res 67:2649–2656

Zhang Q. et al (2010) The role of the intravascular microenvironment in spontaneous metastasis development. Int J Cancer 126:2534–2541

Part II
Gene Properties of Metastatic Cells

Editor:
Jean-Claude Marshall

Chapter 3
Introduction to Metastasis Suppressor Genes

Jean-Claude Marshall, Silvin Bakalian and Claudia Maria de Oliveira Martins

In the past forty to fifty years, clever scientific insight and innovation has rapidly advanced our understanding of the molecular mechanisms of cancer biology. The discoveries of oncogenes and tumor suppressors and the elucidation of their functions has greatly aided our understanding of the molecular etiology of primary tumors. In the last decade, there has been an explosion in the technology available to scientists to study the genetics of cancer cells at several different levels. It is now possible to study a particular cancer at the whole genome, transcriptome, and proteome levels. This vast increase in available information has led to significant advancements in our understanding of the genetic variations and mutations, which can drive the development of a primary tumor in patients.

Despite these advancements, cancer biologists still have relatively little understanding of the molecular aspects of metastasis. Considering that metastasis is the primary cause of mortality in patients who are diagnosed with most types of cancer, it is obvious that this field requires substantially more investigation. Our understanding of the biological role that genes play in metastasis is still in its infancy, with considerable breakthroughs to come based on our current knowledge. In this chapter we will describe areas in which our understanding of metastasis has evolved during the past several decades and where significant advances have already been made.

One of the first landmark findings to be described in understanding the pathways involved in the formation of primary tumors and subsequent formation of metastasis were the tumor suppressor genes. These genes were characterized when it was discovered that their loss of function was a critical step in tumorigenesis. The first of these genes to be described was retinoblastoma (Rb). Prior to its discovery, the prevailing theories of the day was that the oncogenic phenotype was always dominant

J.-C. Marshall (✉)
National Cancer Institute, 37 Convent Blvd, Building 37,
Bethesda, MD, USA
e-mail: jeanclaude.marshall@gmail.com

S. Bakalian · C. M. de O. Martins
Henry C. Witelson Ocular Pathology Laboratory, McGill University,
Montreal, QC, Canada
e-mail: sbakalian@hotmail.com

J. V. Burnier, M. N. Burnier, Jr. (eds.), *Experimental and Clinical Metastasis*,
DOI 10.1007/978-1-4614-3685-0_3,

in cells, meaning that a mutation was required in a single allele of a gene in order for a normal cell to be transformed into a tumor cell. However, not all disease incidence data appeared to fit neatly into this hypothesis. Research into retinoblastoma case history yielded a new hypothesis, that predicted in at least some cancers the need for two mutations to occur, one on each allele, in order to successfully transform a normal cell into a tumor cell (Knudson 1971). The Rb gene would subsequently become known as the first described tumor suppressor. Since this discovery, it has become widely accepted that "two hits" are required, and that these may result from any combination of germ line, and or somatic mutations, mitotic recombinations, gene conversions, and functional inactivation of genes. To date there is an extensive list of tumor suppressors that have been described in the literature, which includes: Rb, p53, APC, PTEN, TSC1, and NF1 among many others. The discovery of Rb opened and entire new field of research for tumor suppressor genes which could regulate the formation of primary tumors.

Translating that discovery into the understanding of metastasis was a more problematic challenge, one that would take several more years to arrive. The prevailing view at the time was that the formation of metastasis was too complex to be dissected mechanistically. Furthermore, it was believed that once cancer cells had escaped from the primary tumor location and entered either the lymphatics or blood stream it became only a matter of time before the patient would succumb to metastatic disease.

This was the scientific thinking before a novel hypothesis was proposed by Steeg et al. in 1988 (Steeg et al. 1988a). They proposed that there existed a set of genes that were analogous to tumor suppressor genes, but which would function in the metastatic process and whose functional loss would contribute to the tumor cells gaining metastatic ability. To test this hypothesis they used a comparative hybridization screen with ^{32}P-labeled mRNA probes generated from cell lines possessing low and high metastatic potential (Steeg et al. b). From this screen they identified a cDNA clone, labeled non-metastatic clone #23 (Nm23), that exhibited higher expression in the low metastatic cell lines versus the highly metastatic ones. Subsequent *in vivo* functional studies showed that both highly metastatic mouse and human cells transfected to express Nm23 physiological expression levels and injected into mice significantly reduced the formation of metastasis at secondary sites, independent of the formation of primary tumors. In particular, pulmonary metastases were reduced by as much as 96 %. This confirmed that Nm23 was the first of what is now an entire field of study of metastasis suppressor genes (Leone et al. 1991, 1993). Perhaps just as importantly, this work provided direct evidence that the formation of a primary tumor and subsequent metastasis were separate events and that the formation of metastasis could therefore be specifically targeted and studied.

Since the discovery of Nm23 the field of metastasis suppressor genes (MSGs) has expanded to include more than 20 (Horak et al. 2008). The current working definition of an MSG is the ability of that gene to suppress spontaneous metastases formation without affecting the growth of the primary tumor *in vivo*. Although it has become possible to study the formation of metastasis and to try to dissect each step a cell must complete in order to metastasize (migration, invasion, extravasation, adhesion, and proliferation at a secondary site) the overall pathways and mechanisms involved in metastasis remain highly complex. To date, a variety of researchers have shown that MSGs are involved in several pathways that regulate multiple steps in metastasis, indicating that MSGs can inhibit metastatic ability at several points throughout the metastatic process. For example three well studied MSGs, MKK4, MKK7 and MKK6 are involved in the stress-activated MAPK pathway that can regulate cell cycle progression and/or apoptosis (Chekmareva et al. 1997). While another MSG, RhoGDI2 regulates cytoskeletal reorganization and motility by inhibiting Rho (Gildea et al. 2002).

3.1 MSG Identification and Validation Strategies

Since the characterization of Nm23, the search for additional candidate MSGs has involved using a wide variety of techniques including subtractive hybridization, differential display, microcell-mediated chromosome transfer (MMCT), and microarray analysis. The latter two in particular have proven to be valuable, giving rise to a large number of putative MSGs in the last decade.

Early on during the search for MSGs, MMCT was widely used to discover candidate genes. In this process, growing cells are blocked in mitosis and then their mitotic spindle is chemically disrupted, allowing the condensed chromosomes to drift freely (McNeill and Brown 1980). The cells were then allowed to re-enter the cell cycle and the free chromosomes would become membrane bound, forming micronuclei that contained single or multiple chromosomes. From these single chromosomes, microcells could be further isolated using chemical treatments, differential centrifugation and filtrations. The microcells containing the chromosome of interest could then be fused to recipient cells, such as metastatic cancer cells. The newly formed hybrid cells were then screened and if they were found to have suppressed metastatic capabilities compared to the parental cell, positional cloning techniques would be used to pinpoint genes of interest on the transferred chromosome. This was quite labor intensive and required significant amounts of time to pinpoint individual genes from the chromosomes that were responsible for the decreased metastatic phenotype.

More recently, the development of microarray technology, especially its refinement over the past decade, has greatly facilitated the search for MSGs. The concept of microarray analysis is simple, although in practice it can become quite complicated by the need for bio-informatic analysis. Oligonucleotide probes corresponding to thousands of gene products are adhered to a substrate, usually either glass or silicon in an ordered array. RNA that has been isolated from the tissue or cells of interest is then labeled and hybridized with the arrayed probe and the fluorescent intensities of the hybridized samples are measured. The intensity is compared to a standardized sample or control, which allows for the determination of if the gene products are either up or down regulated in comparison. This technique allows for the analysis of relative gene product expression from tens of thousands of genes using only picomoles of nucleic acid products. Candidate MSGs may then be identified on the arrays either by their reduced expression in metastatic versus non-metastatic cell lines, or in clinically resected tumors associated with metastatic versus non-metastatic disease.

The presence of thousands of probes poses an informatic problem which includes sorting through the data and separating it from background noise.

Validation of these candidate MSGs are usually done via a variety of *in vitro* and *in vivo* tests. To accomplish this, metastatic cell lines expressing low levels of the candidate MSG are generally used. Stable s of the MSG to force expression of the candidate gene product at physiological levels are then established and these cells are used and compared to the parental cells in the assays. The MSG candidates may display *in vitro* characteristics of metastasis suppression, including decreased motility, invasion, anchorage independent growth and angiogenesis. While the presence of a decreased *in vitro* metastatic phenotype is suggestive of an MSG it is not the gold standard for establishing a new metastasis suppressor gene. These must be carried out with *in vivo* testing, either by a spontaneous or experimental metastasis assay. In the spontaneous assay, cancer cells are implanted into the orthotopic site allowing primary tumors and subsequent metastatic formation and growth. The experimental metastasis assay by-passes the formation of the primary tumor, with tumor cells injected directly into the blood, either intravenously or intracardiacly, from where they will form metastasis. The use of a spontaneous assay is preferable as this allows for measurement of the primary tumor formation as well as characterization of the proposed MSGs affect on metastasis. Experimental assays generally take less time to develop metastases and occasionally orthotopic injection of primary tumor cells is difficult to accomplish. Therefore in order to conform to the definition of an MSG, transfected cells must also be injected to form a measurable primary tumor.

The development of optical and molecular imaging techniques for the assessment of *in vivo* metastasis formation has recently been the source of considerable interest. These techniques, such as fluorescent protein labeled cells (GFP, RFP), bioluminescence such as luciferase tagged cells, and magnetic resonance imaging allow for *in vivo* imaging without the need to sacrifice the animal. While this obviously has its benefits, it is important to recognize the limitations that are inherent to each technique: the imaging data may add to the overall understanding of metastasis formation in these models but they must always be confirmed by pathological examination of the tissue to confirm metastases.

Only after this *in vitro* and *in vivo* confirmation does a MSG gene loose its status as candidate and become accepted as a true metastasis suppressor gene by causing a decrease in the number of quantifiable metastases without affecting primary tumor growth.

3.2 MSG and Metastatic Colonization

Collectively, the steps required for a tumor cell to leave the primary tumor and become an established metastasis have been termed the metastatic cascade. The complex process of the metastatic cascade begins when tumor cells acquire the ability to break away and grow independently from a primary tumor as well as migrating through the complex network of proteins, proteoglycans and collagens of the extracellular matrix. These cells then intravasate into the blood or lymphatic vessels where they survive the shear stress involved in transportation, resist anoikis, and evade immune surveillance.

Following vessel transport, metastatic cells may become lodged in capillary beds due to their size or the size of emboli (both homotypic or heterotypic), or adhere to integrins and other receptors on organ-specific endothelial cells. In response to chemoattractants, extravasation from vessels at a secondary location follows, but is not absolutely essential, to proceed to subsequent steps. Following extravasation, metastatic cells must then complete the most crucial, and perhaps most selective, step of the metastatic cascade, proliferation at the secondary site. This last step or metastatic colonization is defined as the process by which disseminated tumor cells, present as single or small clusters of cells in a second parenchyma (micrometastasis), grow to form a clinically detectable metastatic nodule (macrometastasis).

The fate of cells in this last step of the metastatic cascade is complex and to date poorly studied. They may either extravasate into the surrounding tissue or remain within the vasculature. In either location they can undergo proliferation, apoptosis or remain essentially quiescent for extended periods of time. Work from metastasis suppressor studies supports previous findings that growth in the primary tumor and metastatic site are not identical processes. A number of preclinical drug studies show disparate effects on primary tumor and metastatic growth leading to the conclusion that applying the well-worn principles of primary tumor growth is unlikely to produce a complete understanding of metastatic colonization. Studies are only beginning to tease out the cancer cell-microenvironmental interactions that contribute to cell fate and ultimately metastasis formation. Metastasis suppressors are proving to be an important tool in these *in vivo* mechanistic studies.

Clinically, metastatic colonization may represent an optimal and untapped therapeutic target. In breast cancer, once a patient is diagnosed with a lymph node positive tumor, invasion has already occurred and it is probable that cells have already disseminated into the vasculature. It is also likely that these cells have lodged at secondary sites implying that cells need only to survival and ultimately grow in order to complete the colonization process. The finding that some metastasis suppressors seem to specifically affect metastatic colonization, as described later in this chapter, provides a unanticipated application for their use in developing molecular therapeutics that target their functions/pathways. This may change disease management by extending the dormancy of the disseminated tumor cells making the disease a clinically treatable chronic condition, or perhaps even killing disseminated cell in the adjuvant setting thereby preventing metastasis formation altogether. While these are important clinical goals, current cancer research is only beginning to look at targeting these cells in a mechanistic manner.

References

Chekmareva MA et al (1997) Localization of prostate cancer metastasis-suppressor activity on human chromosome 17. Prostate 33(4):271–280

Gildea JJ et al (2002) RhoGDI2 is an invasion and metastasis suppressor gene in human cancer. Cancer Res 62(22):6418–6423

Horak CE et al (2008) The role of metastasis suppressor genes in metastatic dormancy. APMIS 116(7–8):586–601

Knudson AG Jr. (1971) Mutation and cancer: statistical study of retinoblastoma. Proc Natl Acad Sci U S A 68(4):820–823

Leone A et al (1991) Reduced tumor incidence, metastatic potential, and cytokine responsiveness of nm23-transfected melanoma cells. Cell 65(1):25–35

Leone A et al (1993) Transfection of human nm23-H1 into the human MDA-MB-435 breast carcinoma cell line: effects on tumor metastatic potential, colonization and enzymatic activity. Oncogene 8(9):2325–2333

McNeill CA, Brown RL (1980) Genetic manipulation by means of microcell-mediated transfer of normal human chromosomes into recipient mouse cells. Proc Natl Acad Sci U S A 77(9):5394–5398

Steeg PS et al (1988a) Altered expression of NM23, a gene associated with low tumor metastatic potential, during adenovirus 2 Ela inhibition of experimental metastasis. Cancer Res 48(22):6550–6554

Steeg PS et al (1988b) Evidence for a novel gene associated with low tumor metastatic potential. J Natl Cancer Inst 80(3):200–204

Chapter 4
Metastasis Suppressor Genes

Jean-Claude Marshall, Silvin Bakalian and Claudia Maria de Oliveira Martins

Below is a list of the most extensively studied MSGs, describing their initial characterization as well as what possible mechanism has been characterized for each.

4.1 NM23

Steeg and coworkers discovered and validated the first MSG in 1988, which they named *NM23*. The results of the study showed that the RNA levels of *NM23* were highest in cell lines and tumors with relatively low metastatic potential in two different experimental systems; the first was in murine K-1735 melanoma cell lines and the second was in rat mammary carcinomas. Since this date, eight isotypes of human *NM23* have been described (Nm23-H1 through Nm23-H8) (Lacombe et al. 2000). Among these isotypes, it has been shown that only Nm23-H1 and Nm23-H2 possess anti metastatic abilities. These isotypes have been studied extensively in different types of tumors including melanomas (Hartsough and Steeg 2000). The metastasis-suppressive function of *NM23* was previously correlated with its histidine protein-kinase activity in site-directed mutagenesis experiments (Freije et al. 1997; Wagner et al. 1997). Recently, Steeg et al. reported that *NM23* co-immunoprecipitated with the kinase suppressor of RAS (KSR) protein, which is thought to be a scaffold protein for the extracellular signal regulated kinase–mitogen activated protein kinase (ERK–MAPK) pathway (Hartsough et al. 2002; Morrison 2001). *NM23* was shown to phosphorylate KSR serine (Ser) 392 (a 14-3-3 binding site) and Ser 434, which was phosphorylated *in vivo* (Cacace et al. 1999; Volle et al. 1999). Therefore, it was

J.-C. Marshall (✉)
National Cancer Institute, 37 Convent Blvd, Building 37,
Bethesda, MD, USA
e-mail: jeanclaude.marshall@gmail.com

S. Bakalian · C. M. de O. Martins
Henry C. Witelson Ocular Pathology Laboratory, McGill University,
Montreal, QC, Canada
e-mail: sbakalian@hotmail.com

J. V. Burnier, M. N. Burnier, Jr. (eds.), *Experimental and Clinical Metastasis*,
DOI 10.1007/978-1-4614-3685-0_4, © Springer Science+Business Media New York 2013

hypothesized that the phosphorylation of KSR by *NM23* altered its scaffold function, possibly by altering the docking of proteins or KSR intracellular localization, which lead to reduced ERK activation in response to signaling (Steeg 2003). In agreement with these findings, Steeg et al. showed that MDA-MB-435 breast carcinoma cells that over expressed *NM23* showed reduced ERK activation levels compared with vector-alone control transfectants. In addition, a histidine-kinase-deficient mutant of *NM23* (Nm23-H1P96S) showed high levels of activated ERK, comparable to those of the control transfectants. Combining all this research, the authors concluded that altered levels of *NM23* in metastatic versus non-metastatic tumor cells might impact ERK activation through a complex interaction with the KSR scaffold protein (Steeg 2003).

NM23 represents the most extensively studied and confirmed MSG. The aforementioned data was recently extended by the characterization of Nm23-M1 knockout mouse, where they induced hepatocellular carcinoma in mice that contained Nm23-M1 or lacked Nm23-M1. The results of the study showed that the size of the primary tumor of the knockout mice did not change significantly, but the incidence rate of metastases increased significantly in the knockout mice (Boissan 2005).

Different expression levels of *NM23* gene products have been widely reported in different human tumor cohorts. Reduced *NM23* gene products expression are correlated with aspects of high metastatic potential including reduced overall survival time, the presence of lymph node metastases, and poor tumor differentiation grade in a subset of breast, gastric, ovarian, cervical, hepatocellular carcinomas and melanoma cohorts.

A study performed by Heiman et al. showed that the fifteen-year disease-free survival rate was found to be significantly better in breast cancer patients with high Nm23 immunostaining compared to low Nm23 immunostaining. Moreover, Nm23 was associated with excellent survival, even when there were other unfavorable prognostic markers such as angiogenesis or nuclear grade (Heimann et al. 1998).

Differential colony hybridization between low and high metastatatic murine melanoma cell lines identified different levels of Nm23. The mRNA levels of the Nm23 were ten-fold higher in low metastatic clones compared to high metastatic clones.

Similarly, significantly lower levels of Nm23 mRNA were detected in cell lines that were derived from aggressive primary melanomas. These melanomas showed higher Clark's level and greater Breslow thickness, which are considered to be poor prognostic markers for cutaneous melanoma patients (Caligo et al. 1994). Nm23 protein expression in primary cutaneous melanomas was found to be significantly and inversely correlated with the dermatopathological predictors of poor prognosis in patients with localized melanoma, including thickness, ulceration, level of invasion, and mitotic figures (Ferrari et al. 2007). Using tissue microarray analysis in one hundred and twenty patients with primary cutaneous melanoma an important role for Nm23 assessment in these patients was suggested. The results of the study showed that Nm23 expression was strongly correlated with Clark's level ($P < 0.001$), Breslow depth ($P = 0.002$) and patient age ($P = 0.014$). In addition, Nm23 expression was significantly associated with poor patient outcome ($chi2 = 7.2219$, $P = 0.0072$).

Further analysis revealed that the intensity of Nm23 expression was also correlated with patient outcome (chi2 = 11.3281, P = 0.0035) (Pacifico et al. 2005).

A study performed by Bakalian et al. showed that the invasive abilities of different human uveal melanoma cell lines with different metastatic potentials increased after silencing the expression of Nm23-H1 in these cell lines with small interference RNA. Furthermore, uveal melanoma patients with high immunostaining intensity for Nm23-H1 survived longer as opposed to patients with low immunostaining intensity (Kaplan-Meier test P = 00097). They concluded that Nm23-H1 could be a prognostic marker to predict the survival rate of uveal melanoma patients and could be a potential marker to identify high-risk patients (Bakalian et al. 2007).

4.2 RHOGDI2

Theodorescu and coworkers recently has identified the Rho family GDP dissociation inhibitor 2 (RhoGDI2) protein as a functional metastasis suppressor gene in bladder cancer. RhoGDI2 was originally identified during differential studies of invasive and metastatic properties of isogenic human bladder carcinoma cell lines, where T24 (non-metastatic), and T24T (highly invasive and metastatic) cell lines, using experimental metastasis models and comparative genomic studies (Seraj et al. 2000a; Titus et al. 2005). The results of the studies demonstrated that reduced expression of RhoGDI2 correlated with increasing invasive and metastatic activities in T24T highly invasive and metastatic cells. In human bladder tumors, the RhoGDI2 level inversely correlated with the development of metastatic disease, and multivariate analysis identified RhoGDI2 as an independent prognostic marker of tumor recurrence following radical cystectomy (Theodorescu et al. 2004). Therefore, RhoGDI2 is considered a prognostic marker in bladder cancer patients after cystectomy, where diminished expression is associated with decreased patient survival (Theodorescu et al. 2004). Using DNA microarrays to monitor the changes in gene expression following restoration of RhoGDI2 expression, Titus and coworkers identified several potentially targetable proteins, including the endothelin-1 ligand (ET-1), that were suppressed in the presence of RhoGDI2 protein. The results of the study revealed that loss of RhoGDI2 during the clinical progression of bladder carcinoma might lead to up-regulation of the endothelin axis. The later was confirmed by examining the relationship between RhoGDI2 expression levels and those of ET-1 in human tumor samples and cell lines. These findings suggested that adjuvant trials with endothelin antagonists might be contemplated for patients with advanced bladder carcinoma following the initial therapy (Titus et al. 2005). Lately, RhoGDI2 has been found to suppress the expression of neuromidinU, a molecule that mediates both increased growth of metastases and increased tumor cachexia in animal models (Wu et al. 2007). All these experiments showed a novel approach of identifying downstream therapeutic targets of metastasis suppressor genes. This new therapeutic approach warrants further clinical evaluation.

4.3 Ndrg1

N-myc downstream regulated gene 1(NDRG1) was originally identified by differential displays as being significantly up regulated by induction of *in vitro* differentiation of colon carcinoma cells (van Belzen et al. 1997). NDRG1 has been shown to act as a tumor suppressor as well as a metastasis suppressor depending on cell context (Kovacevic and Richardson 2006). The level of the NDRG1 expression was inversely related with the status of metastasis in breast and prostate carcinoma patients, supporting the notion that NDRG1 is a tumor metastasis suppressor gene (Bandyopadhyay et al. 2003, 2004). Ectopic expression of the NDRG1 gene in a highly metastastic prostate cancer cell line significantly reduced the incidence of lung metastases, suggesting that NDRG1 was able to block the metastatic process without affecting the primary tumor growth (Bandyopadhyay et al. 2003, 2004). NDRG1 significantly suppressed the invasive potential of prostate and breast cancer cells as tested by *in vitro* invasion chamber assay (Bandyopadhyay et al. 2003, 2004). Similar metastasis suppressor effect of NDRG1 was also observed in colon carcinoma cells (Guan et al. 2000).

Studies in which mice injected with SW620 colon cancer cells over expressing Ndrg-1 resulted in only 23 % of these developing liver metastases,compared to 75 % in the control group (Guan et al. 2000). To date, there has been little assessment of the molecular targets of Ndrg-1 that mediate its anti-metastatic activity. The adhesion molecule and metastasis suppressor, E-cadherin was found to be up regulated by Ndrg-1 (Guan et al. 2000). Increased expression of E-cadherin has been shown to reduce the motility of metastatic breast cancer cells *in vitro* (Liu et al. 2005). However, it is widely believed that E-cadherin is not the only molecular target of Ndrg-1 that contributes to metastasis suppression. Recently, it has been shown that Ndrg-1 expression was regulated by cellular iron levels and induced by iron chelators (Kovacevic and Richardson 2006). These latter compounds were identified as potential anticancer agents as they selectively prevent cancer cell proliferation and lead to apoptosis. The discovery that iron chelators increase Ndrg-1 expression further augments their antitumor and anti metastatic activity and offers a potential new strategy for the treatment of cancer and metastases.

4.4 RKIP

It has been shown that RKIP negatively regulates the Raf/MEK/ERK pathway by interfering with the activity of Raf-1. In its phosphorylated state, RKIP dissociates from Raf-1 and inhibits GRK-2, a negative regulator of G-protein coupled receptors (GPCRs). In addition, it has been demonstrated that RKIP is a negative regulator of the NF-kappaB pathway. Recent studies have also shown that phosphorylated RKIP binds to the centrosomal and kinetochore regions of metaphase chromosomes, where it may be involved in regulating the partitioning of chromosomes and the progression through mitosis. Therefore, evidence based research indicates that RKIP regulates the activity and mediates the cross talk between several important cellular signaling pathways of metastasis, angiogenesis, resistance to apoptosis, and genome integrity (Klysik et al. 2008).

The first evidence about RKIP came from cell lines derived from metastatic prostate cancers, which displayed decreased levels of RKIP mRNA and protein as compared with primary tumor cell lines (Fu et al. 2003). Furthermore, studies showed that over-expression of RKIP in metastatic cancer cells decreased their invasive capabilities. Consistent with the notion that RKIP is a potent suppressor of metastases, experiments from several laboratories have demonstrated that malignant melanomas, breast cancer lymph node metastases, colorectal cancer, and hepatocarcinoma cells frequently display a marked decrease in RKIP expression (Klysik et al. 2008).

Recently, measuring the levels of RKIP in the blood has been proposed as a prognostic marker for prostate cancer patients, where RKIP plays a major role (Fu et al. 2006). A study performed by Zhu et al. showed that a small molecule, called locostatin, has the ability to abrogate RKIP's ability to inhibit Raf (Zhu et al. 2005). Interventions capable of enhancing RKIP-1 activity would be particularly useful for the control of metastatic cells that display attenuated steady-state levels of RKIP-1. Therefore, future studies evaluating the drug-induced modulation of RKIP expression may provide a potent means of controlling metastases.

4.5 KISS1

KISS1 is one of the metastasis suppressor genes that appears to function in the dormancy phase of the metastatic cascade. In addition, the gene encodes a protein that is further cleaved (called metastin) that likely exerts its function through the binding of metastin to a G-coupled-receptor. This event makes *KISS1* a possible candidate for therapy.

KISS1 was identified as a metastasis suppressor gene in melanoma cells in 1996 by Lee et al., when transfection of a full-length *KISS1* cDNA into C8161 melanoma cells suppressed metastasis in an expression-dependent way (Lee et al. 1996).

Nash et al. were the first to show that the introduction of *KISS1* into highly metastatic human melanoma cell lines C8161 and MelJuSo suppressed *in vivo* metastases to the lung by more than 95 % (Miele et al. 1996). Interestingly, introduction of *KISS1* into a metastatic breast cancer cell line MDA-MB-435 also showed a > 95 % suppression of metastases to the lung (Lee and Welch 1997).

It was also demonstrated that loss of KISS1 mRNA expression correlated with the conversion from benign to malignant phenotype in human melanoma (Shirasaki et al. 2001). This data strongly suggested *KISS1* metastasis suppression being pertinent in tumors of broadly different origins, a conclusion that was confirmed by later studies (Ikeguchi et al. 2004). Furthermore, reduced KISS1 expression has been shown to be a strong prognostic marker in patients with urinary bladder cancer (Sanchez-Carbayo et al. 2003) and gastric carcinoma (Dhar et al. 2004).

In general, loss or reduction of KISS1 expression in different tumor types negatively affected tumor progression, metastatic potential, and survival (Nash and Welch 2006).

Goldberg et al. showed that when chromosome 6 hybrid cells were injected intravenously into athymic mice, grossly detectable metastases did not form. Despite arriving in the lungs at frequencies comparable to the controls, the *Mkk4* and *KISS1* metastasis suppressor transfectants failed grow (Chekmareva et al. 1998; Goldberg et al. 1999). The results of these studies are responsible for identifying the role of these genes in the dormancy phase of the metastatic disease.

KISS1 encodes a 145-amino acid residue peptide that is further processed posttranslationaly. One of the products, a 54-amino acid peptide is called Metastin or Kisspeptin-54 and is a natural ligand to a G-coupled receptor known as HOT7T175/AXOR12/GPR54 (Ohtaki et al. 2001).

Evidence suggests that KISS1/metastin promotes dormancy of solitary cells (Nash et al. 2007) and acts in the final stage of tumor cell colonization at the metastatic site (Steeg 2004). A potential therapeutic approach involves administering exogenous KISS1 which has been shown to suppress cutaneous melanoma metastasis to multiple organs and enhanced median survival almost three-fold (Steeg and Theodorescu 2008). This has become a possibility due to the advent of small molecule mimetics.

Orsini et al in 2007 reported a molecule in which structure-activity approach may yield pharmacologically useful compounds relevant in defining and modulating metastin receptor function (Orsini et al. 2007).

4.6 KAI1

KAI1 is also known as CD82, R2, C33, IA4, and 4F9. It structurally belongs to tetraspanin family while categorized as metastasis suppressor gene (Malik et al. 2009). Tetraspanins are large group of cell surface transmembrane proteins with four transmembrane structures, which can form complexes with integrins.

KAI1/CD82 was initially identified as a metastasis suppressor of prostate cancer. However, evidence supports KAI1/CD82 as a invasion- and metastasis-suppressor during the progression of a variety of solid tumors (Malik et al. 2009).

The role of KAI1/CD82 in cancer progression was discovered by a genetic screen attempting to identify metastasis suppressor genes. Using microcell-mediated chromosome transfer, human gene(s) responsible for suppressing metastasis of the highly metastatic rat AT6.1 prostate cancer cells was mapped to the short arm of human chromosome 11. Later on, an important progress was made, by cloning the metastasis suppressor gene located on human chromosome 11 p11.2–13, which was named KAI1 (Ichikawa 1992).

KAI1/CD82 expression leads to a marked suppression of lung metastases of AT6.1 prostate cancer cells, with no effect on the growth rate of the primary tumor (Dong et al. 1995).

KAI1 appears to prompt dormancy in solitary tumor cells by binding DARC on the surface of vascular endothelial cells and inducing tumor cell growth arrest.

An inverse correlation between KAI1/CD82 expression and the invasive and metastatic potentials of cancer has been frequently observed in a wide range of malignancies such as prostate, gastric, colon, cervix, breast, skin, bladder, lung, pancreas, liver, and thyroid cancers (Liu and Zhang 2006).

4.7 MKK4 and MKK7

Mitogen-activated protein (MAP) kinase kinase 4 (MKK4) is a component of stress activated MAP kinase signaling modules. It directly phosphorylates and activates the c-Jun N-terminal kinase (JNK) and p38 families of MAP kinases in response to environmental stress, pro-inflammatory cytokines, and developmental cues (Whitmarsh and Davis 2007). The human MKK4 gene is located on chromosome 17 and encodes a protein of 399 amino acids (Yoshida et al. 1999).

MKK7 (also known as JNKK2) and MKK6 are also mitogen-activated protein kinase kinase that specifically phosphorylate JNK and p38, respectively (Vander Griend 2005)

Yoshida et al. first characterized MKK4 as an MSG in 1999 when they reported a reduction of the metastatic potential of prostate cancer cells by 80 % in a spontaneous metastasis assay (Yoshida et al. 1999). These experiments using the highly metastatic rat prostate cancer cell line AT6.1 (which lacks MKK4 expression) as a model system have demonstrated that the overexpression of MKK4 significantly reduces their metastatic ability (Whitmarsh and Davis 2007).

There is strong evidence that MKK4 play a role in dormancy of metastatic cells. In a model of spontaneous metastasis, MKK4 was shown to be required for suppression of overt metastases by inhibiting the ability of disseminated cells to colonize the lung (secondary site) (Vander Griend 2005). Ectopic expression of MKK4 also prolonged survival after surgical resection of the primary tumor from 7–20 days. Metastatic lung cells from mice were then cultured again in plaques and showed viability, stressing the dormant behavior of tumor cells expressing the gene (Vander Griend 2005). MKK-7 also plays an important role in dormancy, since it showed the same results as MKK-4 in these experiments. It was shown that ectopic expression MKK-7 suppresses the formation of overt metastases, whereas MKK6 had no effect (Vander Griend 2005).

A tissue-specific role for MKK7 was indicated when a difference between MKK4 and MKK7's regulation in dormancy was traced to the JNK arm of the MAPK pathway. In prostate cancer, MKK4 functions through the JNK pathway, which is also regulated by MKK7. NK activation leads to inhibition of the pro-survival gene Bcl2 and activation of the apoptotic genes BAX, Cytochrome C, Bim/Bmf, and c-Jun. The kinase activities of MKK4 and MKK7 were functional only in the metastatic site and not the primary tumor as identified using immunoprecipitation from primary and lung metastases.

The impaired expression of MKK4 in prostate and ovarian tumors appears to promote their metastasis (Yoshida et al. 1999; Yoshida et al. 2001), while reduced

MKK4 mRNA levels have been reported in breast cancer to brain metastases (Stark et al. 2005)

In normal prostate tissue there are high levels of MKK4 protein expression in the epithelial compartment but not in the stromal compartment, whereas in neoplastic prostate tissues the levels of MKK4 were reduced and there was in inverse relationship between the reduction of MKK4 expression and metastatic potential (Kim et al. 2001). Also, MKK4 protein expression is also reduced in ovarian metastatic tissues compared to normal ovarian epithelial cells (Yamada et al. 2002).

All these studies suggest that MKK4 functions as a metastasis suppressor that works in the dormancy phase of the metastatic cascade. It is probable that different tissues and organs dictate which MAP kinase pathway is targeted by MKK4 depending on specific stimuli.

4.8 BRMS1

BRMS1 (Breast Cancer Metastasis Suppressor) was identified using a combination of clinical observation and molecular biology. Seraj et al. identified BRMS1 by differential display comparing metastasis-suppressed chromosome 11 hybrids with metastatic, parental MDA-MB-435 human breast carcinoma cells. BRMS1 has subsequently been shown to suppress metastasis, but not tumorigenicity of human melanoma cells (Seraj et al. 2000b). A spontaneous metastasis assay was performed and originally showed to functionally suppress the metastatic capacity of breast cancer cells following injection into immunocompromised, athymic mice (Seraj et al. 2000b). BRMS1-transfected MDA-MB-435 cells demonstrated a decreased incidence and number of metastases to lung and regional lymph nodes when cells were injected orthotopically. These results demonstrated that BRMS1 suppressed metastasis without significantly affecting tumorigenicity, indicating that BRMS1 is a metastasis suppressor gene (Meehan and Welch 2003).

Further studies have proven that BRMS1 is not only a metastasis suppressor gene in breast cancer models but also in various other cancers such as melanoma and ovarian cancer (Meehan and Welch 2003). Recent studies have also demonstrated that low levels of BRMS1 protein correlated with poor prognosis in cancer patients with advanced metastatic disease. In addition, reduced BRMS1 mRNA levels have been shown to correlate with reduced disease-free survival in breast cancer patients.

BRMS1 is thought to possibly regulate metastasis through multiple mechanisms; such as the restoration of gap junctions, influencing phosphoinositide signaling, regulating genes through histone deacetylase (HDAC) interaction, and complex formation and inhibiting NFκB signaling in breast cancer. In particular, BRMS1 has been shown to downregulate osteopontin (OPN) expression by modulating the activity of NFκB signaling in breast cancer. Hedley et al. reported that decreased OPN associated with BRMS1 expression contributes to its metastasis suppression activity (Metge et al. 2010).

BRMS1 suppresses metastasis by inhibiting multiple steps in the metastatic cascade through different regulation mechanisms of many protein-encoding and metastasis-associated genes.

References

Bakalian S et al (2007) Expression of nm23-H1 in uveal melanoma. Melanoma Res 17(5):284–290

Bandyopadhyay S et al (2003) The Drg-1 gene suppresses tumor metastasis in prostate cancer. Cancer Res 63(8):1731–1736

Bandyopadhyay S et al (2004) Role of the putative tumor metastasis suppressor gene Drg-1 in breast cancer progression. Oncogene 23(33):5675–5681

Boissan M et al (2005) Increased lung metastasis in transgenic NM23-Null/SV40 mice with hepatocellular carcinoma. J Natl Cancer Inst 97(11):836–845

Cacace AM et al (1999) Identification of constitutive and ras-inducible phosphorylation sites of KSR: implications for 14-3-3 binding, mitogen-activated protein kinase binding, and KSR overexpression. Mol Cell Biol 19(1):229–240

Caligo MA et al (1994) A low NM23.H1 gene expression identifying high malignancy human melanomas. Melanoma Res 4(3):179–184

Chekmareva MA et al (1998) Chromosome 17-mediated dormancy of AT6.1 prostate cancer micrometastases. Cancer Res 58(21):4963–4969

Dhar DK et al (2004) Downregulation of KiSS-1 expression is responsible for tumor invasion and worse prognosis in gastric carcinoma. Int J Cancer 111(6):868–872

Dong JT et al (1995) KAI1, a metastasis suppressor gene for prostate cancer on human chromosome 11p11.2. Science 268(5212):884–886

Ferrari D et al (2007) Dermatopathological indicators of poor melanoma prognosis are significantly inversely correlated with the expression of NM23 protein in primary cutaneous melanoma. J Cutan Pathol 34(9):705–712

Freije JM et al (1997) Site-directed mutation of Nm23-H1. Mutations lacking motility suppressive capacity upon transfection are deficient in histidine-dependent protein phosphotransferase pathways in vitro. J Biol Chem 272(9):5525–5532

Fu Z et al (2003) Effects of raf kinase inhibitor protein expression on suppression of prostate cancer metastasis. J Natl Cancer Inst 95(12):878–889

Fu Z et al (2006) Metastasis suppressor gene Raf kinase inhibitor protein (RKIP) is a novel prognostic marker in prostate cancer. Prostate 66(3):248–256

Goldberg SF et al (1999) Metastasis-suppressed C8161 melanoma cells arrest in lung but fail to proliferate. Clin Exp Metastasis 17(7):601–607

Guan RJ et al (2000) Drg-1 as a differentiation-related, putative metastatic suppressor gene in human colon cancer. Cancer Res 60(3):749–755

Hartsough MT, Steeg PS (2000) Nm23/nucleoside diphosphate kinase in human cancers. J Bioenerg Biomembr 32(3):301–308

Hartsough MT et al (2002) Nm23-H1 metastasis suppressor phosphorylation of kinase suppressor of Ras via a histidine protein kinase pathway. J Biol Chem 277(35):32389–32399

Heimann R, Ferguson DJ, Hellman S (1998) The relationship between nm23, angiogenesis, and the metastatic proclivity of node-negative breast cancer. Cancer Res 58(13):2766–2771

Ichikawa T et al (1992) Localization of metastasis suppressor gene(s) for prostatic cancer to the short arm of human chromosome 11. Cancer Res 52(12):3486–3490

Ikeguchi M, Yamaguchi K, Kaibara N (2004) Clinical significance of the loss of KiSS-1 and orphan G-protein-coupled receptor (hOT7T175) gene expression in esophageal squamous cell carcinoma. Clin Cancer Res 10(4):1379–1383

Kim HL et al (2001) Mitogen-activated protein kinase kinase 4 metastasis suppressor gene expression is inversely related to histological pattern in advancing human prostatic cancers. Cancer Res 61(7):2833–2837

Klysik J et al (2008) Signaling crossroads: the function of Raf kinase inhibitory protein in cancer, the central nervous system and reproduction. Cell Signal 20(1):1–9

Kovacevic Z, Richardson DR (2006) The metastasis suppressor, Ndrg-1: a new ally in the fight against cancer. Carcinogenesis 27(12):2355–2366

Lacombe ML et al (2000) The human Nm23/nucleoside diphosphate kinases. J Bioenerg Biomembr 32(3):247–258

Lee JH, Welch DR (1997) Suppression of metastasis in human breast carcinoma MDA-MB-435 cells after transfection with the metastasis suppressor gene, KiSS-1. Cancer Res 57(12):2384–2387

Lee JH et al (1996) KiSS-1, a novel human malignant melanoma metastasis-suppressor gene. J Natl Cancer Inst 88(23):1731–1737

Liu WM, Zhang XA (2006) KAI1/CD82, a tumor metastasis suppressor. Cancer Lett 240(2):183–194

Liu YN et al (2005) Regulatory mechanisms controlling human E-cadherin gene expression. Oncogene 24(56):8277–8290

Malik FA, Sanders AJ, Jiang WG (2009) KAI-1/CD82, the molecule and clinical implication in cancer and cancer metastasis. Histol Histopathol 24(4):519–30

Meehan WJ, Welch DR (2003) Breast cancer metastasis suppressor 1: update. Clin Exp Metastasis 20(1):45–50

Metge BJ et al (2010) Elevated Osteopontin Levels in Metastatic Melanoma Correlate with Epigenetic Silencing of Breast Cancer Metastasis Suppressor 1. Oncology 78(1):75–86

Miele ME et al (1996) Metastasis suppressed, but tumorigenicity and local invasiveness unaffected, in the human melanoma cell line MelJuSo after introduction of human chromosomes 1 or 6. Mol Carcinog 15(4):284–299

Morrison DK (2001) KSR: a MAPK scaffold of the Ras pathway? J Cell Sci 114(Pt 9):1609–1612

Nash KT, Welch DR (2006) The KISS1 metastasis suppressor: mechanistic insights and clinical utility. Front Biosci 11:647–659

Nash KT et al (2007) Requirement of KISS1 secretion for multiple organ metastasis suppression and maintenance of tumor dormancy. J Natl Cancer Inst 99(4):309–321

Ohtaki T et al (2001) Metastasis suppressor gene KiSS-1 encodes peptide ligand of a G-protein-coupled receptor. Nature 411(6837):613–617

Orsini MJ et al (2007) Metastin (KiSS-1) mimetics identified from peptide structure-activity relationship-derived pharmacophores and directed small molecule database screening. J Med Chem 50(3):462–471

Pacifico MD et al (2005) nm23 as a prognostic marker in primary cutaneous melanoma: evaluation using tissue microarray in a patient group with long-term follow-up. Melanoma Res 15(5):435–440

Sanchez-Carbayo M, Capodieci P, Cordon-Cardo C (2003) Tumor suppressor role of KiSS-1 in bladder cancer: loss of KiSS-1 expression is associated with bladder cancer progression and clinical outcome. Am J Pathol 162(2):609–617

Seraj MJ et al (2000a) The relationship of BRMS1 and RhoGDI2 gene expression to metastatic potential in lineage related human bladder cancer cell lines. Clin Exp Metastasis 18(6):519–525

Seraj MJ et al (2000b) Functional evidence for a novel human breast carcinoma metastasis suppressor, BRMS1, encoded at chromosome 11q13. Cancer Res 60(11):2764–2769

Shirasaki F et al (2001) Loss of expression of the metastasis suppressor gene KiSS1 during melanoma progression and its association with LOH of chromosome 6q16.3-q23. Cancer Res 61(20):7422–7425

Stark AM et al (2005) Reduced metastasis-suppressor gene mRNA-expression in breast cancer brain metastases. J Cancer Res Clin Oncol 131(3):191–198

Steeg PS (2003) Metastasis suppressors alter the signal transduction of cancer cells. Nat Rev Cancer 3(1):55–63

Steeg PS (2004) Perspectives on classic article: metastasis suppressor genes. J Natl Cancer Inst 96(6):E4

Steeg PS, Theodorescu D (2008) Metastasis: a therapeutic target for cancer. Nat Clin Pract Oncol 5(4):206–219

Theodorescu D et al (2004) Reduced expression of metastasis suppressor RhoGDI2 is associated with decreased survival for patients with bladder cancer. Clin Cancer Res 10(11):3800–3806

Titus B et al (2005) Endothelin axis is a target of the lung metastasis suppressor gene RhoGDI2. Cancer Res 65(16):7320–7327

van Belzen N et al (1997) A novel gene which is up-regulated during colon epithelial cell differentiation and down-regulated in colorectal neoplasms. Lab Invest 77(1):85–92

Vander Griend DJ et al (2005) Suppression of metastatic colonization by the context-dependent activation of the c-Jun NH2-terminal kinase kinases JNKK1/MKK4 and MKK7. Cancer Res 65(23):10984–10991

Volle DJ et al (1999) Phosphorylation of the kinase suppressor of ras by associated kinases. Biochemistry 38(16):5130–5137

Wagner PD, Steeg PS, Vu ND (1997) Two-component kinase-like activity of nm23 correlates with its motility-suppressing activity. Proc Natl Acad Sci U S A 94(17):9000–9005

Whitmarsh AJ, Davis RJ (2007) Role of mitogen-activated protein kinase kinase 4 in cancer. Oncogene 26(22):3172–3184

Wu Y et al (2007) Neuromedin U is regulated by the metastasis suppressor RhoGDI2 and is a novel promoter of tumor formation, lung metastasis and cancer cachexia. Oncogene 26(5):765–773

Yamada SD et al (2002) Mitogen-activated protein kinase kinase 4 (MKK4) acts as a metastasis suppressor gene in human ovarian carcinoma. Cancer Res 62(22):6717–6723

Yoshida BA et al (1999) Mitogen-activated protein kinase kinase 4/stress-activated protein/Erk kinase 1 (MKK4/SEK1), a prostate cancer metastasis suppressor gene encoded by human chromosome 17. Cancer Res 59(21):5483–5487

Yoshida S et al (2001) The c-Jun NH2-terminal kinase3 (JNK3) gene: genomic structure, chromosomal assignment, and loss of expression in brain tumors. J Hum Genet 46(4):182–187

Zhu S et al (2005) A chemical inhibitor reveals the role of Raf kinase inhibitor protein in cell migration. Chem Biol 12(9):981–991

Chapter 5
Metastatic Dormancy and Metastasis Suppressor Genes

Jean-Claude Marshall, Silvin Bakalian and Claudia Maria de Oliveira Martins

To date it is evident that MSGs can suppress metastasis by inhibiting several different steps in the metastatic cascade. Several of the MSGs can inhibit tumor cell motility and invasion, while others can impinge upon tumor cell arrest and extravasation at the secondary site. In addition, a growing list of MSGs that function by inducing dormancy and regulating the final stage of the metastatic cascade, metastatic colonization has been discovered. The idea of metastatic dormancy has become of significant interest to cancer researchers, encouraged by clinical findings similar to those of breasts cancer studies in which up to 45 % of patients with invasive breast cancer will relapse years or even decades after successful treatment for the primary tumor (Aguirre-Ghiso 2007).

Two different types of metastatic dormancy have been studied using experimental model systems. The first involves solitary tumor cells that have survived to arrive at a distant organ and are neither proliferating nor undergoing apoptosis. The second type of tumor dormancy has been characterized as small clusters of tumor cells, known as micrometatstases, which have implanted at a secondary site and either no longer proliferate, or have a balanced rate of proliferation and cell death, resulting in no increase in size of the micrometastases. These dormant, micrometastases may, in part, be explained by their failure to induce angiogenesis and recruit additional nutrients to their location (Naumov et al. 2006a, b). While the phenomenon of metastatic dormancy has become generally accepted, the actual mechanisms of how a metastatic cell becomes dormant are only now beginning to be studied. Recently a possible marker of metastatic dormancy has been described (Aguirre-Ghiso et al. 2003, 2004). In a series of experiments, Aguirro-Ghiso et al. showed that a balance between phosphorylated activated Erk, a component of the MAPK pathway and

J.-C. Marshall (✉)
National Cancer Institute, 37 Convent Blvd, Building 37,
Bethesda, MD, USA
e-mail: jeanclaude.marshall@gmail.com

S. Bakalian · C. M. de O. Martins
Henry C. Witelson Ocular Pathology Laboratory, McGill University,
Montreal, QC, Canada
e-mail: sbakalian@hotmail.com

J. V. Burnier, M. N. Burnier, Jr. (eds.), *Experimental and Clinical Metastasis*,
DOI 10.1007/978-1-4614-3685-0_5,

phosphorylated p38, a stress activated protein kinase, was important for tumor cell dormancy. Increased levels of phosphorylated p38 induced a dormant state in tumor cells that was reversible. This may prove to be of therapeutic benefit as, by using targets regulated by MSGs, such as LPA1 by Nm23 (Horak et al. 2007a, b), it may be possible to induce metastatic dormancy in patients.

To date, four metastasis suppressor genes have been well characterized as having a potential role in dormancy, while evidence for other MSGs continues to be reviewed. KISS1, as previously described in this chapter, was first characterized as an MSG in 1996. It is unique among MSGs as it encodes for secreted polypeptides that are known as kisspeptins. Evidence suggests that secretion of these kisspeptins and binding to the G protein coupled receptor GPR54 can promote dormancy of solitary cells. Fluorescently labeled cutaneous melanoma cells were injected into athymic nude mice via the tail vein and shown to disseminate throughout the body of the mouse. Cells that had been transfected to express an empty vector or a secretion signal deletion variant of kisspeptin formed detectable metastases. In comparison those cells that were transfected to express wild type kisspeptin remained dormant in multiple organs without detectible growth. Interestingly, the authors noted that the role of kisspeptin did not appear to dependent on GPR54, suggesting that another receptor may be implicated in this process.

Another MSG that can induce dormancy is Kai1 (also known as CD82). Although it was first described as inhibiting cancer cell migration and invasion (Ichikawa et al. 1991), recent studies have suggested it can also inhibit tumor cell colonization (Bandyopadhyay et al. 2006). Kai1 interacts with Duffy antigen receptor for chemokines (DARC), a transmembrane protein which is expressed on endothelial cells. Aggressive prostate cancer cells transfected to express Kai1 had a much higher binding affinity for DARC than the non-expressing Kai1 control cells. The binding of these cells to DARC induced growth arrest in the tumor cells and decreased *in vitro* colony formation without detectible apoptosis. Using DARC knockout mice, the authors showed that Kai1 positive cells were able to develop significant lung metastasis in the knockout mice, while they formed only a few large metastases in the wild type DARC expressing mice. The results indicated that Kai1 required DARC for the induction of dormancy at a secondary site.

MKK4 and MKK7 have also been shown to induce dormancy in micrometastatic colonies (Lefter et al. 2003) that was found to be tissue specific. In ovarian cancer, MKK4 activated p38 leading to cell cycle arrest. In addition it was found that MKK4 can also induce an up-regulation of p21, which is a selective cell cycle inhibitor that suppresses CDK and activates RB. No increase in cell death was seen in cells transfected to express MKK4. The cell cycle arrest was shown to be reversible *ex vivo*, as the tumor cells, once removed from secondary sites, were able to overcome the growth inhibition in culture.

As previously described, Nm23-H1 has been shown to cause growth arrest of micrometastatic lesions and has been shown to suppress metastasis in a several different cancer models. To date, two different models have suggested a role for Nm23 in metastatic dormancy. In the first, expression of Nm23-H1 was induced by treatment of cells with medroxyprogesterone acetate (MPA) (Palmieri et al. 2005; Ouatas et al. 2003). The induction of Nm23-H1 was correlated with decreased anchorage-independent growth *in vitro* and also inhibited metastatic colonization *in vivo*. Using an experimental model of metastasis, human breast cancer cells were injected into the tail vein of nude mice. Those mice treated with MPA had significantly smaller pulmonary metastases then those treated with vehicle control. Pervious studies have shown a link between Nm23-H1 and Ksr, an ERK scaffold protein, that may shift the ERK, p38 activation balance. A second model has shown that Nm23-H1 expression is inversely related to LPA1 expression, a cell surface receptor for Lysophosphatidic acid (Horak et al. 2007a, b). Over expression of Nm23-H1 by transfection reduced the expression of LPA1 in breast cancer cell lines, and this reduced expression was found to be crucial for Nm23 mediated suppression of motility, invasion and metastasis. When LPA1 was over expressed in the Nm23-H1 expressing cells they were capable of overcoming Nm23-H1 suppression of tumor cell arrest, adhesion and survival in a secondary site. When these cells were used in an experimental metastasis model, fluorescently labeled cells expressing Nm23-H1 were retained in the lungs of mice ten times less than controls. The expression of LPA1 in the Nm23-H1 expressing cells restored the tumor cell retention in the lungs of mice. Taken together these data indicate that Nm23 can control multiple steps in the metastatic cascade, including motility, invasion, and metastatic colonization at a secondary site.

5.1 Key Points

- Metastasis suppressor genes encode proteins that have the ability to prevent or reduce the development of metastases *in vivo*, without affecting the growth rate of the primary tumor. This is different from tumor suppressor genes that affect the growth rate of the primary tumors.
- Metastasis suppressor genes are lost during cancer progression.
- Metastasis suppressor genes suppress the metastatic colonization
- The function of metastasis suppressor genes can be stored by exogenous gene therapy or by potential therapeutic targets.
- Dormancy can be induced by metastasis suppressor genes and may be a potential therapeutic target.

References

Aguirre-Ghiso JA (2007) Models, mechanisms and clinical evidence for cancer dormancy. Nat Rev Cancer 7(11):834–846

Aguirre-Ghiso JA et al (2003) ERK(MAPK) activity as a determinant of tumor growth and dormancy; regulation by p38(SAPK). Cancer Res 63(7):1684–1695

Aguirre-Ghiso JA, Ossowski L, Rosenbaum SK (2004) Green fluorescent protein tagging of extracellular signal-regulated kinase and p38 pathways reveals novel dynamics of pathway activation during primary and metastatic growth. Cancer Res 64(20):7336–7345

Bandyopadhyay S et al (2006) Interaction of KAI1 on tumor cells with DARC on vascular endothelium leads to metastasis suppression. Nat Med 12(8):933–938

Horak CE et al (2007a) Nm23-H1 suppresses tumor cell motility by down-regulating the lysophosphatidic acid receptor EDG2. Cancer Res 67(15):7238–7246

Horak CE et al (2007b) Nm23-H1 suppresses metastasis by inhibiting expression of the lysophosphatidic acid receptor EDG2. Cancer Res 67(24):11751–11759

Ichikawa T, Ichikawa Y, Isaacs JT (1991) Genetic factors and suppression of metastatic ability of prostatic cancer. Cancer Res 51(14):3788–3792

Lefter LP et al (2003) Inserting chromosome 18 into pancreatic cancer cells switches them to a dormant metastatic phenotype. Clin Cancer Res 9(13):5044–5052

Naumov GN et al (2006a) A model of human tumor dormancy: an angiogenic switch from the nonangiogenic phenotype. J Natl Cancer Inst 98(5):316–325

Naumov GN, Akslen LA, Folkman J (2006b) Role of angiogenesis in human tumor dormancy: animal models of the angiogenic switch. Cell Cycle 5(16):1779–1787

Ouatas T, Halverson D, Steeg PS (2003) Dexamethasone and medroxyprogesterone acetate elevate Nm23-H1 metastasis suppressor gene expression in metastatic human breast carcinoma cells: new uses for old compounds. Clin Cancer Res 9(10 Pt 1):3763–3772

Palmieri D et al (2005) Medroxyprogesterone acetate elevation of Nm23-H1 metastasis suppressor expression in hormone receptor-negative breast cancer. J Natl Cancer Inst 97(9):632–642

Chapter 6
Clinical Implications

Jean-Claude Marshall, Silvin Bakalian and Claudia Maria de Oliveira Martins

The ability to control primary tumor growth with surgery and either radiotherapy, chemotherapy or some combination of the above provides adequate control at the initial site for most patients. For most solid cancers, mortality usually arises due to metastatic disease or as a complication of treatment. Although the metastatic process is complex, the inhibition of even one step of the metastatic cascade will halt the entire process. Therefore, the ability to restore the function of an MSG into cancer cells prior to the completion of the entire metastatic process has great clinical potential. Metastatic colonization may represent the portion of the metastatic process most amenable to therapeutic intervention.

It is an unfortunate reality that most cancer therapeutic trials to date focus on the ability of a therapeutic agent to shrink a large metastatic lesion in a patient. Therapeutic agents which target MSGs would be expected to halt, rather than reverse metastatic progression in patients. These compounds would be unlikely to meet current clinical response standards for early clinical testing. This would necessitate the use of tailored clinical trials to investigate MSG therapeutic compounds in an adjuvant setting. However, the future of study in this field is promising as new techniques allow us to dissect areas of the metastatic cascade that were previously clandestine. The push to introduce these into clinic and targeting them as potential therapeutic targets, currently in the case of NM23 and RHOGDI1, has opened the entire field of study for potential breakthrough into clinical use.

J.-C. Marshall (✉)
National Cancer Institute, 37 Convent Blvd, Building 37,
Bethesda, MD, USA
e-mail: jeanclaude.marshall@gmail.com

S. Bakalian · C. M. de O. Martins
Henry C. Witelson Ocular Pathology Laboratory, McGill University,
Montreal, QC, Canada
e-mail: sbakalian@hotmail.com

J. V. Burnier, M. N. Burnier, Jr. (eds.), *Experimental and Clinical Metastasis*,
DOI 10.1007/978-1-4614-3685-0_6, © Springer Science+Business Media New York 2013

Part III
Molecular Mechanisms of Tumor Growth and Spread

Editor:
Shawn Maloney

Chapter 7
Cell Cycle Control and Growth Factor Systems in Metastasis

Jonathan Cools-Lartigue and Jonathan Spicer

7.1 Introduction

Cancer remains a leading cause of death in industrialized countries despite advances in the detection and treatment of this disease (Heron et al. 2009). Traditional models of cancer posit that neoplastic cells arise through the sequential accumulation of genetic mutations leading to independent and uninhibited replication, the evasion of apoptosis, sustained angiogenesis, and ultimately, invasion and metastasis. The latter is of particular clinical significance as metastasis is the leading cause of cancer related death (Pantel and Brakenhoff 2004; Colotta et al. 2009; Wu and Zhou 2009; Sica et al. 2008).

In recent years, emerging evidence has challenged the previously held notion that metastasis is a late phenomenon in the natural history of malignant disease. The current understanding of the metastatic cascade represents a paradigm shift in which invasion and metastasis represent early occurrences in patients with cancer. Prior to the advent of the molecular characterization of neoplasia, aggressive phenotypes of primary tumors were observed histopathologically. For example, high grade, mitotically active cutaneous melanoma was shown to carry a worse prognosis than a less mitotically active tumor. Similar observations have been made across numerous malignancies including breast, thyroid and gastrointestinal tumors. The modern corollary to these observations is evident in the observation of a molecular metastatic phenotype evident in primary tumors whereby genetic expression profiles of metastatic lesions are mirrored in their primary counterparts (Pantel and Brakenhoff 2004; Colotta et al. 2009; Fidler 2003; Weigelt and Veer 2004).

Further analysis of the genes expressed in these metastatic signatures reveals that many are the same genes and proteins that have been the subject of laborious experimental analysis over the past decade and are not distinct. These genes and their translation products are the same ones implicated in the so called hallmarks of cancer, namely, evasion of apoptosis, self-sufficiency in growth signals, insensitivity

J. C.-Lartigue (✉) · J. Spicer
Department of Surgery, McGill University, Montreal, QC, Canada
e-mail: jonathan.cools-lartigue@mail.mcgill.ca

J. V. Burnier, M. N. Burnier, Jr. (eds.), *Experimental and Clinical Metastasis*, 57
DOI 10.1007/978-1-4614-3685-0_7, © Springer Science+Business Media New York 2013

to anti-growth signals, sustained angiogenesis, limitless replicative potential and tissue invasion and metastasis. In this chapter the basic pathways and some of the molecules involved in dysregulation of cell cycle control and self-sufficiency in growth signals will be reviewed (Weigelt and Veer 2004; Woelfle et al. 2003; Weigelt et al. 2003; Vijver et al. 2002; Ramaswamy et al. 2003).

7.1.1 Evidence for Metastasis as an Early Phenomenon

Emerging evidence supports the notion that metastasis is an inherent property of primary tumors and may arise early in the course of disease. Animal models have demonstrated distinct clonal populations within the primary tumor that display the propensity for metastasis to different sites (Weigelt et al. 2003). Similarly, the in vivo demonstration of circulating malignant cells (CMC's), whose poor prognostic significance has been demonstrated prospectively in a number of malignancies, have been observed in patients decades before the emergence of metastatic disease further supporting the notion of dissemination and metastasis as early events in neoplasia (Cools-Lartigue et al. 2008; Criscitiello et al. 2010; Fleitas et al. 2010). Additionally, the presence of small numbers of malignant cells within distant organs has been demonstrated in animal models prior to the development of clinically evident metastatic disease in several malignancies, including melanoma, breast, lung, and esophageal cancer (Cools-Lartigue et al. 2008; Minn et al. 2005; Lurje et al. 2010).

These observations support the hypothesis that malignancy is a systemic disease early in its evolution. This suggests that the ultimate emergence of clinically overt metastatic disease is the result of a complex interplay between the tumor and the host, which ultimately supports distant metastatic growth.

7.2 The Metastatic Phenotype

Recent evidence has challenged the traditional model of the metastatic cascade. The traditional model posits that within a primary tumor, individual cells undergo successive mutations, which confer a survival advantage, increasing their replicative success (Pantel and Brakenhoff 2004; Bernards and Weinberg 2002). This process continues in successive generations with the eventual emergence of rare cells capable of dissemination and metastasis. This theory implies therefore that the emergence of cells capable of metastasis is infrequent and a relatively late phenomenon in the tumor progression model (Pantel and Brakenhoff 2004; Bernards and Weinberg 2002).

Conceptually, this model has many flaws. Bernards and Weinberg suggest that a different conceptualization of tumor genesis is necessary, given that the emergence of cells capable of metastasizing confers no survival advantage to the primary tumor. The frequency of emergence of cells with metastatic potential in this construct is estimated at one in ten million. Accordingly, the impetus favoring metastasis is difficult to conceptualize in this model. The authors therefore posit that the metastatic potential is inherent to the primary tumor, that the development of metastasis may be an early phenomenon in tumor progression, and the genes responsible for metastasis are not distinct (Bernards and Weinberg 2002).

Experimental evidence supports this hypothesis. Ramsawamy et al. analyzed the gene expression profile of metastatic adenocarcinoma from several tumors, including lung, breast, prostate, colorectal and ovarian, and compared them to primary tumors of the same subtypes (Ramaswamy et al. 2003). The authors demonstrated distinct gene expression patterns in the two groups as would be expected according to the traditional model of metastasis. However, in a subset of tumors, an overlap in the expression profile of primary and metastatic lesions was observed, initially leading the authors to misclassify the primary tumors as metastases. Furthermore, the authors demonstrated that patients exhibiting this metastatic genetic profile in their primary tumors had significantly shorter overall survival compared to patients that did not. Of particular significance, the authors were able to refine this metastatic profile to a group of 17 genes of which 8 were up regulated and 9 were downregulated. This metastatic profile was able to predict outcome across the different malignancies examined in this study. Thus, the authors concluded that this signature is not specific to a particular neoplasm but representative of the processes governing metastasis as a whole.

Weigelt et al. performed a similar study in which the genetic profile of primary breast tumors was compared to samples from metastatic tumors. The authors demonstrated that in 6 of the 8-primary/metastatic pairs analyzed, the gene expression profile of the primary was closer to its metastatic counterpart than to the other primary tumors (Weigelt and veer 2004; Weigelt et al. 2003).

Van de Vijveer et al. demonstrated the presence of a poor outcome expression profile derived from estrogen receptor (ER) positive primary breast tumors in patients with advanced age. These patients demonstrated a different genetic profile than younger patients with ER positivity and a significantly increased propensity to die of metastatic disease than younger patients. This suggests that ER positivity in older patients is a distinct clinical entity, replete with a genetic predisposition for metastasis that is not mirrored in younger individuals with ER positive disease (Vijver et al. 2002).

Bhattacharjee et al. developed a molecular classification of carcinoma of the lung and were able to delineate genetic subtypes, which correlated with overall prognosis and metastatic potential. Collectively, these results support the hypothesis that metastatic potential may be inherent to the primary tumor (Bhattacharjee et al. 2001).

Data also supports the notion that features inherent to the primary tumor govern the site of metastasis. Woelfle et al. examined the gene expression profiles of primary breast tumors. In addition, patient lymph nodes and bone marrow (BM) were analyzed for the presence of metastases (micro- or macroscopic). The authors then compared the gene expression profiles of patients with BM^+ and BM^- disease, and patients with LN^+ and LN^- disease. The authors demonstrated that the gene expression profiles in patients with BM^+ disease were distinct from those with BM^-

disease and did not overlap with the gene expression profiles in patients with LN+ disease (Woelfle et al. 2003).

Minn et al. demonstrated differential tissue tropism among metastases in a mouse model of metastatic breast carcinoma. The authors used cells derived from a primary tumor with a known poor prognosis profile as described by Woelfle et al. Tumor cells were injected systemically into immune deficient mice and single cell progenies were derived after harvesting metastases from different sites, including bone, lung and adrenals. The authors subsequently demonstrated homogeneous expression of the poor prognosis genotype amongst the various metastases. However, the authors also identified a subset of genes unique to progeny cells isolated from different metastatic sites, with cells with a metastatic tropism for bone displaying a distinct metastatic profile, which was not expressed in cells displaying other tissue tropisms. Furthermore, this metastatic genetic profile was distinct from the initial poor prognosis profile. Subsequent genomic analysis of tissue-specific metastatic phenotypes demonstrated that they were preserved in the metastasis of primary tumors that had demonstrated spread to their corresponding tissues. As a whole, this data further supports the postulate that the mechanisms required for dissemination and ultimately metastasis are present in the primary tumor (Woelfle et al. 2003; Minn et al. 2005).

7.2.1 The Genes Involved in Metastasis are Not Novel

Further analysis of the metastatic phenotype identified by Ramsawamy et al. demonstrated a cluster of 17 genes that could reliably predict survival in their cohort of patients. None of the identified genes were individually involved in metastasis and the authors concluded that the signature as a whole was predictive of metastasis. Of these 17 genes, 8 were up regulated and 9 were down regulated. Four of the 8 up regulated genes were members of the protein translational apparatus; one, securin, is involved in sister chromatid separation during the metaphase-anaphase transition, and the remaining three were cytoskeletal and extracellular matrix proteins. Of the 9 down-regulated genes, again, a large number of extracellular matrix proteins and cytoskeletal proteins were identified. These findings suggest that the mediators of metastasis are not novel, but play an already established role in tumor genesis (Ramaswamy et al. 2003).

Along these lines, Hong et al. demonstrated a metastatic signature in patients with left sided colon cancer, which was found to be predictive of metastasis-related mortality. The authors observed that the genes involved in predicting metastasis are indicative of "cell-wide" perturbations in basic cellular functions (Hong et al. 2010).

7.3 Growth Factor Systems in Metastasis

Taken together the above data suggests that the genes mediating metastasis play a role in basic cellular processes. Along these lines, a variety of growth factors have been identified and are known to play key roles in promoting progression of cancer cells through the cell cycle, thus promoting accelerated growth and progression. One of the hallmarks of cancer is the notion of self-sufficiency in growth factor signals (Colotta et al. 2009). Cancer cells must survive within foreign host tissues sometimes under harsh conditions. The metastatic microenvironment must be groomed to offer a fertile soil for cancer cells to thrive. Recent investigations have revealed that growth factor signals arise from numerous sources in the metastatic microenvironment. Contributions arise from numerous mechanisms and cell types in this highly orchestrated and complex process. Additionally, each metastatic signature mentioned implicates conserved pathways with multiple downstream effectors involved in cellular growth, replication and cell cycle regulation. Furthermore, these pathways have been the subject of cancer related study for decades and do not represent exclusively novel metastatic mediators.

7.3.1 Transforming Growth Factor Beta (TGF-β)

Original reports on the effects of TGF-β signaling on cancer cells suggested that it inhibited cell cycle progression and induced apoptosis. However, the tumor suppressive aspects of TGF-β signaling were countered by studies where complete abrogation of TGF-β in cancer cells could also promote metastasis *in vivo* (Bierie and Moses 2006). TGF-β ligands reside in the extracellular matrix and require activation via a number of mechanisms to carry out their signal. Integrins, a number of proteases such as elastase or matrix metalloproteinase 9 and glycoproteins such as thrombospondin can all interact with TGF-β ligands, resulting in activation and eventual intracellular signaling. Indeed many of these 'activators' of TGF-β signaling are known to be involved in the metastatic process and have frequently been described as essential components of the metastatic tumor microenvironment (Bierie and Moses 2009).

TGF-β signaling is a complex affair. Ligation of its receptors TβRI and TβRII leads to transactivation, resulting in signaling through the SMAD pathway. SMAD signaling leads to transcriptional control. In addition, TGF-β can signal through numerous SMAD independent networks (Shi and Massague 2003). The net effect of the TGF-β pathway is highly dependent on the co-activation of parallel pathways. As mentioned, these effects can include such dichotomous anti-tumorigenic and pro metastatic phenotypes as induction of apoptosis and increased motility and invasion. These diametrically opposed effects have been reconciled by recent studies that delineate how inflammatory cells of the tumor microenvironment can modulate the effects of TGF-β signaling (Bierie and Moses 2009). Although TGF-β may suppress entry into the cell cycle, it also has been shown to suppress chemokine production that is largely responsible for the attraction of myeloid-derived suppressor cells (MDSC) to the tumor microenvironment. This host-tumor interaction is increasingly recognized as an essential component of tumor progression. The immune suppression that is effected locally by MDSC has been reported to promote metastatic growth. These findings highlight the importance of studying signaling events within the context of a heterogeneous and complex tumor microenvironment.

7.3.2 Epidermal Growth Factor Receptor

Epidermal growth factor receptor is over-expressed in most epithelial malignancies (Kalyankrishna and Grandis 2006). The downstream effects of EGFR signaling have been extensively studied and its role in cancer progression has been described at many levels (Hynes and Lane 2005). Indeed, EGFR is involved in the pathogenesis of some cancers and is also responsible for some aspects of progression to metastasis. Elevated expression of EGFR correlates with poor prognosis. EGFR can signal through the ERK pathway to promote proliferation in response to TGF-alpha binding (Albanell et al. 2001). Furthermore, signaling through the STAT3 pathway has been shown to promote tumor growth (Grandis et al. 1998; Thomas et al. 2003). Finally, by activating PLC-γ, EGFR activation can promote tumor cell survival (Thomas et al. 2003). Together, these characteristics of the EGFR pathway contribute to a pro-metastatic phenotype in cancer cells that over express this receptor and that are exposed to its ligand.

While EGFR signaling can be triggered by a number of ligands, it can also be triggered by transactivation via receptors like Insulin Growth Factor 1 Receptor (IGF-1R) (Adams et al. 2004). Such a pathway is of particular clinical significance. Trials that have incorporated EGFR inhibitors have yielded inconsistent results. Although such inhibitors may have potent action on the ligand mediated effects of EGFR signaling, transactivation of the pathway via a receptor like IGF-1R may detract from the efficacy of such an inhibitor. The complexity of these systems is at the root of the inefficacy of certain growth factor inhibitors like the EGFR blockers. Similarly to the impact of the tumor microenvironment on cancer cell proliferation, the cross talk between various growth factor pathways is key to robust oncogenic progression. Thus, therapies must be targeted broadly to the cancer cell, the microenvironment and the multiple facets via which growth factors affect the cancer cell cycle.

7.3.3 Inflammatory Cytokines and the Cell Cycle

Perhaps one of the most striking discoveries in recent years for the field of cancer metastasis is the pivotal role played by supporting inflammatory cells (Coussens and Werb 2002). Over a century and half ago, Virchow first drew the parallel between cancer progression and the inflammation present in healing wounds by noting the presence of abundant leukocytes within tumors (Wu and Zhou 2009). Later, cancer was likened to a non-healing wound. Wounds require trophic factors to bridge an epithelial gap. Multiple growth factors are required to induce proliferation of epithelial cells and to promote their migration across the wound. The wound microenvironment is rich with inflammatory cells that orchestrate and drive the process. Many seminal studies over the past 10 years have shown that cells like macrophages, neutrophils and MDSC are very active players in the metastatic process (Sica et al. 2008; Bunt et al. 2006; McDonald et al. 2009). One key aspect of their function is to promote cancer cell proliferation via the production of inflammatory cytokines.

One of the gateways to the production of inflammatory cytokines is NFκB activation. Activation of NFκB in cancer cells has been shown to suppress apoptosis, thus promoting survival and progression (Karin 2006). The result of NFκB activation is the production of inflammatory cytokines like TNF-α, IL-1 and IL-6 to name a few. Production of cytokines like IL-6 in the tumor microenvironment has been shown to cause STAT3 phosphorylation, which is a key signaling step related to metastatic progression (Groner et al. 2008). Indeed, STAT3 activation leads to protection from apoptosis and progression through the cell cycle. Sources of IL-6 can arise from the cancer cell or from the microenvironment. Multiple reports have shown that cancer cells are capable of producing inflammatory cytokines and thus may support their own growth via this mechanism. However, the overwhelming source of inflammatory mediators within the tumor microenvironment appears to be derived from inflammatory cells like tumor-associated macrophages. As alluded to earlier, these cells are key to metastatic progression and act as cytokine factories (Spicer et al. 2010). The effects of cytokines go well beyond cell cycle control as they promote angiogenesis and support stromal cells to create a milieu that is welcoming to cancer progression. Nevertheless, these inflammatory mediators have the net effect of stabilizing cancer cells and favoring their survival in an otherwise harsh metastatic environment.

7.3.4 The PI3-Akt Pathway

This family of lipid kinases has been intensely studied since its discovery in the 1980s and its regulation in diverse cellular processes such as survival, proliferation, and differentiation has been demonstrated. Not surprisingly, dysregulated functioning of this pathway has been linked to many of the processes at play in malignancy, which have been collectively referred to as the hallmarks of cancer (Colotta et al. 2009).

The PI3-Akt pathway is a conserved pathway, which transduces signals from various cytokines and growth factors via the association of the PI3 lipid kinase and activated receptor tyrosine kinases (RTK), G-protein coupled receptors (GPCR) and oncogenes such as RAS (Fig. 7.1) (Vivanco and Sawyers 2002). The PI3 lipid kinase is a heterodimer composed of a regulatory p85 subunit and a catalytic p110 subunit. The p85/p110 complex is capable of participating in multiple protein-protein interactions via its association with phosphorylated tyrosine residues. In the context of RTK initiated signaling, binding of a ligand to its receptor initiates recruitment of PI3k to the plasma membrane via the association of the p85 regulatory subunit with phosphorylated tyrosine residues. The now active p110 subunit subsequently catalyzes the phosphorylation of phosphatidyl inositol 4,5, bisphosphate (PtdIns(4,5)P2) to PtdIns(3,4,5)P3 which, among other processes, recruits the serine threonine kinase Akt to the cell membrane via the association of its pleckstrin homology (PH) domain to PtdIns (3,4,5)P3. This association induces a conformational change in Akt permitting its phosphorylation, and concomitant activation by 3-phosphoinositide dependent kinases (PDK). The major regulatory protein, phosphatase and tensin homologue (PTEN), acts to limit the availability of PtdIns(3,4,5)P3 and active PDK

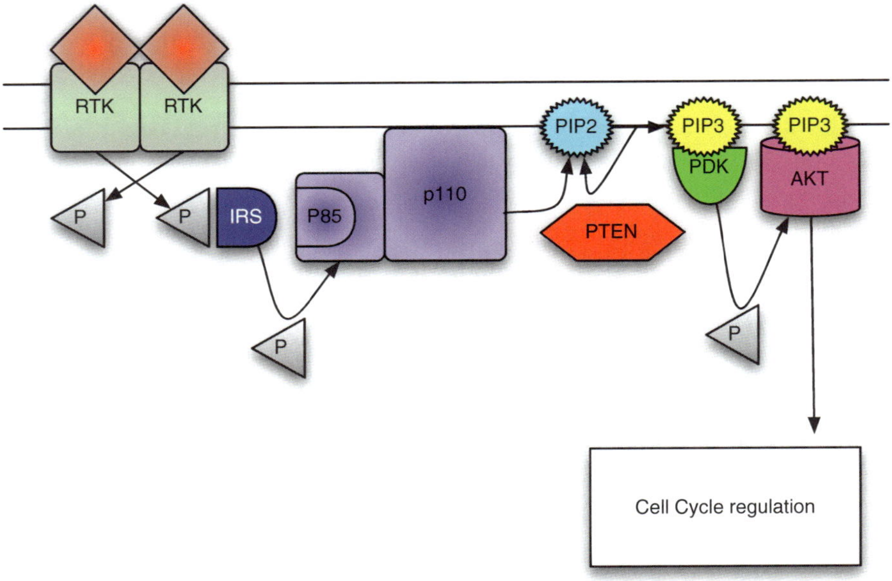

Fig. 7.1 The PI3-Akt Pathway. The PI3 lipid kinase is a heterodimer composed of a regulatory p85 subunit and a catalytic p110 subunit. The p85/p110 complex is capable of participating in multiple protein-protein interactions via its association with phosphorylated tyrosine residues. Binding of a ligand to its receptor initiates recruitment of PI3k to the plasma membrane via the association of p85 with phosphorylated tyrosine residues. Active p110 subsequently catalyzes the phosphorylation PtdIns(4,5)P2 to PtdIns(3,4,5)P3 which recruits the serine threonine kinase Akt to the cell membrane via the association of its PH domain to PtdIns (3,4,5)P3. This association induces a conformational change in Akt permitting its phosphorylation, and concomitant activation by 3-phosphoinositide dependent kinases (PDK). The major regulatory protein, PTEN, acts to limit the availability of PtdIns(3,4,5)P3 and active PDK through the removal of phosphate groups. Activated Akt participates in a broad range of downstream signaling events including regulation of the cell cycle. Figure adapted from Vivanco et al. 2002

through the removal of phosphate groups. Activated Akt participates in a broad range of downstream signaling events (Adams et al. 2004; Kelly-Spratt et al. 2009). In the context of this chapter, its role in cell cycle regulation will be discussed (Fig. 7.2, 7.3).

7.3.4.1 The PI3-Akt Pathway and Proliferation

The insulin growth factor 1 receptor (IGF-1R) can control transition through the cell cycle via multiple signaling pathways. However, the summative evidence would suggest that it causes progression at the G1-S interface via ERK and PI-3K/AKT signaling (Samani et al. 2007). Increased expression of IGF-1R and its ligands IGF-1 and IGF-2 are elevated in a number of malignancies. The coincidental presence of high levels of ligand and receptor in the tumor microenvironment suggest that the

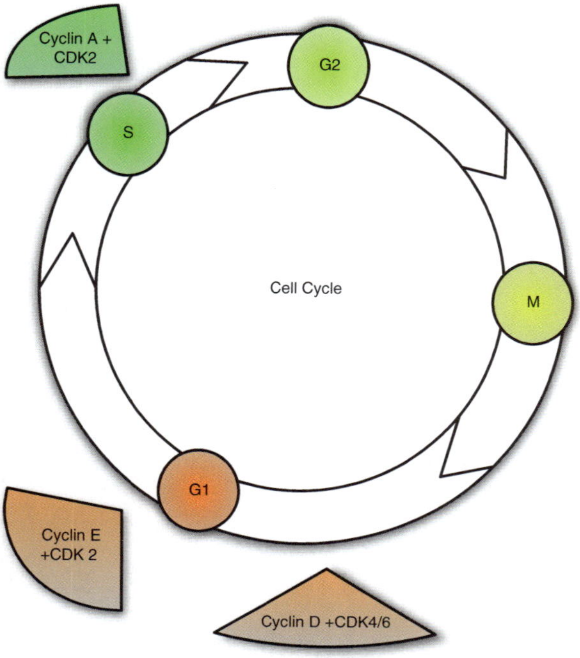

Fig. 7.2 The cell cycle. The progression from G1 to S and through the S phase is a multi-step process mediated by the association of D, E and A type cyclins with CDK4 or 6, and CDK2, respectively. The expression of the D-type cyclins occurs early in G1; as such, the D type cyclins are commonly regarded as nuclear relays of extracellular signaling

IGF axis can function both in an autocrine and paracrine fashion. Indeed, studies that genetically engineered liver metastasizing H-59 Lewis lung carcinoma cells to express the soluble form of IGF-1R had significantly fewer metastases, suggesting that the paracrine effect of IGF-1 liver expression is tumor promoting (Brodt et al. 2001). Confirming this hypothesis was a series of experiments where the size of primary tumor and liver metastases were increased by the addition of exogenous IGF-1 to liver-specific IGF-1 deficient mice in an orthotopic model of colon carcinoma metastasis (Wu et al. 2002). The role of IGF-1 was further delineated in a model of bone metastasis where prostate cancer cells expressed urokinase plasminogen activator (uPA) to degrade IGF-1 binding protein. As a result the bioavailability of IGF-1 in the metastatic microenvironment was bolstered (Koutsilieris and Polychronakos 1992).

These studies highlight the contribution of the host metastatic organ in terms of trophic factors that can promote cancer cell proliferation. Such environmental particularities contribute to the site specificity of certain malignancies. In addition, cancer cells benefit from being equipped with an armament of growth factor receptors and proteolytic enzymes to match the growth factor production line of the metastatic site where they attempt to implant. Metastatic inefficiency is in part attributed to this frequent mismatch. Cells capable of expressing high levels of growth factor in addition to high levels of the corresponding receptor may be more aggressive and metastasize more widely. Cancer cells with a poor match for the eventual metastatic microenvironment may not survive or may require the arrival of supporting inflammatory cells to engage further growth.

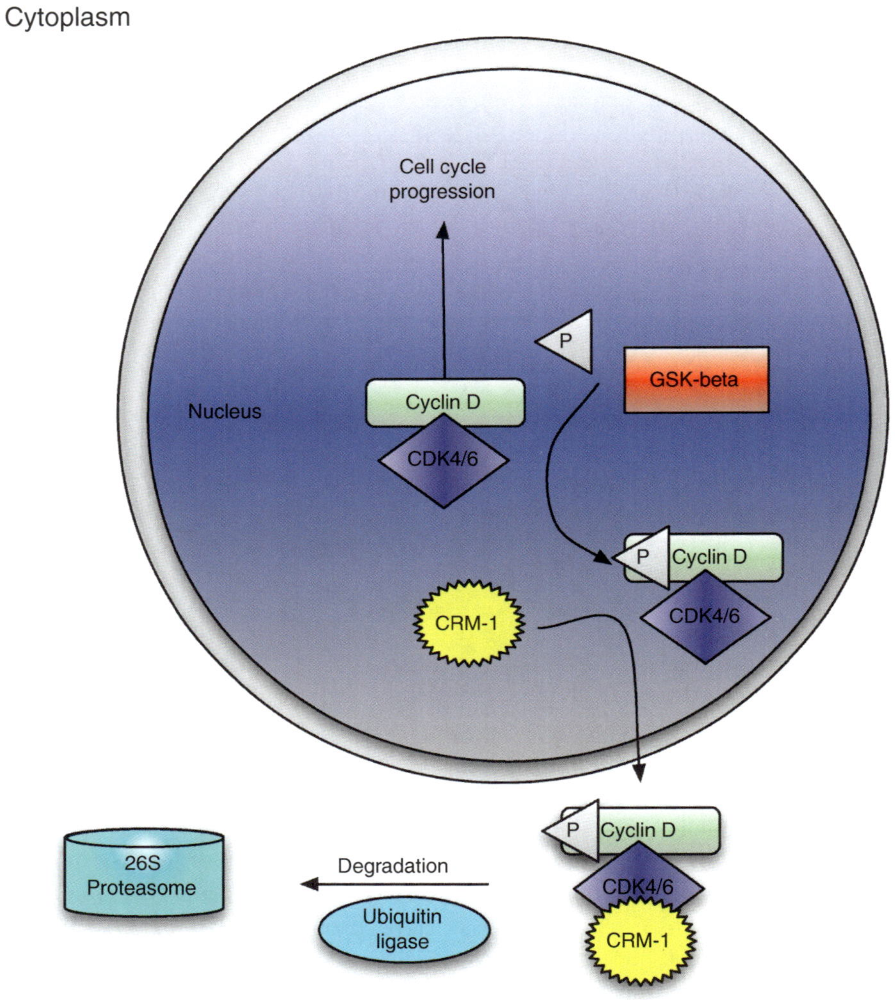

Fig. 7.3 Postranslational regulation of Cyclin D1. Cyclin D1 normally shuttles between the nucleus and the cytoplasm. Within the nucleus, it is able to complex with CDK4/6 and drive cell cycle progression. Its phosphorylation at Threonine 286 by GSK beta renders it amenable to nuclear export in a CRM-1 dependent manner. Within the cytoplasm, it is vulnerable to ubiquitination by the SCF ubiquitin ligase and proteosomal degradation. Figure adapted from Witzle et al. (2010)

Activated Akt appears to promote progression through the cell cycle and thus cellular replication. This is achieved in two general ways. First, activated Akt inhibits the function of the forkhead family of transcription factors, whose production is associated with cell cycle arrest in G1 and at the G2-M transition (Medema et al. 2000). Similarly, Akt mediates the inhibition of glyceraldehyde synthase kinase 3 beta (GSK3b), which is similarly implicated in cell cycle arrest at the G1-S interface via its inhibitory role on cyclin dependent signaling (Burgering and Kops 2002).

7.4 Cell Cycle Control

Dysregulation of the Cell Cycle in Malignancy The cell cycle is a tightly controlled process and its dysregulation is implicated in tumor genesis. Transition from G1-S, progression through the S-phase, G2-M transition and completion of mitosis are processes that are regulated through differential expression of cyclin dependent kinases (CDK) and their binding partners, cyclins. While the expression of the CDK is relatively stable throughout the cell cycle, the cyclins are a diverse group of proteins, which exhibit periodic expression at key phases. These proteins function as allosteric modulators of the CDK (Slingerland and Pagano 2000).

The transition from G1 to S has demonstrated aberrant function in nearly all human malignancies. Under normal conditions, the progression from G1 to S and through the S phase, induced, for example, by exposure to mitogens, is a multi-step process mediated by the association of D, E and A type cyclins with CDK4 or 6, and CDK2, respectively. The expression of the D-type cyclins occurs early in G1; as such, the D type cyclins are commonly regarded as nuclear relays of extracellular signaling (Slingerland and Pagano 2000).

Progression Through the Cell Cycle and Its Regulation In response to mitogen stimulated increased transcription, translation and inhibited proteolysis of Cyclin D takes place via both MAPK and PI3-Akt dependent pathways respectively. Consequently, intra-nuclear accumulation of cyclin D, with its resultant association with CDK4 or 6, results in the phosphorylation of the retinoblastoma (RB) tumor suppressor gene which in turn results in increased E2F mediated transcription. This leads to enhanced transcription and translation of E type cyclins, which, in association with CDK2 promote ongoing E2F mediated transcription and are responsible for progression through the G to S restriction point. Finally, A type cyclins, in conjunction with CDK1 or 2 are responsible for progression through the S phase (Slingerland and Pagano 2000; Witzel et al. 2010).

Regulation of cyclin:CDK complexes is under the control of 2 families of CDK inhibitors; the INK4 and Cip/Kip families. INK4 proteins (p16ink41, p15ink4b, p18ink4c, p19ink4d) bind and inhibit CDK4 and 6 while the Cip/Kip proteins (p21cip1/waf1/sdil, p27kip1, p57kip2) inhibit CDK2/cyclin E and CDK1/2:cylin A. As levels of CDK4/6/Cyclin D rise throughout early G1, these complexes sequester Cip/Kip family CDK inhibitors facilitating CDK2/Cyclin E complex formation and progression from G1-S. Finally, the cyclins are under posttranslational control at the level of sub-cellular localization and proteolysis, all of which have been implicated in malignancy (Witzel et al. 2010; Alt et al. 2000).

7.4.1 D type Cyclins in Malignancy

D-type Cyclins in Human Cancers Demonstrate Translocations, Amplifications, and Subtle Polymorphisms Not surprisingly, increased expression of D type cyclins has been demonstrated in human cancers including, breast, bladder, head and neck, lung and esophageal cancer. A variety of mechanisms for the aberrant expression of Cyclin D have been observed including chromosomal translocations, and amplifications as well as single nucleotide polymorphisms that alter the sensitivity of cyclin D to proteolysis.

In mantle cell lymphoma, the demonstration of the t(11;14)(q13;q32) translocation, which places the cyclin D1 gene CCND1 under the control of the immunoglobulin heavy chain (IgH) promoter has been observed in over 90 % of cases. The postulate here is that cyclin D1 expression is constitutive, thereby driving cellular proliferation (Schmitz et al. 2005).

Cyclin D1 overexpression has also been demonstrated through amplification of the CCND1 locus at 11q13 in multiple human cancers including esophageal squamous cell carcinoma. The study by Shinozaki et al demonstrated over 3-fold amplification of 11q13 in 23 % of 122 primary esophageal squamous cell carcinomas examined. The authors also demonstrated a statistically significant decrease in overall survival as well as an increase in the presence of distant metastasis in patients harboring this genetic abnormality. Thus, the over expression of cyclin D1 in these patients is of clinical significance (Shinozaki et al. 1996).

Finally, cyclin D1 over expression has been linked to more subtle genetic alterations. More than 100 polymorphisms have been identified at the CCND1 locus. One such polymorphism, the G/A substitution at position 870, has been extensively studied. This polymorphism generates a truncated protein known as cyclin D1b, which retains the capacity to associate with CDK4/6 but lacks the GSK b phosphorylation site and PEST sequence necessary for nuclear export and ubiquitin mediated degradation, respectively. This polymorphism has been demonstrated in approximately 5 % of Mantle cell lymphomas and approximately 60 % of human bladder cancers (Krieger et al. 2006; Kim et al. 2009).

Mechanisms of Cyclin D oncogenesis

Cyclin D overexpression alone is insufficient to drive neoplastic transformation The mechanism by which Cyclin D influences tumor progression remains incompletely understood. Its observed over expression among multiple malignancies has led to the postulate that it is a proto-oncogene. However, the ability of cyclin D to transform cells alone has not been supported by experimental data. Over expression of cyclin D1 in 3T3 fibroblasts by itself is unable to induce transformation. Over expression of cyclin D1 alone in murine lymphocytes is similarly unable to elicit transformation unless it is co-transfected with c-myc. A similar observation was made by Rodriguez et al wherein over expression of cyclin D1 and ras results in the formation of skin tumors in mice (Rodriguez-Puebla et al. 1999).

Along these lines, Opitz et al demonstrated that over expression of Cyclin D1 alone is insufficient to generate oral squamous cell carcinoma (OSCC) in mice. The authors, knowing that cyclin D was over expressed and p53 was under expressed in human OSCC, generated mice with differential expression of these proteins. The authors bred mice which over expressed cyclin D1 (L2D1^{+}) and either demonstrated wild type p53 expression (p53$^{+/+}$), were heterozygous for p53 expression (p53$^{+/-}$)

or lacked p53 expression altogether ($p53^{-/-}$). The authors demonstrated tumor formation in only $L2D1^{+}$, $p53^{+/-}$ or $p53^{-/-}$. No L2D1 $p53^{+/+}$ mice exhibited tumor formation (Opitz et al. 2002).

Thus, experimental data suggests that isolated over expression of cyclin D1 is generally insufficient to drive neoplastic transformation. Instead data suggests that it can potentiate ras and myc oncogenesis *in vitro* and can induce tumors efficiently *in vivo* in the absence of additional regulatory mechanisms as evidenced by the generation of OSCC in only those mice lacking appropriate p53 expression. Given the extent to which cyclin D over expression is observed in human cancers, additional mechanisms explaining its oncogenic activity were sought.

Post-Translational Regulation of Cyclin D and Enhanced Oncogenic Potential Experimental evidence supports the hypothesis that the subcellular localization of cyclins influences their role in tumor formation. Cyclin D1 normally shuttles between the nucleus and the cytoplasm. Within the nucleus, it is able to complex with CDK4/6 and drive cell cycle progression. Its phosphorylation at Threonine 286 by GSK beta renders it amenable to nuclear export in a CRM-1 dependent manner. Within the cytoplasm, it is vulnerable to ubiquitination by the SCF ubiquitin ligase and proteosomal degradation. Data supports the hypothesis that excessive intranuclear CDK/cyclinD1 is involved in tumor genesis (Kelly-Spratt et al. 2009; Gladden et al. 2006).

Chul Jang Kim et al. demonstrated increased invasiveness and anchorage independent growth of bladder cancer cell lines transfected with cyclin D1b, a variant not amenable to nuclear export, *in vitro*. Furthermore, this effect was abrogated by siRNA specific for cyclin D1b. The results of their study suggest that the malignant phenotype of urothelial carcinoma is enhanced by the expression of cyclin D1b and may be related to its nuclear localization (Kim et al. 2009).

Experimental data supports this hypothesis. Alt et al. demonstrated that 3T3 fibroblasts transfected with cyclin D T286A, a mutant not amenable to GSK phosphorylation and CRM-1 mediated nuclear export, exhibited contact independent growth and were immortalized. By contrast, 3T3 fibroblasts transfected with wild type Cyclin D constructs exhibited only a shortened G1 phase, consistent with previous reports that over expresion of cyclin D1 alone is not sufficient to effect transformation (Alt et al. 2000).

This phenomenon was demonstrated *in vivo* by Gladden et al. who generated transgenic mice with constitutive expression of cyclin D T286A. These mice exhibited a significantly shorter lifespan compared to controls attributable to disseminated B-cell lymphoma. Of particular interest, however, was the observation that a large proportion of B-cells that were driven to proliferate by the mutant cyclin D1 demonstrated apoptosis, suggesting that S-phase entry in these cells is countered by increased apoptosis (Gladden et al. 2006). Thus, lymphomatous cells that escape apoptosis must acquire a second hit rendering them resistant to apoptosis. Indeed aberrations in the p19ARF-MDM2-p53 pathway were observed in these malignant cells and corroborate the experimental observation that cyclin D over expression in conjunction with p53 under expression is sufficient to drive tumor development.

The above data suggests that cell cycle control is aberrant across a heterogeneous group of malignancies. This deregulation is mediated in part through proliferation driven by increased cyclin D1 activity, which is mediated by multiple mechanisms including amplifications, translocations, and mutations rendering nuclear export and proteolysis less efficient.

7.4.2 Forkhead Transcription Factors in Cell Cycle Control and Malignancy

Cell Cycle Arrest via Forkhead Transcription Factors Forkhead transcription factors, also known as Foxo proteins, are collectively implicated in cell cycle arrest and apoptosis. They belong to a family of transcription factors related through homology in their DNA binding domain. They are important downstream targets of PI3-Akt signaling. Phosphorylation of Foxo proteins by Akt increases their cytoplasmic localization as a result of inhibited interaction with nuclear DNA binding proteins such as 14-3-3. Within the cytoplasm, they are vulnerable to degradation. In the absence of mitogenic stimulation, Foxo proteins are retained within the nucleus and drive transcription of their targets (Medema et al. 2000; Burgering and Kops 2002).

Foxo Proteins Inhibit Cell Cycle Progression via Upregulation of Cip/Kip Cdk Inhibitors Foxo proteins are implicated in increased production of the Cip/Kip family cyclin dependent kinase inhibitors including p27kip1. In the study by Medena et al. the authors demonstrated that over expression of AFX, a forkhead transcription factor, induces G1 arrest in 3T3 fibroblasts. This effect was dependent on the inhibition of cyclin dependent signaling via increased levels of p27kip1, and was independent of downstream effectors of cyclin dependent signaling such as the retinoblastoma (Rb) tumor suppressor (McDonald et al. 2009).

7.4.3 Foxo Proteins As Tumor Suppressors

Abundant evidence suggests that Foxo proteins are bona fide tumor suppressors in mammals. Zou et al. demonstrated that FOXO 1 and 3 inhibit estrogen receptor (ER) mediated signaling in the estrogen-dependent human breast cancer cell line MCF 7, and this effect is associated with reduced proliferation *in vitro*. The authors generated MCF-7 breast cancer cell lines transfected with a FOXO expression vector. The decreased ER signaling observed was mediated through direct contact of FOXO proteins and ER and was associated with increased expression of cyclin dependent kinase (CDK) inhibitors including p27kip1 and reduced expression of cyclin D1. These findings were associated with a significant reduction in proliferation in the transfected MCF-7 cell lines compared to wild-type (Zou et al. 2008).

Furthermore, the authors demonstrated that inhibition of FOXO3 in MCF-7 cells promotes tumor genesis *in vivo*. The authors constructed an MCF-7 FOXO3 knock-down derivative and demonstrated the development of tumors in the mammary fat pad of nude mice in the absence of estrogen stimulation. This effect was not observed with wild-type MCF-7 cells in the absence of exogenous 17-b estradiol.

Further evidence supporting the role of the forkhead transcription factors as tumor suppressors stems from the study by Paik et al. Here, the authors demonstrated the development of a widespread cancer phenotype in mice with FOXO gene deletions. The authors also demonstrated that the tumors were cell lineage specific, with thymic FOXO deletions producing aggressive lymphomas while endothelial cell targeted mutations resulted in a widespread hamartomatous phenotype associated with premature death. With respect to lymphangiogenesis, the authors demonstrated that tumor genesis in this model was mediated in part by increased cell cycle progression, inferred from strong down regulation of p27kip1 in the context of the FOXO null mice (Paik et al. 2007).

Tothova et al. demonstrated similar results. The authors again generated conditional FOXO null mice. This was associated with the development of a non-fatal myeloproliferative phenotype as well as quantitative and qualitative abnormalities of lymphoid cells. These abnormalities were mediated in part by abnormal cell cycle regulation as demonstrated by a two-fold increase of hematopoetic stem cells in S/G2/M in FOXO null mice compared to wild type. This finding was associated with aberrant expression of FOXO target genes including down regulation of p27 and up regulation of cyclin D2 (Tothova et al. 2007).

Dysregulated FOXO Function is Mediated by Akt Dependent and Independent Mechanisms in Humans Aberrant function of Foxo proteins, either through dysregulated PI3-Akt signaling or mutation, has an experimentally established role in tumor genesis. In fact, such a role has been demonstrated in humans as well. Chronic myelogenous leukemia (CML) is characterized by the BCR-ABL translocation, which results in strong Akt activation. This activity is inhibited by the RTK inhibitor imatinib mesylate and is associated with a significant survival benefit. In this model, Akt activity drives the nuclear export and degradation of FOXO proteins, supporting ongoing proliferation. In the presence of RTK inhibitors, nuclear localization of Foxo proteins is restored, driving cell cycle arrest and apoptosis (Naka et al. 2010).

Alveolar rhabdomyosarcoma demonstrates characteristic translocations t(2;13)(q35;q14) and t(1;13)(p36;q14) which generate fusion proteins between PAX and forkhead member transcription factors. These proteins are resistant to Akt mediated cytoplasmic redistribution and are collectively localized to the nucleus where the fusion proteins drive the transcription of genes involved in proliferation, apoptosis and motility (Sumegi et al. 2010).

Kornblau et al. demonstrated that high levels of phosphorylated FOXO3A are an independent marker of poor prognosis in AML. Similarly, Song et al. demonstrated that loss of FOXA1 and FOXA2 are critical steps in the epithelial to mesenchymal transition in pancreatic ductal carcinoma, an important step in tumor genesis and predicted precursory step to metastasis. Along these lines, forkhead family transcription factors have been implicated in invasion and metastasis in multiple other human malignancies including leukemia, breast, thyroid and esophageal cancer (Song et al. 2010; Kornblau et al. 2010).

7.5 CDK Inhibitors are Implicated in Tumor Genesis

7.5.1 P27 and Cell Cycle Progression

P27 is one of the downstream effectors of forkhead family transcription factors implicated in cell cycle control, tumor genesis and metastasis. As alluded to previously, this molecule is extensively involved in the regulation of cell cycle progression particularly in the G1-S transition through its association with cyclin E-CDK2, and its subsequent inhibition of ongoing RB phosphorylation and E2F mediated transcription of genes necessary to complete the G1-S transition. However, further studies implicate p27 in processes including aberrant cell cycle control and metastasis.

The regulation of p27 itself is complex and a full discussion is beyond the scope of this chapter. Briefly, however, early in G1, p27 plays a role in stabilizing cyclin D-cdk4/6 complexes within the cytoplasm, assisting in their localization to the nucleus and hence the phosphorylation of Rb. However, p27 also acts to inhibit cyclin E-CDK 2, thereby keeping levels of cyclin A low and preventing progression through S phase. It is only when levels of p27 drop in late G1, which is believed to be mediated at least in part by phosphorylation, nuclear export and ubiquitin mediated degradation of p27, that the activity of cyclin E-cdk2 increases and progression through the cell cycle occurs (Kelly-Spratt et al. 2009; Alt et al. 2000).

7.5.2 Post-Translational Mechanisms Mediate Aberrant P27 Function in Malignant Disease

This tightly regulated process has been shown to be dysfunctional in a variety of human cancers. Considering the importance of p27 in the regulation of the cell cycle, one would expect mutations of this allele to be common in human cancers. While loss of a single allele has been demonstrated among various malignancies, loss of both alleles has only been rarely observed. Instead, dysregulation appears to occur at the level of p27 protein, not gene transcription. Low levels of p27 protein are independent predictors of poor outcome in multiple malignancies including lung, colon, ovarian, breast, prostate and gastric carcinoma. In fact, it has been estimated that up to 50 % of human cancers lack normal p27 expression. Furthermore, in a variety of these cancers, the low protein levels observed appear to be related to increased ubiquitin mediated proteolytic degradation (Zhou et al. 2003).

Calvisi et al., in a model of hepatocellular carcinoma (HCC), demonstrated that increased ubiquitination of p27 among other cell cycle regulators was associated with increased cellular proliferation. In a separate study, these authors demonstrated that susceptibility to the development of HCC in a rat model was dependent on ubiquitin-mediated degradation of cell cycle regulatory proteins, including p27. The authors examined two rat strains of known divergent susceptibility to the development of HCC induced by exogenous dietary nitrosamine. Only 35 % of Norway Brown (BN) rats exposed to exogenous nitrosamines developed overt HCC in the study, compared to all F344 rats. The authors demonstrated that although no difference in p27 mRNA was observed between the two groups over the course of the study, levels of p27 protein were significantly higher in BN compared to F344 rats. In order to elucidate the posttranslational mechanism responsible for the observed disparity in p27, the authors demonstrated significantly lower levels of SCF ubiquitin ligase components (Skp-2, Cks-1) in the resistant compared to the susceptible rats. Furthermore an inverse correlation between increased levels of cell cycle regulatory proteins, including p27, and proliferation based on Ki67 protein levels was observed. Taken together, this data supports the role of ubiquitin-mediated degradation of p27 in disease progression of HCC (Calvisi et al. 2010).

In keeping with this theme, Liu et al. demonstrated that the anti-neoplastic effects of hinokitiol, which induces G1 cell cycle arrest in human FEM melanoma cell lines is associated with inhibition of ubiquitin driven degradation of p27. This effect was mediated both through decreased phosphorylation of p27 at threonine 187, which targets p27 for proteosomal degradation, and down regulation of skp2, a subunit of the SCF ubiquitin protein ligase. This finding further implicates increased proteolysis as one mechanism whereby p27 activity is reduced (Liu and Yamauchi 2009).

7.5.3 Cytoplasmic Sequestration of P27 is Involved in Tumor Progression and Metastasis

A subset of human cancers has failed to demonstrate markedly reduced levels of p27 protein, prompting the search for alternate modalities of p27 inactivation in these neoplasms. Additional mechanisms for aberrant p27 function and cell cycle regulation have accordingly been observed (Besson et al. 2008).

Akt Independent Mechanisms Active p27 has been shown to be sequestered in cyclinD:CDK complexes in association with Myc mediated proliferation *in vitro* (Yamamoto et al. 2009; Wu et al. 2009). Consequently, p27 is unable to bind and inhibit cyclinE:CDK complexes leading to cell cycle progression (Zhou et al. 2003). *In vivo* cytoplasmic sequestration of p27 in cyclin-D1:CDK4 complexes has been observed in some human lymphomas (Qi et al. 2006). Furthermore, Her-2 over expression in breast cancer is associated with c-myc over expression, upregulation of D-type cyclins and p27 sequestration in cyclinD:Cdk4 complexes (Acosta et al. 2008).

Akt Dependent Mechanisms Akt mediated cytoplasmic accumulation of p27 has been documented in a variety of human cancers including melanoma, breast, colon, thyroid and esophageal cancer. Liang et al. demonstrated impaired nuclear import and cytoplasmic accumulation of p27 in both human mammary epithelial cells (HMECS) and WM35 cell lines transfected with constitutively active Akt *in vitro*. Furthermore, the authors demonstrated an abrogated G1 arrest in response to exogenous TGF-beta in Akt over expressing cell lines. Finally, the authors demonstrated that impaired nuclear import of p27 was the result of Akt phosphorylation at threonine 157 on p27. Furthermore, this shift in p27 compartmentalization is associated with increased cdk2 activity and cell cycle progression. Accordingly, cytoplasmic sequestration of p27 was impaired in cells expressing a mutant p27T157A, not amenable to phosphorylation by Akt at this site. Thus the authors concluded that abnormal progression through G1 may be mediated by aberrant Akt signaling and consequent cytoplasmic sequestration of p27 (Liang et al. 2002). Additional *in vitro* support of this hypothesis is evident in the observation that the pharmacologic PI3K inhibitor LY294002 abrogates this effect, restoring nuclear localization (Motti et al. 2005).

In vivo evidence supporting cytoplasmic accumulation of p27 in tumor genesis has also been demonstrated. Viglietto et al. demonstrated that Akt dependent phosphorylation and cytoplasmic mislocalization functionally inactivates p27 in human breast cancer. They examined the cellular localization of T157 phosphorylated p21 in 54 human primary breast cancers. Furthermore, they classified the primary tumors into three groups based on the ratio of p-Akt:Akt. Group 1 tumors, of which there were 15, had a pAkt:Akt ratio <0.1; group 2 tumors, of which 10 were identified, demonstrated an p-Akt:Akt between 0.1–0.8; group 3 tumors, of which there were 15, demonstrated a p-Akt:Akt >0.8. P27 was absent in 14 tumors. The authors subsequently noted that there was a statistically significant rise of T157 phosphorylated p27 from group 1 to group 3 tumors with 6 % expression in group 1,40 % expression in group 2 and 65 % expression in group 3. Furthermore, T157 phosphorylated Akt was almost exclusively localized to the cytoplasm. Thus, functional inactivation of p27 may occur via Akt mediated cytoplasmic sequestration in human breast cancer (Viglietto et al. 2002).

7.6 Summary

Progression through the cell cycle is a defining characteristic of a cancer cell that wishes to metastasize. Despite metastatic inefficiency, growth factor signals are numerous and redundant. These signals can arise from the cancer cell itself as well as the inflammatory tumor microenvironment and from the host organ tissue. Cross talk between various growth factor pathways like EGFR/IGF-1R transactivation may bypass the need for autocrine or paracrine growth factor stimulation. Mutations in the signaling pathway may lead to constitutive activation. Inflammatory cells of the microenvironment provide a nurturing source of growth signals. These myriad pathways lead to a similar outcome of proliferation. This obvious complexity highlights the importance of improved understanding of these processes. Only tailored therapies that address organ tropism during metastasis and the numerous portals via which cancer cells gain access to the cell cycle and proliferate out of control will yield a healthy therapeutic response.

References

Acosta JC et al (2008) Myc inhibits p27-induced erythroid differentiation of leukemia cells by repressing erythroid master genes without reversing p27-mediated cell cycle arrest. Mol Cell Biol 28(24):7286–7295

Adams TE, McKern NM, Ward CW (2004) Signalling by the type 1 insulin-like growth factor receptor: interplay with the epidermal growth factor receptor. Growth Factors 22(2):89–95

Albanell J et al (2001) Activated extracellular signal-regulated kinases: association with epidermal growth factor receptor/transforming growth factor alpha expression in head and neck squamous carcinoma and inhibition by anti-epidermal growth factor receptor treatments. Cancer Res 61(17):6500–6510

Alt JR et al (2000) Phosphorylation-dependent regulation of cyclin D1 nuclear export and cyclin D1-dependent cellular transformation. Genes Dev 14(24):3102–3114

Bernards R, Weinberg RA (2002) A progression puzzle. Nature 418(6900):823

Besson A, Dowdy SF, Roberts JM (2008) CDK inhibitors: cell cycle regulators and beyond. Dev Cell 14(2):159–169

Bhattacharjee A et al (2001) Classification of human lung carcinomas by mRNA expression profiling reveals distinct adenocarcinoma subclasses. Proc Natl Acad Sci U S A 98(24):13790–13795

Bierie B, Moses HL (2006) Tumour microenvironment: TGFbeta: the molecular Jekyll and Hyde of cancer. Nat Rev Cancer 6(7):506–520

Bierie B, Moses HL (2009) Gain or loss of TGFbeta signaling in mammary carcinoma cells can promote metastasis. Cell Cycle 8(20):3319–3327

Brodt P et al (2001) Cooperative regulation of the invasive and metastatic phenotypes by different domains of the type I insulin-like growth factor receptor beta subunit. J Biol Chem 276(36):33608–33615

Bunt SK et al (2006) Inflammation induces myeloid-derived suppressor cells that facilitate tumor progression. J Immunol 176(1):284–290

Burgering BM, Kops GJ (2002) Cell cycle and death control: long live Forkheads. Trends Biochem Sci 27(7):352–360

Calvisi DF et al (2010) The degradation of cell cycle regulators by SKP2/CKS1 ubiquitin ligase is genetically controlled in rodent liver cancer and contributes to determine the susceptibility to the disease. Int J Cancer 126(5):1275–1281

Colotta F et al (2009) Cancer-related inflammation, the seventh hallmark of cancer: links to genetic instability. Carcinogenesis 30(7):1073–1081

Cools-Lartigue JJ et al (2008) Immunomagnetic isolation and in vitro expansion of human uveal melanoma cell lines. Mol Vis 14:50–55

Coussens LM, Werb Z (2002) Inflammation and cancer. Nature 420(6917):860–867

Criscitiello C, Sotiriou C, Ignatiadis M (2010) Circulating tumor cells and emerging blood biomarkers in breast cancer. Curr Opin Oncol 22(6):552–558

Fidler IJ (2003) The pathogenesis of cancer metastasis: the 'seed and soil' hypothesis revisited. Nature Rev Cancer 3:453–458

Fleitas T et al (2010) Circulating endothelial and endothelial progenitor cells in non-small-cell lung cancer. Clin Transl Oncol 12(8):521–525
Gladden AB et al (2006) Expression of constitutively nuclear cyclin D1 in murine lymphocytes induces B-cell lymphoma. Oncogene 25(7):998–1007
Grandis JR et al (1998) Requirement of Stat3 but not Stat1 activation for epidermal growth factor receptor- mediated cell growth In vitro. J Clin Invest 102(7):1385–1392
Groner B, Lucks P, Borghouts C (2008) The function of Stat3 in tumor cells and their microenvironment. Semin Cell Dev Biol 19(4):341–350
Heron M et al (2009) Deaths: final data for 2006. Natl Vital Stat Rep 57(14):1–134
Hong Y et al (2010) A 'metastasis-prone' signature for early-stage mismatch-repair proficient sporadic colorectal cancer patients and its implications for possible therapeutics. Clin Exp Metastasis 27(2):83–90
Hynes NE, Lane HA (2005) ERBB receptors and cancer: the complexity of targeted inhibitors. Nat Rev Cancer 5(5):341–354
Kalyankrishna S, Grandis JR (2006) Epidermal growth factor receptor biology in head and neck cancer. J Clin Oncol 24(17):2666–2672
Karin M (2006) Nuclear factor-kappaB in cancer development and progression. Nature 441(7092):431–436
Kelly-Spratt KS et al (2009) Inhibition of PI-3K restores nuclear p27Kip1 expression in a mouse model of Kras-driven lung cancer. Oncogene 28(41):3652–3662
Kim CJ et al (2009) Cyclin D1b variant promotes cell invasiveness independent of binding to CDK4 in human bladder cancer cells. Mol Carcinog 48(10):953–964
Kornblau SM et al (2010) Highly phosphorylated FOXO3A is an adverse prognostic factor in acute myeloid leukemia. Clin Cancer Res 16(6):1865–1874
Koutsilieris M, Polychronakos C (1992) Proteinolytic activity against IGF-binding proteins involved in the paracrine interactions between prostate adenocarcinoma cells and osteoblasts. Anticancer Res 12(3):905–910
Krieger S et al (2006) Relevance of cyclin D1b expression and CCND1 polymorphism in the pathogenesis of multiple myeloma and mantle cell lymphoma. BMC Cancer 6:238
Liang J et al (2002) PKB/Akt phosphorylates p27, impairs nuclear import of p27 and opposes p27-mediated G1 arrest. Nat Med 8(10):1153–1160
Liu S, Yamauchi H (2009) p27-Associated G1 arrest induced by hinokitiol in human malignant melanoma cells is mediated via down-regulation of pRb, Skp2 ubiquitin ligase, and impairment of Cdk2 function. Cancer Lett 286(2):240–249
Lurje G et al (2010) Circulating tumor cells in gastrointestinal malignancies: current techniques and clinical implications. J Oncol 2010:392652
McDonald B et al (2009) Systemic inflammation increases cancer cell adhesion to hepatic sinusoids by neutrophil mediated mechanisms. Int J Cancer 125(6):1298–1305
Medema RH et al (2000) AFX-like Forkhead transcription factors mediate cell-cycle regulation by Ras and PKB through p27kip1. Nature 404(6779):782–787
Minn AJ et al (2005) Distinct organ-specific metastatic potential of individual breast cancer cells and primary tumors. J Clin Invest 115(1):44–55
Motti ML et al (2005) Complex regulation of the cyclin-dependent kinase inhibitor p27kip1 in thyroid cancer cells by the PI3K/AKT pathway: regulation of p27kip1 expression and localization. Am J Pathol 166(3):737–749
Naka K et al (2010) TGF-beta-FOXO signalling maintains leukaemia-initiating cells in chronic myeloid leukaemia. Nature 463(7281):676–680
Opitz OG et al (2002) A mouse model of human oral-esophageal cancer. J Clin Invest 110(6):761–769
Paik JH et al (2007) FoxOs are lineage-restricted redundant tumor suppressors and regulate endothelial cell homeostasis. Cell 128(2):309–323
Pantel K, Brakenhoff RH (2004) Dissecting the metastatic cascade. Nat Rev Cancer 4(6):448–456

Qi CF et al (2006) Expression of the cyclin-dependent kinase inhibitor p27 and its deregulation in mouse B cell lymphomas. Leuk Res 30(2):153–163

Ramaswamy S et al (2003) A molecular signature of metastasis in primary solid tumors. Nat Genet 33(1):49–54

Rodriguez-Puebla ML, Robles AI, Conti CJ (1999) Ras activity and cyclin D1 expression: an essential mechanism of mouse skin tumor development. Mol Carcinog 24(1):1–6

Samani AA et al (2007) The role of the IGF system in cancer growth and metastasis: overview and recent insights. Endocr Rev 28(1):20–47

Schmitz R et al (2005) Insights into the multistep transformation process of lymphomas: IgH-associated translocations and tumor suppressor gene mutations in clonally related composite Hodgkin's and non-Hodgkin's lymphomas. Leukemia 19(8):1452–1458

Shi Y, Massague J (2003) Mechanisms of TGF-beta signaling from cell membrane to the nucleus. Cell 113(6):685–700

Shinozaki H et al (1996) Cyclin D1 amplification as a new predictive classification for squamous cell carcinoma of the esophagus, adding gene information. Clin Cancer Res 2(7):1155–1161

Sica A et al (2008) Macrophage polarization in tumour progression. Semin Cancer Biol 18(5):349–355

Slingerland J, Pagano M (2000) Regulation of the cdk inhibitor p27 and its deregulation in cancer. J Cell Physiol 183(1):10–17

Song Y, Washington MK, Crawford HC (2010) Loss of FOXA1/2 is essential for the epithelial-to-mesenchymal transition in pancreatic cancer. Cancer Res 70(5):2115–2125

Spicer JD, Brodt P, Ferri LE (2010) Role of inflammation in the early stages of liver metastasis. In: Brodt P (Ed) Liver metastasis – Biology and Clinical Management. Spinger, Berlin

Sumegi J et al (2010) Recurrent t(2;2) and t(2;8) translocations in rhabdomyosarcoma without the canonical PAX-FOXO1 fuse PAX3 to members of the nuclear receptor transcriptional coactivator family. Genes Chromosomes Cancer 49(3):224–236

Thomas SM et al (2003) Epidermal growth factor receptor-stimulated activation of phospholipase Cgamma-1 promotes invasion of head and neck squamous cell carcinoma. Cancer Res 63(17):5629–5635

Tothova Z et al (2007) FoxOs are critical mediators of hematopoietic stem cell resistance to physiologic oxidative stress. Cell 128(2):325–339

van de Vijver MJ et al (2002) A gene-expression signature as a predictor of survival in breast cancer. N Engl J Med 347(25):1999–2009

Viglietto G (2002) Cytoplasmic relocalization and inhibition of the cyclin-dependent kinase inhibitor p27(Kip1) by PKB/Akt-mediated phosphorylation in breast cancer. Nat Med 8(10):1136–1144

Vivanco I, Sawyers CL (2002) The phosphatidylinositol 3-Kinase AKT pathway in human cancer. Nat Rev Cancer 2(7):489–501

Weigelt B et al (2003) Gene expression profiles of primary breast tumors maintained in distant metastases. Proc Natl Acad Sci U S A 100(26):15901–15905

Weigelt B, van't Veer LJ (2004) Hard-wired genotype in metastatic breast cancer. Cell Cycle 3(6):756–757

Witzel II, Koh LF, Perkins ND (2010) Regulation of cyclin D1 gene expression. Biochem Soc Trans 38(Pt 1):217–222

Woelfle U et al (2003) Molecular signature associated with bone marrow micrometastasis in human breast cancer. Cancer Res 63(18):5679–5684

Wu Y, Zhou BP (2009) Inflammation: a driving force speeds cancer metastasis. Cell Cycle 8(20):3267–3273

Wu Y et al (2002) Circulating insulin-like growth factor-I levels regulate colon cancer growth and metastasis. Cancer Res 62(4):1030–1035

Wu GQ et al (2009) Cell cycle-related kinase supports ovarian carcinoma cell proliferation via regulation of cyclin D1 and is a predictor of outcome in patients with ovarian carcinoma. Int J Cancer 125(11):2631–2642

Yamamoto S et al (2009) Aberrant expression of p27(Kip1)-interacting cell-cycle regulatory proteins in ovarian clear cell carcinomas and their precursors with special consideration of two distinct multistage clear cell carcinogenetic pathways. Virchows Arch 455(5):413–422

Zhou Q, He Q, Liang LJ (2003) Expression of p27, cyclin E and cyclin A in hepatocellular carcinoma and its clinical significance. World J Gastroenterol 9(11):2450–2454

Zou Y et al (2008) Forkhead box transcription factor FOXO3a suppresses estrogen-dependent breast cancer cell proliferation and tumorigenesis. Breast Cancer Res 10(1):R21

Chapter 8
Regulation of Angiogenesis by Tumour Suppressor Pathways

Karen J. Lefebvre, Sarah Assadian, Wissal El-Assaad and Jose G. Teodoro

8.1 Introduction to Angiogenesis

During the process of tumour formation, mutations and epigenetic effects allow cancer cells to acquire capabilities that promote uncontrolled growth. Such capabilities include insensitivity to negative growth signals, resistance to apoptosis, uncontrolled cell cycle progression, and enhanced angiogenic potential. Cancer cells are no different from normal tissues in that they require a vascular system to provide oxygen and nutrients that are critical for survival and growth. As a general rule most cell types in the human body exist within 100–200 μm of a capillary blood vessel—the diffusion limit of oxygen (Carmeliet and Jain 2000). During embryogenesis, blood vessels are formed from endothelial precursor cells through the process of vasculogenesis. Subsequently, angiogenesis, the process of formation of new blood vessels from the existing vasculature, expands this network (Carmeliet and Jain 2000). In adults, new blood vessels are produced exclusively through angiogenesis (Hanahan and Folkman 1996). Physiological angiogenesis occurs in adults only in very specific situations such as during the female reproductive cycle and wound healing. However, several human diseases have been associated with inappropriate induction of angiogenesis including psoriasis, macular degeneration and cancer (Hanahan and Folkman 1996). The concept that tumour formation involves the pathological stimulation of angiogenesis has now become an accepted tenet in cancer biology, after first being proposed by the late Judah Folkman in 1971 (Folkman et al. 1971).

Angiogenesis involves a complex set of steps and cellular interactions. In the first step, pericytes surrounding existing blood vessels detach resulting in vessel dilation. Next, the basement membrane surrounding the existing blood vessels is degraded to allow endothelial cells to invade into the perivascular space. The endothelial cells then proliferate and form a migrating column that moves through the perivascular space toward the angiogenic stimuli produced by the tumour cells or stromal cells.

J. G. Teodoro (✉) · K. J. Lefebvre · S. Assadian
Goodman Cancer Research Centre and Department of Biochemistry,
McGill University, 1160 Pine Avenue, Montreal, QC H3A 1A3, Canada
e-mail: jose.teodoro@mcgill.ca

W. El-Assaad
Goodman Cancer Research Centre, McGill University, 1160 Pine Avenue,
Montreal, QC H3A 1A3, Canada

J. V. Burnier, M. N. Burnier, Jr. (eds.), *Experimental and Clinical Metastasis*,
DOI 10.1007/978-1-4614-3685-0_8, © Springer Science+Business Media New York 2013

Behind the migrating column, endothelial cells change shape and adhere to each other to form a new capillary tube. This is accompanied by basement membrane formation and pericyte attachment. Lastly, the newly formed sprouts fuse with other vessels, thereby beginning to circulate blood to the newly vascularized region (Hanahan and Folkman 1996; Bergers and Benjamin 2003).

Pathological tumour angiogenesis is similar to that in normal tissues except that the resulting blood vessels are abnormal in terms of their structure and function. In contrast to the highly ordered network of venules, arterioles and capillaries of the normal vasculature, the tumour vasculature is very disorganized (Bergers and Benjamin 2003). Tumour vessels are dilated and tortuous, have uneven diameters, and exhibit excessive branching (Carmeliet and Jain 2000). Furthermore, tumour blood vessels have high vascular permeability due to abnormalities in the vessel walls. Together, these abnormalities cause irregular blood flow through the tumour, which leads to hypoxic and acidic regions (Carmeliet and Jain 2000).

Since angiogenesis does not actively occur in adults, tumours must acquire the capacity to induce blood vessel formation through mutation and/or epigenetic effects. Once tumour cells develop the capacity to stimulate angiogenesis, they are able to enter a rapid stage of growth. The transition from small, avascular lesions less than 2 mm in diameter to large, vascularized tumours is known as the "angiogenic switch" and is now viewed as a necessary transition in tumour progression (Bergers and Benjamin 2003). In the avascular phase, tumour cells proliferate but this proliferation is counteracted by apoptosis; thus, the tumour remains dormant (Ribatti et al. 2007). The molecular events that underlie the angiogenic switch are not well understood and remain a topic of intense research but some of the key players have emerged. Overall, the angiogenic switch is thought to be triggered by a change in the balance of pro- and anti-angiogenic factors found in the extracellular space (Hanahan and Folkman 1996). Endogenous pro- and anti-angiogenic factors signal to endothelial cells to either promote or inhibit proliferation and migration. An emerging theme in angiogenesis research has been that many of the pathways that promote cell autonomous growth also promote the non-cell autonomous pathways that control angiogenesis (Fig. 8.1). During normal growth conditions, such as embryonic development, the production of pro-angiogenic factors is potently induced by physiological stimuli such as hypoxia and growth factor signaling pathways. During oncogenesis, activating mutations in proto-oncogenes such as Ras, Myc and PI3K induce expression of pro-angiogenic factors, while repressing anti-angiogenic ones (reviewed in, Rak and Yu 2004; Folkman 2006). Conversely, just as oncogenes can promote angiogenesis, tumour suppressor genes (TSGs) are able to negatively regulate the process by shutting down production of pro-angiogenic factors and stimulating anti-angiogenic ones (Fig. 8.1, Tables 8.1 and 8.2). Therefore, as cancerous cells accumulate mutations, amplifications, or epigenetic modifications activating oncogenic pathways and inactivating tumour suppressor pathways, these effects concomitantly lead to increasing angiogenic output. The rest of this chapter will focus on the mechanisms by which TSGs have been shown to negatively regulate angiogenesis. Inactivating mutations of TSGs including VHL, p53, RB, and PTEN have all been shown to increase angiogenic potential (Bergers and Benjamin 2003; Ribatti et al. 2007). In each case these

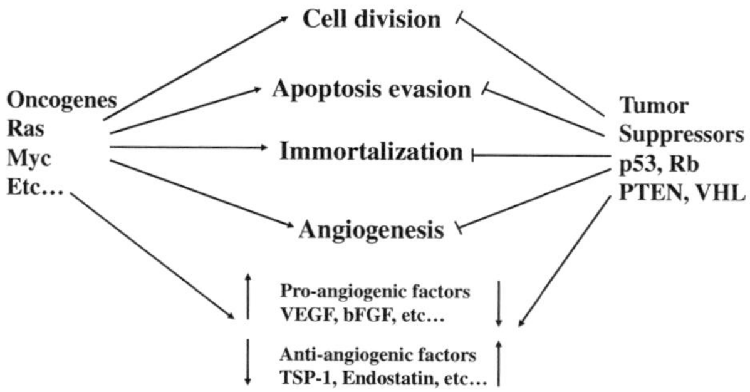

Fig. 8.1 Cancer and Angiogenesis. Cancer cells acquire several cell autonomous capabilities in the process of becoming tumours. These include enhanced cell division, apoptosis evasion, and immortalization. In addition, oncogenes can also promote the non-cell autonomous process of angiogenesis. Conversely, tumour suppressor pathways function to antagonize oncogene driven processes including angiogenesis. There are two basic mechanisms by which oncogenes and tumour suppressor proteins modulate angiogenesis. Oncogenes can stimulate production of pro-angiogenic factors and inhibit anti-angiogenic ones. The opposite holds true for tumour suppressor pathways

Table 8.1 Anti-angiogenic factors upregulated by tumour suppressor genes

Factor name	p53	PTEN	VHL	Rb
Arresten	Wei et al. (2006)			
BAI1	Nishimori et al. (1997)			
Endostatin	Miled et al. (2005)			
Ephrin A1	Dohn et al. (2001)			
Ephrin Receptor A2	Dohn et al. (2001)			
Maspin	Eitel et al. (2009); Chenau et al. (2009)	Eitel et al. (2009)		
TSP-1	Dameron et al. (1994)	Wen et al. (2001)		
Tumstatin	Teodoro et al. (2006)			

BAI1 brain-specific angiogenesis inhibitor 1; *TSP-1* thrombospondin-1

tumour suppressors use a variety of molecular mechanisms, both transcriptional and post-transcriptional, to shift the production of angiogenic factors towards a state that limits angiogenesis.

8.2 Tumour Suppressor Pathways and Angiogenesis

8.2.1 Von Hippel-Lindau (VHL)

Von Hippel-Lindau (VHL) syndrome is an inherited autosomal dominant disorder characterized by susceptibility to a variety of tumours, both benign and malignant (Latif et al. 1993). The most frequent tumours observed in VHL are hemangioblastomas, pheochromocytomas and renal-cell carcinomas of the clear cell type. The genetics of VHL follow the classical "two-hit hypothesis" pattern in which individuals with VHL disease carry a germline mutation in one VHL allele and then acquire a

Table 8.2 Pro-angiogenic factors downregulated by tumour suppressor genes

Factor name	p53	PTEN	VHL	Rb
Adrenomedullin		Betchen et al. (2006); Matsushima-Nishiu et al. (2001)		
bFGF	Ueba et al. (1994)			
bFGF-BP	Sherif et al. (2001)			
COX-2	Subbaramaiah et al. (1999)			
Osteopontin		Wang et al. (2003); Shao et al. (2007); Packer et al. (2006)		
Pleiotrophin		Li et al. (2006)		
VEGF	Pal et al. (2001)	Zundel et al. (2000); Jiang et al. (2001); Zhong et al. (2000)	Ohh et al. (2000)	Chellappan et al. (1991); Claudio et al. (2001)

bFGF basic fibroblast growth factor; *bFGF-BP* basic fibroblast growth factor binding protein; *COX-2* cyclooxygenase-2; *VEGF* vascular endothelial growth factor

second somatic inactivation of the second allele. The critical nature of angiogenesis in tumour formation is underscored by the function of the VHL tumour suppressor gene, which encodes a component of a ubiquitin ligase complex that negatively regulates hypoxia inducible factor 1 (HIF-1) (Ohh et al. 2000). HIF-1 is a heterodimeric transcription factor consisting of α and β subunits. Under conditions of normal oxygen levels, a family of enzymes called prolylhydroxylases (PHDs) hydroxylates HIF-1α on a conserved proline residue. The hydroxylated proline moiety of HIF-1α creates a binding site for the VHL protein (pVHL), which then targets HIF-1α for polyubiquitination and proteosomal degradation (Fig. 8.2). Under hypoxic conditions, PHD activity is low because the enzyme uses molecular oxygen as a substrate; therefore, the HIF-1α protein is stabilized since it is not hydroxylated and cannot bind VHL. Upon stabilization, HIF-1α heterodimerizes with its partner HIF-1β and regulates the expression of several genes involved in angiogenesis, cell proliferation, and metastasis. Cells lacking functional pVHL are unable to downregulate the HIF-1 system and therefore have constitutively activated HIF-1 transcription. Transcriptional activation by HIF-1 drives the expression of several genes that create a favourable environment for angiogenesis and tumour growth (reviewed in, Semenza 2003). A major target gene of HIF-1 is the pro-angiogenic factor vascular endothelial growth factor (VEGF).

VEGF is secreted from tumour or stromal cells and binds to VEGF receptor-1 or VEGF receptor-2 on endothelial cells. These VEGF receptors are receptor tyrosine kinases, which undergo dimerization and autophosphorylation upon VEGF binding, thus triggering a downstream signaling cascade that promotes endothelial cell proliferation (Carmeliet 2005). VEGF promotes angiogenesis in several different ways. VEGF increases vascular permeability and promotes migration of endothelial cells (Carmeliet 2005). Furthermore, VEGF protects endothelial cells from apoptosis by inducing expression of the anti-apoptotic proteins Bcl-2 and survivin (Carmeliet

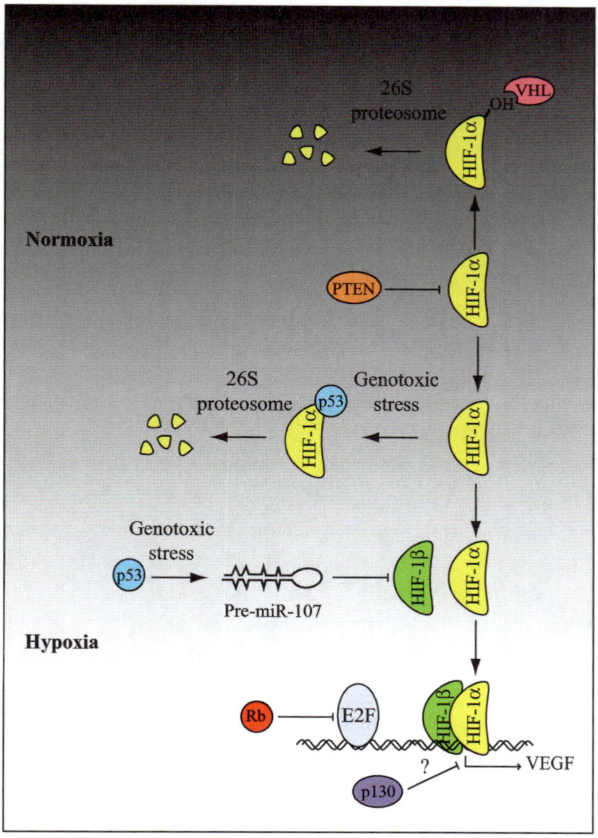

Fig. 8.2 Interactions of tumour suppressor pathways with the HIF-1 pathway. The HIF-1 pathway is the central regulator of angiogenesis that is activated in response to hypoxia. HIF-1 is a heterodimeric transcription factor composed of the subunits HIF-1α and HIF-1β. Under conditions of normoxia, HIF-1α is degraded by a process requiring the VHL tumour suppressor (see text for details). Under hypoxic conditions, HIF-1α is stabilized and activates transcription of numerous genes required for angiogenesis including VEGF. Each of the major tumour suppressor pathways discussed in this chapter are able to prevent HIF-1 activity and hence production of VEGF. In the case of p53, two redundant mechanisms have been shown to inhibit HIF-1. P53 can target HIF-1α for degradation and also stimulates production of a microRNA that prevents HIF-1β production. PTEN can prevent the translation of HIF-1α. The Rb tumour suppressor family also inhibits VEGF production by inhibiting the E2F transcription factor or, in the case of p130, through an unknown E2F independent mechanism

2005). VEGF is currently the only pro-angiogenic factor that is targeted directly in cancer therapy. The drug Bevacizumab (Avastin) is now approved for the treatment of several types of cancers, including colorectal, lung and breast, and trials are underway for other cancers as well. As will be discussed in the following sections, VEGF is negatively regulated by several of the major tumour suppressor pathways, highlighting the necessity of keeping this factor under tight control in order to prevent tumour formation.

8.2.2 PTEN

Phosphatase and tensin homologue deleted on chromosome 10 (PTEN) is the second most frequently mutated gene in human cancer after TP53. PTEN, also known as MMAC1 or TEP1, was first identified on human chromosome 10q23 as a region that is homozygously mutated in many clinical cancer samples and tumour cell lines (Li et al. 1997; Steck et al. 1997). Functionally, the PTEN protein acts as both a lipid and protein phosphatase. The major lipid substrate for PTEN is phosphatidylinositol (3,4,5) triphosphate (PIP_3) (Maehama and Dixon 1998). This lipid phosphatase activity, which directly antagonizes phosphatidylinositol 3-kinase (PI3K), is the main tumour suppressive function of PTEN (Myers et al. 1998; Stambolic et al. 1998). The PI3K pathway is a major driver of cell growth and survival. PI3K is a lipid kinase that is activated by various receptor tyrosine kinases upon binding of their extracellular growth factor ligands (Carracedo and Pandolfi 2008). PI3K converts the lipid second messenger phosphatidylinositol (4,5) bisphosphate (PIP_2) into PIP_3. PIP_3 then recruits phosphatidylinositol-dependent kinase 1 (PDK1) and Akt to the membrane, where Akt is phosphorylated. Akt is a serine/threonine kinase that phosphorylates many downstream targets and thus acts as a central node in the PI3K pathway. Akt phosphorylates mammalian target of rapamycin (mTOR), which in turn phosphorylates and activates the ribosomal protein S6K and inactivates the eIF4E inhibitory factor 4E-BP (Hay and Sonenberg 2004). Thus phosphorylation of mTOR by Akt activates protein synthesis and thereby promotes cell growth. Moreover, active Akt inhibits apoptosis by phosphorylating and inactivating the forkhead transcription factors, thereby inhibiting the transcription of pro-apoptotic genes including Bim (Manning and Cantley 2007).

Over the last ten years, it has become clear that PI3K and PTEN signaling regulate tumour angiogenesis. Loss of function of PTEN in clinical prostate cancer samples was found to be associated with increased microvessel number and density (Giri and Ittmann 1999). Jiang and colleagues were the first to directly link PI3K signaling to angiogenesis. Their 2000 study showed that overexpression of PI3K in the chorioallantoic membrane (CAM) of the chicken embryo led to sprouting of new blood vessels and enlargement of existing vessels (Jiang et al. 2000). Furthermore, overexpression of PTEN or dominant negative mutants of PI3K inhibited angiogenesis (Jiang et al. 2000). More recently, PTEN has been shown to regulate several pro- and anti-angiogenic factors.

PTEN and PI3K regulate VEGF production by controlling protein levels of HIF-1α. Reintroduction of PTEN into PTEN-null U373 glioblastoma cells inhibited the stabilization of HIF-1α and thereby blocked the transcription of VEGF and other HIF-1α-regulated genes (Zundel et al. 2000). PTEN and PI3K were shown to affect protein levels of HIF-1α but not mRNA levels (Jiang et al. 2001). HIF-1α-dependent transcriptional activity was inhibited by expression of wild-type PTEN or dominant negative mutants of PI3K in prostate cancer cells (Jiang et al. 2001). Moreover, treatment of prostate cancer cells with the PI3K inhibitor LY294002 or the mTOR inhibitor rapamycin inhibited transcription of VEGF (Jiang et al. 2001; Zhong et al.

2000). Overexpression of PTEN inhibited VEGF transcription, whereas overexpression of a lipid phosphatase mutant of PTEN increased VEGF transcription (Zhong et al. 2000).

More recently, two studies have demonstrated that PTEN's ability to inhibit VEGF transcription mediates its anti-angiogenic activity. Knockdown of the PI3K catalytic subunit (p110α) using siRNAs decreased HIF-1α levels and VEGF expression, and also resulted in decreased tumour growth and angiogenesis, as measured in the CAM model (Xia et al. 2006). Moreover, introduction of PTEN into PTEN-null prostate cancer cells blocked angiogenesis by decreasing expression levels of HIF-1α and VEGF (Fang et al. 2007). Altogether these studies suggest that PI3K promotes angiogenesis by regulating VEGF levels through HIF-1α, and that the lipid phosphatase activity of PTEN reverses this effect.

In addition to VEGF, PTEN has been demonstrated to affect other regulators of angiogenesis such as maspin (Table 8.1). Maspin is a secreted protein previously shown to have anti-angiogenic and anti-metastatic activity. PTEN reconstitution in PTEN-null glioblastoma cells resulted in increased protein levels of maspin in response to hypoxia (Eitel et al. 2009). PTEN controls maspin expression through a complex network with p53 (Eitel et al. 2009). Cytoplasmic PTEN activity blocks Akt-induced phosphorylation of Mdm2, thereby preventing its translocation to the nucleus (Mayo and Donner 2002). Mdm2 is a ubiquitin ligase which degrades p53 only in the nucleus; by preventing its translocation to the nucleus, PTEN stabilizes p53 (Mayo and Donner 2002). In turn, p53 transcriptionally regulates PTEN, thus forming a feedback loop. Interestingly, both PTEN and p53 activity were necessary to activate maspin expression in glioblastoma cells (Eitel et al. 2009).

Pleiotrophin is a secreted growth factor with oncogenic and pro-angiogenic activity (Mikelis and Papadimitriou 2008). Pleiotrophin mRNA and protein levels were increased in PTEN-null mouse embryonic fibroblasts (Li et al. 2006). Expression of constitutively active mutants of Akt increased pleiotrophin levels, while treatment with the PI3K inhibitor LY294002 or expression of PTEN decreased pleiotrophin levels (Li et al. 2006). Together these results suggest that PTEN inhibits pleiotrophin expression through its ability to antagonize PI3K signaling.

Osteopontin (OPN) is a secreted glycophosphoprotein that is commonly overexpressed in human cancers (Rangaswami et al. 2006). OPN is known to promote tumour angiogenesis and metastasis (Rangaswami et al. 2006). OPN mRNA levels were elevated in PTEN-null prostate cancer and colon cancer cells (Wang et al. 2003; Shao et al. 2007). Additionally, PTEN has been shown to decrease mRNA and protein levels of OPN in melanoma cells (Packer et al. 2006). Treatment with the PI3K inhibitor LY294002 produced a similar effect, suggesting that PTEN's lipid phosphatase activity mediates its inhibitory effects on OPN (Packer et al. 2006).

Adrenomedullin is a secreted peptide that promotes tumour angiogenesis (Nikitenko et al. 2006). PTEN decreases adrenomedullin mRNA levels in glioma cells and endometrial cancer cells (Betchen et al. 2006; Matsushima-Nishiu et al. 2001). Adrenomedullin expression is induced by hypoxia, and its promoter has several putative hypoxia response elements (Nikitenko et al. 2006); thus, PTEN may control adrenomedullin expression through its effects on HIF-1α.

In addition to its important function in tumour cells, PI3K signaling also plays a role in endothelial cells to regulate angiogenesis. PI3K is activated in endothelial cells by binding of growth factors such as VEGF and angiopoietins, and subsequently promotes endothelial cell proliferation and migration (Jiang and Liu 2009). Conversely, overexpression of PTEN in cultured endothelial cells inhibited vessel sprouting and tube formation induced by VEGF (Huang and Kontos 2002).

In an endothelial cell-specific PTEN knockout mouse model, mice with a homozygous deletion of PTEN died by embryonic day 11.5 due to excessive bleeding and cardiac failure (Hamada et al. 2005). In heterozygotes, partial loss of PTEN made the endothelial cells hypersensitive to growth factors including VEGF, and led to enhanced angiogenesis and more rapid tumour growth (Hamada et al. 2005). Similarly, mice with endothelial cell-specific knockout of the p85 regulatory subunit of PI3K also died during embryonic development due to excessive bleeding (Yuan et al. 2008). However, mice with a heterozygous deletion of PI3K-p85 in endothelial cells had smaller vessel size and decelerated tumour growth compared to control mice (Yuan et al. 2008). Together these two mouse models indicate that expression of both PI3K and PTEN in endothelial cells is essential for vessel formation during embryogenesis, but that the two proteins play opposite roles during tumour progression.

8.2.3 The Retinoblastoma Tumour Suppressor Gene Family

The retinoblastoma tumour suppressor gene (Rb) was first identified in pediatric cancers arising from retinal cells. Several types of human tumours show mutations or deletions of the Rb gene. Like the other tumour suppressors described above, inherited allelic loss of Rb increases susceptibility to cancer formation (Dunn et al. 1988). The Rb protein (pRb) is a component of the G1 checkpoint, which blocks S-phase entry and cell proliferation. pRb and its closely related proteins, p107 and p130, regulate cell cycle by inhibiting the activity of E2F transcription factors (Weinberg 1995; Chellappan 2009). E2Fs bind to the promoter regions of many genes required for S-phase entry, allowing the progression of the cell cycle from G1 to S phase. The Rb family of proteins is regulated by the cyclin-dependent kinases (CDKs)-cyclins, which phosphorylate Rb proteins in a cell cycle dependent manner (Grana et al. 1998; Mittnacht 1998). Rb is hyperphosphorylated during most of the cell cycle while the hypophosphorylated form is present only during G1 phase. Sequential phosphorylation of Rb leads to dissociation of Rb-E2F complexes, which allows E2F to bind promoters of genes required for S-phase entry (Harbour and Dean 2000).

Several lines of experimental evidence have demonstrated that at least part of the tumour suppressive effects of the Rb family function through inhibition of angiogenesis. Significantly, in addition to S-phase promoting genes, E2F was shown to activate several genes involved in processes such as angiogenesis, invasion and metastasis, including fibroblast growth factor 2 (FGF2), fibroblast growth factor receptor 3 (FGFR3), matrix metalloproteinase 16 (MMP16) and VEGF-B (Stanelle et al. 2002). Thus, by globally suppressing E2F-dependent transcription, the Rb family can inhibit production of such angiogenesis promoting factors. p130 has been shown to downregulate VEGF expression both at the RNA and protein levels in different cell types and also to downregulate the activity of the VEGF promoter through an unknown mechanism that does not involve E2F (Claudio et al. 2001).

The hypophosphorylated form of Rb is targeted by several viral transforming proteins such as E1A of adenovirus, large T antigen of simian virus 40 (SV40) (reviewed in, DeCaprio 2009) and E7 of human papilloma virus (HPV) (Munger and Howley 2002). It has been shown that HPV E6 and E7 oncoproteins enhance angiogenesis by increasing the expression of many pro-angiogenic factors and decreasing the levels of anti-angiogenic factors. In this study, VEGF and interleukin 8 (IL-8) were shown to increase whereas thrombospondin-1 (TSP-1) was decreased (Toussaint-Smith et al. 2004). Therefore, viral oncogene mediated deregulation of Rb may contribute to promoting angiogenesis of tumours such as HPV-induced cervical carcinoma.

8.2.4 The p53 Tumour Suppressor Gene (TP53)

The p53 tumour suppressor protein is arguably the most important factor limiting tumour development in metazoans. One of the many tumour suppressive functions of p53 is the inhibition of angiogenesis. The gene encoding p53 (TP53) is mutated in half of all human tumours, which makes it the most frequently altered gene in all cancers (Hollstein et al. 1991; Vogelstein et al. 2000). The importance of the tumour inhibiting functions of p53 is best demonstrated in mouse models, where deletion of p53 results in spontaneous tumours at a very early age (Attardi and Donehower 2005). Under normal conditions, the steady-state level of p53 is maintained low due to a negative feedback loop involving the E3 ubiquitin ligase MDM2 (Momand et al. 2000). Only following genotoxic stress, DNA damage or aberrant growth signals resulting from the activation of oncogenes do p53 protein levels become stabilized. This then allows p53 to mediate several cellular stress responses to allow for repair of damaged DNA, eliminate defective cells from the replicative pool, and create an environment unsuitable for the growth of tumours (Vousden and Lu 2002). The structure of p53 is that of a prototypical transcription factor and cancer associated alterations in p53 primarily arise from point mutations within its DNA-binding domain (Vogelstein and Kinzler 1992). For these reasons, much attention has been focused on the identification of p53 transcriptional targets in order to understand the mechanism through which p53 exerts its effects. Most of the well-characterized p53 functions, including cell cycle arrest, DNA damage repair and apoptosis, have been primarily attributed to its ability to directly upregulate expression of such genes as the CDK inhibitor, $p21^{WAF1/CIP1}$ to inhibit cell cycle progression, and a plethora of pro-apoptotic genes including Bax and NOXA (Vousden and Lu 2002). However, p53 can also execute some of its biological functions, including its inhibitory role on angiogenesis, independent of its transcription factor activity (reviewed in Yee and Vousden 2005).

Initial clues suggesting a role for p53 in angiogenesis came from clinical studies correlating the status of p53 in tumours with their microvessel density (MVD). In prostate (Yu et al. 1997), colon (Kang et al. 1997; Takahashi et al. 1998; Faviana et al. 2002), head and neck (Gasparini et al. 1993), and breast cancers (Gasparini et al. 1994), significantly higher MVDs were observed in tumours with mutated p53 than in those carrying the wild-type gene. The anti-angiogenic role of p53 was further highlighted in studies where reconstitution of p53 in vivo resulted in avascular dormant tumours, independent of its anti-proliferative and pro-apoptotic effects (Holmgren et al. 1998; Gautam et al. 2002).

Three basic mechanisms have been found to mediate the inhibitory effect of p53 on angiogenesis. These mechanisms include: transcriptional repression of pro-angiogenic genes, inhibition of HIF-1, and transcriptional activation of anti-angiogenic genes. Thus far, four genes encoding pro-angiogenic factors have been found to be negatively regulated by p53 through several different mechanisms (Table 8.2). Perhaps most intriguing is the ability of p53 to impede the transcription of VEGF under hypoxic conditions. This effect is partly mediated by the ability of p53 to bind to the Sp1 transcription factor and to thus prevent it from activating the VEGF promoter (Pal et al. 2001). P53 also represses the expression of cyclooxygenase-2 (COX-2), a key enzyme involved in prostanoid-mediated angiogenesis, by competing with the TATA-box binding protein for binding to its promoter (Subbaramaiah et al. 1999). Basic fibroblast growth factor (bFGF) and its activator, the bFGF-binding protein (bFGF-BP), are also downregulated in response to p53. Although the mechanism of bFGF-BP inhibition has not been defined, p53 was shown to repress the expression of bFGF itself by directly binding to core promoter elements (Sherif et al. 2001; Ueba et al. 1994).

The second mechanism through which p53 inhibits angiogenesis is by impeding the activity of HIF-1. As previously described, HIF-1 is a major regulator of angiogenesis in response to hypoxia. The inhibitory effect of p53 on HIF-1 is partly mediated by its ability to bind to the HIF-1α subunit and to target it for proteosomal degradation under hypoxic conditions (Ravi et al. 2000). Recently, p53 was also found to inhibit the expression of HIF-1β by directly upregulating miR-107, a microRNA encoded in an intron of the pantothenate kinase enzyme 1 (PANK1) (Yamakuchi et al. 2010). miR-107 targets the 3′ untranslated region of HIF-1β and reduces its expression under both normoxic and hypoxic conditions (Yamakuchi et al. 2010). The result of these inhibitory effects on both HIF-1α and HIF-1β is that HIF-1 is unable to stabilize and upregulate VEGF; consequently, the pro-angiogenic output of the tumour is markedly reduced. Interestingly, p53 does not inhibit the activity of HIF-1α under normal physiological conditions (Rempe et al. 2007) and expression of miR-107 under normoxic conditions does not affect the levels of VEGF produced by the cell (Yamakuchi et al. 2010). Also, the inhibitory effect of p53 on HIF-1 necessitates p53 itself to stabilize in the cell either in response to DNA damage (Kaluzova et al. 2004) or acidosis and nutrient deprivation secondary to hypoxia (Pan et al. 2004). As such, this mechanism only operates in an environment commonly found in small tumours where extreme hypoxic conditions and genotoxic stress both exist.

The third way by which p53 inhibits angiogenesis is by transcriptional upregulation of endogenous anti-angiogenic factors (Table 8.1). TSP-1 was the first of such p53 targets to be identified (Dameron et al. 1994) and was also the first characterized example of an endogenous anti-angiogenic factor (Good et al. 1990). TSP-1 and the related factor, TSP-2, are large glycoproteins that localize to the extracellular matrix (ECM). Overexpression of TSP-1 inhibits angiogenesis and tumour growth, while loss of TSP-1 leads to increased angiogenesis (Nyberg et al. 2005). Furthermore, TSP-1 and TSP-2-null mice both display enhanced tumour angiogenesis (Nyberg et al. 2005). The upregulation of TSP-1 by p53, along with its downregulation in response to the activation of src (Slack and Bornstein 1994), myc (Tikhonenko et al. 1996; Janz et al. 2000) and ras (Watnick et al. 2003; Rak et al. 2000), demonstrate the opposing effects of oncogenes and tumour suppressors on angiogenic factors (Fig. 8.1).

Other anti-angiogenic factors upregulated by p53 include the brain-specific angiogenesis inhibitor (BAI1) (Nishimori et al. 1997) and maspin (Eitel et al. 2009; Chenau et al. 2009; Yu et al. 2006), as well as the ephrin receptor A2 (EPHA2) and its ligand ephrin A1 (Brantley et al. 2002; Dohn et al. 2001). The coupled regulation of EPHA2 and its ligand ephrin A1 by p53 also demonstrates that p53 can trigger an entire transcriptional program in order to inhibit angiogenesis. This phenomenon is also highlighted in the mechanism through which p53 induces the release of collagen-derived anti-angiogenic factors (CDAFs) in the ECM (Teodoro et al. 2006, 2007; Assadian and Teodoro 2008).

8.2.4.1 Collagen-Derived Anti-Angiogenic Factors (CDAFs) and p53

Whereas pro-angiogenic factors are mostly growth factors secreted by the tumour or the stroma, many of the endogenous anti-angiogenic factors are components or proteolytic fragments derived from the ECM. The basement membrane of blood vessels is a specialized, collagen-rich ECM that provides structural support to the endothelium (Kalluri 2003). Several collagen isoforms in the basement membrane contain C-terminal peptides that, when proteolytically cleaved, have anti-angiogenic activity. These CDAFs include arresten, derived from the $\alpha 1$ collagen IV chain, tumstatin, derived from the $\alpha 3$ collagen IV chain, and endostatin, derived from the $\alpha 1$ collagen XVIII chain. CDAFs have been shown to inhibit endothelial cell proliferation, migration, and tube formation as well as inducing apoptosis (Assadian and Teodoro 2008). Through these complex inhibitory mechanisms, CDAFs have potent anti-angiogenic effects.

To activate CDAFs, p53 directly upregulates the transcription of: 1) collagen genes containing CDAFs in their C-terminal noncollagenous-1 domain (NC1), 2) the enzyme necessary to stabilize and assemble collagens for secretion, and 3) the proteolytic enzymes necessary to cleave CDAFs from the full-length protein. Out of seven collagen chains identified to contain CDAFs in their NC1 domains, two have been identified as p53 targets: $\alpha 1$-collagen XVIII (COL18A1) and $\alpha 1$-collagen IV

(COL4A1) (Miled et al. 2005; Wei et al. 2006). However, p53 has also been shown to stabilize the expression of other CDAF parent proteins, such as α3-collagen IV, by directly upregulating α(II)-prolyl-4-hydroxylase (PH4A2), a rate limiting enzyme crucial to collagen stability and assembly (Teodoro et al. 2006). The same study also demonstrated that p53 was able to induce the cleavage of CDAFs from the NC1 domains of α1-collagen XVIII and α3-collagen IV. Although the exact mechanism through which p53 executes the proteolytic cleavage of the CDAFs from their parent collagens remains unknown, MMP-2, a p53 target with collagenase activity, may potentially mediate this effect (Bian and Sun 1997).

Overall these effects seem to strongly support a model where p53 acts to alter the angiogenic output of the tumour. By upregulating the endogenous inhibitors of angiogenesis and limiting the production of pro-angiogenic factors, p53 creates an environment non-permissive to the growth and migration of endothelial cells and prevents the angiogenic switch. Much effort is now being devoted to understanding these changes on a larger scale and identifying novel secreted targets of p53 and other tumour suppressors. The therapeutic use of such factors may allow tumours to be maintained in a dormant, non-aggressive state.

8.3 Clinical Perspectives

From the survey of the literature presented above it is apparent that a significant function of the major tumour suppressor pathways is inhibition of pathological angiogenesis. Functional loss of one or more of these tumour suppressor pathways occurs in essentially all cancers. Therefore, the ultimate objective of anti-angiogenic therapy is the pharmacological replacement of tumour suppressor function to maintain tumours in the dormant, avascular state that exists before the angiogenic switch occurs. Each of the tumour suppressor proteins discussed above has the capacity to inhibit the production of VEGF (Fig. 8.2) and, not surprisingly, this factor has also been the major pharmaceutical target in anti-angiogenic cancer therapy in recent years. Currently there are more than 10 angiogenesis inhibitors approved for clinical use against a variety of cancers that each target some aspect of VEGF biology (Folkman 2007). Bevacizumab (Avastin), a humanized monoclonal antibody against VEGF, was the first anti-angiogenic molecule approved by the FDA in 2004. Bevacizumab has become the major anti-angiogenic treatment and is now used in combination with conventional chemotherapy for late stages of colon cancer, non-small cell lung cancer, breast cancer, glioblastoma, and metastatic renal cell carcinoma. Small molecule inhibitors of the VEGF receptor are also now in use. Sorafenib (Nexavar) and Sunitinib (Sutent) are tyrosine kinase inhibitors that target VEGF as well as other angiogenic receptors including platelet derived growth factor (PDGF). Sorafenib and Sunitinib are approved by the FDA to treat metastatic renal cell carcinoma as single agents. Sorefenib is also approved for treatment of hepatocellular carcinoma, and Sunitinib for gastrointestinal tumours.

Despite the ability of drugs such as Bevacizumab to completely inhibit VEGF activity, patient treatment generally results in only modest extension of overall survival by a matter of months (Hurwitz et al. 2004; Miller et al. 2007). Because of the inherent genetic instability and heterogeneity of tumour cells, inhibition of a single angiogenic factor such as VEGF likely results in resistance through expression of other angiogenic factors (Relf et al. 1997). Experimental evidence supporting this notion has shown that some tumours may evade the inhibition of VEGF signaling by upregulation of additional pro-angiogenic factors such as bFGF (Relf et al. 1997; Dorrell et al. 2007). In these studies, it was shown that blocking compensatory angiogenic signals via treatment with combination therapy could significantly reduce tumour angiogenesis (Dorrell et al. 2007; Casanovas et al. 2005). Interestingly, as was discussed above, p53 is able to inhibit both the bFGF and VEGF pathways, suggesting that blocking both of these factors is required for effective angiogenesis blockade. Further identification of mechanisms by which tumour suppressor pathways inhibit angiogenesis may therefore provide insights towards the design of combination therapies in order to limit acquired resistance.

8.3.1 The Relationship Between Angiogenesis and Metastasis

The final, and perhaps most devastating, capability that tumour cells acquire is metastatic potential. The angiogenic and metastatic processes are often discussed as two completely different processes; however, recent results emerging from both basic research and the clinic have suggested that these processes are inextricably linked. Under some conditions, pharmacologically inhibiting either angiogenesis or metastasis alone can result in acceleration of the other process and thereby complicate treatment strategies.

An example of the complex relationship between metastasis and angiogenesis has come from the efforts to target MMPs as a therapeutic strategy to prevent tumour metastasis. MMPs are essential regulators of the cell's microenvironment through their control of extracellular proteolysis (Egeblad and Werb 2002). The importance of MMPs during cancer progression was initially highlighted during tumour progression owing to their ability to degrade the ECM, break natural barriers and allow tumour cells to spread in surrounding tissues and metastasize (Egeblad and Werb 2002; Freije et al. 2003). This represented a key therapeutic target during tumorigenesis, which led to the development of small-molecule inhibitors for the treatment of metastatic cancer, in particular of molecules targeting MMPs and plasminogen activators (Turk 2006). Unfortunately, results from the clinical trials showed that MMP inhibitors had either no effect or, in some cases, even accelerated tumour growth. This forced a re-evaluation of the prevailing concepts and suggested the possibility that some proteases might have anti-tumour roles (Coussens et al. 2002; Overall and Kleifeld 2006). Recent studies have provided evidence for the existence of extracellular proteases with anti-tumour properties based on the generation of loss-of-function animal models (Overall and Kleifeld 2006; Balbin et al. 2003;

McCawley et al. 2004). These results support an emerging and paradoxical role for proteases in tumour progression.

The likely cause of the failure of MMP inhibitors in the clinic is that several members of the MMP family have tumour suppressor activities. Collagenase 2 (MMP8), for example, was the first protease to be described in vivo as having anti-tumour activity (Balbin et al. 2003). It is mainly produced by neutrophils and is associated with inflammation. Its expression has been linked to a decrease in metastasis of breast cancer cells (Montel et al. 2004). Macrophage metalloelastase, also known as MMP12, is produced by macrophages. Its role in human cancer is still unclear because of its anti- and pro-tumour activities. It has been reported to have a protective role against tumour growth in lungs by inhibiting angiogenesis (Gorrin-Rivas et al. 2000). It has also been shown to have anti-metastatic activities in experimental metastasis models (Houghton et al. 2006). The anti-tumour effects of MMP12 could be derived from cleaving plasminogen to release angiostatin, an anti-angiogenic peptide (Dong et al. 1997). Gelatinase B (MMP9) is another example of a protease with opposite effects in cancer. It has been associated with tumour growth (Egeblad and Werb 2002) but studies have also reported it as having a protective role, which is derived, similar to MMP12, from its ability to cleave and release endogenous anti-angiogenic inhibitors such as angiostatin, tumstatin and endostatin (Hamano et al. 2003; Pozzi et al. 2002). Stromelysin 3 (MMP11) (Andarawewa et al. 2003) and MMP19 (Pendas et al. 2004; Jost et al. 2006) were originally recognized as pro-tumorigenic proteases, however, a protective role has also been reported.

Of particular significance has been the demonstration that various MMPs are necessary for releasing ECM-sequestered endogenous anti-angiogenic factors. The CDAF molecules, which were introduced above, are proteolytic fragments of the NC1 domain of several collagens that possess potent anti-angiogenic activity (Kalluri 2003). These include endostatin, released from the $\alpha1$ collagen XVIII chain by the action of several MMPs, including MMP-3, 9, 12, 13 and 20 (Ferreras et al. 2000). Endostatin binds to cell surface proteoglycans, to VEGFR-2 and to integrin $\alpha5\beta1$, to inhibit VEGF and bFGF-induced endothelial cell migration and to induce apoptosis (Kalluri 2003; Sudhakar et al. 2003). Tumstatin, a CDAF generated from $\alpha3$ collagen IV, can be released by MMP9. Tumstatin inhibits endothelial cell proliferation and promotes apoptosis via signaling through integrin $\alpha v\beta3$ (Hamano et al. 2003; Sudhakar et al. 2003). Decreased levels of tumstatin in MMP9 knockout mice were shown to be responsible for increased growth of Lewis lung carcinoma compared to wild-type mice (Hamano et al. 2003). Arresten, released from $\alpha1$ collagen IV, binds to $\alpha1\beta1$ integrin. Canstatin, released from $\alpha2$ collagen IV, binds both $\alpha v\beta3$ and $\alpha3\beta1$ integrins. Binding of arresten and canstatin to integrins presumably mediates their anti-angiogenic activities (Kalluri 2003). MMP-2, 7, 9, and 12 all have the capacity to hydrolyze plasminogen and release the anti-angiogenic peptide angiostatin (Dong et al. 1997; O'Reilly et al. 1999; Patterson and Sang 1997). Thus we find that the MMPs are very much like double-edged swords with the capacity to promote cell motility and metastasis, but at the same time liberate anti-angiogenic peptides that can keep tumour growth in check. Since anti-angiogenic molecules such as CDAFs have been shown to be effectors in tumour suppressor pathways such as p53 (see above), inhibiting the MMPs that liberate these peptides would have the effect of crippling anti-tumour responses.

Just as inhibition of metastasis by targeting MMPs may result in enhanced angiogenesis and tumour growth, there is also experimental evidence showing that inhibition of angiogenesis alone can accelerate metastasis. Two recent high-profile studies investigated the effects of anti-VEGF therapy on tumour growth and metastasis (Ebos et al. 2009; Paez-Ribes et al. 2009). These studies used two different animal models to show that, under some circumstances, anti-VEGF treatment could result in enhanced metastasis. The first study showed that short-term treatment of healthy mice with the VEGFR/PDGFR kinase inhibitor, Sunitinib, even prior to injection of tumour cells, resulted in accelerated metastasis and shorter survival as compared to control mice that did not receive anti-angiogenic therapy (Ebos et al. 2009). The second study came to similar conclusions using either DC101, a VEGFR-2-blocking monoclonal antibody, or by using continuous Sunitinib treatment or tumour-specific deletion of VEGF-A in a β-VEGF knockout background (Paez-Ribes et al. 2009). Taken together, these results suggest that metastasis and angiogenesis are intimately linked and treatment for one of these processes cannot be undertaken without taking into account what may be happening to the other.

8.3.2 Mimicking Tumour Suppressor Function as a Treatment Paradigm

Loss of tumour suppressor functions is one of the main driving forces of tumour development. Rational design of therapies to target tumour growth through angiogenesis inhibition can benefit greatly from understanding the basic mechanisms used by tumour suppressor pathways. With respect to angiogenesis, several mechanistic trends emerge by which tumour suppressor genes (TSGs) inhibit this pathway effectively. The first mechanism is to effectively control VEGF. All of the major tumour suppressor proteins discussed above have evolved capabilities to control VEGF on a transcriptional or post-transcriptional level. However, the resistance seen in the clinic to VEGF inhibitors conclusively shows that inhibition of VEGF is not sufficient. The emergence of resistance to cancer therapy poses the same problems that are observed in the treatment of infectious disease. For example, developing a drug regimen that could maintain HIV as a stable infection required administration of a drug cocktail that targets multiple aspects of viral biology. The same approach is likely required for effective clinical inhibition of angiogenesis and is an approach that tumour suppressor proteins have evolved to exploit. The second trend is therefore to utilize multiple pathways to target tumour angiogenesis to limit possibility of resistance. This could be through inhibiting secondary pro-angiogenic molecules such as bFGF or by actively producing endogenous anti-angiogenic factors such as TSP-1 or CDAFs. This approach has not yet been translated to the clinical setting for a variety of reasons. Perhaps the major reason why anti-angiogenic factors, including CDAFs and TSP-1, have not been successfully translated to the clinic is because a single mechanism of action has not emerged for these agents. Although these proteins display potent anti-angiogenic activity both in vitro and in vivo, the mechanism of action is complex and poorly understood, which makes clinical application problematic. Nonetheless, an extensive clinical trial using the CDAF endostatin was carried out in China for treatment of lung cancer. The results of the trial were excellent and resulted in approval of the drug in combination with conventional chemotherapy (Sun et al. 2005). The search for new approaches to prevent angiogenesis that do not rely on VEGF blockade is imperative if sustained angiogenesis inhibition is to be achieved in the clinic.

A final trend that is observed in tumour suppressors is that angiogenesis and metastasis are inhibited simultaneously. Tumour suppressor pathways often increase expression of factors that are able to inhibit metastasis as well as angiogenesis. An excellent example of such a mechanism is the protein maspin, which is upregulated by both the PTEN and p53 pathways. The maspin protein is a potent inhibitor of both angiogenesis and metastasis. This may be a critical aspect to inhibit tumour growth since inhibiting only angiogenesis can result in metastasis acceleration and vice versa. In addition, the trend between MMP expression and tumorigenesis is not as straightforward as was initially thought. The fact that several proteases have opposing effects in cancer, depending on tissue type and tumour microenvironment, introduces an additional level of difficulty and represents a challenge in designing specific inhibitors. It is possible that the use of anti-angiogenic agents may prove to be effective in combination with the metastasis-targeting MMP inhibitors that were ineffective as a monotherapy.

In most individuals, the action of tumour suppressor pathways can maintain the body free of life-threatening cancers for an entire lifetime. Part of the effectiveness of tumour suppressor pathways seems to be derived from preventing small cancerous lesions from becoming vascularized. Thus, further study of how these proteins function to prevent tumour angiogenesis in vivo will continue to provide insights towards achieving sustained angiogenesis inhibition in the clinic.

Acknowledgments Research in the lab of J.G.T. is supported by funding from the Canadian Institute of Health Research (CIHR) and the Natural Science and Engineering Council of Canada. K.J.L. and S.A. are both supported by studentship from the CIHR. W.E. is the recipient of a post-doctoral training award form the McGill Integrated Cancer Research Training Program.

References

Andarawewa KL et al (2003) Dual stromelysin-3 function during natural mouse mammary tumor virus-ras tumor progression. Cancer Res 63:5844–5849

Assadian S, Teodoro JG (2008) Regulation of collagen-derived antiangiogenic factors by p53. Expert Opin Biol Ther 8:941–950

Attardi LD, Donehower LA (2005) Probing p53 biological functions through the use of genetically engineered mouse models. Mutat Res 576:4–21

Balbin M et al (2003) Loss of collagenase-2 confers increased skin tumor susceptibility to male mice. Nat Genet 35:252–257

Bergers G, Benjamin LE (2003) Tumorigenesis and the angiogenic switch. Nat Rev Cancer 3:401–410

Betchen SA, Musatov S, Roberts J, Pena J, Kaplitt MG (2006) PTEN inhibits adrenomedullin expression and function in brain tumor cells. J Neurooncol 79:117–123

Bian J, Sun Y (1997) Transcriptional activation by p53 of the human type IV collagenase (gelatinase A or matrix metalloproteinase 2) promoter. Mol Cell Biol 17:6330–6338

Brantley DM et al (2002) Soluble Eph A receptors inhibit tumor angiogenesis and progression in vivo. Oncogene 21:7011–7026

Carmeliet P (2005) VEGF as a key mediator of angiogenesis in cancer. Oncology 69(Suppl 3):4–10

Carmeliet P, Jain RK (2000) Angiogenesis in cancer and other diseases. Nature 407:249–257

Carracedo A, Pandolfi PP (2008) The PTEN-PI3K pathway: of feedbacks and cross-talks. Oncogene 27:5527–5541

Casanovas O, Hicklin DJ, Bergers G, Hanahan D (2005) Drug resistance by evasion of antiangiogenic targeting of VEGF signaling in late-stage pancreatic islet tumors. Cancer Cell 8:299–309

Chellappan SP, Hiebert S, Mudryj M, Horowitz JM, Nevins JR (1991) The E2F transcription factor is a cellular target for the RB protein. Cell 65:1053–1061

Chenau J et al (2009) The cell line secretome, a suitable tool for investigating proteins released in vivo by tumors: application to the study of p53-modulated proteins secreted in lung cancer cells. J Proteome Res 8:4579–4591

Claudio PP et al (2001) RB2/p130 gene-enhanced expression down-regulates vascular endothelial growth factor expression and inhibits angiogenesis in vivo. Cancer Res 61:462–468

Coussens LM, Fingleton B, Matrisian LM (2002) Matrix metalloproteinase inhibitors and cancer: trials and tribulations. Science 295:2387–2392

Dameron KM, Volpert OV, Tainsky MA, Bouck N (1994) Control of angiogenesis in fibroblasts by p53 regulation of thrombospondin-1. Science 265:1582–1584

DeCaprio JA (2009) How the Rb tumor suppressor structure and function was revealed by the study of Adenovirus and SV40. Virology 384:274–284

Dohn M, Jiang J, Chen X (2001) Receptor tyrosine kinase EphA2 is regulated by p53-family proteins and induces apoptosis. Oncogene 20:6503–6515

Dong Z, Kumar R, Yang X, Fidler IJ (1997) Macrophage-derived metalloelastase is responsible for the generation of angiostatin in Lewis lung carcinoma. Cell 88:801–810

Dorrell MI, Aguilar E, Scheppke L, Barnett FH, Friedlander M (2007) Combination angiostatic therapy completely inhibits ocular and tumor angiogenesis. Proc Natl Acad Sci U S A 104:967–972

Dunn JM, Phillips RA, Becker AJ, Gallie BL (1988) Identification of germline and somatic mutations affecting the retinoblastoma gene. Science 241:1797–1800

Ebos JM et al (2009) Accelerated metastasis after short-term treatment with a potent inhibitor of tumor angiogenesis. Cancer Cell 15:232–239

Egeblad M, Werb Z (2002) New functions for the matrix metalloproteinases in cancer progression. Nat Rev Cancer 2:161–174

Eitel JA et al (2009) PTEN and p53 are required for hypoxia induced expression of maspin in glioblastoma cells. Cell Cycle 8:896–901

Fang J, Ding M, Yang L, Liu LZ, Jiang BH (2007) PI3K/PTEN/AKT signaling regulates prostate tumor angiogenesis. Cell Signal 19:2487–2497

Faviana P et al (2002) Neoangiogenesis in colon cancer: correlation between vascular density, vascular endothelial growth factor (VEGF) and p53 protein expression. Oncol Rep 9:617–620

Ferreras M, Felbor U, Lenhard T, Olsen BR, Delaisse J (2000) Generation and degradation of human endostatin proteins by various proteinases. FEBS Lett 486:247–251

Folkman J (2006) Angiogenesis. Annu Rev Med 57:1–18

Folkman J (2007) Angiogenesis: an organizing principle for drug discovery? Nat Rev Drug Discov 6:273–286

Folkman J, Merler E, Abernathy C, Williams G (1971) Isolation of a tumor factor responsible for angiogenesis. J Exp Med 133:275–288

Freije JM et al (2003) Matrix metalloproteinases and tumor progression. Adv Exp Med Biol 532:91–107

Gasparini G et al (1993) Intratumoral microvessel density and p53 protein: correlation with metastasis in head-and-neck squamous-cell carcinoma. Int J Cancer 55:739–744

Gasparini G et al (1994) Tumor microvessel density, p53 expression, tumor size, and peritumoral lymphatic vessel invasion are relevant prognostic markers in node-negative breast carcinoma. J Clin Oncol 12:454–466

Gautam A, Densmore CL, Melton S, Golunski E, Waldrep JC (2002) Aerosol delivery of PEI-p53 complexes inhibits B16-F10 lung metastases through regulation of angiogenesis. Cancer Gene Ther 9:28–36

Giri D, Ittmann M (1999) Inactivation of the PTEN tumor suppressor gene is associated with increased angiogenesis in clinically localized prostate carcinoma. Hum Pathol 30:419–424

Good DJ et al (1990) A tumor suppressor-dependent inhibitor of angiogenesis is immunologically and functionally indistinguishable from a fragment of thrombospondin. Proc Natl Acad Sci U S A 87:6624–6628

Gorrin-Rivas MJ et al (2000) Mouse macrophage metalloelastase gene transfer into a murine melanoma suppresses primary tumor growth by halting angiogenesis. Clin Cancer Res 6:1647–1654

Grana X, Garriga J, Mayol X (1998) Role of the retinoblastoma protein family, pRB, p107 and p130 in the negative control of cell growth. Oncogene 17:3365–3383

Hamada K et al (2005) The PTEN/PI3K pathway governs normal vascular development and tumor angiogenesis. Genes Dev 19:2054–2065

Hamano Y et al (2003) Physiological levels of tumstatin, a fragment of collagen IV alpha3 chain, are generated by MMP-9 proteolysis and suppress angiogenesis via alphaV beta3 integrin. Cancer Cell 3:589–601

Hanahan D, Folkman J (1996) Patterns and emerging mechanisms of the angiogenic switch during tumorigenesis. Cell 86:353–364

Harbour JW, Dean DC (2000) The Rb/E2F pathway: expanding roles and emerging paradigms. Genes Dev 14:2393–2409

Hay N, Sonenberg N (2004) Upstream and downstream of mTOR. Genes Dev 18:1926–1945

Hollstein M, Sidransky D, Vogelstein B, Harris CC (1991) p53 mutations in human cancers. Science 253:49–53

Holmgren L, Jackson G, Arbiser J (1998) p53 induces angiogenesis-restricted dormancy in a mouse fibrosarcoma. Oncogene 17:819–824

Houghton AM et al (2006) Macrophage elastase (matrix metalloproteinase-12) suppresses growth of lung metastases. Cancer Res 66:6149–6155

Huang J, Kontos CD (2002) PTEN modulates vascular endothelial growth factor-mediated signaling and angiogenic effects. J Biol Chem 277:10760–10766

Hurwitz H et al (2004) Bevacizumab plus irinotecan, fluorouracil, and leucovorin for metastatic colorectal cancer. N Engl J Med 350:2335–2342

Janz A, Sevignani C, Kenyon K, Ngo CV, Thomas-Tikhonenko A (2000) Activation of the myc oncoprotein leads to increased turnover of thrombospondin-1 mRNA. Nucleic Acids Res 28:2268–2275

Jiang BH et al (2001) Phosphatidylinositol 3-kinase signaling controls levels of hypoxia-inducible factor 1. Cell Growth Differ 12:363–369

Jiang BH, Liu LZ (2009) PI3K/PTEN signaling in angiogenesis and tumorigenesis. Adv Cancer Res 102:19–65

Jiang BH, Zheng JZ, Aoki M, Vogt PK (2000) Phosphatidylinositol 3-kinase signaling mediates angiogenesis and expression of vascular endothelial growth factor in endothelial cells. Proc Natl Acad Sci U S A 97:1749–1753

Jost M et al (2006) Earlier onset of tumoral angiogenesis in matrix metalloproteinase-19-deficient mice. Cancer Res 66:5234–5241

Kalluri R (2003) Basement membranes: structure, assembly and role in tumour angiogenesis. Nat Rev Cancer 3:422–433

Kaluzova M, Kaluz S, Lerman MI, Stanbridge EJ (2004) DNA damage is a prerequisite for p53-mediated proteasomal degradation of HIF-1alpha in hypoxic cells and downregulation of the hypoxia marker carbonic anhydrase IX. Mol Cell Biol 24:5757–5766

Kang SM et al (1997) Combined analysis of p53 and vascular endothelial growth factor expression in colorectal carcinoma for determination of tumor vascularity and liver metastasis. Int J Cancer 74:502–507

Latif F et al (1993) Identification of the von Hippel-Lindau disease tumor suppressor gene. Science 260:1317–1320

Li G et al (2006) PTEN deletion leads to up-regulation of a secreted growth factor pleiotrophin. J Biol Chem 281:10663–10668

Li J et al (1997) PTEN, a putative protein tyrosine phosphatase gene mutated in human brain, breast, and prostate cancer. Science 275:1943–1947

Maehama T, Dixon JE (1998) The tumor suppressor, PTEN/MMAC1, dephosphorylates the lipid second messenger, phosphatidylinositol 3,4,5-trisphosphate. J Biol Chem 273:13375–13378

Manning BD, Cantley LC (2007) AKT/PKB signaling: navigating downstream. Cell 129:1261–1274

Matsushima-Nishiu M et al (2001) Growth and gene expression profile analyses of endometrial cancer cells expressing exogenous PTEN. Cancer Res 61:3741–3749

Mayo LD, Donner DB (2002) The PTEN, Mdm2, p53 tumor suppressor-oncoprotein network. Trends Biochem Sci 27:462–467

McCawley LJ, Crawford HC, King LE Jr, Mudgett J, Matrisian LM (2004) A protective role for matrix metalloproteinase-3 in squamous cell carcinoma. Cancer Res 64:6965–6972

Mikelis C, Papadimitriou E (2008) Heparin-binding protein pleiotrophin: an important player in the angiogenic process. Connect Tissue Res 49:149–152

Miled C, Pontoglio M, Garbay S, Yaniv M, Weitzman JB (2005) A genomic map of p53 binding sites identifies novel p53 targets involved in an apoptotic network. Cancer Res 65:5096–5104

Miller K et al (2007) Paclitaxel plus bevacizumab versus paclitaxel alone for metastatic breast cancer. N Engl J Med 357:2666–2676

Mittnacht S (1998) Control of pRB phosphorylation. Curr Opin Genet Dev 8:21–27

Momand J, Wu HH, Dasgupta G (2000) MDM2–master regulator of the p53 tumor suppressor protein. Gene 242:15–29

Montel V et al (2004) Altered metastatic behavior of human breast cancer cells after experimental manipulation of matrix metalloproteinase 8 gene expression. Cancer Res 64:1687–1694

Munger K, Howley PM (2002) Human papillomavirus immortalization and transformation functions. Virus Res 89:213–228

Myers MP et al (1998) The lipid phosphatase activity of PTEN is critical for its tumor supressor function. Proc Natl Acad Sci U S A 95:13513–13518

Nikitenko LL, Fox SB, Kehoe S, Rees MC, Bicknell R (2006) Adrenomedullin and tumour angiogenesis. Br J Cancer 94:1–7

Nishimori H et al (1997) A novel brain-specific p53-target gene, BAI1, containing thrombospondin type 1 repeats inhibits experimental angiogenesis. Oncogene 15:2145–2150

Nyberg P, Xie L, Kalluri R (2005) Endogenous inhibitors of angiogenesis. Cancer Res 65:3967–3979

Ohh M et al (2000) Ubiquitination of hypoxia-inducible factor requires direct binding to the beta-domain of the von Hippel-Lindau protein. Nat Cell Biol 2:423–427

O'Reilly MS, Wiederschain D, Stetler-Stevenson WG, Folkman J, Moses MA (1999) Regulation of angiostatin production by matrix metalloproteinase-2 in a model of concomitant resistance. J Biol Chem 274:29568–29571

Overall CM, Kleifeld O (2006) Tumour microenvironment—opinion: validating matrix metalloproteinases as drug targets and anti-targets for cancer therapy. Nat Rev Cancer 6:227–239

Packer L et al (2006) Osteopontin is a downstream effector of the PI3-kinase pathway in melanomas that is inversely correlated with functional PTEN. Carcinogenesis 27:1778–1786

Paez-Ribes M et al (2009) Antiangiogenic therapy elicits malignant progression of tumors to increased local invasion and distant metastasis. Cancer Cell 15:220–231

Pal S, Datta K, Mukhopadhyay D (2001) Central role of p53 on regulation of vascular permeability factor/vascular endothelial growth factor (VPF/VEGF) expression in mammary carcinoma. Cancer Res 61:6952–6957

Pan Y, Oprysko PR, Asham AM, Koch CJ, Simon MC (2004) p53 cannot be induced by hypoxia alone but responds to the hypoxic microenvironment. Oncogene 23:4975–4983

Patterson BC, Sang QA (1997) Angiostatin-converting enzyme activities of human matrilysin (MMP-7) and gelatinase B/type IV collagenase (MMP-9). J Biol Chem 272:28823–28825

Pendas AM et al (2004) Diet-induced obesity and reduced skin cancer susceptibility in matrix metalloproteinase 19-deficient mice. Mol Cell Biol 24:5304–5313

Pozzi A, LeVine WF, Gardner HA (2002) Low plasma levels of matrix metalloproteinase 9 permit increased tumor angiogenesis. Oncogene 21:272–281

Rak J, Yu JL (2004) Oncogenes and tumor angiogenesis: the question of vascular "supply" and vascular "demand". Semin Cancer Biol 14:93–104

Rak J et al (2000) Oncogenes and tumor angiogenesis: differential modes of vascular endothelial growth factor up-regulation in ras-transformed epithelial cells and fibroblasts. Cancer Res 60:490–498

Rangaswami H, Bulbule A, Kundu GC (2006) Osteopontin: role in cell signaling and cancer progression. Trends Cell Biol 16:79–87

Ravi R et al (2000) Regulation of tumor angiogenesis by p53-induced degradation of hypoxia-inducible factor 1alpha. Genes Dev 14:34–44

Relf M et al (1997) Expression of the angiogenic factors vascular endothelial cell growth factor, acidic and basic fibroblast growth factor, tumor growth factor beta-1, platelet-derived endothelial cell growth factor, placenta growth factor, and pleiotrophin in human primary breast cancer and its relation to angiogenesis. Cancer Res 57:963–969

Rempe DA, Lelli KM, Vangeison G, Johnson RS, Federoff HJ (2007) In cultured astrocytes, p53 and MDM2 do not alter hypoxia-inducible factor-1alpha function regardless of the presence of DNA damage. J Biol Chem 282:16187–16201

Ribatti D, Nico B, Crivellato E, Roccaro AM, Vacca A (2007) The history of the angiogenic switch concept. Leukemia 21:44–52

Semenza GL (2003) Targeting HIF-1 for cancer therapy. Nat Rev Cancer 3:721–732

Shao J, Washington MK, Saxena R, Sheng H (2007) Heterozygous disruption of the PTEN promotes intestinal neoplasia in APCmin/ +mouse: roles of osteopontin. Carcinogenesis 28:2476–2483

Sherif ZA, Nakai S, Pirollo KF, Rait A, Chang EH (2001) Downmodulation of bFGF-binding protein expression following restoration of p53 function. Cancer Gene Ther 8:771–782

Slack JL, Bornstein P (1994) Transformation by v-src causes transient induction followed by repression of mouse thrombospondin-1. Cell Growth Differ 5:1373–1380

Stambolic V et al (1998) Negative regulation of PKB/Akt-dependent cell survival by the tumor suppressor PTEN. Cell 95:29–39

Stanelle J, Stiewe T, Theseling CC, Peter M, Putzer BM (2002) Gene expression changes in response to E2F1 activation. Nucleic Acids Res 30:1859–1867

Steck PA et al (1997) Identification of a candidate tumour suppressor gene, MMAC1, at chromosome 10q23.3 that is mutated in multiple advanced cancers. Nat Genet 15:356–362

Subbaramaiah K et al (1999) Inhibition of cyclooxygenase-2 gene expression by p53. J Biol Chem 274:10911–10915

Sudhakar A et al (2003) Human tumstatin and human endostatin exhibit distinct antiangiogenic activities mediated by alpha v beta 3 and alpha 5 beta 1 integrins. Proc Natl Acad Sci U S A 100:4766–4771

Sun Y, Wang J, Liu Y, Song X, Zhang Y, Li K, Zhu Y, Zhou Q, You L, Yao C (2005) Results of phase III trial of rh-endostatin (YH-16) in advanced non-small cell lung cancer (NSCLC) patients. J Clin Oncol 23:7138

Takahashi Y, Bucana CD, Cleary KR, Ellis LM (1998) p53, vessel count, and vascular endothelial growth factor expression in human colon cancer. Int J Cancer 79:34–38

Teodoro JG, Parker AE, Zhu X, Green MR (2006) p53-mediated inhibition of angiogenesis through up-regulation of a collagen prolyl hydroxylase. Science 313:968–971

Teodoro JG, Evans SK, Green MR (2007) Inhibition of tumor angiogenesis by p53: a new role for the guardian of the genome. J Mol Med 85:1175–1186

Tikhonenko AT, Black DJ, Linial ML (1996) Viral Myc oncoproteins in infected fibroblasts down-modulate thrombospondin-1, a possible tumor suppressor gene. J Biol Chem 271:30741–30747

Toussaint-Smith E, Donner DB, Roman A (2004) Expression of human papillomavirus type 16 E6 and E7 oncoproteins in primary foreskin keratinocytes is sufficient to alter the expression of angiogenic factors. Oncogene 23:2988–2995

Turk B (2006) Targeting proteases: successes, failures and future prospects. Nat Rev Drug Discov 5:785–799

Ueba T et al (1994) Transcriptional regulation of basic fibroblast growth factor gene by p53 in human glioblastoma and hepatocellular carcinoma cells. Proc Natl Acad Sci U S A 91:9009–9013

Vogelstein B, Kinzler KW (1992) p53 function and dysfunction. Cell 70:523–526

Vogelstein B, Lane D, Levine AJ (2000) Surfing the p53 network. Nature 408:307–310

Vousden KH, Lu X (2002) Live or let die: the cell's response to p53. Nat Rev Cancer 2:594–604

Wang S et al (2003) Prostate-specific deletion of the murine Pten tumor suppressor gene leads to metastatic prostate cancer. Cancer Cell 4:209–221

Watnick RS, Cheng YN, Rangarajan A, Ince TA, Weinberg RA (2003) Ras modulates Myc activity to repress thrombospondin-1 expression and increase tumor angiogenesis. Cancer Cell 3:219–231

Wei CL et al (2006) A global map of p53 transcription-factor binding sites in the human genome. Cell 124:207–219

Weinberg RA (1995) The retinoblastoma protein and cell cycle control. Cell 81:323–330

Wen S et al (2001) PTEN controls tumor-induced angiogenesis. Proc Natl Acad Sci U S A 98:4622–4627

Xia G et al (2006) Expression and significance of vascular endothelial growth factor receptor 2 in bladder cancer. J Urol 175:1245–1252

Yamakuchi M et al (2010) P53-induced microRNA-107 inhibits HIF-1 and tumor angiogenesis. Proc Natl Acad Sci U S A 107:6334–6339

Yee KS, Vousden KH (2005) Complicating the complexity of p53. Carcinogenesis 26:1317–1322

Yu EY, Yu E, Meyer GE, Brawer MK (1997) The relation of p53 protein nuclear accumulation and angiogenesis in human prostatic carcinoma. Prostate Cancer Prostatic Dis 1:39–44

Yu X, Harris SL, Levine AJ (2006) The regulation of exosome secretion: a novel function of the p53 protein. Cancer Res 66:4795–4801

Yuan TL et al (2008) Class 1A PI3K regulates vessel integrity during development and tumorigenesis. Proc Natl Acad Sci U S A 105:9739–9744

Zhong H et al (2000) Modulation of hypoxia-inducible factor 1alpha expression by the epidermal growth factor/phosphatidylinositol 3-kinase/PTEN/AKT/FRAP pathway in human prostate cancer cells: implications for tumor angiogenesis and therapeutics. Cancer Res 60:1541–1545

Zundel W et al (2000) Loss of PTEN facilitates HIF-1-mediated gene expression. Genes Dev 14:391–396

Chapter 9
Inflammatory Mediators in Tumorigenesis and Metastasis

Jeremy Dupaul-Chicoine and Maya Saleh

9.1 Introduction

The intimate link between chronic inflammation and tumorigenesis was first recognized by the 19th century scientist Rudolf Virchow (Balkwill and Mantovani 2001). More than a century later, his initial hypothesis is being explored in greater detail. It is now clear that inflammation is a double-edged sword in cancer: it mediates tumor promotion and progression while activating immunity against the tumor. Collectively, this chapter provides a comprehensive view of the crosstalk between tumors and their microenvironment, specifically the dual role of the immune system in cancer development. We describe the chemokine network and discuss its role in recruiting immune cells to the tumor site and in the homing of tumors to metastatic niches. We follow by presenting the cellular players of the immune system, their pathways and cytokines and their contributions to tumor promotion and dissemination versus tumor immune surveillance. Throughout, we review current immunotherapies and discuss future therapeutic strategies aimed at fighting cancer.

M. Saleh (✉) · J. Dupaul-Chicoine
Department of Biochemistry, McGill University, 3655 William Olser,
Rm 905, Montreal, QC H3G 1Y6, Canada

M. Saleh
Department of Medicine, McGill University, 687 Pine Ave W. Rm A3:09,
Montreal, H3A 1A1, Canada

Department of Microbiology and Immunology, McGill University, 3775 University Street,
Rm 511, Montreal, QC H3A 2B4, Canada

J. Dupaul-Chicoine
e-mail: maya.saleh@mcgill.ca

J. V. Burnier, M. N. Burnier, Jr. (eds.), *Experimental and Clinical Metastasis,*
DOI 10.1007/978-1-4614-3685-0_9,

9.2 Inflammation

Inflammation is a physiological response to the presence of "danger" that is required for host defense. The sensing of "non-self" or "altered self" by the immune system induces the production of cascades of pro-inflammatory cytokines, chemokines and lipid mediators that act synergistically to restore homeostasis. Indeed, physiological levels of inflammation are salutary, however, excessive or chronic inflammation is associated with pathogenesis. It is widely recognized that diseases that exert considerable burden on human health, including cancer, infectious diseases and inflammatory disorders, have both an intrinsic genetic susceptibility component and an extrinsic environmental component (chemical factors, physical factors, infectious agents etc.). The complex interaction between these two interfaces determines the time of disease onset, progression and pathogenic outcome. Inflammation can arise in response to environmental triggers, such as cigarette smoke or infection, or because of a genetic defect, and its contribution to tumorigenesis is paramount (Grivennikov et al. 2010; Mantovani et al. 2008). Chronic infection with Hepatitis B or C virus increases the risk of hepatocellular carcinoma (Sherman 2010); and ulcerative colitis, a form of inflammatory bowel disease, augments the odds of developing gastrointestinal cancer (Clevers 2004). Oncoproteins such as K-RAS and MYC activate pro-inflammatory transcription factors such as NF-κB, STAT3 and AP-1 and contribute to tumorigenesis by promoting a smoldering form of inflammation that presents without clinical manifestations (Grivennikov et al. 2010; Mantovani et al. 2008). The first evidence that an oncogene directly affects inflammation in clinical settings was demonstrated in papillary thyroid carcinoma (PTC). This cancer occurs following rearrangement of the *RET* gene with that of a receptor tyrosine kinase creating the *RET/PTC* oncogene that encodes a constitutively activate tyrosine kinase receptor. This chromosomal rearrangement results in reprogramming of thyrocytes and the expression of pro-inflammatory cytokines, chemokines and factors involved in promoting metastasis (Borrello et al. 2005).

Tumor biopsies are frequently infiltrated with several populations of immune cells including neutrophils, mast cells, natural killer (NK) cells, macrophages, dendritic cells (DCs), myeloid-derived suppressor cells (MDSCs), as well as T and B cells. Although initially recruited to attack the tumor, experimental evidence indicates that these cells are later subverted by the tumor to favor its growth and aggressiveness (Qian and Pollard 2010; DeNardo et al. 2010; Porta et al. 2009). In particular, a subset of macrophages, designated as Tumor-Associated Macrophages (TAMs), are pro-tumorigenic and their level of infiltration in tumor biopsies correlates with poor prognosis. In a mouse model of aggressive breast cancer, mice lacking macrophages have delayed primary tumor growth and are devoid of lung metastasis (Lin et al. 2001). High serum concentrations of pro-inflammatory cytokines and chemokines are associated with poor prognosis. In colorectal cancer, high levels of Interleukin (IL)-6 and soluble gp130 (a chain of the IL-6 receptor) correlate directly with bad prognosis (Sharma et al. 2008) and elevated expression of CXCL8 (IL-8) is linked to the progression of several cancers including hepatocellular carcinoma, prostate and colorectal cancer (Aggarwal and Gehlot 2009). Consistently, single nucleotide polymorphisms (SNP) in several pro-inflammatory cytokine genes are associated with increased probability of developing cancer. Polymorphisms in the gene encoding IL-1β, which lead to increased production of this cytokine, are linked to increased chances of developing *Helicobacter pylori*-induced gastric cancer (Sugimoto et al. 2010). These findings are corroborated by results from transgenic mice showing that over-expression of human IL-1β in the stomach results in spontaneous development of gastric cancer (Tu et al. 2008). Other cytokines involved in gastric cancer include Tumor necrosis factor (TNF)α and the IL-1 receptor antagonist (IL1RN) (Sugimoto et al. 2010). In particular, TNFα is also associated with bad prognosis in melanoma, prostate, breast and pancreatic cancers and both $Tnfr1^{-/-}$ (TNF Receptor1) and $Tnf\alpha^{-/-}$ mice are resistant to tumorigenesis in experimental cancer models (Balkwill 2006). Recently, TNFα antagonists have been used in cancer clinical trials. Infliximab, a monoclonal antibody against TNFα, and etanercept, a soluble TNF receptor, have yielded promising results (Balkwill 2009). Moreover, epidemiologic studies have supported experimental findings and revealed that patients treated prophylactically for 10–15 years with non-steroidal anti-inflammatory drugs (NSAIDs) that target the cyclooxygenase enzymes, COX1 and COX2, have reduced risk of cancer development (Rostom et al. 2007; Harris 2009). Below, we dwell on the dual role of the immune system in promoting versus restricting cancer growth and provide seminal examples from the recent literature that impacted on our understanding of the key role of immunity in this elusive disease.

9.3 Chemokines and Tumorigenesis

9.3.1 The Chemokine Network

To create a suitable microenvironment that supports cell survival, proliferation and growth, tumors recruit inflammatory tumor-promoting cells into their stroma. This is achieved through the use of small chemotactic peptides named chemokines. Indeed, the chemokine network is the major system used to control hematopoietic and non-hematopoietic cell migration and trafficking. It is also critical for cell activation and differentiation, and plays a critical role during organogenesis, embryogenesis and angiogenesis. Chemokines and their receptors are subdivided into 4 different families depending on the cysteine motifs present in the mature chemokine. The four subgroups consist of CC, CXC, XC and CX3C chemokines. CC and CXC chemokines are the most common, consisting of 28 and 17 members, respectively. The CXC subfamily is further subdivided into the Glu-Leu-Arg -positive (ELR+) and ELR- chemokines. The ELR motif precedes the CXC motif and this subdivision will be important later on in the discussion as the ELR+ chemokines are angiogenic whereas the ELR- are angiostatic. The chemokine receptors are G-protein coupled receptors that signal through a wide range of transduction pathways involved in chemotaxis, cell survival and proliferation (Lazennec and Richmond 2010; Mantovani et al. 2010). The chemokine system is very redundant and most chemokines of the CC and CXC subfamilies can interact with several different chemokine receptors. Similarly, one chemokine receptor interacts with more than one ligand. Furthermore, chemokines can be sub-divided into inflammatory and homeostatic factors. The inflammatory chemokines are inducible and are mainly involved in the recruitment of hematopoietic cells. These are critical to induce tissue repair and are therefore important in the context of tumor promotion. The homeostatic chemokines, on the other hand, are constitutively produced and are important for organ development and hematopoiesis. Recently, decoy receptors of the chemokine network have been identified, namely D6, Duffy Antigen Receptor for Chemokines (DARC) and Chemo Centryx ChemoKine Receptor (CCX-CKR). The common link between these 3 decoy receptors is their inability to signal following ligand binding. Thus, their primary function is to neutralize the chemokine response and maintain homeostasis. D6 and DARC are required for the clearance of inflammatory CC chemokines. DARC can also sequester ELR + CXC chemokines. On the other hand, CCX-CKR scavenges homeostatic chemokines (Lazennec and Richmond 2010; Mantovani et al. 2010).

9.3.2 Decoy Chemokine Receptors and Cancer

Because of the significant redundancy in the chemokine network, decoy receptors constitute important regulatory nodes and their role in cancer and metastasis is now emerging. The role of D6 has been investigated in experimental mouse models of colitis-associated colorectal cancer and inflammation-induced skin carcinogenesis. In both cases, *D6*$^{-/-}$ mice are more susceptible to cancer development, mainly due to increased inflammatory chemokines in the tumor microenvironment that lead to greater infiltration of leukocytes (Nibbs et al. 2007; Vetrano et al. 2010). In breast cancer, D6 is negatively correlated with lymph node metastasis; and in a nude mouse xenograft model, transplantation of a breast cancer cell line over-expressing D6 decreases metastatic potential (Wu et al. 2008). DARC also plays a critical role in regulating both primary tumor growth and metastasis. Transgenic mice over-expressing DARC in their endothelial cells are resistant to melanoma formation due to decreased angiogenesis (Horton et al. 2007). Similarly, *DARC*$^{-/-}$ mice present with enhanced prostate cancer because of greater concentrations of angiogenic chemokines (Shen et al. 2006). Interestingly, African-American individuals have a 60 % greater chance of developing prostate cancer, possibly because the majority of the African-American population does not express DARC. Loss of DARC is a result of a genetic selection against infection with *Plasmodium vivax*, one of the agents of malaria (Lentsch 2002). In addition to its function in primary tumors, DARC expression negatively correlates with lymph node metastasis in breast cancer patients (Wang et al. 2006b). DARC controls metastasis partly through its interaction with the membrane-associated protein KAI1. Tumor cells expressing KAI1 interact with DARC on blood vessel endothelial cells leading to senescence of the circulating tumor cell (Bandyopadhyay et al. 2006).

As for DARC, expression of CCX-CKR decreases the odds of lymph node metastasis in breast cancer (Feng et al. 2009). Furthermore, in a multivariate analysis, all three decoy receptors were shown to be associated with relapse-free survival suggesting that loss of these receptors in the tumor microenvironment could be critical for the development of invasive cancer (Zeng et al. 2010).

9.3.3 Chemokines and Homing

Chemokines were initially investigated in the context of metastasis due to their role in mediating cellular homing. Several different chemokines and chemokine receptors have been shown to play a critical role in mediating metastasis. Each tumor has a different migration pattern, which seems to be highly dependent on the set of chemokine receptors that it expresses. One of the best-studied chemokine/chemokine receptor pairs in metastasis is the CXCL12 (Stromal Derived Factor-1 (SDF-1))/CXCR4 pair because of its role in mediating stem cell migration (Teicher and Fricker 2010). Both CXCL12- and CXCR4-deficient mice are embryonic lethal and share a very similar phenotype (Ma et al. 1998). CXCL12 is expressed in the liver, bone, lungs, adrenal glands and lymph nodes and its expression gradient determines attraction of metastatic cells. This is observed in several cancers ranging from hepatocellular carcinoma (Schimanski et al. 2006), prostate (Du et al. 2008), breast (Muller et al. 2001), ovarian (Hall and Korach 2003), thyroid (Hwang et al. 2003) and small cell lung cancers (Burger et al. 2003) to hematological cancers (Javelaud et al. 2007). Interestingly, CXCL12 was recently found to bind to another receptor, CXCR7 (Burns et al. 2006). The exact role of CXCR7 is still controversial, and it seems to play a role both independently and in combination with CXCR4. In some cell-lines it promotes tumor growth and metastasis, while in others it has no effect (Lazennec and Richmond 2010). In both breast and lung cancer cell lines that do not express CXCR4, knockdown of CXCR7 leads to decreased tumor growth (Miao et al. 2007). Consistently, injection of Severe Combined ImmunoDeficiency (SCID) mice with a prostate cancer cell line over-expressing CXCR7 leads to increased tumor growth, presumably through increased angiogenesis (Wang et al. 2008). Conversely, expression of CXCR7 has no effect on the growth of colon carcinoma (CT26) or lung cancer (KEPI) *in vivo* (Meijer et al. 2008). There is strong evidence suggesting that CXCR7 serves as a decoy receptor, which neutralizes both CXCL12 and CXCL11 (Boldajipour et al. 2008; Luker et al. 2010; Naumann et al. 2010). How then does CXCR7 enhance tumorigenesis in some settings? Currently, one hypothesis is that CXCR4 and CXCR7 heterodimerize leading to increased signaling through CXCR4 (Lazennec and Richmond 2010). CXCR7 could also mediate cellular adhesion with endothelial cells (Burns et al. 2006). However, additional experimental evidence is needed to support these hypotheses.

Because of their high metastatic potential, melanomas have been extensively investigated to determine which chemokine/chemokine receptor pairs mediate homing of metastatic cells. Three receptors seem to be major determining factors, namely

CXCR4, CCR7 and CCR9. CXCR4-expressing melanomas tend to home to the liver, the bone marrow (Javelaud et al. 2007) and the lungs (Murakami et al. 2002), whereas CCR7 expression directs to the lymph nodes (Fang et al. 2008) and that of CCR9 to the small intestine (Amersi et al. 2008). In all cases, homing is due to high levels of chemokine expression in secondary sites. In breast cancer, CXCL1 is critical in primary tumor growth and in mediating metastasis to the lungs (Minn et al. 2005), which is in agreement with the phenotype of *Cxcr2*$^{-/-}$ mice that are resistant to lung metastasis (Singh et al. 2009). Another receptor involved in metastasis is CX3CR1. Pancreatic ductal adenocarcinomas have a very unique metastatic pattern, in that they home to intra- and extra-pancreatic nerves, which express the CX3CR1 ligand, CX3CL1 (Marchesi et al. 2008). Surprisingly, in colorectal cancer CX3CL1 has anti-tumorigenic effects (Vitale et al. 2007). CCR6 and CCL20, on the other hand, promote colorectal cancer metastasis to the liver (Rubie et al. 2006), as does CXCR4 (Zeelenberg et al. 2003).

9.3.4 Chemokines and Angiogenesis

Chemokines do more than increase tumor growth and determine metastatic sites. Indeed, several ELR + CXC chemokines, through interaction with their cognate receptors CXCR1 and 2, also play a critical role in angiogenesis. CXCL1, for instance, triggers angiogenesis in colorectal cancer (Wang et al. 2006a) and anti-CXCR2 treatment decreases angiogenesis and tumor growth (Matsuo et al. 2009). In non-small cell lung cancer, up-regulation of CXCL8 and CXCL5 is important for angiogenesis (Yanagawa et al. 2009). Other chemokines, which are not themselves angiogenic, can mediate the recruitment of different cell types to induce angiogenesis. For example, CXCL12 induces angiogenesis through MDSCs in a breast cancer model (Liu et al. 2010), and CCL2 stimulates the recruitment of TAMs to induce angiogenesis in prostate cancer (Loberg et al. 2007).

9.3.5 Immunosuppression Through Chemokines

A new aspect of chemokine tumor biology is the role of chemokines in converting the tumor microenvironment into a tolerogenic state. Recently, CCL21-over-expressing melanomas were shown to induce the formation of a lymphoid-like structure around the tumor. Specifically, CCL21 leads to the recruitment of MDSCs and regulatory T cells (Tregs), which suppress immune-surveillance (Shields et al. 2010). The recruitment of Tregs is also observed in response to high levels of CCL22 (Qin et al. 2009). Similarly, in gastric cancer, CCL17 and CCL22 recruit Tregs leading to immunosuppression (Mizukami et al. 2008).

9.4 The Role of Immune Cells and Immunity in Tumorigenesis

The tumor microenvironment is composed of a dynamic cellular network that shapes tumorigenecity and determines its outcome. In general, transformed epithelial cells form the core of solid tumors and are surrounded by stromal cells including fibroblasts, endothelial cells, pericytes, and immune cells (Pietras and Ostman 2010). Here we focus our discussion on immune cells and examine their complex role in cancer development (Fig. 9.1).

The immune system is divided into innate and adaptive immune systems. Innate immunity provides first line defenses against invading microbial pathogens and endogenous "danger" signals by activating pathways that mediate inflammation and pathogen clearance. It also serves as a sentinel that alerts and primes adaptive immunity, which eliminates any remaining pathogens and builds memory against re-challenge. Specific activation of innate immune responses is orchestrated by evolutionarily conserved germline-encoded "Pattern Recognition Receptors" (PRRs) that discriminate between self and non-self or altered self. PRRs recognize conserved motifs expressed by microbes or exposed by host cells under stress, termed Microbe- and Danger-Associated Molecular Patterns (MAMPs and DAMPs) (Iwasaki and Medzhitov 2010). Various classes of innate immunity recognition systems have been discovered and their function in cancer is discussed below. The innate immune system is composed of several cell types, including granulocytes (neutrophils, eosinophils, basophils), NK cells, macrophages, MDSCs and dendritic cells (DCs) (Murdoch et al. 2008). On the other hand, T and B cells direct specific adaptive immunity. T cells differentiate into CD4+ T cells (or T helper (Th) cells) or CD8+ T cells (or cytotoxic T cells (CTLs)), and the CD4+ lineage is further sub-divided into Th1, Th2, Th17 and Treg sub-lineages. Interestingly, it has been recently demonstrated that lineage fate determination is under epigenetic control and is more plastic than previously estimated (Zhu and Paul 2010; Wei et al. 2009).

The concept of immunosurveillance, or elimination of cancers by immune attack, was, for a long time, under appreciated due to lack of experimental data. The first evidence came from mice deficient in key molecules, such as InterFeroN (IFN)γ or perforin, required for mounting a proper adaptive immune response. These knockout animals were more susceptible to the induction of tumorigenesis (Street et al. 2001). It is now clear that both the innate and adaptive immune systems are involved in immunosurveillance (Dunn et al. 2004). In addition, they exert a pressure on tumor antigenicity, a process termed immune editing, with one of three consequences: elimination (the net outcome of immunosurveillance), equilibrium or escape (Dunn et al. 2004) (Fig. 9.2). Consistently, tumors grown in $Rag2^{-/-}$ (Recombinase Activator Gene) mice, which lack all T and B cells, are more immunogenic when transplanted into WT mice (Shankaran et al. 2001), which suggests that the immunogenicity of a tumor is constantly being sculpted by the immune system. This persistent editing process is conducive to tumor equilibrium or dormancy that precedes malignancy and results in the rise of a tumor's most fit clone. Tumor equilibrium is not necessarily followed by tumor escape; it could lead to elimination or persist indefinitely (Dunn

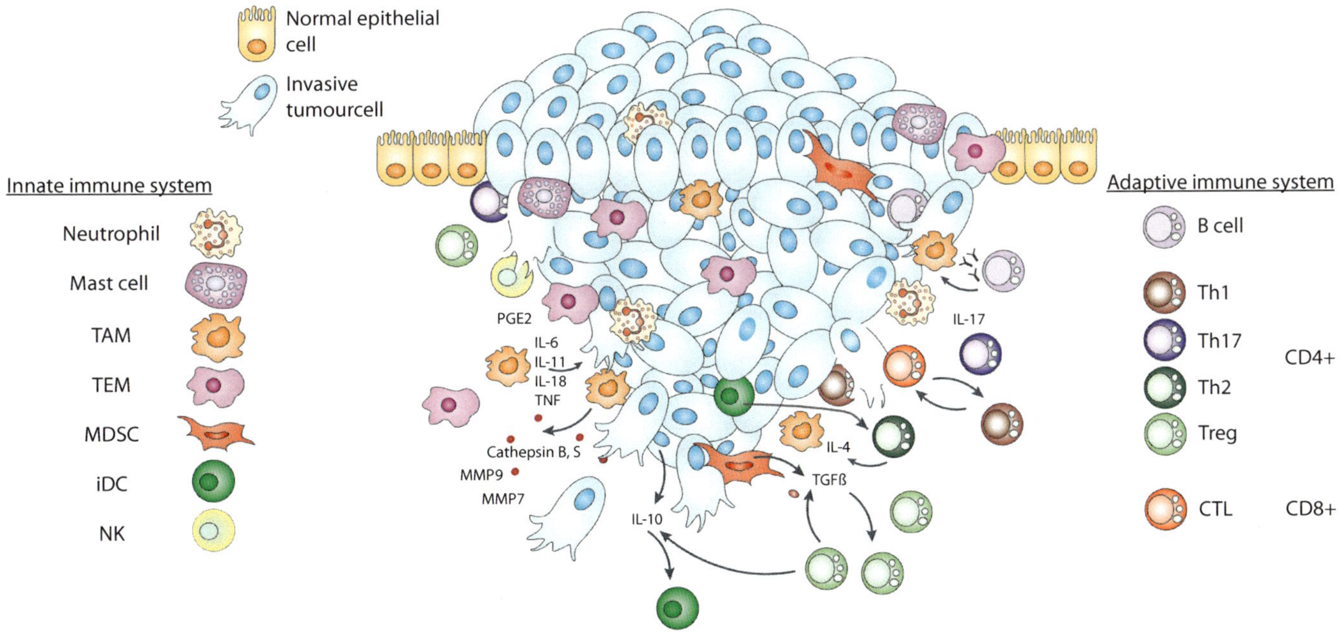

Fig. 9.1 The multifaceted role of the immune system in cancer. The crosstalk between the tumor and the stroma involves several different cell lineages of both the innate and adaptive immune systems. Tumors employ multiple strategies to evade immune surveillance including functional skewing of immune cells from pro-inflammatory into immunosuppressive. The innate and adaptive immune systems are highly plastic in their response against cancer and can play both tumor-promoting and inhibitory functions. (Adapted by permission from Macmillan Publishers Ltd: Joyce, J.A. & Pollard, J.W. Microenvironmental regulation of metastasis. Nat Rev Cancer 9, 239–52 (2009). Copyright 2010.)

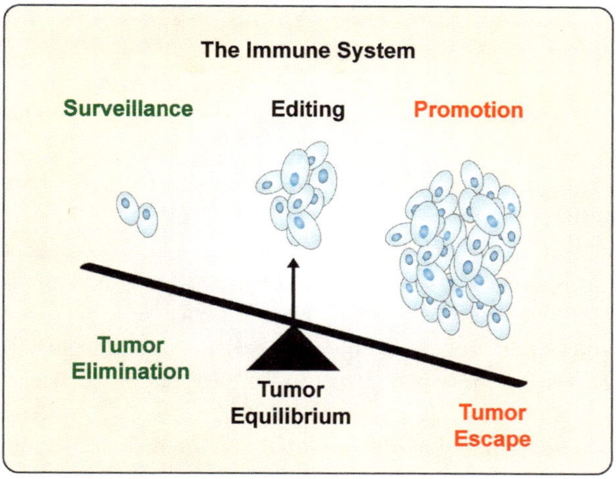

Fig. 9.2 The cancer immunoediting hypothesis. This hypothesis proposes that cancer growth is under constant antigenic pressure, whereby the immune system senses "altered self" or de novo tumor antigens and responds to them by stunting tumor growth and maintaining it in equilibrium. This process can last for years and is often referred to as tumor dormancy. However, this phase is dynamic and the cell growth balance is often tipped towards tumor elimination or escape. The elimination phase is the net result of active immune surveillance, whereas tumor escape results when the microenvironment is successfully modulated by the tumor to accommodate its unrestricted growth. In this case, immune cells promote, rather than curb, tumorigenesis

et al. 2004). For instance, in a model of sarcoma, treatment of mice harboring stable tumors with monoclonal antibodies against CD4 and CD8 or IFNγ led to relapse in tumor growth, indicating that tumor equilibrium is maintained by the immune system (Koebel et al. 2007) Tumor escape is the tumor's most favorable outcome, as it permits its growth without immunological restrictions (Dunn et al. 2004).

9.4.1 Innate Immunity and Promotion of Tumorigenesis

The role of innate immune cells in cancer and metastasis appears to be tissue specific, with both pro-tumorigenic and anti-tumorigenic functions reported in different contexts. NK cells are the exception as they play a universal anti-tumorigenic role. Macrophages are phagocytic cells and have a wide variety of functions from scavenging cellular debris, microbes and apoptotic cells to presenting antigens to T cells. The macrophage lineage is highly plastic but two distinct macrophage types have been described, M1 and M2-type cells. M1 macrophages are involved in clearing pathogens and help mount a Th1 response. They are potent phagocytes and are efficient at producing anti-microbial substances including pro-inflammatory cytokines, anti-microbial peptides and reactive oxygen and nitrogen species. M1 macrophages are often referred to as the classically-activated macrophage type. On the other hand,

M2 or alternatively-activated macrophages prime Th2 responses and are generally immunosuppressive. They are needed for wound healing and are closely related to TAMs (Qian and Pollard 2010; Murdoch et al. 2008). The role of TAMs in tumorigenesis was first demonstrated in a mouse model of breast cancer, where macrophage deficiency reduced breast cancer aggressiveness and metastasis to the lung (Lin et al. 2001). Consistently, depletion of macrophages, either genetically or using clodronate liposomes, decreases tumor growth in several cancer models (Qian and Pollard 2010). TAMs are involved in the angiogenic switch (Lin et al. 2006) and facilitate tumor dissemination by secreting various proteases. More specifically, depletion of cathepsin S and B from macrophages leads to reduced invasiveness (Gocheva et al. 2010). Another subtype of hematopoietic cells related to TAMs is that of Tie2-Expressing Monocytes (TEMs). TEMs specialize in promoting angiogenesis and seem to be recruited to hypoxic areas (De Palma et al. 2005). *Stat6*$^{-/-}$ mice, which are only capable of producing M1-polarized macrophages, are resistant to tumorigenesis and metastasis (Ostrand-Rosenberg et al. 2000), suggesting that in contexts where only M1 macrophages are found, the innate immune system is anti-tumorigenic. On the other hand, SHIP-deficient mice in which macrophage differentiation is skewed towards M2 have increased tumor growth (Rauh et al. 2005). This suggests that macrophages recruited to the tumor site are initially anti-tumorigenic but are reprogrammed into M2 cells by the tumor microenvironment. This has significant therapeutic implications as it suggests that manipulation of macrophage differentiation could induce tumor regression. A famous example to illustrate this is that of Coley's mixed toxin. William Coley had noticed that some patients recovered from sarcomas following infections. Therefore, by developing a cocktail containing bacterial extracts and injecting it into sarcomas, he was able to cure some patients (Coley 1893). A more recent example is the treatment of bladder cancer with Bacillus Calmette-Guérin (BCG), an attenuated form of *Mycobacterium bovis*. This treatment leads to localized inflammation and a Th1 response (Rosevear et al. 2009). Although the exact mechanism is not completely understood, it seems to be largely Toll-Like Receptor (TLR)-dependent (Rakoff-Nahoum and Medzhitov 2009). This approach has been further refined with the use of vaccine adjuvants such as CpG or IL-12 that have been shown to reprogram TAMs reducing their tumor-supporting activities and metastasis (Stout et al. 2009; Vollmer and Krieg 2009). Altogether, these examples provide compelling evidence, which indicate that rewiring of the innate inflammatory response in cancer could lead to immunotherapy. The M1 to M2 switch is believed to be a function of MDSCs. MDSCs are a heterogeneous population of immature myeloid cells and myeloid progenitor cells. Under homeostatic conditions, MDSCs would differentiate into DCs, macrophages and mature granulocytes but under pathological conditions such as in cancer they remain undifferentiated and exert immunosuppressive effects (Gabrilovich and Nagaraj 2009). MDSCs are recruited to the tumor site in response to pro-inflammatory cytokines and lipid mediators including IL-1β[14], IL-6 (Bunt et al. 2007) and ProstaGlandin E2 (PGE2) (Sinha et al. 2007). Once at the tumor site, MDSCs mediate immune suppression through the production of Reactive Oxygen Species (ROS) and peroxynitrite and the modulation of the levels of arginine, an essential amino acid needed for T cell activation (Ostrand-Rosenberg and Sinha 2009).

Similarly to macrophages, neutrophils can be functionally polarized into N1 or N2-types or Tumor-Associated Neutrophils (TANs). Tumor Growth Factor (TGF)β is one of the factors important for the generation of N2 neutrophils (Fridlender et al. 2009). Neutrophils can also contribute to angiogenesis, as demonstrated in a mouse model of pancreatic cancer, through the production of specific proteases such as Matrix MetalloProteinase (MMP) 9 (Nozawa et al. 2006). Interestingly, in a model of ovarian cancer, $Ccr2^{-/-}$ mice that fail to attract TAMs to the tumor site have equivalent tumor growth as compared to wild-type animals due to recruitment of TANs (Pahler et al. 2008). These results have important therapeutic implications since they suggest that depletion of TAMs could potentially lead to a compensatory mechanism involving TANs.

NK cells are cytolytic, non-phagocytic cells that discriminate between self and non-self, or altered-self, through a series of stimulatory and inhibitory receptors (Sutlu and Alici 2009). NK cells play an important role in immunosurveillance and are generally associated with good cancer prognosis (Smyth et al. 2005). However, they are infrequently found in tumors and their receptors are often down-regulated in cancer, inhibiting immunoediting. Transgenic expression of the NKG2D ligand ubiquitously results in decreased immunosurveillance via a mechanism that involves down-regulation of the NKG2D receptor (Oppenheim et al. 2005). Thus, overexpression of an NK activating ligand could lead to inhibition of NK cell cytotoxicity, and tumors often secrete a soluble form of the NK cell receptor ligand to inhibit NK cell function (Nausch and Cerwenka 2008).

DCs are professional Antigen Presenting Cells (APCs) that link innate responses to adaptive immunity (Murdoch et al. 2008). They are critical for priming immunity as well as inducing tolerance to self. One of the tumor's immune escape strategies is to maintain DCs in an immature state (iDCs) through signals such as Vascular Endothelial Growth Factor (VEGF) and IL-10 (Lin et al. 2010). Similar to MDSCs, iDCs are immunosuppressive and favor angiogenesis. They recruit Tregs by producing TGFβ (Ghiringhelli et al. 2005) and promote angiogenesis by undergoing endothelialization (Conejo-Garcia et al. 2004). In a breast cancer model, iDCs were shown to induce a Th2 polarized response and accelerate tumor development (Aspord et al. 2007).

Altogether, these studies illustrate the subversive mechanisms employed by tumors to achieve immunosuppression and ensure survival. As discussed above, immune cells are generally plastic and most can play both pro- and anti-tumorigenic roles. What dictates the outcome of tumor growth is the integration of the cytokine milieu. This knowledge provides a therapeutic strategy to rewire the immune system to mount a response against cancer.

9.4.2 The Adaptive Immune System and Immunosurveillance

Much like innate immunity, the adaptive immune system plays an important role in immunoediting as well as cancer progression. For example, in a mouse model of sarcomas, T and B cell deficiency, such as in *Rag1*$^{-/-}$ or *Rag2*$^{-/-}$ mice, leads to enhanced tumor growth. Moreover, and as mentioned earlier, anti-CD4, -CD8, -IFNγ or -IL-12 antibodies have been shown to break tumor dormancy and induce relapse in tumor growth (Koebel et al. 2007). Indeed, a Th1 (but not Th2) response and CD8+ T cells are associated with good cancer prognosis (DeNardo et al. 2010; Daniel et al. 2005; Sato et al. 2005). The role of Th17 cells in tumorigenesis is more controversial. In a mouse model of melanoma, transfer of Th17 cells was reported to confer protection, presumably through recruitment of DCs and activation of CD8+ T cells (Martin-Orozco et al. 2009). Conversely, others have shown, both in models of melanoma and bladder carcinoma, that *Il-17*$^{-/-}$ mice have decreased tumorigenesis compared to wild-type animals (Wang et al. 2009). Clearly, further experiments are needed to clarify the role of Th17 cells in cancer. In contrast, there is more of an accord as to the role of Tregs in tumorigenesis. In a variety of cancer models including breast cancer, renal cell carcinoma and non-small cell lung cancer, Tregs were shown to be tumor promoting (DeNardo et al. 2010). They modulate the tumor microenvironment by producing immunosuppressive cytokines such as IL-10 and TGFβ (Strauss et al. 2007) and are thought to be directly cytotoxic to CD8+ T cells and NK cells through a mechanism involving granzyme B and perforin (Cao et al. 2007).

The crosstalk between innate and adaptive immunity in cancer is bidirectional. Indeed, it has been recently demonstrated that adaptive immune cells modulate cancer progression through a feedback mechanism that involves further stimulation of innate immune responses and the consequent instatement of chronic inflammation. In a mouse model of breast cancer, CD4+ T cells were shown to be critical for M2 cell polarization and metastasis to the lung through the production of IL-4 (DeNardo et al. 2009). IL-4 is also needed for the up-regulation of cathepsin B and S in TAMs, factors essential for angiogenesis and tumor dissemination (Gocheva et al. 2010). B cells and humoral immunity also regulate innate immunity through the secretion of immunoglobulins. In a transgenic model of squamous cell carcinoma, *Rag1*$^{-/-}$ mice but not *CD4*$^{-/-}$ or *CD8*$^{-/-}$ mice were resistant to tumorigenesis. Transfer of B cells or serum from wild-type mice into *Rag1*$^{-/-}$ mice restored skin cancer susceptibility (Visser et al. 2005). In this context, B cells regulated innate immunity through activating Fcgamma Receptors (FcγRs) on resident and recruited myeloid cells (Andreu et al. 2010). These studies caution on the use of antibodies to treat cancer as it would potentially induce chronic inflammation that promotes de novo carcinogenesis. B cells were also implicated in a model of castration-resistant metastatic carcinoma, through the production of lymphotoxin beta, a TNF related cytokine (Ammirante et al. 2010). Therefore, the intricate crosstalk within the immune system increases the complexity of the understanding of the immune control of tumorigenesis, and dissection of these interactions is hoped to provide an advance to tailor personalized cancer and metastasis treatments.

9.5 Master Molecular Orchestrators of Inflammation in Cancer

9.5.1 Toll-Like Receptors and Nod-Like Receptors

The innate immune system is equipped with several PRRs, which could be grouped into three classes: secreted, transmembrane and cytosolic receptors. Ficolins, collectins and pentrataxins are secreted receptors useful for opsonization and activation of phagocytosis. Transmembrane PRRs include TLRs and lectins that are expressed on the cell surface or on endosomes (Fig. 9.3). The cytosolic class of PRRs encompasses Nod-like receptors (NLRs) and Retinoic acid-Inducible Gene-I (RIG-I)-like receptors (Iwasaki and Medzhitov 2010). Of these, TLRs and NLRs have been the most studied in the context of cancer. A spectrum of MAMPs is recognized by TLRs; TLR4 recognizes lipopolysaccharide, TLR2 heterodimerizes with both TLR1 or TLR6 and senses lipoteichoic acid and peptidoglycan (PGN), TLR5 recognizes flagellin and TLR11 profilin. These TLRs are expressed on the plasma membrane, whereas TLR3, 7 and 9 are found on endolysosomes and recognize double stranded RNA, single stranded RNA and CpG DNA, respectively (Rakoff-Nahoum and Medzhitov 2009). TLRs also sense DAMPs released from necrotic cells such as the High-Mobility Group Box 1 protein (Branco-Madeira and Lambrecht 2010), or from carcinomas such as the extracellular matrix proteoglycan versican (Kim et al. 2009). Following ligand sensing by TLRs, the activating signal is generally transduced via the common adaptor molecule Myeloid Differentiation primary response gene 88 (MyD88), except for TLR3 that signals through TRIF. Eventually, the TLR signal converges on master transcription factors, predominantly NF-κB, IFN-Response Factors and AP-1 that induce pro-inflammatory and pro-survival transcription programs. TLRs play a central role in the maintenance of tissue homeostasis, recruitment of inflammatory cells to the site of injury and priming of adaptive immunity (Rakoff-Nahoum and Medzhitov 2009). Their crucial role in tumorigenesis was investigated mainly using *MyD88*$^{-/-}$ mice. In a model of spontaneous intestinal cancer, *MyD88*$^{-/-}$ mice were significantly more resistant to the development of polyps compared to wild-type animals. Several factors involved in tumor growth were down-regulated in the absence of MyD88 including COX2 and MMP7 (Rakoff-Nahoum and Medzhitov 2007). In carcinogen-induced cancer models such as DiEthyl Nitrosamine (DEN)-induced hepatocellular carcinoma or 7,12-DiMethylBenz (a) Anthracene (DMBA)-induced skin cancer, MyD88-deficiency also resulted in resistance to tumor formation (Naugler et al. 2007; Swann et al. 2008). Similarly, *MyD88*$^{-/-}$ mice were less susceptible to the formation of sarcomas (Swann et al. 2008). It is noteworthy that MyD88 functions not only downstream of TLRs, but

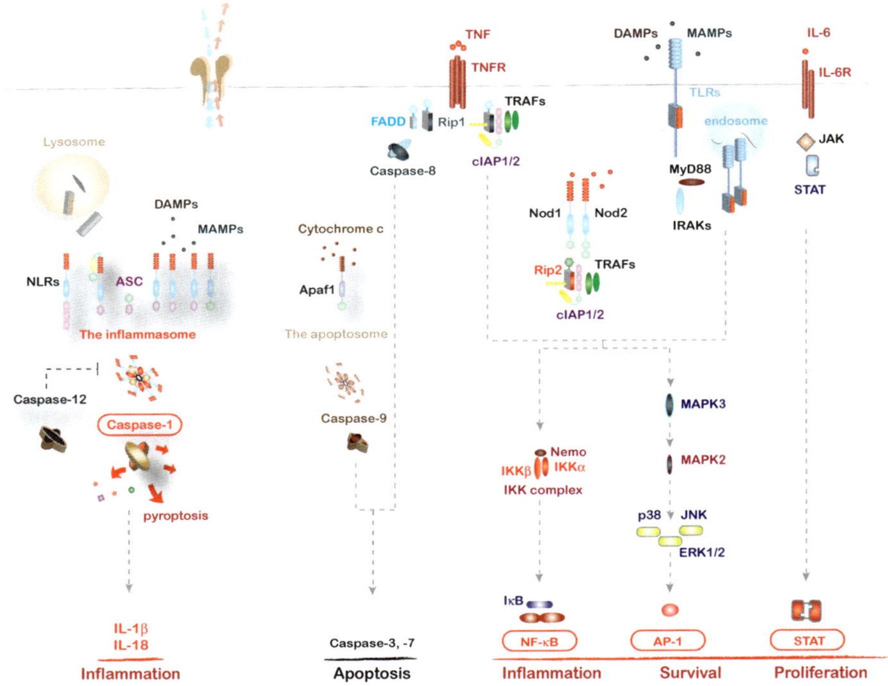

Fig. 9.3 Master regulators of inflammation, cell survival and cell death. Innate immune cells sense the presence of danger (MAMPs and DAMPs) through evolutionarily conserved receptors termed PRRs (TLRs and NLRs are shown) that trigger inflammation by converging on central proteases and transcription factors (red rectangles). TLRs and some NLRs activate the NF-κB and MAPK pathways leading to the production of cytokine, chemokine and lipid mediator cascades. Other NLRs assemble "inflammasomes" that recruit and activate caspase-1, which cleaves IL-1β and IL-18 into their mature active cytokine forms. Inflammation and cell death are often intertwined. Excessive caspase-1 activation leads to an inflammatory form of cell death termed pyroptosis, and TNFα can induce both inflammation and survival or apoptosis. The MAPK pathways that converge on the AP-1 family of transcription factors are also involved in determining cell fate in inflammatory contexts. IL-6 and IL-11 bind to their cognate receptors on the cell surface and activate the JAK-STAT3 pathway that controls cell survival and proliferation

is additionally the adaptor of the IL-1 and IL-18 receptors (Rakoff-Nahoum and Medzhitov 2009). Therefore, the phenotype of $MyD88^{-/-}$ mice in some instances is independent of TLR function.

NLRs, cytosolic PRRs, are further grouped into 5 different sub-families: NLRA (CIITA), NLRB (NAIP), NLRC (including NOD1/2 and IPAF), NLRP (NALP) and NLRX (NOD9) (Ting et al. 2008). These proteins are characterized by an N-terminal CAspase-Recruitment Domain (CARD) or PYrin Domain (PYD), involved in homotypic protein-protein interactions, a central Nucleotide-binding and Oligomerization Domain (NOD) and a C-terminal Leucine Rich Repeat (LRR) domain that recognizes the ligand. The LRR domain is believed to auto-repress NLR proteins in the absence of their cognate ligands. NOD1 and NOD2 recognize PGN derivatives, namely meso-DiAminoPimelic acid (DAP) and Muramyl DiPeptide (MDP), respectively, and elicit inflammation by oligomerizing, through CARD-CARD interactions, with the Receptor-Interacting Protein 2 (RIP2), which engages the MAPK and NF-κB pathways (Geddes et al. 2009) (Fig. 9.3). NLRPs are sensors of danger and are thus activated by a wide variety of stress signals. For example, NLRP3 is activated by various microbial molecules as well as by particulate matter including monosodium urate crystals found in joints of gout patients, irritants like asbestos and silica and protein aggregates such as amyloid beta. Once activated, NLRPs associate with the adaptor molecule Apoptosis -associated Speck-like protein containing a CARD (ASC) and recruit and activate the inflammatory caspase, caspase-1, to form a macromolecular complex dubbed the "inflammasome" (Schroder and Tschopp 2010) (Fig. 9.3). Inflammatory caspases include caspase-1, -4 -5 and -12 in humans and caspases-1, -11 and -12 in mice. Caspase-1 is the prototypical inflammatory caspase that cleaves pro-IL-1β and pro-IL-18 into their mature biologically active cytokine forms. Caspases-5 and -11 are recruited to select inflammasomes and act as co-activators of caspase-1 (Mc Intire et al. 2009). On the other hand, caspase-12 is an inhibitor of the inflammasome, as well as the NF-κB pathway, and its expression has been linked to severe sepsis in the clinic (Saleh et al. 2006; Saleh et al. 2004). The role of the inflammasome in tissue repair and tumorigenesis has been recently investigated. In colitis and colitis-associated colorectal cancer, the NLRP3 inflammasome has been shown to be protective. A recent report has identified SNPs in a regulatory region downstream of the human *NLRP3* gene, which were found to be associated with Crohn's disease susceptibility in individuals of European descent. SNPs in this region result in decreased NLRP3 expression and dampened IL-1 family cytokine production (Villani et al. 2009). Of these cytokines, IL-18 is the most relevant as it contributes to intestinal epithelial cell regeneration as well as to chronic inflammation in inflammatory bowel disease. In response to Dextran Sulfate Sodium (DSS)-induced injury, deficiency in IL-18, IL-18 Receptor (IL-18R) or the IL-18R adaptor MyD88 results in severe colitis (Pizarro et al. 1999; Reuter and Pizarro 2004; Salcedo et al. 2010; Sivakumar et al. 2002; Takagi et al. 2003). On the other hand, Autophagy-related protein 16-L1 (ATG16L1), which is implicated in Crohn's disease, negatively regulates the inflammasome, and mice that lack ATG16L1 in hematopoietic cells hyper-produce IL-1β and IL-18 and are susceptible to DSS colitis (Saitoh et al. 2008). Thus, it appears that IL-18 exerts a dual role in intestinal homeostasis and colitis. Early in the mucosal immune response, its expression by intestinal epithelial cells and lamina propria mononuclear cells mediates a cytoprotective role but under chronic inflammation its excessive production results in deleterious effects (Pizarro et al. 1999; Siegmund 2010). Consistently, others and we have recently demonstrated that the inflammasome is required for intestinal epithelial cell regeneration and tissue repair following injury (Dupaul-Chicoine et al. 2010; Zaki et al. 2010). Caspase-1 deficient mice are extremely susceptible to DSS-induced injury of the intestinal mucosa, succumbing very early on compared to wild-type animals. This phenotype is primarily ascribed to lack of IL-18 production by the intestinal epithelium in *Casp1*$^{-/-}$ mice, as it is completely reversed by exogenous administration of this cytokine (Dupaul-Chicoine et al. 2010; Zaki et al. 2010). In conjunction with the pro-carcinogen AzOxyMethane (AOM), chronic administration of DSS promotes tumorigenesis in the colon, and deficiency in the inflammasome pathway has been shown to result in enhanced tumorigenesis, presumably promoted by exaggerated tissue damage and colitis (Salcedo et al. 2010; Allen et al. 2010). Interestingly, we have recently demonstrated that modulation of caspase-1 function by caspase-12 is necessary for immune tolerance in the gut. *Casp12*$^{-/-}$ mice, in which the inflammasome is derepressed, are resistant to acute colitis but are highly susceptible to AOM-DSS-induced colorectal cancer due to excessive tissue repair and enhanced inflammatory response (Dupaul-Chicoine et al. 2010). Excessive inflammasome activation is also associated with metastatic melanomas, *in vitro* chemotaxis of macrophages and angiogenesis (Okamoto et al. 2010). Moreover, the NLRP3 inflammasome bridges innate to adaptive immunity through DCs production and is essential for priming CD8+ T cells and mounting immunity against dying tumor cells in response to chemotherapy (Ghiringhelli et al. 2009).

9.5.2 Nuclear Factor-Kappa-Light-Chain-Enhancer of Activated B Cells (Nf-κB)

NF-κB is a central regulator of inflammation. TLRs, NLRs and some cytokine receptors, including the TNFR1 and IL1R1/IL-18R, converge on NF-κB to trigger inflammation (Fig. 9.3). NF-κB is sequestered in the cytosol by IκB inhibitory proteins and translocates to the nucleus in response to phosphorylation, consequent ubiquitination and proteosomal degradation of IκB. IκB phosphorylation is executed by the central IκB Kinase (IKK) complex, which consists of two kinase subunits, IKKα and IKKβ, and a regulatory subunit NEMO (IKKγ). NF-κB plays a central role in tumorigenesis, primarily because of its functions in inflammation (transcriptional control of COX-2, IL-6, and TNF) and cell survival pathways (Bcl-Xl, cIAP2, cFLIP) (Bollrath and Greten 2009; Grivennikov and Karin 2010). Using tissue specific *Ikkb*$^{-/-}$ mice, Greten et al. investigated colitis-associated colorectal cancer and demonstrated a requirement for NF-κB activation, in both the myeloid and epithelial compartments, in tumor promotion; NF-κB induced inflammation in myeloid cells and inhibited apoptosis of intestinal epithelial cells (Greten et al. 2004). Similarly, deletion of *Ikkb* from the myeloid compartment led to diminished tumor growth in a cigarette-induced lung cancer model (Takahashi et al. 2010). In the DEN model of hepatocellular carcinoma, compensatory proliferation in response to DEN-induced hepatocyte cell death is NF-κB-dependent. Accordingly, deletion of *Ikkb* in both hepatocytes and Kupffer cells resulted in decreased tumorigenesis (Maeda et al. 2005), and blockade of the NF-κB pathway through inducible expression of an IκBα super-repressor transgene inhibited hepatocellular carcinoma in *Mdr2*$^{-/-}$ (Multi-Drug Resistance) mice (Pikarsky et al. 2004).

Tumor necrosis factor or TNF is an NF-κB target, and as its name implies, was initially thought to induce tumor cell death. This was subsequently refuted when *Tnfα*$^{-/-}$ mice were generated and found to be resistant to skin cancer (Moore et al. 1999). This paradigm-shifting paper demonstrated that expression of pro-inflammatory cytokines promotes tumor growth. TNFα signals through TNFR1 or TNFR2 to induce one of two opposite cell fates: survival and inflammation versus cell death. The extent of NF-κB activation downstream of TNF determines the outcome (Balkwill 2009). The pro-tumorigenic activity of TNFα is mediated by TNFR1, but not TNFR2, as *Tnfr1*$^{-/-}$mice phenocopy *Tnfα*$^{-/-}$ mice (Arnott et al. 2004). In addition, reconstitution of wild-type mice with bone marrow from *Tnfr1*$^{-/-}$ mice markedly reduced the number and size of tumors in the AOM-DSS model of colorectal cancer (Popivanova et al. 2008). TNF-α is also required for the development of lung and liver metastasis (Kitakata et al. 2002; Tomita et al. 2004).

COX2 is another NF-κB target that is key in tumor promotion. As mentioned previously, the impact of COX2 in colorectal cancer is undeniable, as prophylactic treatment with NSAIDs decreases colorectal cancer risk (Rostom et al. 2007). COX1 and COX2 convert arachidonic acid into the pro-inflammatory lipid mediators, prostaglandins, prostacyclins and thrombaxane. One of the major metabolites produced by COX2 is PGE2, which plays an important role in tumor survival, growth and invasion (Lee et al. 2008). COX2-deficiency or inhibition with pharmacological agents decreases tumor growth in models of skin (Tiano et al. 2002), breast (Howe et al. 2005) and lung cancer (Stolina et al. 2000). Interestingly, a recent meta-analysis has suggested that NSAIDs have a wider breadth on cancers in addition to colon cancer, reducing the relative risk of breast, lung and prostate cancers (Harris 2009).

In addition to its role in inflammation and survival, the NF-κB pathway regulates macrophage polarization, response to hypoxia, angiogenesis and metastasis. Co-culture of macrophages with an ovarian cancer cell-line known to induce M2 polarization failed to switch NF-κB-deficient macrophages from M1 to M2. This was also reproduced *in vivo* and the decreased tumor growth was dependent on IL-12 and the recruitment of NK cells (Hagemann et al. 2008). The role of NF-κB in metastasis is partly mediated by TNFα and involves the stabilization of SNAIL, a transcription factor required for epithelial-mesenchymal transition (EMT) and invasiveness (Wu et al. 2009). Interestingly, the role of the NF-κB pathway in cancer is not confined to NF-κB's transcriptional function. Indeed, it has been recently demonstrated that nuclear IKKα controls metastasis, independently of NF-κB, through epigenetic control of Maspin expression (Luo et al. 2007).

9.5.3 *Janus Kinase-Signal Transducer and Activator of Transcription (JAK-STAT)*

A number of cytokines employ the JAK-STAT pathway to elicit inflammation. Binding of a cytokine to its cognate receptor leads to the recruitment of JAK, which phosphorylates the cytoplasmic tail of the receptor. This initial phosphorylation step allows for the recruitment of STAT and its subsequent phosphorylation by JAK. Phosphorylated STATs dimerize and translocate to the nucleus to activate transcription (Li 2008) (Fig. 9.3). In cancer research, a particular attention has been paid to the role of IL-6, an NF-κB target, and STAT3. The IL-6 receptor is heterodimeric and consists of two chains, gp80 and gp130. IL-6 binds to gp80 and signals through gp130. Activating somatic mutations are often found in *GP130* in hepatocellular adenomas, delineating the critical function of this pathway in cancer development (Rebouissou et al. 2009). This is supported by resistance of $STAT3^{-/-}$ mice to experimental induction of cancer and metastasis (He et al. 2010; Maeda et al. 2009). In AOM-induced colorectal cancer, enterocyte-specific deletion of *Stat3* or full deletion of *Il-6* diminishes tumorigenesis (Grivennikov et al. 2009). STAT3 was also shown to be required in a model of spontaneous intestinal tumorigenesis (Musteanu et al. 2010). Altogether, these results portray the tight link between NF-κB and STAT3 in cancer, whereby IL-6, produced by NF-κB in myeloid cells, induces the proliferation of tumor epithelial cells in a STAT3-dependent manner. Similar to IL-6, IL-11 also signals through gp130, while binding to IL-11Rα determines the specificity. Constitutive activation of gp130 induces spontaneous development of gastric carcinoma (Jenkins et al. 2005; Tebbutt et al. 2002). Interestingly, in this model, IL-11 is the key cytokine promoting cancer (Ernst et al. 2008).

9.5.4 Activating Protein-1 (AP-1)

AP-1 is a dimeric transcription factor composed predominantly of members of the Fos (FOS, FOSB, FRA1 and FRA2) and Jun (JUN, JUNB and JUND) families, but also ATF2 or MAF, and is activated downstream of the MAPK cascades (Lopez-Bergami et al. 2010; Shaulian 2010) (Fig. 9.3). AP-1 is highly up-regulated in response to stress such as UVB and was initially investigated in the context of skin cancer. C-Jun mediates tumorigenesis in the skin (Zenz et al. 2003) and intestine (Nateri et al. 2005), but appears not to be involved in colitis-associated colorectal cancer (Hasselblatt et al. 2008). Another important protein in the AP-1 complex is JunB. This factor is needed for myeloid cell homeostasis, as its myeloid-specific deletion resulted in a myeloproliferative disease similar to myeloid leukemia (Passegue et al. 2001). Consistently, epigenetic silencing of JunB is observed in patients with chronic myeloid leukemia (Yang et al. 2003) and JunB is transcriptionally repressed in acute myeloid leukemia (Steidl et al. 2006). Similar to Jun, c-Fos controls tumorigenesis in the skin, and c-Fos-deficient mice are resistant to the induction of papillomas (Saez et al. 1995). Conversely, overexpression of c-Fos induces apoptosis, which is linked to reduced tumorigenesis, in a model of hepatocellular carcinoma (Mikula et al. 2003). Taken together, these studies demonstrate that tissue-specificity of each of these factors determines their effects on tumor growth. In humans, Jun and Fos overexpression is often observed in cancer and generally correlates with poor prognosis (Lopez-Bergami et al. 2010). The complexity of the role of AP-1 in cancer is probably due to the diversity of its dimerization possibilities as well as the breadth of cellular processes it governs.

9.6 Summary

The link between inflammation and cancer has been firmly established in the last decade and what has recently emerged is that inflammatory mediators play an important part throughout the process of tumorigenesis. Chemokines are tightly linked to homing of tumors to secondary sites but they also have a role in promoting angiogenesis and immunosuppression. Furthermore, the plasticity of the immune response in the tumor microenvironment has been demonstrated. Both axes of the immune system have the ability to protect the host and to promote tumor growth. Understanding the impact of the inflammatory milieu and how it induces the polarization of different cell lineages will have important therapeutic consequences. Finally, several transcription factors have an impact on regulating inflammation and by the same token tumor growth. The role of each pathway is tissue-specific, which underlines the complexity involved in tumorigenesis. Overall, each cancer is unique and understanding the regulatory intricacies of each pathway could lead to important pharmacological discoveries.

References

Aggarwal BB, Gehlot P (2009) Inflammation and cancer: how friendly is the relationship for cancer patients? Curr Opin Pharmacol 9:351–369. doi:S1471-4892(09)00090-3 [pii] 10.1016/j.coph.2009.06.020

Allen IC et al (2010) The NLRP3 inflammasome functions as a negative regulator of tumorigenesis during colitis-associated cancer. J Exp Med 207:1045–1056. doi:jem.20100050 [pii] 10.1084/jem.20100050

Amersi FF et al (2008) Activation of CCR9/CCL25 in cutaneous melanoma mediates preferential metastasis to the small intestine. Clin Cancer Res 14:638–645. doi:14/3/638 [pii] 10.1158/1078-0432.CCR-07-2025

Ammirante M, Luo JL, Grivennikov S, Nedospasov S, Karin M (2010) B-cell-derived lymphotoxin promotes castration-resistant prostate cancer. Nature 464:302–305. doi:nature08782 [pii] 10.1038/nature08782

Andreu P et al (2010) FcRgamma activation regulates inflammation-associated squamous carcinogenesis. Cancer Cell 17:121–134. doi:S1535-6108(09)00431-0 [pii] 10.1016/j.ccr.2009.12.019

Arnott CH et al (2004) Expression of both TNF-alpha receptor subtypes is essential for optimal skin tumour development. Oncogene 23:1902–1910. doi:10.1038/sj.onc.1207317 1207317 [pii]

Aspord C et al (2007) Breast cancer instructs dendritic cells to prime interleukin 13-secreting CD4+ T cells that facilitate tumor development. J Exp Med 204:1037–1047. doi:jem.20061120 [pii] 10.1084/jem.20061120

Balkwill F (2006) TNF-alpha in promotion and progression of cancer. Cancer Metastasis Rev 25:409–416. doi:10.1007/s10555-006-9005-3

Balkwill F (2009) Tumour necrosis factor and cancer. Nat Rev Cancer 9:361–371. doi:nrc2628 [pii] 10.1038/nrc2628

Balkwill F, Mantovani A (2001) Inflammation and cancer: back to Virchow? Lancet 357:539–545
Bandyopadhyay S et al (2006) Interaction of KAI1 on tumor cells with DARC on vascular endothelium leads to metastasis suppression. Nature medicine 12:933–938. doi:nm1444 [pii] 10.1038/nm1444
Boldajipour B et al (2008) Control of chemokine-guided cell migration by ligand sequestration. Cell 132:463–473. doi:S0092-8674(08)00055-X [pii] 10.1016/j.cell.2007.12.034
Bollrath J, Greten FR (2009) IKK/NF-kappaB and STAT3 pathways: central signalling hubs in inflammation-mediated tumour promotion and metastasis. EMBO Rep 10:1314–1319. doi:embor2009243 [pii] 10.1038/embor.2009.243
Borrello MG et al (2005) Induction of a proinflammatory program in normal human thyrocytes by the RET/PTC1 oncogene. Proc Natl Acad Sci U S A 102:14825–14830. doi:0503039102 [pii] 10.1073/pnas.0503039102
Branco-Madeira F, Lambrecht BN (2010) High mobility group box-1 recognition: the beginning of a RAGEless era? EMBO Mol Med 2:193–195. doi:10.1002/emmm.201000077
Bunt SK et al (2007) Reduced inflammation in the tumor microenvironment delays the accumulation of myeloid-derived suppressor cells and limits tumor progression. Cancer Res 67:10019–10026. doi:67/20/10019 [pii] 10.1158/0008-5472.CAN-07-2354
Burger M et al (2003) Functional expression of CXCR4 (CD184) on small-cell lung cancer cells mediates migration, integrin activation, and adhesion to stromal cells. Oncogene 22:8093–8101. doi:10.1038/sj.onc.1207097 1207097 [pii]
Burns JM et al (2006) A novel chemokine receptor for SDF-1 and I-TAC involved in cell survival, cell adhesion, and tumor development. J Exp Med 203:2201–2213. doi:jem.20052144 [pii] 10.1084/jem.20052144
Cao X et al (2007) Granzyme B and perforin are important for regulatory T cell-mediated suppression of tumor clearance. Immunity 27:635–646. doi:S1074-7613(07)00444-X [pii] 10.1016/j.immuni.2007.08.014
Clevers H (2004) At the crossroads of inflammation and cancer. Cell 118:671–674
Coley WB (1893) The treatment of malignant tumors by repeated inoculations of erysipelas: with a report of ten original cases. Am J Med Sci 105:487–511
Conejo-Garcia JR et al (2004) Tumor-infiltrating dendritic cell precursors recruited by a beta-defensin contribute to vasculogenesis under the influence of Vegf-A. Nat Med 10:950–958. doi:10.1038/nm1097 nm1097 [pii]
Daniel D et al (2005) CD4+ T cell-mediated antigen-specific immunotherapy in a mouse model of cervical cancer. Cancer Res 65:2018–2025. doi:65/5/2018 [pii] 10.1158/0008-5472.CAN-04-3444
De Palma M et al (2005) Tie2 identifies a hematopoietic lineage of proangiogenic monocytes required for tumor vessel formation and a mesenchymal population of pericyte progenitors. Cancer Cell 8:211–226. doi:S1535-6108(05)00260-6 [pii] 10.1016/j.ccr.2005.08.002
de Visser KE, Korets LV, Coussens LM (2005) De novo carcinogenesis promoted by chronic inflammation is B lymphocyte dependent. Cancer Cell 7:411–423. doi:S1535-6108(05)00125-X [pii] 10.1016/j.ccr.2005.04.014
DeNardo DG et al (2009) CD4(+) T cells regulate pulmonary metastasis of mammary carcinomas by enhancing protumor properties of macrophages. Cancer Cell 16:91–102. doi:S1535-6108(09)00216-5 [pii] 10.1016/j.ccr.2009.06.018
DeNardo DG, Andreu P, Coussens LM (2010) Interactions between lymphocytes and myeloid cells regulate pro- versus anti-tumor immunity. Cancer Metastasis Rev 29:309–316. doi:10.1007/s10555-010-9223-6
Du YF, Shi Y, Xing YF, Zeng FQ (2008) Establishment of CXCR4-small interfering RNA retrovirus vector driven by human prostate-specific antigen promoter and its biological effects on prostate cancer in vitro and in vivo. J Cancer Res Clin Oncol 134:1255–1264. doi:10.1007/s00432-008-0394-2

Dunn GP, Old LJ, Schreiber RD (2004) The immunobiology of cancer immunosurveillance and immunoediting. Immunity 21:137–148. doi:10.1016/j.immuni.2004.07.017 S1074761304002092 [pii]

Dupaul-Chicoine J et al (2010) Control of intestinal homeostasis, colitis, and colitis-associated colorectal cancer by the inflammatory caspases. Immunity 32:367–378. doi:S1074-7613(10)00082-8 [pii] 10.1016/j.immuni.2010.02.012

Ernst M et al (2008) STAT3 and STAT1 mediate IL-11-dependent and inflammation-associated gastric tumorigenesis in gp130 receptor mutant mice. J Clin Invest 118:1727–1738. doi:10.1172/JCI34944

Fang L, Lee VC, Cha E, Zhang H, Hwang ST (2008) CCR7 regulates B16 murine melanoma cell tumorigenesis in skin. J Leukoc Biol 84:965–972. doi:jlb.1107776 [pii] 10.1189/jlb.1107776

Feng LY, Ou ZL, Wu FY, Shen ZZ, Shao ZM (2009) Involvement of a novel chemokine decoy receptor CCX-CKR in breast cancer growth, metastasis and patient survival. Clin Cancer Res 15:2962–2970. doi:1078-0432.CCR-08-2495 [pii] 10.1158/1078-0432.CCR-08-2495

Fridlender ZG et al (2009) Polarization of tumor-associated neutrophil phenotype by TGF-beta: "N1" versus "N2" TAN. Cancer Cell 16:183–194. doi:S1535-6108(09)00215-3 [pii] 10.1016/j.ccr.2009.06.017

Gabrilovich DI, Nagaraj S (2009) Myeloid-derived suppressor cells as regulators of the immune system. Nature reviews 9:162–174. doi:nri2506 [pii] 10.1038/nri2506

Geddes K, Magalhaes JG, Girardin SE (2009) Unleashing the therapeutic potential of NOD-like receptors. Nat Rev Drug Discov 8:465–479. doi:nrd2783 [pii] 10.1038/nrd2783

Ghiringhelli F et al (2005) Tumor cells convert immature myeloid dendritic cells into TGF-beta-secreting cells inducing CD4+CD25+ regulatory T cell proliferation. J Exp Med 202:919–929. doi:jem.20050463 [pii] 10.1084/jem.20050463

Ghiringhelli F et al (2009) Activation of the NLRP3 inflammasome in dendritic cells induces IL-1beta-dependent adaptive immunity against tumors. Nat Med 15:1170–1178. doi:nm.2028 [pii] 10.1038/nm.2028

Gocheva V et al (2010) IL-4 induces cathepsin protease activity in tumor-associated macrophages to promote cancer growth and invasion. Genes Dev 24:241–255. doi:gad.1874010 [pii] 10.1101/gad.1874010

Greten FR et al (2004) IKKbeta links inflammation and tumorigenesis in a mouse model of colitis-associated cancer. Cell 118:285–296. doi:10.1016/j.cell.2004.07.013 S0092867404006713 [pii]

Grivennikov SI, Karin M (2010) Dangerous liaisons: STAT3 and NF-kappaB collaboration and crosstalk in cancer. Cytokine Growth Factor Rev 21:11–19. doi:S1359-6101(09)00112-9 [pii] 10.1016/j.cytogfr.2009.11.005

Grivennikov S et al (2009) IL-6 and Stat3 are required for survival of intestinal epithelial cells and development of colitis-associated cancer. Cancer Cell 15:103–113. doi:S1535-6108(09)00002-6 [pii] 10.1016/j.ccr.2009.01.001

Grivennikov S I, Greten F R, Karin M (2010) Immunity, inflammation, and cancer. Cell 140:883–899. doi:S0092-8674(10)00060-7 [pii] 10.1016/j.cell.2010.01.025

Hagemann T et al (2008) "Re-educating" tumor-associated macrophages by targeting NF-kappaB. J Exp Med 205:1261–1268. doi:jem.20080108 [pii] 10.1084/jem.20080108 (2008)

Hall JM, Korach KS (2003) Stromal cell-derived factor 1, a novel target of estrogen receptor action, mediates the mitogenic effects of estradiol in ovarian and breast cancer cells. Mol Endocrinol 17:792–803. doi:10.1210/me.2002-0438 me.2002-0438 [pii]

Harris RE (2009) Cyclooxygenase-2 (cox-2) blockade in the chemoprevention of cancers of the colon, breast, prostate, and lung. Inflammopharmacology 17:55–67. doi:10.1007/s10787-009-8049-8

Hasselblatt P, Gresh L, Kudo H, Guinea-Viniegra J, Wagner EF (2008) The role of the transcription factor AP-1 in colitis-associated and beta-catenin-dependent intestinal tumorigenesis in mice. Oncogene 27:6102–6109. doi:onc2008211 [pii] 10.1038/onc.2008.211

He G et al (2010) Hepatocyte IKKbeta/NF-kappaB inhibits tumor promotion and progression by preventing oxidative stress-driven STAT3 activation. Cancer Cell 17:286–297. doi:S1535-6108(10)00063-2 [pii] 10.1016/j.ccr.2009.12.048

Horton LW, Yu Y, Zaja-Milatovic S, Strieter RM, Richmond A (2007) Opposing roles of murine duffy antigen receptor for chemokine and murine CXC chemokine receptor-2 receptors in murine melanoma tumor growth. Cancer Res 67:9791–9799. doi:67/20/9791 [pii] 10.1158/0008-5472.CAN-07-0246

Howe LR et al (2005) HER2/neu-induced mammary tumorigenesis and angiogenesis are reduced in cyclooxygenase-2 knockout mice. Cancer Res 65:10113–10119. doi:65/21/10113 [pii] 10.1158/0008-5472.CAN-05-1524

Hwang JH et al (2003) CXC chemokine receptor 4 expression and function in human anaplastic thyroid cancer cells. J Clin Endocrinol Metab 88:408–416

Iwasaki A, Medzhitov R (2010) Regulation of adaptive immunity by the innate immune system. Science (New York, N.Y.) 327:291–295. doi:327/5963/291 [pii] 10.1126/science.1183021

Javelaud D et al (2007) Stable overexpression of Smad7 in human melanoma cells impairs bone metastasis. Cancer Res 67:2317–2324. doi:67/5/2317 [pii] 10.1158/0008-5472.CAN-06-3950

Jenkins BJ et al (2005) Hyperactivation of Stat3 in gp130 mutant mice promotes gastric hyperproliferation and desensitizes TGF-beta signaling. Nat Med 11:845–852. doi:nm1282 [pii] 10.1038/nm1282

Kim S et al (2009) Carcinoma-produced factors activate myeloid cells through TLR2 to stimulate metastasis. Nature 457:102–106. doi:nature07623 [pii] 10.1038/nature07623

Kitakata H et al (2002) Essential roles of tumor necrosis factor receptor p55 in liver metastasis of intrasplenic administration of colon 26 cells. Cancer Res 62:6682–6687

Koebel CM et al (2007) Adaptive immunity maintains occult cancer in an equilibrium state. Nature 450:903–907. doi:nature06309 [pii] 10.1038/nature06309

Lazennec G, Richmond A (2010) Chemokines and chemokine receptors: new insights into cancer-related inflammation. Trends Mol Med 16:133–144. doi:S1471-4914(10)00009-2 [pii] 10.1016/j.molmed.2010.01.003

Lee JM et al (2008) Inflammation in lung carcinogenesis: new targets for lung cancer chemoprevention and treatment. Crit Rev Oncol Hematol 66:208–217. doi:S1040-8428(08)00015-2 [pii] 10.1016/j.critrevonc.2008.01.004

Lentsch AB (2002) The Duffy antigen/receptor for chemokines (DARC) and prostate cancer. A role as clear as black and white? FASEB J 16:1093–1095. doi:10.1096/fj.02-0066hyp 16/9/1093 [pii]

Li WX (2008) Canonical and non-canonical JAK-STAT signaling. Trends Cell Biol 18:545–551. doi:S0962-8924(08)00237-7 [pii] 10.1016/j.tcb.2008.08.008

Lin EY, Nguyen AV, Russell RG, Pollard JW (2001) Colony-stimulating factor 1 promotes progression of mammary tumors to malignancy. J Exp Med 193:727–740

Lin EY et al (2006) Macrophages regulate the angiogenic switch in a mouse model of breast cancer. Cancer Res 66:11238–11246. doi:0008-5472.CAN-06-1278 [pii] 10.1158/0008-5472.CAN-06-1278

Lin A, Schildknecht A, Nguyen LT, Ohashi PS (2010) Dendritic cells integrate signals from the tumor microenvironment to modulate immunity and tumor growth. Immunol Lett 127:77–84. doi:S0165-2478(09)00232-6 [pii] 10.1016/j.imlet.2009.09.003

Liu BY et al (2010) Stromal cell-derived factor-1/CXCL12 contributes to MMTV-Wnt1 tumor growth involving Gr1+CD11b+ cells. PloS one 5:e8611. doi:10.1371/journal.pone.0008611

Loberg RD et al (2007) CCL2 as an important mediator of prostate cancer growth in vivo through the regulation of macrophage infiltration. Neoplasia 9:556–562

Lopez-Bergami P, Lau E, Ronai Z (2010) Emerging roles of ATF2 and the dynamic AP1 network in cancer. Nat Rev Cancer 10:65–76. doi:nrc2681 [pii] 10.1038/nrc2681

Luker KE, Steele JM, Mihalko LA, Ray P, Luker GD (2010) Constitutive and chemokine-dependent internalization and recycling of CXCR7 in breast cancer cells to degrade chemokine ligands. Oncogene 29(32):4599–4610

Luo JL et al (2007) Nuclear cytokine-activated IKKalpha controls prostate cancer metastasis by repressing Maspin. Nature 446:690–694. doi:nature05656 [pii] 10.1038/nature05656

Ma Q et al (1998) Impaired B-lymphopoiesis, myelopoiesis, and derailed cerebellar neuron migration in CXCR4- and SDF-1-deficient mice. Proc Natl Acad Sci U S A 95:9448–9453

Maeda S et al (2009) Ikappa B kinasebeta/nuclear factor-kappaB activation controls the development of liver metastasis by way of interleukin-6 expression. Hepatology 50:1851–1860. doi:10.1002/hep.23199

Maeda S, Kamata H, Luo JL, Leffert H, Karin M (2005) IKKbeta couples hepatocyte death to cytokine-driven compensatory proliferation that promotes chemical hepatocarcinogenesis. Cell 121:977–990. doi:S0092-8674(05)00394-6 [pii] 10.1016/j.cell.2005.04.014

Mantovani A, Allavena P, Sica A, Balkwill F (2008) Cancer-related inflammation. Nature 454:436–444. doi:nature07205 [pii] 10.1038/nature07205

Mantovani A et al (2010) The chemokine system in cancer biology and therapy. Cytokine Growth Factor Rev 21:27–39. doi:S1359-6101(09)00114-2 [pii] 10.1016/j.cytogfr.2009.11.007

Marchesi F et al (2008) The chemokine receptor CX3CR1 is involved in the neural tropism and malignant behavior of pancreatic ductal adenocarcinoma. Cancer Res 68:9060–9069. doi:68/21/9060 [pii] 10.1158/0008-5472.CAN-08-1810

Martin-Orozco N et al (2009) T helper 17 cells promote cytotoxic T cell activation in tumor immunity. Immunity 31:787–798. doi:S1074-7613(09)00451-8 [pii] 10.1016/j.immuni.2009.09.014

Matsuo Y et al (2009) CXC-chemokine/CXCR2 biological axis promotes angiogenesis in vitro and in vivo in pancreatic cancer. Int J Cancer 125:1027–1037. doi:10.1002/ijc.24383

McIntire CR, Yeretssian G, Saleh M (2009) Inflammasomes in infection and inflammation. Apoptosis 14:522–535

Meijer J, Ogink J, Roos E (2008) Effect of the chemokine receptor CXCR7 on proliferation of carcinoma cells in vitro and in vivo. Br J Cancer 99:1493–1501. doi:6604727 [pii] 10.1038/sj.bjc.6604727

Miao Z et al (2007) CXCR7 (RDC1) promotes breast and lung tumor growth in vivo and is expressed on tumor-associated vasculature. Proc Natl Acad Sci U S A 104:15735–15740. doi:0610444104 [pii] 10.1073/pnas.0610444104

Mikula M et al (2003) The proto-oncoprotein c-Fos negatively regulates hepatocellular tumorigenesis. Oncogene 22:6725–6738. doi:10.1038/sj.onc.1206781 1206781 [pii]

Minn AJ et al (2005) Genes that mediate breast cancer metastasis to lung. Nature 436:518–524. doi:nature03799 [pii] 10.1038/nature03799

Mizukami Y et al (2008) CCL17 and CCL22 chemokines within tumor microenvironment are related to accumulation of Foxp3+ regulatory T cells in gastric cancer. Int J Cancer 122:2286–2293. doi:10.1002/ijc.23392

Moore RJ et al (1999) Mice deficient in tumor necrosis factor-alpha are resistant to skin carcinogenesis. Nat Med 5:828–831. doi:10.1038/10552

Muller A et al (2001) Involvement of chemokine receptors in breast cancer metastasis. Nature 410:50–56. doi:10.1038/35065016 35065016 [pii]

Murakami T et al (2002) Expression of CXC chemokine receptor-4 enhances the pulmonary metastatic potential of murine B16 melanoma cells. Cancer Res 62:7328–7334

Murdoch C, Muthana M, Coffelt SB, Lewis CE (2008) The role of myeloid cells in the promotion of tumour angiogenesis. Nat Rev Cancer 8:618–631. doi:nrc2444 [pii] 10.1038/nrc2444

Musteanu M et al (2010) Stat3 is a negative regulator of intestinal tumor progression in Apc(Min) mice. Gastroenterology 138:1003–1011 (e1001-1005). doi:S0016-5085(09)02101-5 [pii] 10.1053/j.gastro.2009.11.049

Nateri AS, Spencer-Dene B, Behrens A (2005) Interaction of phosphorylated c-Jun with TCF4 regulates intestinal cancer development. Nature 437:281–285. doi:nature03914 [pii] 10.1038/nature03914

Naugler WE et al (2007) Gender disparity in liver cancer due to sex differences in MyD88-dependent IL-6 production. Science (New York, N.Y.) 317:121–124. doi:317/5834/121 [pii] 10.1126/science.1140485

Naumann U et al (2010) CXCR7 functions as a scavenger for CXCL12 and CXCL11. PloS one 5:e9175. doi:10.1371/journal.pone.0009175

Nausch N, Cerwenka A (2008) NKG2D ligands in tumor immunity. Oncogene 27:5944–5958. doi:onc2008272 [pii] 10.1038/onc.2008.272

Nibbs RJ et al (2007) The atypical chemokine receptor D6 suppresses the development of chemically induced skin tumors. J Clin Invest 117:1884–1892. doi:10.1172/JCI30068

Nozawa H, Chiu C, Hanahan D (2006) Infiltrating neutrophils mediate the initial angiogenic switch in a mouse model of multistage carcinogenesis. Proc Natl Acad Sci U S A 103:12493–12498. doi:0601807103 [pii] 10.1073/pnas.0601807103

Okamoto M et al (2010) Constitutively active inflammasome in human melanoma cells mediating autoinflammation via caspase-1 processing and secretion of interleukin-1beta. J Biol Chem 285:6477–6488. doi:M109.064907 [pii] 10.1074/jbc.M109.064907

Oppenheim DE et al (2005) Sustained localized expression of ligand for the activating NKG2D receptor impairs natural cytotoxicity in vivo and reduces tumor immunosurveillance. Nat Immunol 6:928–937. doi:ni1239 [pii] 10.1038/ni1239

Ostrand-Rosenberg S, Sinha P (2009) Myeloid-derived suppressor cells: linking inflammation and cancer. J Immunol 182:4499–4506. doi:182/8/4499 [pii] 10.4049/jimmunol.0802740

Ostrand-Rosenberg S, Grusby MJ, Clements VK (2000) Cutting edge: STAT6-deficient mice have enhanced tumor immunity to primary and metastatic mammary carcinoma. J Immunol 165:6015–6019

Pahler JC et al (2008) Plasticity in tumor-promoting inflammation: impairment of macrophage recruitment evokes a compensatory neutrophil response. Neoplasia 10:329–340

Passegue E, Jochum W, Schorpp-Kistner M, Mohle-Steinlein U, Wagner EF (2001) Chronic myeloid leukemia with increased granulocyte progenitors in mice lacking junB expression in the myeloid lineage. Cell 104:21–32. doi:S0092-8674(01)00188-X [pii]

Pietras K, Ostman A (2010) Hallmarks of cancer: interactions with the tumor stroma. Exp Cell Res 316:1324–1331. doi:S0014-4827(10)00108-4 [pii] 10.1016/j.yexcr.2010.02.045

Pikarsky E et al (2004) NF-kappaB functions as a tumour promoter in inflammation-associated cancer. Nature 431:461–466. doi:10.1038/nature02924 nature02924 [pii]

Pizarro TT et al (1999) IL-18, a novel immunoregulatory cytokine, is up-regulated in Crohn's disease: expression and localization in intestinal mucosal cells. J Immunol 162:6829–6835

Popivanova BK et al (2008) Blocking TNF-alpha in mice reduces colorectal carcinogenesis associated with chronic colitis. J Clin Invest 118:560–570. doi:10.1172/JCI32453

Porta C et al (2009) Cellular and molecular pathways linking inflammation and cancer. Immunobiology 214:761–777. doi:S0171-2985(09)00105-3 [pii] 10.1016/j.imbio.2009.06.014

Qian BZ, Pollard J W (2010) Macrophage diversity enhances tumor progression and metastasis. Cell 141:39–51. doi:S0092-8674(10)00287-4 [pii] 10.1016/j.cell.2010.03.014

Qin XJ et al (2009) CCL22 recruits CD4-positive CD25-positive regulatory T cells into malignant pleural effusion. Clin Cancer Res 15:2231–2237. doi:1078-0432.CCR-08-2641 [pii] 10.1158/1078–0432.CCR-08-2641

Rakoff-Nahoum S, Medzhitov R (2007) Regulation of spontaneous intestinal tumorigenesis through the adaptor protein MyD88. Science (New York, N.Y.) 317:124–127

Rakoff-Nahoum S, Medzhitov R (2009) Toll-like receptors and cancer. Nat Rev Cancer 9:57–63. doi:nrc2541 [pii] 10.1038/nrc2541

Rauh MJ et al (2005) SHIP represses the generation of alternatively activated macrophages. Immunity 23:361–374. doi:S1074-7613(05)00276-1 [pii] 10.1016/j.immuni.2005.09.003

Rebouissou S et al (2009) Frequent in-frame somatic deletions activate gp130 in inflammatory hepatocellular tumours. Nature 457:200–204. doi:nature07475 [pii] 10.1038/nature07475

Reuter BK, Pizarro TT (2004) Commentary: the role of the IL-18 system and other members of the IL-1R/TLR superfamily in innate mucosal immunity and the pathogenesis of inflammatory bowel disease: friend or foe? Eur J Immunol 34:2347–2355

Rosevear HM, Lightfoot AJ, O'Donnell MA, Griffith TS (2009) The role of neutrophils and TNF-related apoptosis-inducing ligand (TRAIL) in bacillus Calmette-Guerin (BCG) immunotherapy for urothelial carcinoma of the bladder. Cancer Metastasis Rev 28:345–353. doi:10.1007/s10555-009-9195-6

Rostom A et al (2007) Nonsteroidal anti-inflammatory drugs and cyclooxygenase-2 inhibitors for primary prevention of colorectal cancer: a systematic review prepared for the U.S. Preventive Services Task Force. Ann Intern Med 146:376–389. doi:146/5/376 [pii]

Rubie C, Oliveira-Frick V, Rau B, Schilling M, Wagner M (2006) Chemokine receptor CCR6 expression in colorectal liver metastasis. J Clin Oncol 24:5173–5174; author reply 5174, doi:24/32/5173-a [pii] 10.1200/JCO.2006.07.9095

Saez E et al (1995) c-fos is required for malignant progression of skin tumors. Cell 82:721–732. doi:0092-8674(95)90469-7 [pii]

Saitoh T et al (2008) Loss of the autophagy protein Atg16L1 enhances endotoxin-induced IL-1beta production. Nature 456:264–268

Salcedo R et al (2010) MyD88-mediated signaling prevents development of adenocarcinomas of the colon: role of interleukin 18. J Exp Med 207(8):1625–1636

Saleh M et al (2004) Differential modulation of endotoxin responsiveness by human caspase-12 polymorphisms. Nature 429:75–79

Saleh MMJC, Wolinski MK, Bensinger SJ, Fitzgerald P, Droin N, Ulevitch RJ, Green DR, Nicholson DW (2006) Enhanced bacterial clearance and sepsis resistance in caspase-12 deficient mice. Nature 440:1064–1068

Sato E et al (2005) Intraepithelial CD8+ tumor-infiltrating lymphocytes and a high CD8+/regulatory T cell ratio are associated with favorable prognosis in ovarian cancer. Proc Natl Acad Sci U S A 102:18538–18543. doi:0509182102 [pii] 10.1073/pnas.0509182102

Schimanski CC et al (2006) Dissemination of hepatocellular carcinoma is mediated via chemokine receptor CXCR4. Br J Cancer 95:210–217. doi:6603251 [pii] 10.1038/sj.bjc.6603251

Schroder K, Tschopp J (2010) The inflammasomes. Cell 140:821–832. doi:S0092-8674(10)00075-9 [pii] 10.1016/j.cell.2010.01.040

Shankaran V et al (2001) IFNgamma and lymphocytes prevent primary tumour development and shape tumour immunogenicity. Nature 410:1107–1111. doi:10.1038/35074122 35074122 [pii]

Sharma R et al (2008) Systemic inflammatory response predicts prognosis in patients with advanced-stage colorectal cancer. Clin Colorectal Cancer 7:331–337. doi:452T0P35288LJG78 [pii] 10.3816/CCC.2008.n.044

Shaulian E (2010) AP-1-The Jun proteins: Oncogenes or tumor suppressors in disguise? Cell Signal 22:894–899. doi:S0898-6568(10)00003-3 [pii] 10.1016/j.cellsig.2009.12.008

Shen H, Schuster R, Stringer KF, Waltz SE, Lentsch A B (2006) The Duffy antigen/receptor for chemokines (DARC) regulates prostate tumor growth. FASEB J 20, 59–64, doi:20/1/59 [pii] 10.1096/fj.05-4764com

Sherman M (2010) Hepatocellular carcinoma: New and emerging risks. Dig Liver Dis 42(Suppl 3):S215–222. doi:S1590-8658(10)60508-7 [pii] 10.1016/S1590-8658(10)60508-7 (2010)

Shields JD, Kourtis IC, Tomei AA, Roberts JM, Swartz MA (2010) Induction of lymphoidlike stroma and immune escape by tumors that express the chemokine CCL21. Science (New York, N.Y) 328:749–752. doi:science.1185837 [pii] 10.1126/science.1185837

Siegmund B (2010) Interleukin-18 in intestinal inflammation: friend and foe? Immunity 32:300–302. doi:S1074-7613(10)00093-2 [pii] 10.1016/j.immuni.2010.03.010

Singh S, Varney M, Singh RK (2009) Host CXCR2-dependent regulation of melanoma growth, angiogenesis, and experimental lung metastasis. Cancer Res 69:411–415. doi:69/2/411 [pii] 10.1158/0008-5472.CAN-08-3378

Sinha P, Clements VK, Fulton AM, Ostrand-Rosenberg S (2007) Prostaglandin E2 promotes tumor progression by inducing myeloid-derived suppressor cells. Cancer Res 67:4507–4513. doi:67/9/4507 [pii] 10.1158/0008-5472.CAN-06-4174

Sivakumar PV et al (2002) Interleukin 18 is a primary mediator of the inflammation associated with dextran sulphate sodium induced colitis: blocking interleukin 18 attenuates intestinal damage. Gut 50:812–820

Smyth MJ et al (2005) NKG2D function protects the host from tumor initiation. J Exp Med 202:583–588. doi:jem.20050994 [pii] 10.1084/jem.20050994

Steidl U et al (2006) Essential role of Jun family transcription factors in PU.1 knockdown-induced leukemic stem cells. Nat Genet 38:1269–1277. doi:ng1898 [pii] 10.1038/ng1898

Stolina M et al (2000) Specific inhibition of cyclooxygenase 2 restores antitumor reactivity by altering the balance of IL-10 and IL-12 synthesis. J Immunol 164:361–370. doi:ji_v164n1p361 [pii]

Stout RD, Watkins SK, Suttles J (2009) Functional plasticity of macrophages: in situ reprogramming of tumor-associated macrophages. J Leukoc Biol 86:1105–1109. doi:jlb.0209073 [pii] 10.1189/jlb.0209073

Strauss L et al (2007) A unique subset of CD4+CD25highFoxp3+ T cells secreting interleukin-10 and transforming growth factor-beta1 mediates suppression in the tumor microenvironment. Clin Cancer Res 13:4345–4354. doi:13/15/4345 [pii] 10.1158/1078-0432.CCR-07-0472

Street SE, Cretney E, Smyth MJ (2001) Perforin and interferon-gamma activities independently control tumor initiation, growth, and metastasis. Blood 97:192–197

Sugimoto M, Yamaoka Y, Furuta T (2010) Influence of interleukin polymorphisms on development of gastric cancer and peptic ulcer. World J Gastroenterol 16:1188–1200

Sutlu T, Alici E (2009) Natural killer cell-based immunotherapy in cancer: current insights and future prospects. J Intern Med 266:154–181. doi:JIM2121 [pii] 10.1111/j.1365-2796.2009.02121.x

Swann JB et al (2008) Demonstration of inflammation-induced cancer and cancer immunoediting during primary tumorigenesis. Proc Natl Acad Sci U S A 105:652–656. doi:0708594105 [pii] 10.1073/pnas.0708594105

Takagi H et al (2003) Contrasting action of IL-12 and IL-18 in the development of dextran sodium sulphate colitis in mice. Scand J Gastroenterol 38:837–844

Takahashi H, Ogata H, Nishigaki R, Broide DH, Karin M (2010) Tobacco smoke promotes lung tumorigenesis by triggering IKKbeta- and JNK1-dependent inflammation. Cancer Cell 17:89–97. doi:S1535-6108(09)00430-9 [pii] 10.1016/j.ccr.2009.12.008

Tebbutt NC et al (2002) Reciprocal regulation of gastrointestinal homeostasis by SHP2 and STAT-mediated trefoil gene activation in gp130 mutant mice. Nat Med 8:1089–1097. doi:10.1038/nm763 nm763 [pii]

Teicher BA, Fricker SP (2010) CXCL12 (SDF-1)/CXCR4 pathway in cancer. Clin Cancer Res 16:2927–2931. doi:1078-0432.CCR-09-2329 [pii] 10.1158/1078-0432.CCR-09-2329

Tiano HF et al (2002) Deficiency of either cyclooxygenase (COX)-1 or COX-2 alters epidermal differentiation and reduces mouse skin tumorigenesis. Cancer Res 62:3395–3401

Ting JP et al (2008) The NLR gene family: a standard nomenclature. Immunity 28:285–287. doi:S1074-7613(08)00076-9 [pii] 10.1016/j.immuni.2008.02.005

Tomita Y et al (2004) Spontaneous regression of lung metastasis in the absence of tumor necrosis factor receptor p55. Int J Cancer 112:927–933. doi:10.1002/ijc.20493

Tu S et al (2008) Overexpression of interleukin-1beta induces gastric inflammation and cancer and mobilizes myeloid-derived suppressor cells in mice. Cancer Cell 14:408–419. doi:S1535-6108(08)00334-6 [pii] 10.1016/j.ccr.2008.10.011

Vetrano S et al (2010) The lymphatic system controls intestinal inflammation and inflammation-associated Colon Cancer through the chemokine decoy receptor D6. Gut 59:197–206. doi:gut.2009.183772 [pii] 10.1136/gut.2009.183772

Villani AC et al (2009) Common variants in the NLRP3 region contribute to Crohn's disease susceptibility. Nat Genet 41:71–76

Vitale S et al (2007) Tissue-specific differential antitumour effect of molecular forms of fractalkine in a mouse model of metastatic colon cancer. Gut 56:365–372. doi:gut.2005.088989 [pii] 10.1136/gut.2005.088989

Vollmer J, Krieg AM (2009) Immunotherapeutic applications of CpG oligodeoxynucleotide TLR9 agonists. Adv Drug Deliv Rev 61:195–204. doi:S0169-409X(09)00003-9 [pii] 10.1016/j.addr.2008.12.008

Wang D et al (2006a) CXCL1 induced by prostaglandin E2 promotes angiogenesis in colorectal cancer. J Exp Med 203:941–951. doi:jem.20052124 [pii] 10.1084/jem.20052124

Wang J et al (2006b) Enhanced expression of Duffy antigen receptor for chemokines by breast cancer cells attenuates growth and metastasis potential. Oncogene 25:7201–7211. doi:1209703 [pii] 10.1038/sj.onc.1209703

Wang J et al (2008) The role of CXCR7/RDC1 as a chemokine receptor for CXCL12/SDF-1 in prostate cancer. J Biol Chem 283:4283–4294. doi:M707465200 [pii] 10.1074/jbc.M707465200

Wang L et al (2009) IL-17 can promote tumor growth through an IL-6-Stat3 signaling pathway. J Exp Med 206:1457–1464. doi:jem.20090207 [pii] 10.1084/jem.20090207

Wei G et al (2009) Global mapping of H3K4me3 and H3K27me3 reveals specificity and plasticity in lineage fate determination of differentiating CD4+ T cells. Immunity 30:155–167. doi:S1074-7613(08)00555-4 [pii] 10.1016/j.immuni.2008.12.009

Wu FY et al (2008) Chemokine decoy receptor d6 plays a negative role in human breast cancer. Mol Cancer Res 6:1276–1288. doi:6/8/1276 [pii] 10.1158/1541-7786.MCR-07-2108

Wu Y et al (2009) Stabilization of snail by NF-kappaB is required for inflammation-induced cell migration and invasion. Cancer Cell 15:416–428. doi:S1535-6108(09)00085-3 [pii] 10.1016/j.ccr.2009.03.016

Yanagawa J et al (2009) Snail promotes CXCR2 ligand-dependent tumor progression in non-small cell lung carcinoma. Clin Cancer Res 15:6820–6829. doi:1078–0432.CCR-09-1558 [pii] 10.1158/1078-0432.CCR-09-1558

Yang MY, Liu TC, Chang JG, Lin PM, Lin SF (2003) JunB gene expression is inactivated by methylation in chronic myeloid leukemia. Blood 101:3205–3211. doi:10.1182/blood-2002-05-1598 2002-05-1598 [pii]

Zaki MH et al (2010) The NLRP3 inflammasome protects against loss of epithelial integrity and mortality during experimental colitis. Immunity 32:379–391. doi:S1074-7613(10)00086-5 [pii] 10.1016/j.immuni.2010.03.003

Zeelenberg IS, Ruuls-Van Stalle L, Roos E (2003) The chemokine receptor CXCR4 is required for outgrowth of colon carcinoma micrometastases. Cancer Res 63:3833–3839

Zeng XH et al (2010) Coexpression of atypical chemokine binders (ACBs) in breast cancer predicts better outcomes. Breast Cancer Res Treat. doi:10.1007/s10549-010-0875-2

Zenz R et al (2003) c-Jun regulates eyelid closure and skin tumor development through EGFR signaling. Dev Cell 4:879–889. doi:S1534580703001618 [pii]

Zhu J, Paul WE (2010) Heterogeneity and plasticity of T helper cells. Cell Res 20:4–12. doi:cr2009138 [pii] 10.1038/cr.2009.138

Chapter 10
Role of Stroma in Disease Progression

Nicholas R. Bertos and Morag Park

10.1 Introduction

10.1.1 Role of the Microenvironment in Cancer

In the past, most research into cancer initiation and development, as well as into the progression from local to systemic disease, has focused on the tumor tissue *per se*. However, it is becoming increasingly evident that the configuration of the local microenvironment, and the nature of dynamic interactions occurring between cellular and structural elements of the stroma (generally defined as those tissue components distal to the basement membrane in normal tissue) and the tumor, can play significant roles. An understanding of these interactions will thus facilitate the development of strategies to manipulate the microenvironment, which are likely to represent the next important set of additions to the therapeutic armamentarium. Here, we describe the processes occurring in tumor stroma, using breast cancer as a model system.

10.1.2 Breast Cancer

Most breast cancers arise from the epithelial cells that line the ducts and lobules of the breast under physiological conditions. Classically, three classes of such tumors have been defined by differential expression of marker proteins as assessed by immuno-

N. R. Bertos (✉) · M. Park
Rosalind & Morris Goodman Cancer Research Centre, McGill University,
1160 Ave. des Pins O., Montreal, QC H3A 1A3, Canada
e-mail: nicholas.bertos@mcgill.ca

Department of Medicine, McGill University, Montreal, QC, Canada

M. Park
Departments of Oncology and Biochemistry, McGill University,
Montreal, QC, Canada

Department of Medicine, McGill University Health Centre,
Montreal, QC, Canada

J. V. Burnier, M. N. Burnier, Jr. (eds.), *Experimental and Clinical Metastasis*,
DOI 10.1007/978-1-4614-3685-0_10, © Springer Science+Business Media New York 2013

histochemistry techniques. These markers comprise receptors, which, upon ligand binding, activate signaling pathways to promote cellular survival and proliferation, namely the estrogen receptor (ER), the progesterone receptor (PR) and the human epidermal growth factor-2 receptor (HER2). The classes include the ER-positive group (members of which often exhibit co-expression of the PR), the HER2-positive group, in which the HER2 gene is generally amplified at the genomic level, and the "triple-negative" (ER-/PR-/HER2-) group, which appears to use alternate pathways to drive survival and proliferation. Standardized treatments are directed towards these receptors; ER-positive patients generally receive estrogen antagonists or aromatase inhibitors, which reduce estrogen biosynthesis (Patel et al. 2007; Jordan and Brodie 2007; Eneman et al. 2004). HER2-positive patients are treated with regimens including therapies targeting HER2 activity, such as the monoclonal anti-HER2 antibody trastuzumab (Lewis et al. 1993), while there is currently no standard targeted therapy for the triple-negative patient cohort (Rakha and Ellis 2009).

Not only do the three breast cancer subtypes differ at the level of their biologies, but subtype membership also impacts overall survival. ER-positive disease is associated with the best prognosis; HER2-positive disease bears an intermediate overall prognosis, while triple-negative cases have the poorest overall outcome among the three variants (Nishimura and Arima 2008). How much of this is due to intrinsic differences in the aggressivity of the tumors within each subtype, and how much is due to the effects of targeted therapies, is not completely clear; however, it is interesting to note that prior to the introduction of HER2-targeted therapies, HER2-positive disease exhibited the worst overall outcome.

Breast cancer is one of the most intensively studied members of the solid tumor family. It has a relatively high prevalence, and while a significant proportion of those affected go on to die of this disease, the majority do not; both of these characteristics render it easier to identify prognostic factors. Most patients undergo surgery for primary tumor removal, and therefore tissue samples can be obtained for study without necessitating additional procedures. This focus on breast cancer research has led to several gene expression profiling studies being conducted in an attempt to elucidate the molecular underpinnings of this disease, using microarray technology. Earlier studies using this approach have generally used whole-tumor samples as the source of genetic material (primarily RNA). Since the tumor itself represents the vast majority of the cells in such samples, and especially since many of these studies have utilized a minimum tumor content threshold of greater than 50 % for sample selection (Sorlie et al. 2001; Vijver 2002), the strongest signals obtained in these investigations chiefly reflect the expression profiles of the tumor cells *per se*. Interestingly, the results have tended to confirm the classical classification scheme of breast cancer (Sorlie et al. 2001; Veer 2002; Perou et al. 2000). The basal molecular subtype mostly contains triple-negative cases, although some samples exhibit expression of ER or HER2 at the immunohistochemical level. The luminal A and luminal B molecular subtypes contains ER positive patients, while the HER2-positive cohort also forms a separate group upon clustering of gene expression data.

The characterization of tumor subtypes, both at the protein and gene expression levels, has led to the development of specific treatments that target processes important for the survival and proliferation of tumor cells within each group, as well as the generation of schemes for appropriate patient stratification, emphasizing the importance of identifying classification schemes and key subtype-defining elements. Interaction with the microenvironment are known to play important roles in the normal development of breast tissue (Xu et al. 2009), and the importance of the tumor microenvironment and of tumor-stromal interactions in breast cancer initiation and progression are now being recognized. Therefore, the development of a comprehensive catalog of stromal processes associated with breast cancer, and of methods that permit the assignment of a specific patient to a point within this landscape, holds the promise of informing the development of novel therapeutic approaches to target key elements of these interactions in a highly individualized manner.

In order to understand the influence of the microenvironment on the progression of breast cancer, we must first understand the individual elements comprising the stroma, and the role that each of these plays vis-à-vis the tumor *per se*.

10.2 The Stroma

In the normal breast, non-stromal tissues, consisting of cuboidal epithelial cells (responsible for postpartum secretion of milk) surrounded by contractile myoepithelial cells, are embedded in an extracellular matrix (ECM) that contains organized cellular structures (e.g., lymphatic and blood vessels), individual cells (e.g., fibroblasts and immune cells, including macrophages, T cells and mast cells) and collections of adipocytes, as well as the components of the ECM itself.

Upon tumor development, the stromal landscape is altered in several ways. Firstly, the definition of invasive disease requires that epithelial tumor cells be present on the distal side of the basement membrane, which, under physiological conditions, represents the boundary between epithelial and stromal compartments. This process brings tumor cells into close proximity to the cells previously present in the stroma. Secondly, the phenotype of stromal cells already present in the local microenvironment can be altered by interactions with the tumor cells. Thirdly, the presence of the tumor and tumor-associated signaling leads to the recruitment of additional cells from other sites of the body to tumor-adjacent locations, including additional immune cells as well as bone marrow-derived mesenchymal stem cells which can then differentiate into a variety of other cell types, including fibroblasts (Mishra et al. 2008). Such specific recruitment can then enhance the metastatic potential of the original tumor via tumor-stromal cell signaling (Karnoub et al. 2007). Additionally, changes in the non-cellular elements of the ECM itself can affect tumor progression.

10.3 The Extracellular Matrix

The part of the ECM in closest apposition to the tumor prior to the invasive phase is the basement membrane, primarily composed of laminins secreted by myoepithelial cells, which is disrupted as the tumor progresses from a benign to a malignant phase.

There is evidence that perturbations in this component can impact tumor behavior—myoepithelial cells isolated from breast tumors do not express laminin-1, which, when elaborated by myoepithelial cells isolated from normal mammary glands, is necessary for the formation of double-layered breast acini with correct epithelial cell polarity under tissue culture conditions (Gudjonsson et al. 2002). On the other hand, coinjection of myoepithelial cells from normal mammary glands blocked the transition from DCIS (ductal carcinoma *in situ*) towards invasive disease in a model system of progressive disease (Hu et al. 2008).

The non-basement membrane components of the ECM consist primarily of macromolecules (e.g., collagens) and polysaccharides (e.g., hyaluronan), which are elaborated by local fibroblasts. The levels of some of these elements can change in cancer; for example, collagen α (XI) is present at lower levels in tumor-associated vs. normal stroma, and levels further decrease upon tumor progression (Halsted et al. 2008). Chemotherapy can also affect ECM composition, as seen in a study reporting increased basement membrane protein collagen IV levels and decreased syndecan-1 levels following neoadjuvant treatment (Tokes et al. 2009). Interestingly, the same study identified differences in ECM composition between the responder and non-responder patient subsets; tenascin-C was present at lower levels in patients who responded to treatment. In agreement with these results, a study comparing the ECM matrices deposited by tumor-associated vs. normal fibroblasts reported that tumor cell lines reacted differently to the two matrices (Castello-Cros et al. 2009).

An attempt has been made to derive information regarding ECM component status from gene expression profiles of whole tumors (Bergamaschi et al. 2008). Using a list of genes known to be associated with ECM from previous studies, the authors detected four ECM subtypes in multi-sample datasets and established that subtype membership is correlated with differences in overall disease outcome. As has previously been suggested, key differences between good- and poor-outcome classes included changes in the balance between proteases and their inhibitors; the expression of serpin family members (i.e., protease inhibitors) was elevated in good-outcome subtypes, while poor-outcome subtypes demonstrated increased expression of integrins and matrix metallopeptidases (MMPs). This supports the hypothesis that the ability to break down ECM components via the action of MMPs is an essential element in the ability of tumor cells to invade and spread. Interestingly, laminin chain expression was decreased in poor-outcome cases, in agreement with previous reports.

Mechanical properties of the ECM also play a role in tumor development. High breast density is considered to be a risk factor for development of breast cancer in humans (Boyd et al. 2002), while the increased stiffness observed in breast tumor tissue (Huang and Ingber 2005; Paszek et al. 2005) induces β1-integrin clustering with concomitant activation of Rho GTPase and ERK pathways, leading to a DCIS-like phenotype in normal epithelial cells (Paszek et al. 2005; Kass et al. 2007). On the other hand, deletion of β1-integrin in a mouse model can reduce tumor formation (White et al. 2004), while increased levels of collagen in mammary stroma leads to enhanced tumorigenesis and progression in another mouse model (Provenzano et al. 2008).

Beyond the effects of ECM composition and mechanical properties on breast tumor behavior, the overall organization of the ECM can influence and be influenced by the tumor. Existing fibers in the ECM are used as "tracks" along which invading tumor cells can migrate in response to chemotactic gradients (Condeelis and Segall 2003; Provenzano et al. 2006; Wang et al. 2002), while transplanted tumors organize the surrounding collagen matrix into a radial pattern that facilitates further tumor cell dispersion along the fibers (Provenzano et al. 2006).

Thus, the ECM plays multiple roles in the progression of breast tumors. Both individual components thereof and its overall mechanical properties influence tumor cell behavior, while the intimate contact between tumor cells and ECM elements allows tumor cells to both exploit and shape the ECM structure as a determinant of invasion. In this context, it is important to note that experiments conducted using cultured breast cancer cells reveal that responses to targeted therapeutic agents can vary significantly depending on whether cells are grown as two-dimensional monolayers or as three-dimensional colonies (Weigelt et al. 2010), further accentuating the importance of taking the microenvironment into consideration.

10.4 Stroma-Resident Cells

The breast tumor-associated stroma harbors a multiplicity of cell types, including those previously present in this compartment, which may experience functional alterations as a consequence of tumor presence, as well as those recruited to the tumor microenvironment.

10.4.1 Fibroblasts

In the normal breast, fibroblasts are primarily responsible for ECM deposition and remodeling, both in development and in acute situations such as wound healing. As a tumor develops and progresses, however, cancer-associated fibroblasts, or CAFs, take on a myofibroblast phenotype and play multiple additional roles. Their abundance and activity increases (Sappino et al. 1988), as can be visualized by increased expression of the proliferation marker Ki-67 (Hawsawi et al. 2008), leading to the generation of fibrotic ECM with attendant loss of the original tissue organization and enhanced tumor proliferation (Kalluri and Zeisberg 2006).

Changes in CAF phenotype result in increased expression of tumor-associated cytokines and matrix-associated proteins (Singer et al. 2008), as well as MMPs and other factors important for tumor progression. These include stromal-derived factor 1, or SDF (also known as CXCL12); aside from promoting endothelial progenitor cell recruitment and therefore angiogenesis (Orimo and Weinberg 2006), binding of this cytokine to its cognate receptor, CXCR4, which is expressed on tumor cells (Orimo et al. 2005), promotes tumor metastasis to distant sites, especially bone and lung (Muller et al. 2001).

Altered expression and activation of MMPs and other ECM-degrading enzymes by CAFs is another mechanism through which tumor progression is promoted. The broad-spectrum protease plasmin exists as an inactive precursor, known as plasminogen, which requires the action of urokinase plasminogen activator, or uPA (also known as PLAU), to assume its active form. Activation of uPA requires binding to its cognate receptor, uPAR (also known as PLAUR), which appears to be expressed by both tumor and stroma cells, although this has been a subject of debate (Nielsen et al. 2007; Hurd et al. 2007; Meng et al. 2006; Giannopoulou et al. 2007). Plasmin subsequently can activate MMPs and degrade the ECM, resulting in the release of latent bioactive peptides, including TGFß (transforming growth factor ß).

The uPA-uPAR axis also serves as an illustration of the complexity of tumor-stroma interactions. Tumor cells express the glycoprotein EMMPRIN (extracellular MMP inducer) (Quemener et al. 2007), which stimulates uPA production by cells in the stroma. On the other hand, signaling downstream of uPAR in tumor cells enhances their response to epidermal growth factor (EGF). Elevated expression of both uPA and uPAR, leading to increased generation of plasmin, can be driven by signaling downstream of activation of the hepatocyte growth factor (HGF) receptor, Met; Met is overexpressed in poor-outcome breast cancers, especially those belonging to the basal molecular subtype (Garcia et al. 2007a, b), and its actions have been linked to enhanced tumorigenicity and invasiveness of overexpressing cells (Jeffers et al. 1996a, b; Rong et al. 1993, 1994).

Interestingly, fibroblasts possess inducible aromatase activity (Santen et al. 1997, 1998; Santner et al. 1997). This activity is significant as aromatase is a key enzyme in the biosynthesis of estrogen. Therefore, estrogen-dependent breast tumors may form part of a paracrine loop with fibroblasts. Also, phosphoinositide-3-kinase (PI3K) pathway alterations are involved in the generation of activated stroma in proximity to tumors – disruption of Pten, a key negative regulator of this pathway, in stromal fibroblasts leads to increased stroma remodeling, immune cell recruitment and enhanced malignancy, which can be abrogated by concomitant inactivation of the transcription factor Ets2 (Trimboli et al. 2009). Interestingly, it has also been demonstrated that in a model system for the progression of DCIS to invasive disease, coinjection of fibroblasts promoted invasion, presumably via paracrine factors (Hu et al. 2008).

The question of whether CAFs, or stromal cells in general, undergo genomic changes during tumor progression has long been a subject of debate (Orimo and Weinberg 2006; Fukino et al. 2004; Kurose et al. 2002; Moinfar et al. 2000; Hill et al. 2005; Allinen et al. 2004; Hu et al. 2005; Lafkas et al. 2008; Fukino et al. 2007). The current consensus is that CAFs likely do not differ from normal fibroblasts at the genomic level; however, it is clear that gene and protein expression in CAFs is altered with respect to normal fibroblasts (Hawsawi et al. 2008; Singer et al. 2008; Sadlonova et al. 2009). The specificity of these alterations is illustrated by the results of a gene expression profiling study from our group, in which tumor-associated stroma was compared to morphologically normal regions of stroma more distal (> 2 mm) from the tumor site (Finak et al. 2006). The normal-appearing stroma from breast cancer cases was indistinguishable at the gene expression level from stroma samples isolated from non-cancer (breast reduction mammoplasty) cases, suggesting that tumor-specific alterations in stroma configuration are restricted to those regions in intimate contact with the tumor mass.

The phenotype observed for CAFs has been reported to be similar to that seen for fibroblasts in areas of inflammation. Interestingly, a gene expression signature derived from fibroblasts exposed to serum (Chang et al. 2004), termed the "wound-response signature", was found to have prognostic value when applied to whole-tumor gene expression profiles from breast cancer cases (Chang et al. 2005). This further supports the link between inflammation, as reflected in altered fibroblast status, and cancer progression, and highlights the importance of immune responses in modulating tumor progression, as discussed in the following section.

10.4.2 Immune Cells

Multiple types of immune cells populate the breast tumor stroma – however, the most numerous are the tumor-associated macrophages, or TAMs (Balkwill and Mantovani 2001; Coussens and Werb 2002; Balkwill et al. 2005). While, under physiological conditions, macrophages generally act as positive effectors of immune function, elevated numbers of macrophages are often associated with poor outcome in breast and other solid tumors (Bingle et al. 2002; Leek and Harris 2002). This is likely due to the multiple roles that macrophages can play; their activities under these conditions are directed towards their role in promoting wound healing, which can be co-opted by the tumor to enhance its growth and spread.

Macrophages are recruited to the tumor site by the secretion of chemoattractants, which can originate from either the tumor itself or from associated stromal cells. These include chemokines, such as CCL2, CCL5 and CXCL1, among others (Bottazzi et al. 1983; Matsushima et al. 1989; Arenberg et al. 2000; Balkwill 2004; Mantovani et al. 2004a, 2004b), as well as other factors released at tumor sites, such as TGFß, platelet-derived growth factor (PDGF), vascular endothelial growth factor (VEGF), and macrophage colony-stimulating factor (M-CSF), and other bioactive peptides released from the ECM via protease action (Coussens and Werb 2002).

At the tumor site, TAMs have been shown to be polarized towards the M2 phenotype (Sica et al. 2008; Mantovani et al. 2002) by local factors, including IL-10 and hypoxia (Mantovani et al. 2004b; Sica et al. 2008); this promotes their actions in immunosuppression (via polarization of T-cell responses towards a Th2 phenotype), wound healing and tissue remodeling. This process, which has been termed "immunoediting" (Lewis and Pollard 2006), can be reinforced via secretion of IL-10 by M2-activated macrophages (Anderson Mosser 2002). The link between inflammation and cancer is further highlighted by studies demonstrating that persistent activation of STAT3 (Yu et al. 2009) and NF-κB (Karin 2009), as observed in tumor cells, can both promote and be promoted by an inflammatory microenvironment.

Tumor promotion by macrophages occurs via multiple mechanisms. One of their chief roles is to promote invasion, both through the basement membrane in early-stage disease and into the circulatory system in the later stages, as has been demonstrated using mouse models in which macrophages are absent (Lin et al. 2001, 2002). Furthermore, TAMs act to stimulate angiogenesis, remodel the ECM, secrete growth factors and also engage in a paracrine loop with tumor cells, leading to their migration towards and invasion of elements of the circulatory system (Condeelis and Pollard 2006). Tumor cells bear EGF receptors and secrete CSF-1 (colony-stimulating factor 1), while macrophages bear receptors for CSF-1 and secrete EGF. Since each secreted protein is a chemoattractant for the other cell type (Wyckoff et al. 2004), this results in a scenario where macrophages migrate from blood vessels towards the tumor mass, while tumor cells engage in a reciprocal migration towards the vasculature (Goswami et al. 2005). Blockade of either EGF or CSF-1 leads to a reduction in the number of tumor cells released into the circulation, while tumor cell migration and entry into the vasculature is increased in regions where TAMs are present in the vicinity of blood vessels (Wyckoff et al. 2007).

T-cells also play an important role in breast cancer progression. As has been described for TAMs, these cells can play different roles under normal conditions; however, in their case, it is the balance between their potential activities that has important implications for tumor progression. T-cells are generally polarized along either the Th1 or the Th2 axis, where Th1-type cells are involved in the activation of cytotoxic responses (Knutson and Disis 2005). The presence of these cells is associated with good outcome in multiple solid tumor types (Pages et al. 2005; Hiraoka et al. 2006; Finak et al. 2008), and decreased prosurvival signaling for T lymphocytes is seen in stroma from a poor-outcome patient subset (Finak et al. 2008).

However, tumors can also recruit another population of T-cells to evade the cytotoxic response. Under physiological conditions, the function of regulatory T cells, or Tregs, is to mediate immune self-tolerance. These cells reduce the activity of other immune effectors (Lan et al. 2005), and it has been shown that their presence in the tumor mass is correlated with factors prognostic for poor outcome (Bohling and Allison 2008) and with shorter relapse-free and overall survival times (Bates et al. 2006), as well as with a decreased response to neoadjuvant chemotherapy (Ladoire et al. 2008).

Recently, the role of Th17-polarized T cells in the tumor microenvironment has also been investigated. This T cell subset, originally identified as being implicated in autoimmune disease, is involved in mediating inflammation and tissue injury (Steinman 2007; Tesmer et al. 2008). While factors released by tumor cells and cancer-associated fibroblasts can mediate Th17 cell recruitment in solid tumors (Su et al. 2010), their role in influencing tumor progression and disease outcome is currently unclear. Th17 cells have been reported to promote tumorigenesis (Wu et al. 2009), as well as to enhance activation of effector T-cells with anti-tumor activity (Martin-Orozco et al. 2009; Muranski et al. 2008).

Gene expression profiling studies of breast tumors have revealed that an immune response signature can be associated with high grade (generally associated with poor outcome) (Ma et al. 2009) or with good outcome (Teschendorff et al. 2006, 2007). It is likely that an explanation for this discrepancy lies in differential activation of the immune system, which can act as a friend or foe to tumors of multiple types

(Grivennikov et al. 2010); this emphasizes the necessity of characterizing these responses more precisely.

10.4.3 Adipocytes

A significant proportion of the normal human breast consists of fatty tissue, or adipocytes. However, the role of these cells in breast tumor progression has frequently been overlooked. Adipose tissue is an important source of estrogen, especially in the postmenopausal context; however, the relative contributions of local estrogen production vs. synthesis at other body sites to the promotion of estrogen-dependent tumor growth is not clear, and both stromal and tumor cells can produce estrogen in the tumor setting (Miki et al. 2007; Suzuki et al. 2008). The fact that growth of estrogen-dependent tumor cell lines requires the presence of adipocytes in three-dimensional culture (Manabe et al. 2003) and in mouse models (Elliott et al. 1992), however, suggests that the local presence of adipocytes is sufficient for promotion of tumor growth.

Adipocytes also secrete other factors that can act on tumor cells, including adiponectin (Landskroner-Eiger et al. 2009; Dos Santos et al. 2008; Dieudonne et al. 2006), collagen VI (Iyengar et al. 2003, 2005) and lectin (Catalano et al. 2009; Catalano et al. 2003, 2004; Mauro et al. 2007, Cirillo 2008). Tumor cells can also exert reciprocal effects on adipocytes, including induction of MMP11 expression (Andarawewa et al. 2005). Thus, the tumor cell-adipocyte relationship recapitulates many of the themes seen in tumor cell-stromal cell interactions; multiple signals are exchanged between the components, leading to the dynamic modification of the configuration of each.

10.5 Angiogenesis

Pathways related to this topic are the subject of a separate chapter of this work (Chap. 8), and therefore it will not be examined in detail here. However it is important to note that many of the cell types and features described in this chapter interact intimately with elements of the angiogenic process.

10.6 Stroma at the Metastatic Site

Primary breast cancer in itself is generally not a fatal disease. Most disease-associated mortality is due to the effects of distant metastases in more vital organs, including bone, brain, lung and liver. In order for metastases to become established and to proliferate, many of the adaptations described above for the primary tumor must presumably be re-established within a novel microenvironment, although it is also possible that some cellular elements of the stroma may travel with tumor cells in the circulation and be co-embedded at distant sites. One of the factors governing tumor dormancy may be the time required to modify the metastatic stroma so that it can support tumor cell proliferation. This suggests that manipulation of the microenvironment at the metastatic site may be a potential approach to inhibiting the growth of distant metastases—one example of this has been seen in the case of bisphosphonates, classically used to reduce bone remodeling activity. In breast cancer, bisphosphonate treatment results in a reduction in active metastases (Lipton 2008; Coleman 2009), suggesting that the induction of a non-proliferative microenvironment may render tumor cells quiescent even after implantation.

Interactions between tumor cells and the stroma at the metastatic site may be important in determining the location of metastases. For example, homing to bone is enhanced via the chemokine receptor CXCR4 (Lu and Kang 2007), while metastases to lung may be at least partially mediated through metadherin (Brown and Ruoslahti 2004). The relationship between potential metastatic sites and primary tumors can also be reciprocal, as evidenced by a report that osteopontin secretion from actively growing tumors can mobilize bone marrow cells and induce their migration to the sites of non-proliferating tumors, which leads to their renewed proliferation (McAllister et al. 2008).

10.7 The "Macroenvironment"

As well as interacting with each other, both tumor cells and stromal elements are exposed to common environmental conditions. While both compartments react to these stimuli, the specific mechanism of these reactions may differ between them. For example, hypoxia or changes in local estrogen levels would be experienced by both components, while systemic therapeutic interventions also affect both compartments. Administration of Tamoxifen, used as endocrine therapy for ER-positive breast cancer and thought to act through inhibition of estrogen-dependent signaling in tumor cells, led to decreased ECM turnover and changes in ECM protein composition in a mouse model system. ECM isolated from these mice inhibited the motility of both macrophages and cultured tumor cells (Hattar et al. 2009), suggesting that stromal fibroblasts may also be targets for Tamoxifen. Moreover, it has been reported that the HER2-targeted agent trastuzumab can affect the ability of stroma cells to support tumor growth and secrete VEGF (Corsini et al. 2003), as well as potentially target HER2-expressing tumor cells for destruction via antibody-dependent cellular cytotoxicity (Cooley et al. 1999; Clynes et al. 2000; Gennari et al. 2004). Thus, the potential effects of systemic agents on components of the stroma should be taken into account as possible modifiers of their anti-tumor activity or as sources of resistance to treatment (Pontiggia et al. 2009). In addition, the common responses of the tumor and stromal compartments to externally regulated factors may act as confounders in analyses of specific interactions between the two, since the coordinate responses of each to external stimuli would be difficult to distinguish from mutual regulation.

10.8 Tumor-Stroma Interactions in Very Early-Stage Disease

It has been suggested that metastasis is not necessarily associated with a late-stage event in breast cancer, but that it can occur at prior points during progression and that systemic dissemination may occur even before the basement membrane is substantially disrupted (Husemann et al. 2008). Therefore, investigations into stromal-epithelial interactions in early disease may uncover processes that program tumor cells for successful dissemination. Gene expression profiling studies have demonstrated that most gene expression changes in breast tumors occur prior to the transition from DCIS to invasive disease. Interestingly, a similar pattern has been shown to occur in the associated stroma, although more changes accompany the transition to a situation where tumor cells are in direct contact with stromal elements (Ma et al. 2009; Schedin and Borges 2009). While more than 90 % of stromal gene expression changes (with respect to normal tissue) occur prior to the DCIS-IDC (invasive ductal carcinoma) transition, MMPs and ECM components are over-represented in the set of genes differentially expressed between DCIS and IDC stromal samples. An analysis of existing breast cancer signature gene set members across a panel of matched DCIS and IDC samples suggests that signatures are conserved during the DCIS-IDC transition (Sharma et al. 2009). These findings indicate that tumor-stromal interactions likely occur early in breast cancer, and that these may set the stage for the future course of the disease by "locking in" specific conformations of the two compartments. This also suggests that manipulation of the stroma may be a potential approach in breast cancer prevention.

10.9 Global Characterization of the Stromal Microenvironment

Gene expression profiling has been used to specifically examine the role played by stromal components in cancer and such studies have confirmed that information encoded within the tumor stroma is correlated with multiple aspects of breast cancer, including type, outcome, and resistance to treatment (Allinen et al. 2004; Finak et al. 2008; Ma et al. 2009; Casey et al. 2009; Boersma et al. 2008; Farmer et al. 2009).

In one study, breast cancer cell lines were co-cultured with fibroblasts, and the gene expression profiles of each component were analyzed (Buess et al. 2007). It was found that there was a set of genes differentially induced in fibroblasts by ER-positive vs. ER-negative cell lines, and that this signature correlated with outcome in external datasets. However, since the signature obtained here is closely associated with ER positivity, which in itself is highly predictive of outcome, a chief conclusion to be drawn is that tumor subtype can influence stroma configuration. The wound response signature (Chang et al. 2004, 2005) has been described in a previous section. Interestingly, this signature was correlated with a basal (i.e., intrinsically poor-outcome) phenotype in the associated tumors, although the wound response signature displayed additive prognostic value when combined with predictors derived from tumor tissue alone.

Our group utilized laser capture microdissection (LCM) to purify stroma from a set of 53 primary breast tumors, and generated a 26-gene predictor of outcome from the resulting gene expression profiles (Finak et al. 2008). The genes comprising this stroma-derived prognostic predictor, or SDPP, reflect many of the processes previously described here. Th1-type T cell markers (e.g., CD8A, CD247, CD3D and GZMA) were a hallmark of the good-outcome patient class, while chemokines promoting NK and T cell recruitment and survival were reduced in the poor-outcome class, which also exhibited increased expression of genes associated with angiogenesis, hypoxia, matrix remodeling and the presence of TAMs. This signature demonstrates that the integration of multiple stromal processes is essential for enhancing prognostic accuracy, and the finding that it possesses additive value when combined with tumor-derived predictors further argues that breast cancer outcome is driven by the integrated output of processes occurring within both the tumor and in adjacent compartments.

Bioinformatics-based analyses also suggest that resistance to therapy can be influenced by stromal configuration. A gene set characteristic of reactive stroma, which is chiefly encoded by fibroblasts, was overexpressed in tumors resistant to neoadjuvant chemotherapy (Farmer et al. 2009), emphasizing the functional significance of stromal features in governing tumor cell behavior and responses to specific conditions.

One caveat when assessing data from gene expression profiling studies is that not all changes at the mRNA level correlate with alterations at the protein level; also, there exist multiple levels of regulation beyond those that can be identified from mRNA levels alone (e.g., post-translational modification, intracellular localization, etc.). As an example, a study comparing fibroblasts isolated from different regions (interlobular vs. intralobular) of normal mammary stroma identified no differences at the gene expression level; however, immunohistochemical approaches identified several differentially expressed proteins (Fleming et al. 2008). This emphasizes that data obtained at the mRNA level, while useful for identification of overall pathways and processes, may not always be a reliable indicator of the level or activity of individual proteins.

10.10 Summary

As previously mentioned, cells in the tumor stroma are thought to not possess significant alterations at the genomic level, and specific components and processes of stromal origin appear to play crucial roles in tumor progression (Fig. 10.1). Therefore, the stroma has been thought to represent a stable target for therapeutic intervention (Orimo and Weinberg 2006; Micke and Ostman 2004: Joyce 2005; Jain 2005; Howell et al. 2009). Given the range of cell types and interactions possible, however, it is becoming clear that there will be no "one-size-fits-all" approach to targeting the

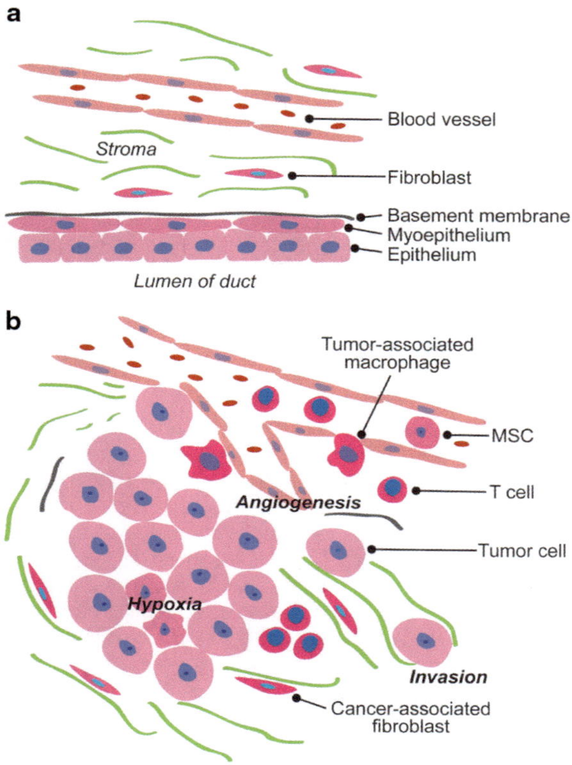

Fig. 10.1 **a** The normal breast microenvironment, depicting cell types present *(normal font)* as well as compartments *(italic font)*. **b** The microenvironment in breast cancer, depicting tumor-associated cell types; processes are indicated in bold italic font (note that not all cell types and processes necessarily co-occur in the same patient or at the same time). MSC, mesenchymal stem cell.

tumor stroma, and that individualized treatment regiments will have to be designed as carefully as, if not more carefully than, those currently utilized to address the tumor *per se*.

Although some stromal processes appear to be associated with specific tumor subtypes, many appear to be independent of this variable. Therefore, a precise definition of a given tumor may require assignment to points along multiple axes, representing tumor, stromal and "macroenvironmental" parameters. Investigations into whether and how stromal configurations impact upon resistance to specific therapies is also an area that warrants further investigation, holding the promise of enhancing the patient-specific selection of treatment options. Given the interdependence of the two compartments, we also suggest that carefully targeted combinations of therapies directed against features of both the tumor and the supporting microenvironment may lead to increased success in breast cancer treatment, and that such a holistic approach may circumvent the development of resistance to approaches directed against the tumor alone.

Acknowledgments Many studies have addressed the various components of the breast cancer stroma and their interactions with each other, and with the tumor *per se*. Therefore space limitations render it impossible to adequately acknowledge all of the contributions by the many key individuals and groups who have studied different aspects of this research area in detail, and have made it necessary to refer the reader to reviews in many cases where the primary literature is very large. The authors apologize in advance for any omissions.

Work on this area in our group has been supported by grants from multiple agencies, including the Québec Breast Cancer Foundation, Genome Canada–Génome Québec, Valorisation-Recherche Québec, the Fonds de la Récherche en Santé du Québec, the Canadian Institutes of Health Research and the Terry Fox Foundation (to M.P.). M.P. holds the Diane and Sal Guerrera Chair in Cancer Genetics at McGill University.

References

Allinen M et al (2004) Molecular characterization of the tumor microenvironment in breast cancer. Cancer Cell 6:17–32

Andarawewa KL et al (2005) Stromelysin-3 is a potent negative regulator of adipogenesis participating to cancer cell-adipocyte interaction/crosstalk at the tumor invasive front. Cancer Res 65:10862–10871

Anderson CF, Mosser DM (2002) A novel phenotype for an activated macrophage: the type 2 activated macrophage. J Leukoc Biol 72:101–106

Arenberg DA et al (2000) Macrophage infiltration in human non-small-cell lung cancer: the role of CC chemokines. Cancer Immunol Immunother 49:63–70

Balkwill F (2004) Cancer and the chemokine network. Nat Rev Cancer 4:540–550

Balkwill F, Mantovani A (2001) Inflammation and cancer: back to Virchow? Lancet 357:539–545

Balkwill F, Charles KA, Mantovani A (2005) Smoldering and polarized inflammation in the initiation and promotion of malignant disease. Cancer Cell 7:211–217

Bates GJ et al (2006) Quantification of regulatory T cells enables the identification of high-risk breast cancer patients and those at risk of late relapse. J Clin Oncol 24:5373–5380

Bergamaschi A et al (2008) Extracellular matrix signature identifies breast cancer subgroups with different clinical outcome. J Pathol 214:357–367

Bingle L, Brown NJ, Lewis CE (2002) The role of tumour-associated macrophages in tumour progression: implications for new anticancer therapies. J Pathol 196:254–265

Boersma BJ et al (2008) A stromal gene signature associated with inflammatory breast cancer. Int J Cancer 122:1324–1332

Bohling SD, Allison KH (2008) Immunosuppressive regulatory T cells are associated with aggressive breast cancer phenotypes: a potential therapeutic target. Mod Pathol 21:1527–1532

Bottazzi B et al (1983) Regulation of the macrophage content of neoplasms by chemoattractants. Science 220:210–212

Boyd NF et al (2002) Heritability of mammographic density, a risk factor for breast cancer. N Engl J Med 347:886–894

Brown DM, Ruoslahti E (2004) Metadherin, a cell surface protein in breast tumors that mediates lung metastasis. Cancer Cell 5:365–374

Buess M et al (2007) Characterization of heterotypic interaction effects in vitro to deconvolute global gene expression profiles in cancer. Genome Biol 8:R191

Casey T et al (2009) Molecular signatures suggest a major role for stromal cells in development of invasive breast cancer. Breast Cancer Res Treat 114:47–62

Castello-Cros R, Khan DR, Simons J, Valianou M, Cukierman E (2009) Staged stromal extracellular 3D matrices differentially regulate breast cancer cell responses through PI3K and beta1-integrins. BMC Cancer 9:94

Catalano S et al (2003) Leptin enhances, via AP-1, expression of aromatase in the MCF-7 cell line. J Biol Chem 278:28668–28676

Catalano S et al (2004) Leptin induces, via ERK1/ERK2 signal, functional activation of estrogen receptor alpha in MCF-7 cells. J Biol Chem 279:19908–19915

Catalano S et al (2009) Evidence that leptin through STAT and CREB signaling enhances cyclin D1 expression and promotes human endometrial cancer proliferation. J Cell Physiol 218:490–500
Chang HY et al (2004) Gene expression signature of fibroblast serum response predicts human cancer progression: similarities between tumors and wounds. PLoS Biol 2:E7
Chang HY et al (2005) Robustness, scalability, and integration of a wound-response gene expression signature in predicting breast cancer survival. Proc Natl Acad Sci U S A 102:3738–3743
Cirillo D, Rachiglio AM, la Montagna R, Giordano A, Normanno N (2008) Leptin signaling in breast cancer: an overview. J Cell Biochem 105:956–964
Clynes RA, Towers TL, Presta LG, Ravetch JV (2000) Inhibitory Fc receptors modulate in vivo cytoxicity against tumor targets. Nat Med 6:443–446
Coleman RE (2009) Adjuvant bisphosphonates in breast cancer: are we witnessing the emergence of a new therapeutic strategy? Eur J Cancer 45:1909–1915
Condeelis J, Pollard JW (2006) Macrophages: obligate partners for tumor cell migration, invasion, and metastasis. Cell 124:263–266
Condeelis J, Segall JE (2003) Intravital imaging of cell movement in tumours. Nat Rev Cancer 3:921–930
Cooley S, Burns LJ, Repka T, Miller JS (1999) Natural killer cell cytotoxicity of breast cancer targets is enhanced by two distinct mechanisms of antibody-dependent cellular cytotoxicity against LFA-3 and HER2/neu. Exp Hematol 27:1533–1541
Corsini C et al (2003) Stroma cells: a novel target of herceptin activity. Clin Cancer Res 9:1820–1825
Coussens LM, Werb Z (2002) Inflammation and cancer. Nature 420:860–867
Dieudonne MN et al (2006) Adiponectin mediates antiproliferative and apoptotic responses in human MCF7 breast cancer cells. Biochem Biophys Res Commun 345:271–279
Dos Santos E et al (2008) Adiponectin mediates an antiproliferative response in human MDA-MB 231 breast cancer cells. Oncol Rep 20:971–977
Elliott BE, Tam SP, Dexter D, Chen ZQ (1992) Capacity of adipose tissue to promote growth and metastasis of a murine mammary carcinoma: effect of estrogen and progesterone. Int J Cancer 51:416–424
Eneman JD, Wood ME, Muss HB (2004) Selecting adjuvant endocrine therapy for breast cancer. Oncology (Williston Park) 18:1733–1744 (discussion 1744–5, 1748, 1751–4)
Farmer P et al (2009) A stroma-related gene signature predicts resistance to neoadjuvant chemotherapy in breast cancer. Nat Med 15:68–74
Finak G et al (2006) Gene expression signatures of morphologically normal breast tissue identify basal-like tumors. Breast Cancer Res 8:R58
Finak G et al (2008) Stromal gene expression predicts clinical outcome in breast cancer. Nat Med 14:518–527
Fleming JM et al (2008) Interlobular and intralobular mammary stroma: genotype may not reflect phenotype. BMC Cell Biol 9:46
Fukino K et al (2004) Combined total genome loss of heterozygosity scan of breast cancer stroma and epithelium reveals multiplicity of stromal targets. Cancer Res 64:7231–7236
Fukino K, Shen L, Patocs A, Mutter GL, Eng C (2007) Genomic instability within tumor stroma and clinicopathological characteristics of sporadic primary invasive breast carcinoma. JAMA 297:2103–2111
Garcia S et al (2007a) Overexpression of c-Met and of the transducers PI3K, FAK and JAK in breast carcinomas correlates with shorter survival and neoangiogenesis. Int J Oncol 31:49–58
Garcia S et al (2007b) Poor prognosis in breast carcinomas correlates with increased expression of targetable CD146 and c-Met and with proteomic basal-like phenotype. Hum Pathol 38:830–841
Gennari R et al (2004) Pilot study of the mechanism of action of preoperative trastuzumab in patients with primary operable breast tumors overexpressing HER2. Clin Cancer Res 10:5650–5655
Giannopoulou I et al (2007) The prognostic value of the topographic distribution of uPAR expression in invasive breast carcinomas. Cancer Lett 246:262–267
Goswami S et al (2005) Macrophages promote the invasion of breast carcinoma cells via a colony-stimulating factor-1/epidermal growth factor paracrine loop. Cancer Res 65:5278–5283

Grivennikov SI, Greten FR, Karin M (2010) Immunity, inflammation, and cancer. Cell 140:883–899
Gudjonsson T et al (2002) Normal and tumor-derived myoepithelial cells differ in their ability to interact with luminal breast epithelial cells for polarity and basement membrane deposition. J Cell Sci 115:39–50
Halsted KC et al (2008) Collagen alpha1(XI) in normal and malignant breast tissue. Mod Pathol 21:1246–1254
Hattar R et al (2009) Tamoxifen induces pleiotrophic changes in mammary stroma resulting in extracellular matrix that suppresses transformed phenotypes. Breast Cancer Res 11:R5
Hawsawi NM et al (2008) Breast carcinoma-associated fibroblasts and their counterparts display neoplastic-specific changes. Cancer Res 68:2717–2725
Hill R, Song Y, Cardiff RD, Van Dyke T (2005) Selective evolution of stromal mesenchyme with p53 loss in response to epithelial tumorigenesis. Cell 123:1001–1011
Hiraoka K et al (2006) Concurrent infiltration by CD8+ T cells and CD4+ T cells is a favourable prognostic factor in non-small-cell lung carcinoma. Br J Cancer 94:275–280
Howell A, Landberg G, Bergh J (2009) Breast tumour stroma is a prognostic indicator and target for therapy. Breast Cancer Res 11(Suppl 3):S16
Hu M et al (2005) Distinct epigenetic changes in the stromal cells of breast cancers. Nat Genet 37:899–905
Hu M et al (2008) Regulation of in situ to invasive breast carcinoma transition. Cancer Cell 13:394–406
Huang S, Ingber DE (2005) Cell tension, matrix mechanics, and cancer development. Cancer Cell 8:175–176
Hurd TC et al (2007) Plasminogen activator system localization in 60 cases of ductal carcinoma in situ. Ann Surg Oncol 14:3117–3124
Husemann Y et al (2008) Systemic spread is an early step in breast cancer. Cancer Cell 13:58–68
Iyengar P et al (2003) Adipocyte-secreted factors synergistically promote mammary tumorigenesis through induction of anti-apoptotic transcriptional programs and proto-oncogene stabilization. Oncogene 22:6408–6423
Iyengar P et al (2005) Adipocyte-derived collagen VI affects early mammary tumor progression in vivo, demonstrating a critical interaction in the tumor/stroma microenvironment. J Clin Invest 115:1163–1176
Jain RK (2005) Normalization of tumor vasculature: an emerging concept in antiangiogenic therapy. Science 307:58–62
Jeffers M, Rong S, Anver M, Vande Woude GF (1996a) Autocrine hepatocyte growth factor/scatter factor-Met signaling induces transformation and the invasive/metastastic phenotype in C127 cells. Oncogene 13:853–856
Jeffers M, Rong S, Woude GF (1996b) Hepatocyte growth factor/scatter factor-Met signaling in tumorigenicity and invasion/metastasis. J Mol Med 74:505–513
Jordan VC, Brodie AM (2007) Development and evolution of therapies targeted to the estrogen receptor for the treatment and prevention of breast cancer. Steroids 72:7–25
Joyce JA (2005) Therapeutic targeting of the tumor microenvironment. Cancer Cell 7:513–520
Kalluri R, Zeisberg M (2006) Fibroblasts in cancer. Nat Rev Cancer 6:392–401
Karin M (2009) NF-kappaB as a critical link between inflammation and cancer. Cold Spring Harb Perspect Biol 1:a000141
Karnoub AE et al (2007) Mesenchymal stem cells within tumour stroma promote breast cancer metastasis. Nature 449:557–563
Kass L, Erler JT, Dembo M, Weaver VM (2007) Mammary epithelial cell: influence of extracellular matrix composition and organization during development and tumorigenesis. Int J Biochem Cell Biol 39:1987–1994
Knutson KL, Disis ML (2005) Tumor antigen-specific T helper cells in cancer immunity and immunotherapy. Cancer Immunol Immunother 54:721–728
Kurose K et al (2002) Frequent somatic mutations in PTEN and TP53 are mutually exclusive in the stroma of breast carcinomas. Nat Genet 32:355–357

Ladoire S et al (2008) Pathologic complete response to neoadjuvant chemotherapy of breast carcinoma is associated with the disappearance of tumor-infiltrating foxp3+ regulatory T cells. Clin Cancer Res 14:2413–2420

Lafkas D, Trimis G, Papavassiliou AG, Kiaris H (2008) P53 mutations in stromal fibroblasts sensitize tumors against chemotherapy. Int J Cancer 123:967–971

Lan RY, Ansari AA, Lian ZX, Gershwin ME (2005) Regulatory T cells: development, function and role in autoimmunity. Autoimmun Rev 4:351–363

Landskroner-Eiger S et al (2009) Proangiogenic contribution of adiponectin toward mammary tumor growth in vivo. Clin Cancer Res 15:3265–3276

Leek RD, Harris AL (2002) Tumor-associated macrophages in breast cancer. J Mammary Gland Biol Neoplasia 7:177–189

Lewis CE, Pollard JW (2006) Distinct role of macrophages in different tumor microenvironments. Cancer Res 66:605–612

Lewis GD et al (1993) Differential responses of human tumor cell lines to anti-p185HER2 monoclonal antibodies. Cancer Immunol Immunother 37:255–263

Lin EY, Nguyen AV, Russell RG, Pollard JW (2001) Colony-stimulating factor 1 promotes progression of mammary tumors to malignancy. J Exp Med 193:727–740

Lin EY, Gouon-Evans V, Nguyen AV, Pollard JW (2002) The macrophage growth factor CSF-1 in mammary gland development and tumor progression. J Mammary Gland Biol Neoplasia 7:147–162

Lipton A (2008) Emerging role of bisphosphonates in the clinic–antitumor activity and prevention of metastasis to bone. Cancer Treat Rev 34(Suppl 1):S25–30

Lu X, Kang Y (2007) Organotropism of breast cancer metastasis. J Mammary Gland Biol Neoplasia 12:153–162

Ma XJ, Dahiya S, Richardson E, Erlander M, Sgroi DC (2009) Gene expression profiling of the tumor microenvironment during breast cancer progression. Breast Cancer Res 11:R7

Manabe Y, Toda S, Miyazaki K, Sugihara H (2003) Mature adipocytes, but not preadipocytes, promote the growth of breast carcinoma cells in collagen gel matrix culture through cancer-stromal cell interactions. J Pathol 201:221–228

Mantovani A, Sozzani S, Locati M, Allavena P, Sica A (2002) Macrophage polarization: tumor-associated macrophages as a paradigm for polarized M2 mononuclear phagocytes. Trends Immunol 23:549–555

Mantovani A et al (2004a) Chemokines in the recruitment and shaping of the leukocyte infiltrate of tumors. Semin Cancer Biol 14:155–160

Mantovani A et al (2004b) The chemokine system in diverse forms of macrophage activation and polarization. Trends Immunol 25:677–686

Martin-Orozco N et al (2009) T helper 17 cells promote cytotoxic T cell activation in tumor immunity. Immunity 31:787–798

Matsushima K, Larsen CG, DuBois GC, Oppenheim JJ (1989) Purification and characterization of a novel monocyte chemotactic and activating factor produced by a human myelomonocytic cell line. J Exp Med 169:1485–1490

Mauro L et al (2007) Evidences that leptin up-regulates E-cadherin expression in breast cancer: effects on tumor growth and progression. Cancer Res 67:3412–3421

McAllister SS et al (2008) Systemic endocrine instigation of indolent tumor growth requires osteopontin. Cell 133:994–1005

Meng S et al (2006) uPAR and HER-2 gene status in individual breast cancer cells from blood and tissues. Proc Natl Acad Sci U S A 103:17361–17365

Micke P, Ostman A (2004) Tumour-stroma interaction: cancer-associated fibroblasts as novel targets in anti-cancer therapy? Lung Cancer 45(Suppl 2):S163–75

Miki Y, Suzuki T, Sasano H (2007) Controversies of aromatase localization in human breast cancer–stromal versus parenchymal cells. J Steroid Biochem Mol Biol 106:97–101

Mishra PJ et al (2008) Carcinoma-associated fibroblast-like differentiation of human mesenchymal stem cells. Cancer Res 68:4331–4339

Moinfar F et al (2000) Concurrent and independent genetic alterations in the stromal and epithelial cells of mammary carcinoma: implications for tumorigenesis. Cancer Res 60:2562–2566
Muller A et al (2001) Involvement of chemokine receptors in breast cancer metastasis. Nature 410:50–56
Muranski P et al (2008) Tumor-specific Th17-polarized cells eradicate large established melanoma. Blood 112:362–373
Nielsen BS, Rank F, Illemann M, Lund LR, Dano K (2007) Stromal cells associated with early invasive foci in human mammary ductal carcinoma in situ coexpress urokinase and urokinase receptor. Int J Cancer 120:2086–2095
Nishimura R, Arima N (2008) Is triple negative a prognostic factor in breast cancer? Breast Cancer 15:303–308
Orimo A, Weinberg RA (2006) Stromal fibroblasts in cancer: a novel tumor-promoting cell type. Cell Cycle 5:1597–1601
Orimo A et al (2005) Stromal fibroblasts present in invasive human breast carcinomas promote tumor growth and angiogenesis through elevated SDF-1/CXCL12 secretion. Cell 121:335–348
Pages F et al (2005) Effector memory T cells, early metastasis, and survival in colorectal cancer. N Engl J Med 353:2654–2666
Paszek MJ et al (2005) Tensional homeostasis and the malignant phenotype. Cancer Cell 8:241–254
Patel RR, Sharma CG, Jordan VC (2007) Optimizing the antihormonal treatment and prevention of breast cancer. Breast Cancer 14:113–22
Perou CM et al (2000) Molecular portraits of human breast tumours. Nature 406:747–752
Pontiggia O et al (2009) Establishment of an in vitro estrogen-dependent mouse mammary tumor model: a new tool to understand estrogen responsiveness and development of tamoxifen resistance in the context of stromal-epithelial interactions. Breast Cancer Res Treat 116:247–255
Provenzano PP et al (2006) Collagen reorganization at the tumor-stromal interface facilitates local invasion. BMC Med 4:38
Provenzano PP et al (2008) Collagen density promotes mammary tumor initiation and progression. BMC Med 6:11
Quemener C et al (2007) Extracellular matrix metalloproteinase inducer up-regulates the urokinase-type plasminogen activator system promoting tumor cell invasion. Cancer Res 67:9–15
Rakha EA, Ellis IO (2009) Triple-negative/basal-like breast cancer: review. Pathology 41:40–47
Rong S et al (1993) Tumorigenesis induced by coexpression of human hepatocyte growth factor and the human met protooncogene leads to high levels of expression of the ligand and receptor. Cell Growth Differ 4:563–569
Rong S, Segal S, Anver M, Resau JH, Vande Woude GF (1994) Invasiveness and metastasis of NIH 3T3 cells induced by Met-hepatocyte growth factor/scatter factor autocrine stimulation. Proc Natl Acad Sci U S A 91:4731–4735
Sadlonova A et al (2009) Identification of Molecular Distinctions Between Normal Breast-Associated Fibroblasts and Breast Cancer-Associated Fibroblasts. Cancer Microenviron 2:9–21
Santen RJ et al (1997) Estrogen production via the aromatase enzyme in breast carcinoma: which cell type is responsible? J Steroid Biochem Mol Biol 61:267–271
Santen RJ et al (1998) Demonstration of aromatase activity and its regulation in breast tumor and benign breast fibroblasts. Breast Cancer Res Treat 49 (Suppl 1):S93–99; (discussion S109–19)
Santner SJ, Pauley RJ, Tait L, Kaseta J, Santen RJ (1997) Aromatase activity and expression in breast cancer and benign breast tissue stromal cells. J Clin Endocrinol Metab 82:200–208
Sappino AP, Skalli O, Jackson B, Schurch W, Gabbiani G (1988) Smooth-muscle differentiation in stromal cells of malignant and non-malignant breast tissues. Int J Cancer 41:707–712
Schedin P, Borges V (2009) Breaking down barriers: the importance of the stromal microenvironment in acquiring invasiveness in young women's breast cancer. Breast Cancer Res 11:102
Sharma M et al (2009) Analysis of stromal signatures in the tumor microenvironment of ductal carcinoma in situ. Breast Cancer Res Treat. 2010 Sep;123(2):397–404. Epub 2009 Dec 1
Sica A et al (2008) Macrophage polarization in tumour progression. Semin Cancer Biol 18:349–355

Singer CF et al (2008) Differential gene expression profile in breast cancer-derived stromal fibroblasts. Breast Cancer Res Treat 110:273–281

Sorlie T et al (2001) Gene expression patterns of breast carcinomas distinguish tumor subclasses with clinical implications. Proc Natl Acad Sci U S A 98:10869–10874

Steinman L (2007) A brief history of T(H)17, the first major revision in the T(H)1/T(H)2 hypothesis of T cell-mediated tissue damage. Nat Med 13:139–145

Su X et al (2010) Tumor microenvironments direct the recruitment and expansion of human Th17 cells. J Immunol 184:1630–1641

Suzuki T et al (2008) Aromatase in human breast carcinoma as a key regulator of intratumoral sex steroid concentrations. Endocr J 55:455–463

Teschendorff AE, Naderi A, Barbosa-Morais NL, Caldas C (2006) PACK: Profile Analysis using Clustering and Kurtosis to find molecular classifiers in cancer. Bioinformatics 22:2269–2275

Teschendorff AE, Miremadi A, Pinder SE, Ellis IO, Caldas C (2007) An immune response gene expression module identifies a good prognosis subtype in estrogen receptor negative breast cancer. Genome Biol 8:R157

Tesmer LA, Lundy SK, Sarkar S, Fox DA (2008) Th17 cells in human disease. Immunol Rev 223:87–113

Tokes AM et al (2009) Stromal matrix protein expression following preoperative systemic therapy in breast cancer. Clin Cancer Res 15:731–739

Trimboli AJ et al (2009) Pten in stromal fibroblasts suppresses mammary epithelial tumours. Nature 461:1084–1091

van 't Veer LJ et al (2002) Gene expression profiling predicts clinical outcome of breast cancer. Nature 415:530–536

van de Vijver, M.J. et al (2002) A gene-expression signature as a predictor of survival in breast cancer. N Engl J Med 347:1999–2009

Wang W et al (2002) Single cell behavior in metastatic primary mammary tumors correlated with gene expression patterns revealed by molecular profiling. Cancer Res 62:6278–6288

Weigelt B, Lo AT, Park CC, Gray JW, Bissell MJ (2010) HER2 signaling pathway activation and response of breast cancer cells to HER2-targeting agents is dependent strongly on the 3D microenvironment. Breast Cancer Res Treat 122:35–43

White DE et al (2004) Targeted disruption of beta1-integrin in a transgenic mouse model of human breast cancer reveals an essential role in mammary tumor induction. Cancer Cell 6:159–170

Wu S et al (2009) A human colonic commensal promotes colon tumorigenesis via activation of T helper type 17T cell responses. Nat Med 15:1016–1022

Wyckoff J et al (2004) A paracrine loop between tumor cells and macrophages is required for tumor cell migration in mammary tumors. Cancer Res 64:7022–7029

Wyckoff JB et al (2007) Direct visualization of macrophage-assisted tumor cell intravasation in mammary tumors. Cancer Res 67:2649–2656

Xu R, Boudreau A, Bissell MJ (2009) Tissue architecture and function: dynamic reciprocity via extra- and intra-cellular matrices. Cancer Metastasis Rev 28:167–176

Yu H, Pardoll D, Jove R (2009) STATs in cancer inflammation and immunity: a leading role for STAT3. Nat Rev Cancer 9:798–809

Part IV
Methods of Tumor Dissemination

Editor:
Bruno Fernandes

Chapter 11
Local Invasion

Patricia Rusa Pereira

11.1 Introduction

Tumor invasion is the hallmark of malignancy. The concept of invasion consists on translocation of tumoral cells from the primary focus into neighboring host tissues, further penetration of vessel endothelium and access to the circulation to form distant metastasis (Guarino et al. 2007). Therefore, invasion and metastases are connected comprising the major causes of morbidity and mortality related to cancer. They consist of multiple steps and complex processes, including cellular detachment and motility within the local microenvironment, degradation of the surrounding extracellular matrix, and cellular movement, all of which must be successfully completed to permit the growth of metastatic tumors in a new location (Ruan et al. 2009; Liotta et al. 1991).

Within a tumor, it is known that multiple signal-transduction pathways changes the adhesive and migratory capabilities of tumor cells, and tumor microenvironment have critical roles in forming an invasive front that is responsible for malignant tumor progression. At this stage of tumor development, tumor cells migrate into and invade the surrounding tissue either as single cells or in collective clusters (Christofori 2006).

The importance of changes in cell phenotype between epithelial and mesenchymal states, defined as epithelial–mesenchymal (EMT) and mesenchymal–epithelial (MET) transitions, has been increasingly recognized in the pathogenesis of cancer (Polyak and Weinberg 2009). The main characteristic of EMT is the disruption of intercellular contacts and the enhancement of cell motility. The resulting mesenchymal-like phenotype is suitable for migration. Although the molecular bases of EMT have not been completely elucidated, several interconnected transduction pathways and a number of potentially involved signaling molecules have been identified (Guarino et al. 2007).

P. R. Pereira (✉)
Henry C. Witelson Ocular Pathology Laboratory, McGill University, Montreal, Canada

J. V. Burnier, M. N. Burnier, Jr. (eds.), *Experimental and Clinical Metastasis*, 151
DOI 10.1007/978-1-4614-3685-0_11, © Springer Science+Business Media New York 2013

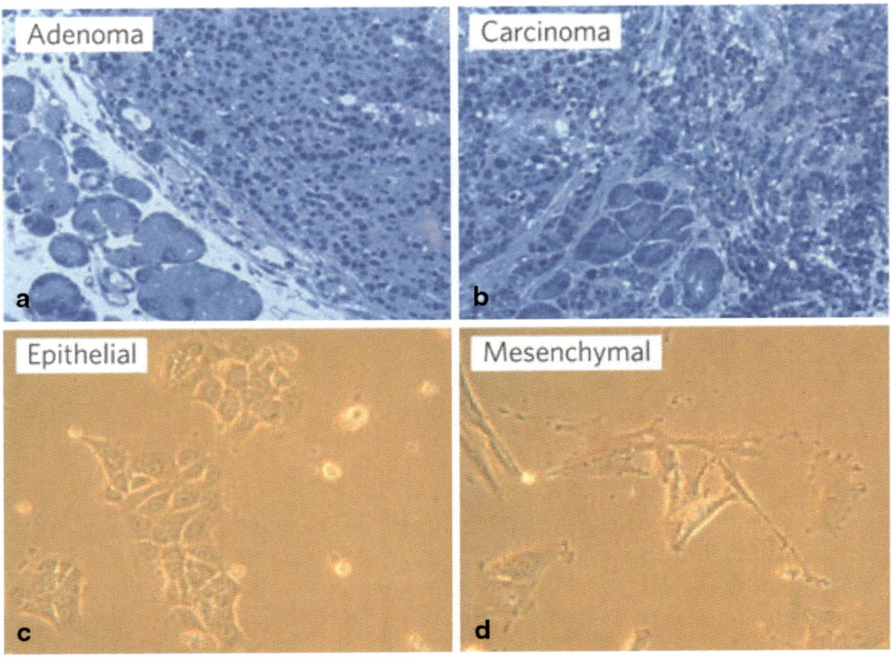

Fig. 11.1 Histopathology of tumours from a transgenic mouse model of pancreatic β-cell carcinogenesis (Rip1Tag)25. Note the differences between the epithelial organization of a benign adenoma (**a**) and the cell invasion and nuclear atypia of a malignant carcinoma (**b**) This transition coincides with partial epithelial–mesenchymal transition (EMT)—that is, loss of E-cadherin but not cytokeratin expression, and gain of N-cadherin but not vimentin expression (not shown). (**c, d**) Cultured normal murine mammary gland (NMuMG) epithelial cells express E-cadherin and grow in epithelial-like sheets. On stimulation with TGF-β, the cells undergo full EMT—that is, they change to a mesenchymal, migratory phenotype through the loss of epithelial and the gain of mesenchymal gene expression, including the cadherin switch. (Christofori, G. New signals from the invasive front. Nature 441, 444–450, doi:nature04872 [pii]10.1038/nature04872 (2006))

Also, in the hypoxic environment, tumor cells undertake a series of changes not only to survive and grow in hypoxic microenvironments but also to subsequently expand and promote invasion and metastasis (Ruan et al. 2009).

11.2 Epithelial–Mesenchymal Transition (EMT) and Invasion

It is well known that epithelial cells are tight and closely related to each other, compounding an unmovable structure. On the other hand, mesenchymal cells are loosely-associated cells with a high capability of movement. The concept of epithelial-mesenchymal transition is related to the change of the phenotype of a malignant cell (in carcinomas) and acquisition of an ability of movement. For example, at the histological level, the invasive front of a solid carcinoma differs from the more central parts by showing a less differentiated and less cohesive architecture, where invading elements appear as individual cells or groups of very few cells in intimate connection with the peritumoural stroma (Gatenby et al. 2007) (Fig. 11.1).

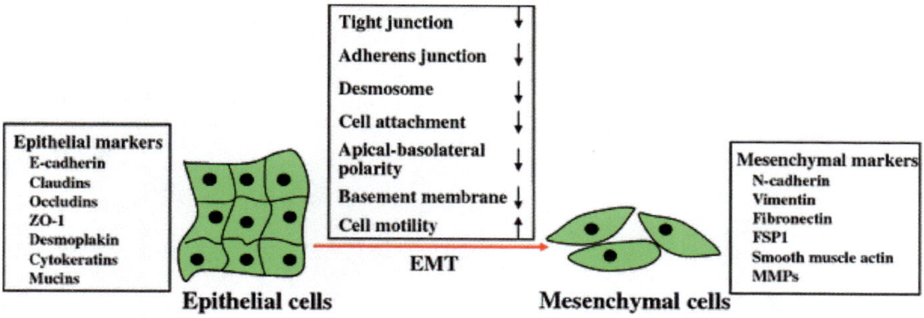

Fig. 11.2 Overview of molecular markers and cellular changes during the epithelial-mesenchymal transition (*EMT*). EMT is a well-coordinated event during embryonic development and a pathological feature in tumorigenesis. During the EMT process, epithelial cells undergo dramatic phenotypic changes, lose expression of E-cadherin and other components of epithelial cell junctions, adopt a mesenchymal cell phenotype, and acquire motility and invasive properties that allow them to migrate through the extracellular matrix. (Ouyang, G., Wang, Z., Fang, X., Liu, J. & Yang, C. J. Molecular signaling of the epithelial to mesenchymal transition in generating and maintaining cancer stem cells. Cell Mol Life Sci, doi:10.1007/s00018-010-0338-2 (2010)

EMT is a process, among other things, related to the invasiveness potential of the cell, which includes: disruption of intercellular adhesion mediated by cadherins at adherens junction, the loss of apicobasal polarity, cytoskeletal architecture reorganization, and the degradation of the basement membrane. At the end, the well-polarized, adhesive epithelial cells are converted to non-polarized mesenchymal cells (Ruan et al. 2009).

In fact, EMT is a physiological process seen in tissue morphogenesis during embryonic development and in some tissue fibrosis in response to injury (Guarino et al. 1999, 2007). Interestingly, many tumors have embryonic characteristics and it is hypothesized that EMT can be considered an embryonic feature acquired by tumor cells that enables them to metastasize. Carcinoma cells become more motile and able to invade by acquiring characteristics similar to embryonic mesenchymal cells, thereby allowing penetration of the stroma adjacent to the initial neoplastic focus (Gatenby et al. 2007).

The molecular mechanisms by which the cells acquire a mesenchymal phenotype are complex and involve multiple steps related to degradation and formation of some crucial proteins. The main type of adhesion system in epithelia is E-cadherin mediated cell-cell interaction. In turn, the mesenchymal cells are surrounded by an extracellular matrix and the adhesion system comprises an integrin-mediated cell-matrix interaction that allows the motility of single elements (Gatenby et al. 2007).

The pathways related to EMT-inducing includes TGF-b, Wnt, Notch, Hh, and other tumor microenvironmental signals via the activation of multiple EMT transcription factors such as Twist 1, Twist 2, Snail, Slug, ZEB1 and ZEB2 (Ouyang et al. 2010).

The most important molecular mechanisms involved in the tumoral invasion are summarized above (Fig. 11.2).

11.3 Invasion and Signaling Pathways

Several cellular proteins implicated in invasion and metastastic activities belong to larger families, members of which serve different activities and which may switch from one isotype to another during tumor progression (Mareel et al. 2009). On this section we will summarize only the most significant ones for invasion (Fig. 11.3).

11.3.1 TGF-β

Transforming growth factor β (TGF-β) is a multifunctional polypeptide signaling, which regulates multiple cellular processes including proliferation, apoptosis, and differentiation. It plays an important but incompletely understood role in normal and cancerous tissues (Chung et al. 2009). Actually, it has a dual role during tumour progression: as a suppressor of tumour growth during the early phases of tumorigenesis by inducing cell-cycle arrest and apoptosis; But during the late phases of carcinogenesis, it promotes EMT, tumour invasion and metastatic dissemination of tumour cells (Christofori 2006).

TGF-β signals through serine/threonine kinase receptor complexes. When activated, it regulates the transcriptional activation of various TGF-β responsive genes. In addition, TGF-β activates cellular mitogen-activated protein kinase signaling pathways, which regulate growth, survival and motility of cells. During tumorigenesis, malignantly transformed cells often lose the response to the tumor suppressive effects of TGF-β, which, in turn, starts to act as an autocrine tumor promoting factor by enhancing cancer invasion and metastasis (Nagaraj and Datta 2010). Moreover, it induces angiogenesis by upregulating the expression of angiogenic factors, such as vascular endothelial growth factor-A (VEGF-A) and angiopoietin-1 (Christofori 2006).

In breast cancer cells, a protein that belongs to the TGF-β family called bone morphogenetic protein seems to be implicated in cell growth, cell migration and invasion, and possesses both tumor suppressive and oncogenic properties in breast cancer cells (Ketolainen et al. 2010). Another *in vitro* studied showed that TGF-β signaling is transiently and locally activated in motile single cells. TGF-β1 switches cells from cohesive to single cell motility through a transcriptional program involving Smad4, EGFR, Nedd9, M-RIP, FARP and RhoC. Blockade of TGF-β signaling prevented cells moving singly *in vivo* but did not inhibit cells moving collectively. Cells restricted to collective invasion were capable of lymphatic invasion but not blood-borne metastasis (Giampieri et al. 2009).

In lung carcinoma, dysregulation of TGF-β signaling was identified as an important mediator of tumor invasion seen by microarray gene expression profiling of human tumors (Toonkel et al. 2010). Also, in prostate cancer, increased production of TGF-β causes immunosuppression, extracellular matrix degradation, EMT and angiogenesis that promotes tumor cell invasion and metastasis (Jones et al. 2009).

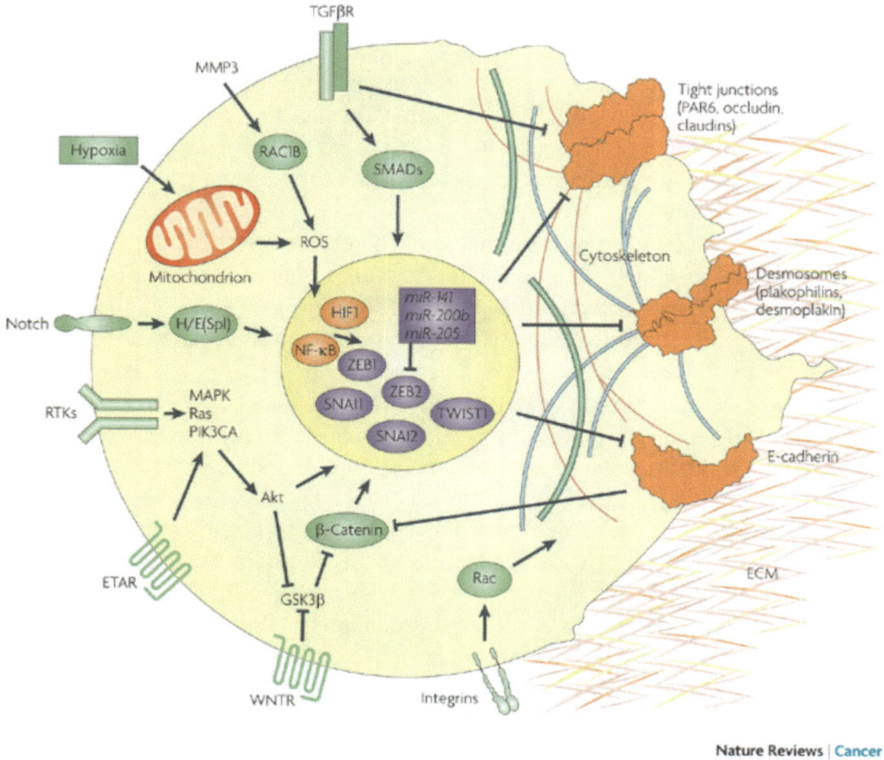

Fig. 11.3 Selected signalling pathways and some of their downstream effects and interactions are depicted. Receptor tyrosine kinases (RTKs), transforming growth factor-β (TGFβ), Notch, endothelin A receptor (ETAR), integrins, Wnt, hypoxia and matrix metalloproteinases (MMPs) can induce EMTs through multiple different signalling pathways, and the relative importance of each of these may depend on the particular cellular context. EMTs and mesenchymal–epithelial transitions (METs) are associated with dramatic changes in the cytoskeleton and extracellular matrix (ECM) composition and attachment that act together to alter cell morphology. EMT-inducing signals can lead to the disruption of tight junctions and desmosomes through protein phosphorylation (for example PAR6A phosphorylation by TGFβ signalling (Ketolainen et al. 2010)) or by repressing protein levels (for example ZEB1 represses plakophilin 3 (Ref. 83)). EMT also results in the dramatic reorganization of the ECM as many EMT-inducing factors upregulate the expression of ECM proteins (such as fibronectin and collagens), proteases (such as MMPs) and other remodelling enzymes (such as lysyl oxidase). Hypoxia, RAC1B activation and activation of certain kinase pathways (such as Akt) may lead to increased mitochondrial production of reactive oxygen species (ROS) that elicit pleiotropic effects, including activation of hypoxia-inducible factor 1α (HIF1α) and nuclear factor-κB (NF-κB) (orange circles), signalling and inactivation of glycogen synthase kinase-3β (GSK3β). Besides the interaction among the various signalling pathways, there is also extensive crosstalk among the EMT-inducing transcription factors (purple circles) and the microRNAs (miRNAs) regulating them. E-cadherin, epithelial cadherin; H/E(Spl), hairy and enhancer of split; WNTR, Wnt receptor. (Polyak, K. & Weinberg, R. A. Transitions between epithelial and mesenchymal states: acquisition of malignant and stem cell traits. Nat Rev Cancer 9, 265–273, doi:nrc2620 [pii]10.1038/nrc2620 (2009)

11.3.2 E-cadherin

E-cadherin, a single-span transmembrane glycoprotein of five repeats and cytoplasmic domain, is expressed primarily in epithelial cells. Its extracellular region has a Ca^{2+}-dependent homophilic adhesion function and the cytoplasmic domain interacts with catenins. It is a tumor suppressor protein of many tumors, including breast cancer (Baranwal and Alahari 2009).

As said, epithelial cells are attached to each other by e-cadherin mediated cell-cell interaction, sustaining an immovable structure (Gatenby et al. 2007). It has been proposed that in malignant tumors, hypermethylation can down-regulate e-cadherin allowing dissociation of cells from the primary tumor enhancing the invasive capability of cells. Subsequently, a decrease in methylation with re-expression of e-cadherin in the metastatic site would restore cell-cell adhesion allowing establishment of secondary colonization (Graff et al. 2000). Moreover, experimental studies have shown that expression of e-cadherin reduces the progressiveness and invasion of tumoral cells, as well as formation of metastasis (Kowalski et al. 2003).

In several cancers, loss of e-cadherin is accompanied by a gain in the expression of n-cadherin, in a process known as 'cadherin switch'. N-cadherin, a cadherin typically expressed in mesenchymal cells, enhances tumour cell motility and migration and exerts a dominant effect over E-cadherin function (Guarino et al. 2007). It is not a surprise that this mechanism seems to be related to the EMT of tumoral cells, in breast (Baranwal and Alahari 2009; Lester et al. 2007), prostate (Gravdal et al. 2007) and other cancers. By various mechanisms, expression of n-cadherin promotes the aggressive behavior of tumor cells, ranging from interacting with receptor tyrosine kinases at the cell surface to influencing the activation levels of Rho-GTPases in the cytosol (Baranwal and Alahari 2009).

In sporadic breast cancer, inactivation of e-cadherins is important for the cancer progression and it is completely lost in infiltrative lobular breast cancer, which suggests its function as a tumor suppressor (Baranwal and Alahari 2009). Morphologically, breast lobular carcinoma cells are more loosely infiltrative compared to others breast carcinomas. Also, abnormal expression of e-cadherins has been correlated to poor prognostic survival in patients with non-small cell lung carcinoma (Miao et al. 2009; Tseng et al. 2010; Liu et al. 2009).

In prostate cancer, loss of e-cadherin has been shown to be correlated to worse prognosis and bone metastasis (Pontes et al. 2010; Oort et al. 2007), the most common site of prostate metastatic growth. Moreover, it was demonstrated an association of the concurrent expression of unmethylated E-cadherin gene and E-cadherin protein with metastatic prostate cancer cells in bone, showing that its expression may have a role in the intercellular adhesion in the formation of metastatic lesions in bone (Saha et al. 2008).

11.3.3 Tyrosine-kinase receptors

Activation of tyrosine-kinase receptors is a molecular feature that leads to the migratory phenotype implicated in EMT/invasion. These receptors, located on the cell surface, are activated by growth factors (Eg.: EGF, FGF, HGF and IGF) that are related to cell proliferation differentiation and invasion (Guarino et al. 2007).

11.3.4 Src

Src is the prototypic member of a family of non-receptor membrane-associated tyrosine kinases including Fyn, Yes, Blk, Yrk, Fgr, Hck, Lck, and Lyn (Guarino 2010), present in several normal tissues including neurons, platelets and osteoclasts (Yeatman 2004). It translate signals from the extracellular environment into intracellular biochemical pathways that either activate nuclear factors ensuing in transcriptional responses, or target cytoplasmic components resulting in a reorganization of the cytoskeleton. Important physiological functions related to Src include cell proliferation and survival, regulation of the cytoskeleton, cell shape control, maintenance of normal intercellular contacts, cell–matrix adhesion dynamics, motility, and migration (Guarino 2010; Thomas and Brugge 1997). Src can affect cell adhesion and migration via interaction with integrins, actins, GTPase-activating proteins, scaffold proteins, such as p130(CAS) and paxillin, and kinases such as focal adhesion kinases (Kim et al. 2009). Also, Src is known to promote the expression of matrix-degrading proteases, such as metalloproteinases (MMPs), by diverse mechanisms (Guarino 2010).

It was demonstrated that in several tumors, the Src family kinases are over expressed or highly activated, and they are central mediators in multiple signaling pathways that are important in oncogenesis. Moreover, Src have a critical role in cell adhesion, invasion, proliferation, survival, and angiogenesis during tumor development. Moreover, it is involved in tumor cell proliferation and angiogenesis (Kim et al. 2009).

In prostate cancer cells, *in vitro* studies have shown that the chemopreventive bioflavonoid apigenin inhibits cell motility through decreasing the activation of Focal Adhesion Kinase/Src signaling (Franzen et al. 2009). Src has been shown to have a role in breast cancer, as a key co-regulator of Estrogen receptor-α, but further studies are necessary to define the potential diagnostic and prognostic value of this protein and as a possible therapeutic target (Gojis et al. 2010). It was also demonstrated that activation of Src in breast carcinoma is related to bone metastasis (Zhang et al. 2009).

Innumerous other signaling pathways exist regarding invasion and many of them are interlinked. For example, Tumor necrosis factor-α (TNF-α) also induces tumor cell invasion through NF-κB- and JNK-mediated upregulation of migration-inhibitor factor (MIF) in macrophages, through enhanced matrix metaloproteinases (see below) production or α2β1 integrin in tumour cells. Furthermore, TNF-α enhances the invasive property of cancer cells by inducing EMT through Snail- or ZEB1/ZEB2-dependent mechanisms (Wu and Zhou 2010).

11.4 The Relation of Hypoxia in Metastatic Signalling Pathways

As one of the most pervasive microenvironmental stresses and common features of solid tumors, hypoxia plays an important but complex role in mediating or regulating some hallmarks in the progression of human tumors from microinvasive to metastatic cancers *in vivo* (Ruan et al. 2009). Hypoxia induces cancer cells to adopt mechanisms that promote proliferation, induce or evade apoptosis, obtain unlimited replication potential and genomic instability, evade immune attack, induce angiogenesis, and invade and metastasize (Ruan et al. 2009).

Clinical studies have shown that tumor hypoxia is one of the important microenvironmental determinants for tumor cell dissemination (Ruan et al. 2009). In breast cancer, Gatenby et al. showed that adaptation to hypoxia may represent one of the key events during the transition from *in situ* to invasive breast cancer (Gatenby et al. 2007).

Hypoxia is known to activate a protein called HIF (Hypoxia Inducible Factor Protein) by regulating two major switches that converge on α subunits (Kaluz et al. 2008). In human colon carcinoma cells, hypoxia or HIF-1α over expression promotes matrigel invasion, whereas this process is inhibited by HIF-1α siRNA (Krishnamachary et al. 2003). In human pancreatic cancer cells, HIF-1α inhibition can enhance apoptosis, and restrain the invasion and metastasis (Chang et al. 2006).

It was shown that hypoxia and over expression of HIF-1 can promote EMT (see above) and metastatic phenotypes (Ruan et al. 2009; Krishnamachary et al. 2006) by upregulation of several proteins including Snail 1, Twist 1, Zeb 1 and 2 (Yang et al. 2008; Pouyssegur et al. 2006). It has been hypothesized that hypoxia within tumors, resulting in tumor necrosis, causes down regulation of E-cadherin, and ultimately sets the metastatic cascade in motion. This dysfunction of the E-cadherin–catenin complex would carry out an accumulation of β-catenin in the nucleus which is accompanied by a more invasive phenotype of tumor cells at the tumour front (Demir et al. 2009). Hypoxia may attenuate the expression of E-cadherin via activation of the lysyl oxidase (LOX)-Snail pathway, indicating that hypoxia-induced LOX and HIFs may be important factors that regulate tumor microenvironments to favor metastasis (Ruan et al. 2009).

All these data indicate that tumor hypoxia and/or HIF signaling are strongly associated with malignant progression. However, the mechanisms that result in the increased metastatic potential of tumor cells exposed to hypoxia and the exact role of HIF-1α in the metastasis still have not been well defined (Ruan et al. 2009).

Tumor hypoxia also induces tumor angiogenesis, and modulates the expression of several genes that have been implicated in tumor metastasis. For example is the hypoxic induction of c-*met* gene expression, which amplifies HGF signaling by sensitizing cells to HGF signaling. Thus, hypoxia seems to affect tumor cells in two ways: it induces angiogenesis (for instance, through hypoxia-inducible factor (HIF)-1α- and HIF-2α-driven expression of the angiogenic factor VEGF-A) and locally adapts the tumor environment for optimal tumor growth (Demir et al. 2009).

Tumor hypoxia can be now widely recognized as a cause of treatment failure and poor outcome for a wide variety of adult malignancies and, thus, needs to be taken into account when evaluating prognostic and therapeutic options for cancer patients. HIF-1 inhibition may represent a global strategy for targeting the hypoxic tumor microenvironment and there is an extensive effort involved in identifying more potent and specific HIF-1 inhibitors (Ruan et al. 2009).

11.5 Matrix Metalloproteinase (MMP) and Tumor Invasion

Degradation of the basement membrane and invasion of the underlying connective tissue by neoplastic cells are recognized as fundamental steps in the development of many epithelial cancers. Degradation of extracellular matrix (ECM) components is primarily controlled by a balance among the proteolytic enzymes called matrix metalloproteinases (MMPs) and the corresponding tissue inhibitors of MMPs (TIMPs) (Chuang et al. 2008), which are also commonly expressed in tumor sites.

Several studies suggest that MMP, a family of zinc-dependent endopeptidases, play a significant role in extracellular matrix invasion. The 23 MMPs expressed in humans are categorized by their architectural features (Kessenbrock et al. 2010). Two members of the MMP family, MMP-2 (gelatinase A, 72-kDa type IV collagenase) and MMP-9 (gelatinase B, 92-kDa type IV collagenase), are primarily responsible for invasion of the ECM and basement membrane. The expression of these gelatinases is relatively low in normal tissues and is induced when ECM remodeling is required. While gelatinase expression is primarily controlled at the transcriptional level, its activity is also regulated by post-translational factors, including proenzyme activation by membrane-type MMPs and inhibition of enzyme activity by naturally occurring TIMP (O-charoenrat et al. 2008). Because MMPs including MMP-2 are secreted as an inactive zymogen, activation is another key regulatory step for MMP function *in vivo*. The molecular environment in tumors appears conducive to MMP activation. Activated MMP-2 was specifically observed in a variety of tumor tissues, suggesting the presence of pro-MMP-2 activator(s) in tumor tissues (Sato and Takino 2010). Indeed, aberrant expression or activation of MMP-2 and MMP-9 has been reported in many different human tumors and has been linked to enhanced tumor invasion or metastasis in in vitro and in vivo model systems (O-charoenrat et al. 2008). Also, there are macrophage-derived MMP-2 and -9 that could act as tumor-associated macrophages that might contribute to intravasation of cancer cells into the blood stream (Kessenbrock et al. 2010).

Studies using high-resolution multimodal microscopy have showed the importance of ECM remodeling by another MMP member, the MMP-14-driven pericellular proteolysis, which potently modeled the tissue to facilitate single-cell and collective-cell migration and invasion (Kessenbrock et al. 2010; Wolf et al. 2007). A number of ECM degrading proteolytic enzymes, such as MMP-1, -2, -13, and -14 and cathepsins B, K, and L have been also implicated in this process; however MMP-14 may be critical and rate limiting in collagen turnover (Kessenbrock et al. 2010; Friedl and Wolf 2008).

In summary, MMPs have been implicated in cancer for more than 40 years, and the notion that MMP-mediated ECM degradation leads to cancer cell invasion and metastasis has been a guiding principle in MMP research (Kessenbrock et al. 2010). MMP has been asssociated to tumor invasion in breast (Hancox et al. 2009; Sun et al. 2009; Mizuma et al. 2008), lung (Lin et al. 2009), colorrectal (Kitamura et al. 2009), pancreatic (Han and Zhu 2010) and endometrial carcinoma (Wang et al. 2010), astroglial tumors (Lettau et al. 2010) and several other types of cancer, and diverse anti-MMP compounds are experimentally being tested as therapeutic drugs. Besides tissue invasion and intravasation, MMPs also affects growth signals, regulate apoptosis, tumor vasculature, and initiation of the neoplastic progression (Kessenbrock et al. 2010).

11.6 Contribution of the Tumor Stroma Microenvironment

In addition to the genetic, epigenetic, or somatic changes that occur in cancer, the tumor microenvironment is now considered to be a critical factor in malignant progression and metastasis, and it influences the response to conventional anti-tumor therapies (Ruan et al. 2009).

The background of the tumor microenvironment is similar to the inflammatory response in a healing wound, which promotes angiogenesis, turnover of the ECM, and tumor cell motility. Understanding the molecular mechanisms of this complex interplay between malignant cancer cells and the surrounding nonmalignant stroma represents one of the major challenges in cancer research (Kessenbrock et al. 2010).

Maintenance of epithelial tissues needs the stroma and when there is an epithelial change, the stroma also changes (Wever and Mareel 2003). The main stromal cells on this process are fibroblasts, also termed myofibroblasts or cancer-associated fibroblasts (CAFs) (Micke and Ostman 2004). In fact, the term fibroblast encompasses a number of stromal cells with a broadly similar phenotype. These cells have received increased attention because of their participation in tumor development, including invasion and metastasis (Franco et al. 2010). CAFs directly stimulate cell proliferation as they produce growth factors, hormones and cytokines such as hepatocyte growth factor, members of the epidermal growth factor, fibroblast growth factor, stromal-derived factor-1α and IL-6 (Pietras and Ostman 2010a; Kalluri and Zeisberg 2006). Moreover, CAFs are known to produce insulin-like growth factor-1 and 2, which appear to impart tumor growth by transmitting survival signals. Additionally, CAFs produces high quantities of pro-angiogenic factors, apart from VEGF-A (Pietras and Ostman 2010b).

Interestingly, in colon cancer myofibroblasts were preferentially located at the tumour–stroma border, and in invasive breast cancer, myofibroblasts were found in a much higher proportion than in *in situ* carcinomas, and predominantly at the invasive front (Micke and Ostman 2004). Moreover, it has been proposed that CAFs could be a new target of the cancer therapy, as shown in the Fig. 11.4.

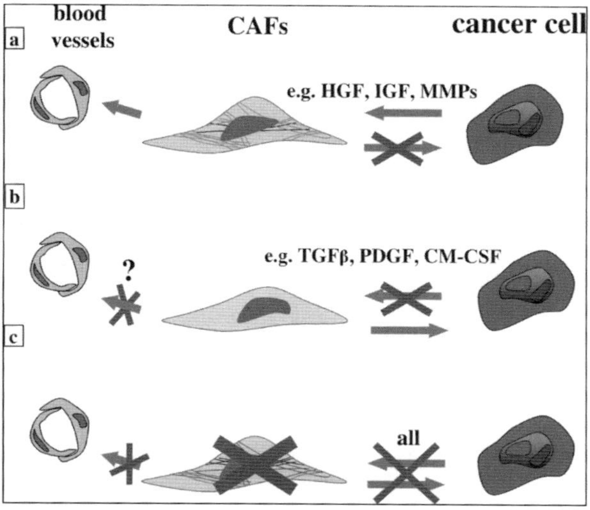

Fig. 11.4 Strategies for targeting tumour–stroma interaction. **a** Signals from CAFs that initiate or promote tumour growth, invasion and metastases can be inhibited. **b** Signals from the cancer cells that are responsible for the recruitment of CAFs can be blocked and inhibit myofibroblastic differentiation or angiogenesis. **c** CAF eradication leads to elimination of signals in both directions and additionally abolishes CAF effects on other stromal cells. (Micke and Ostman 2004)

11.7 Summary

Cancer invasion into adjacent tissue as well as vessels is a complex process mediated by diverse signaling pathways, which are usually interlinked. EMT of the cancer cells as well as degradation of the stromal proteins by MMPs are important features related to cancer invasion. The microenvironment characteristics such as hypoxia and presence of CAFs also contribute to the more invasive phenotype of cancer cells. Innumerous compounds to block these pathways are currently being studied as promising future therapies.

References

Baranwal S, Alahari SK (2009) Molecular mechanisms controlling E-cadherin expression in breast cancer. Biochem Biophys Res Commun 384:6–11

Chang Q, Qin R, Huang T, Gao J, Feng Y (2006) Effect of antisense hypoxia-inducible factor 1alpha on progression, metastasis, and chemosensitivity of pancreatic cancer. Pancreas 32:297–305

Christofori G (2006) New signals from the invasive front. Nature 441:444–450

Chuang HC et al (2008) Active matrix metalloproteinase-7 is associated with invasion in buccal squamous cell carcinoma. Mod Pathol 21:1444–1450

Chung SW et al (2009) Quantitative modeling and analysis of the transforming growth factor beta signaling pathway. Biophys J 96:1733–1750

De Wever O, Mareel M (2003) Role of tissue stroma in cancer cell invasion. J Pathol 200:429–447

Demir R et al (2009) Malignant progression of invasive tumour cells seen in hypoxia present an accumulation of beta-catenin in the nucleus at the tumour front. Exp Mol Pathol 87:109–116

Franco OE, Shaw AK, Strand DW, Hayward SW (2010) Cancer associated fibroblasts in cancer pathogenesis. Semin Cell Dev Biol 21:33–39

Franzen CA et al (2009) The chemopreventive bioflavonoid apigenin inhibits prostate cancer cell motility through the focal adhesion kinase/Src signaling mechanism. Cancer Prev Res (Phila Pa) 2:830–841

Friedl P, Wolf K (2008) Tube travel: the role of proteases in individual and collective cancer cell invasion. Cancer Res 68:7247–7249

Gatenby RA et al (2007) Cellular adaptations to hypoxia and acidosis during somatic evolution of breast cancer. Br J Cancer 97:646–653

Giampieri S et al (2009) Localized and reversible TGFbeta signalling switches breast cancer cells from cohesive to single cell motility. Nat Cell Biol 11:1287–1296

Gojis O et al (2010) The role of SRC-3 in human breast cancer. Nat Rev Clin Oncol 7:83–89

Graff JR, Gabrielson E, Fujii H, Baylin SB, Herman JG (2000) Methylation patterns of the E-cadherin 5' CpG island are unstable and reflect the dynamic, heterogeneous loss of E-cadherin expression during metastatic progression. J Biol Chem 275:2727–2732

Gravdal K, Halvorsen OJ, Haukaas SA, Akslen LA (2007) A switch from E-cadherin to N-cadherin expression indicates epithelial to mesenchymal transition and is of strong and independent importance for the progress of prostate cancer. Clin Cancer Res 13:7003–7011

Guarino M (2010) Src signaling in cancer invasion. J Cell Physiol 223:14–26

Guarino M, Micheli P, Pallotti F, Giordano F (1999) Pathological relevance of epithelial and mesenchymal phenotype plasticity. Pathol Res Pract 195:379–389

Guarino M, Rubino B, Ballabio G (2007) The role of epithelial-mesenchymal transition in cancer pathology. Pathology 39:305–318

Han F, Zhu HG (2010) Caveolin-1 regulating the invasion and expression of matrix metalloproteinase (MMPs) in pancreatic carcinoma cells. J Surg Res 159:443–450

Hancox RA et al (2009) Tumour-associated tenascin-C isoforms promote breast cancer cell invasion and growth by matrix metalloproteinase-dependent and independent mechanisms. Breast Cancer Res 11:R24

Jones E, Pu H, Kyprianou N (2009) Targeting TGF-beta in prostate cancer: therapeutic possibilities during tumor progression. Expert Opin Ther Targets 13:227–234

Kalluri R, Zeisberg M (2006) Fibroblasts in cancer. Nat Rev Cancer 6:392–401

Kaluz S, Kaluzova M, Stanbridge EJ (2008) Does inhibition of degradation of hypoxia-inducible factor (HIF) alpha always lead to activation of HIF? Lessons learnt from the effect of proteasomal inhibition on HIF activity. J Cell Biochem 104:536–544

Kessenbrock K, Plaks V, Werb Z (2010) Matrix metalloproteinases: regulators of the tumor microenvironment. Cell 141:52–67

Ketolainen JM, Alarmo EL, Tuominen VJ, Kallioniemi A (2010) Parallel inhibition of cell growth and induction of cell migration and invasion in breast cancer cells by bone morphogenetic protein 4. Breast Cancer Res Treat

Kim LC, Song L, Haura EB (2009) Src kinases as therapeutic targets for cancer. Nat Rev Clin Oncol 6:587–595

Kitamura T, Biyajima K, Aoki M, Oshima M, Taketo MM (2009) Matrix metalloproteinase 7 is required for tumor formation, but dispensable for invasion and fibrosis in SMAD4-deficient intestinal adenocarcinomas. Lab Invest 89:98–105

Kowalski PJ, Rubin MA, Kleer CG (2003) E-cadherin expression in primary carcinomas of the breast and its distant metastases. Breast Cancer Res 5:R217–222

Krishnamachary B et al (2003) Regulation of colon carcinoma cell invasion by hypoxia-inducible factor 1. Cancer Res 63:1138–1143

Krishnamachary B et al (2006) Hypoxia-inducible factor-1-dependent repression of E-cadherin in von Hippel-Lindau tumor suppressor-null renal cell carcinoma mediated by TCF3, ZFHX1A, and ZFHX1B. Cancer Res 66:2725–2731

Lester RD, Jo M, Montel V, Takimoto S, Gonias SL (2007) uPAR induces epithelial-mesenchymal transition in hypoxic breast cancer cells. J Cell Biol 178:425–436

Lettau I et al (2010) Matrix metalloproteinase-19 is highly expressed in astroglial tumors and promotes invasion of glioma cells. J Neuropathol Exp Neurol 69:215–223

Lin SS et al (2009) Curcumin inhibits the migration and invasion of human A549 lung cancer cells through the inhibition of matrix metalloproteinase-2 and −9 and Vascular Endothelial Growth Factor (VEGF). Cancer Lett 285:127–133

Liotta LA, Steeg PS, Stetler-Stevenson WG (1991) Cancer metastasis and angiogenesis: an imbalance of positive and negative regulation. Cell 64:327–336

Liu Y et al (2009) Abnormal expression of p120-catenin, E-cadherin, and small GTPases is significantly associated with malignant phenotype of human lung cancer. Lung Cancer 63:375–382

Mareel M, Oliveira MJ, Madani I (2009) Cancer invasion and metastasis: interacting ecosystems. Virchows Arch 454:599–622

Miao Y et al (2009) p120ctn isoform 1 expression significantly correlates with abnormal expression of E-cadherin and poor survival of lung cancer patients. Med Oncol

Micke P, Ostman A (2004) Tumour-stroma interaction: cancer-associated fibroblasts as novel targets in anti-cancer therapy? Lung Cancer 45(Suppl 2):S163–175

Mizuma M et al (2008) Up-regulated p27Kip1 reduces matrix metalloproteinase-9 and inhibits invasion of human breast cancer cells. Anticancer Res 28:2669–2677

Nagaraj NS, Datta PK (2010) Targeting the transforming growth factor-beta signaling pathway in human cancer. Expert Opin Investig Drugs 19:77–91

O-charoenrat P et al (2008) SCCRO (DCUN1D1) induces extracellular matrix invasion by activating matrix metalloproteinase 2. Clin Cancer Res 14:6780–6789

Ouyang G, Wang Z, Fang X, Liu J, Yang CJ (2010) Molecular signaling of the epithelial to mesenchymal transition in generating and maintaining cancer stem cells. Cell Mol Life Sci 67:2605–2618

Pietras K, Ostman A (2010a) Hallmarks of cancer: Interactions with the tumor stroma. Exp Cell Res

Pietras K, Ostman A (2010b) Hallmarks of cancer: Interactions with the tumor stroma. Exp Cell Res 316:1324–1331

Polyak K, Weinberg RA (2009) Transitions between epithelial and mesenchymal states: acquisition of malignant and stem cell traits. Nat Rev Cancer 9:265–273

Pontes J Jr et al (2010) E-cadherin and beta-catenin loss of expression related to bone metastasis in prostate cancer. Appl Immunohistochem Mol Morphol 18:179–184

Pouyssegur J, Dayan F, Mazure NM (2006) Hypoxia signalling in cancer and approaches to enforce tumour regression. Nature 441:437–443

Ruan K, Song G, Ouyang G (2009) Role of hypoxia in the hallmarks of human cancer. J Cell Biochem 107:1053–1062

Saha B et al (2008) Unmethylated E-cadherin gene expression is significantly associated with metastatic human prostate cancer cells in bone. Prostate 68:1681–1688

Sato H, Takino T (2010) Coordinate action of membrane-type matrix metalloproteinase—1 (MT1-MMP) and MMP-2 enhances pericellular proteolysis and invasion. Cancer Sci

Sun Y et al (2009) Oroxylin A suppresses invasion through down-regulating the expression of matrix metalloproteinase-2/9 in MDA-MB-435 human breast cancer cells. Eur J Pharmacol 603:22–28

Thomas SM, Brugge JS (1997) Cellular functions regulated by Src family kinases. Annu Rev Cell Dev Biol 13:513–609

Toonkel RL, Borczuk AC, Powell CA (2010) Tgf-beta signaling pathway in lung adenocarcinoma invasion. J Thorac Oncol 5:153–157

Tseng RC et al (2010) SLIT2 attenuation during lung cancer progression deregulates beta-catenin and E-cadherin and associates with poor prognosis. Cancer Res 70:543–551

van Oort IM et al (2007) The prognostic value of E-cadherin and the cadherin-associated molecules alpha-, beta-, gamma-catenin and p120ctn in prostate cancer specific survival: a long-term follow-up study. Prostate 67:1432–1438

Wang FQ et al (2010) Lysophosphatidic acid (LPA) effects on endometrial carcinoma in vitro proliferation, invasion, and matrix metalloproteinase activity. Gynecol Oncol 117:88–95

Wolf K et al (2007) Multi-step pericellular proteolysis controls the transition from individual to collective cancer cell invasion. Nat Cell Biol 9:893–904

Wu Y, Zhou BP (2010) TNF-alpha/NF-kappaB/Snail pathway in cancer cell migration and invasion. Br J Cancer 102:639–644

Yang MH et al (2008) Direct regulation of TWIST by HIF-1alpha promotes metastasis. Nat Cell Biol 10:295–305

Yeatman TJ (2004) A renaissance for SRC. Nat Rev Cancer 4:470–480

Zhang XH et al (2009) Latent bone metastasis in breast cancer tied to Src-dependent survival signals. Cancer Cell 16:67–78

Chapter 12
Lymphatic Dissemination

Alexandre Nakao Odashiro

12.1 Introduction

Lymphatics compose the second vascular system found in higher vertebrates in addition to the blood vasculature. It has several vital functions including the regulation of tissue pressure, immune surveillance and the absorption of dietary fat in the intestine (Cueni and Detmar 2008).

The lymphatic vasculature is considered an important route of tumoral spread, as metastatic spread to lymph nodes is an early and common event in human cancer, especially carcinomas (Achen and Stacker 2008), and has gained the attention of the research community. Metastases can be detected in draining lymph nodes before they are detected in distant organs, and for most tumors, the clinical record suggests that lymph node metastases progress to distant metastases (Leong et al. 2006).

In fact, lymph node metastasis is of major prognostic significance for many types of cancer, although lymph node metastases are themselves rarely life-threatening (Sleeman and Thiele 2009). This importance led to the development of techniques to discern the sentinel lymph node (SLN). Currently, these techniques are used in the clinical practice in several tumors including breast carcinoma (Harris et al. 1992) and melanoma (Balch et al. 2001).

For a long time, it has been demonstrated no survival difference between patients who undergo regional node dissection and those who undergo more conservative dissections or no dissection at all, for melanoma, head and neck cancers, gastric, colorectal cancers, and particularly breast cancers. Thus, the purpose of a sentinel node biopsy or regional node dissection was not to improve survival, but to collect diagnostic and prognostic information to help select systemic therapy to improve prognosis (Leong et al. 2006).

Lymphatic metastasis was previously thought to be a passive process by which detached tumor cells enter lymph nodes via pre-existing lymphatic vessels in the

A. N. Odashiro (✉)
Département de Pathologie & Cytologie du Centre Hospitalier,
Affilié universitaire de Québec (CHA) Hôpital l'Enfant-Jésus,
local C-1210 1401 18e rue, Québec, QC G1J 1Z4, Canada

J. V. Burnier, M. N. Burnier, Jr. (eds.), *Experimental and Clinical Metastasis*, 165
DOI 10.1007/978-1-4614-3685-0_12,

vicinity of a primary tumor (Achen and Stacker 2008; Pepper 2001). This process would be facilitated by the thin walls and incomplete basement membrane of lymphatics (Achen and Stacker 2008; Swartz and Skobe 2001). Moreover, the main function of the lymphatic system is to collect interstitial fluid from peripheral tissues and to return it to the blood circulation. Therefore, tumor-associated lymphatic vessels can drain interstitial fluid containing tumor cells and tumor-derived proteins away from the tumor into the lymphatics and then to the lymph node that drains the tissue (Sleeman et al. 2009). In head and neck carcinoma, for example, some studies have showed a significant correlation between intratumoral lymphatic density and increased metastatic potential towards regional lymph nodes (Maula et al. 2003). But others did not find such correlation and also no differences in survival rates (Maula et al. 2003; Franchi et al. 2004; Munoz-Guerra et al. 2004).

Clinical and experimental data suggest that migration of tumor cells into the lymph nodes is greatly facilitated by lymphangiogenesis, a process that generates new lymphatic vessels from pre-existing lymphatics (Ran et al. 2009), both locally and in regional lymph nodes (Sleeman and Thiele 2009). Nevertheless, the importance of lymphangiogenesis in metastasis may vary, depending on parameters such as the tumor type, and the position of the primary tumor relative to the lymphatic network (Achen and Stacker 2008). Pathways involved in lymphangiogenesis and molecular control of lymphatic metastasis have been studied and described, and some receptors of the Vascular Endothelial Growth Factors (VEGFs) family seem to be the most relevant to this process (Achen and Stacker 2008; Ran et al. 2009).

12.2 Brief Histology and Anatomy of the Lymphatics and Sentinel Lymph node

Lymphatic capillaries start blind-ended in the tissue, where they take up lymph. They are lined by a single layer of overlapping endothelial cells and lack a continuous basement membrane as well as pericyte or smooth muscle cell coverage (Cueni and Detmar 2008). This architecture is related to their function in absorbing interstitial fluid and allowing immune cells to traffic, which makes them intrinsically more amenable to the entry of invasive tumor cells in comparison to blood vessels (Sleeman and Thiele 2009). Via larger collecting lymphatic vessels and ultimately the thoracic duct, the lymph returns to the blood vasculature through the lymphatic-venous connections at the junction of the jugular and subclavian veins. Lymphatic capillaries are present in almost all tissues, except for avascular structures such as epidermis, hair, nails, cartilage and cornea, and some vascularized organs including the brain and the intraocular tissue. Together with lymphatic capillaries, other structures comprise the lymphatic system, such as lymph nodes, thymus, tonsils, spleen and Peyer's patches. They are essential for the immune function of the lymphatic system (Cueni and Detmar 2008). Not only the lymphatic vessels, but also the lymph nodes are remarkably related to tumors and their dissemination.

Metastasis is known to be responsible directly or indirectly for more than 90 % of all cancer deaths, and lymph node are often the first organs in which metastasis occur (Sleeman and Thiele 2009). For the majority types of carcinoma, the presence of lymph node metastasis is the most important predictor of poor prognosis and form the basis for staging schemes in many tumors (Balch et al. 2001; Compton et al. 2000; Yarbro et al. 1999).

Compared with blood vessels, a lymphatic vessel offers many advantages for invasion and transport of malignant cells, such as: (1) discontinuous basement membrane and loose cell–cell junctions; (2) a much lower flow rate that increases survival by minimizing shear stress; and (3) a 1000-fold higher lymph concentration of hyaluronic acid, a molecule with potent cell-protecting and pro-survival properties (Ran et al. 2009; Laurent et al. 1992).

Azzali et al. (2006) called attention to the term tumor-associated absorbing lymphatic (TAAL) vessel, that is the lymphatic vessel associated with a tumor. It has the same ultrastructural characteristics as the absorbing lymphatic vessel in normal organs. However, they demonstrated the transendothelial passage of tumor cells into the TAAL vessel lumen, which takes place by means of the intraendothelial channel ($\sim$ 1.8–2.1 μm in diameter and 6.8–7.2 μm in length). This channel is to be considered a transient morphological entity organized by TAAL vessel endothelium by means of still unidentified molecular mechanisms.

Usually, the lymphatic fluid from peripheral tissues is channeled into lymphatic vessels that drain into one (or occasionally more) lymph node (Sleeman et al. 2009). The SLN is defined as the first node in the lymphatic basin that drains the location in which the primary tumor is. Therefore, the status (compromised or not by tumoral cells) of the SLN(s) accurately reflects the status of the entire basin. In other words, if the SLN is not involved with metastatic disease, the remainder of the lymph nodes should also be negative (Moroi et al. 2009).

Analysis of the SLN for the presence of metastases is highly prognostically significant. Nowadays, intra-operative analysis of the SLN as a means of determining appropriate clinical treatments is widely used clinically as a means of determining future therapy regimes for a variety of cancers (Sleeman et al. 2009) including breast (de Boer et al. 2010; Salem 2009; Iwase et al. 2009) and melanoma (Pasquali et al. 2010; Uhara et al. 2009; van Akkooi et al. 2009). The use of SLN biopsy in breast carcinoma increased dramatically from 1998 and decreased the proportion of women (particularly older women) who received no axillary surgery (Rescigno et al. 2009). However, some studies of cutaneous melanoma demonstrated that there are some patients with histologically negative SNL that develops recurrence during follow-up (De Giorgi et al. 2007).

Histologic parameters of SLN metastases have been assessed to predict which SLN-positive patients are likely to have tumor in regional non-SLNs. They include the size of metastases, tumor penetrative depth, also known as maximal subcapsular depth and centripetal thickness), the location of SLN tumor deposits in the SLN, the percentage cross-sectional area of the SLN involved, and the presence of extracapsular spread (Murali et al. 2009).

In fact, within the lymph node, malignant metastatic cells initially arrive in the subcapsular sinuses through an afferent capsular lymph vessel. Later, there is subcapsular spread of malignant cells in the marginal sinuses and into the immediately adjacent cortical parenchyma. Finally, these cells infiltrate the deeper zones of the lymph node parenchyma, frequently following the medullary sinuses and eventually reaching the efferent lymphatics (Starz et al. 2001; Govindarajan et al. 2007).

12.3 Intratumoral Versus Peritumoral Lymphatic Vessels and Lymphatic Vessel Density

Several tumors show proliferation of intratumoral lymphatic vessels which has been implicated in worse prognosis and increased metastatic potential in melanoma (Dadras et al. 2003), colon (Wang et al. 2005), prostate carcinoma (Zeng et al. 2005), and head and neck carcinomas (Maula et al. 2003). However, it has been proposed that intratumoral lymphatics are not able to transport tumor cells because the elevated hydrostatic pressure within a tumor that may compress these vessels (Padera et al. 2002; Shayan et al. 2006).

On the other hand, peritumoral lymphatics are the vessels located adjacent to the tumor and may represent pre-existing vessels compressed by the tumoral mass (Shayan et al. 2006). Some studies suggests that these vessels can also arise due to lymphangiogenesis and were correlated to poor prognosis in malignant melanoma (Shayan et al. 2006; Valencak et al. 2004), non-small lung cancer (Renyi-Vamos et al. 2005), breast carcinoma (Schoppmann et al. 2004), gastric carcinoma (Kitadai et al. 2005) and others.

Although the relative importance of intratumoral versus peritumoral lymphatics for metastatic spread remains a subject of debate, it is a consensus that the lymphatic vessels associated with a tumor can be important for metastasis and patient outcome (Shayan et al. 2006). Several studies of different cancer types have found correlations between lymphatic vessel density (LVD) and lymphatic metastases and overall survival, suggesting that LVD contains important information about the degree of tumor lymphatic vasculature. In breast carcinoma, for example, studies showed a significant correlation among higher LVD, lymph node metastasis, and high TNM clinical stage (Gu et al. 2008). Also, it was shown that LVD correlates with bad outcome in patients with head and neck squamous carcinoma (Kyzas et al. 2005), lung cancer (Renyi-Vamos et al. 2005), colorectal cancer (Matsumoto et al. 2007), skin squamous carcinoma (Sedivy et al. 2003), prostate cancer (Zeng et al. 2005) and urothelial carcinoma (Bolenz et al. 2009). Nevertheless, the role of LVD in the prognosis in prostate cancer is still a matter of debate (Bolenz et al. 2009).

It has been proposed that the target vessels for invasion by lymph-metastasizing tumor cells include preexisting tissue lymphatics abutting the tumor mass either through coincidence or mutual chemoattraction, as well as new lymphatic vessels that proliferate either within or around the tumor as a result of lymphangiogenesis (Clasper et al. 2008).

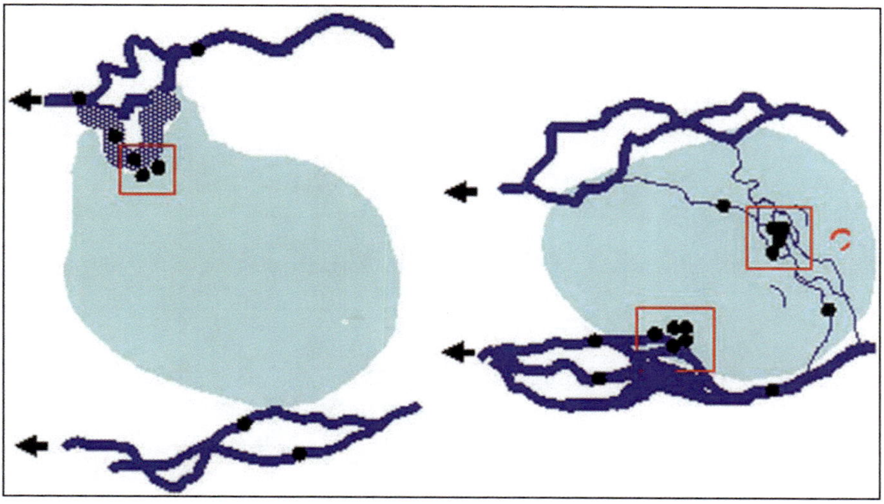

Fig. 12.1 In the first mode (*left panel*) the tumor induces proliferation of pre-existing peritumoral vessels (*stippled shading*), leading to invasion by tumor cells (*filled black circles*) detaching from the main tumor mass. In the second mode (*right panel*), tumor or host-derived factors induce lymph vessel proliferation within the tumor body (intratumoral lymphangiogenesis), leading to invasion by tumor cells (*filled black circles*) deeper within the tumor. However, both modes may operate as shown, and are not mutually exclusive. Arrows indicate the direction of lymph flow (Witte et al. 2006)

Witte et al demonstrated by scheme the two alternative models to explain tumor metastasis via the lymphatics (Witte et al. 2006) (Fig. 12.1).

12.4 Lymphangiogenesis

To date, there is great debate about whether cancer cells can metastasize by expansion and invasion of pre-existing peritumoral lymphatics, or by the formation and invasion of new lymphatics within tumours. Lymphangiogenesis is a mechanism in which lymphatic vessels arise from a pre-existing lymphatic vessel (Mandriota et al. 2001). Evidence of lymphangiogenesis was reported by some studies in melanoma (Rinderknecht and Detmar 2008), head and neck squamous cell (Kyzas et al. 2005), breast carcinoma (Gu et al. 2008) and others cancers (Amioka et al. 2002). Surprisingly, even uveal melanoma, a tumor known to have no relationship to lymphatics as the intraocular environment is devoid of those vessels, has been demonstrated to have lymphangiogenesis when there is extraocular extension. Moreover, this lymphangiogenesis seems to be correlated to poor prognosis (Amioka et al. 2002; Heindl et al. 2010; Heindl et al. 2009).

But the mechanisms of lymphatic invasion and metastasis to regional lymph nodes are not completely known (Massi et al. 2009) for many tumors. Lymphangiogenesis

Table 12.1 Molecules that have been used as markers for lymphatic endothelium. (Witte et al. 2006)

VEGFR-3	Tyrosine kinase receptor for VEGF-C/VEGF-D
Podoplanin (T1á/E11)	Integral membrane sialomucoprotein
Prox-1	Homeobox domain transcription factor
D-6	Endocytic 7 TM receptor for CC chemokines
LYVE-1	Sialoglycoprotein receptor for hyaluronan
Neuropilin-2	Co-receptor for VEGFs and ligand for semaphorins involved in axonal guidance
CCL-21 (Secondary Lymphoid Chemokine)	Chemoattractant for migration of dendritic cells in lymphatic channels

is not exclusively associated with malignancies or metastatic dissemination, but also with several pathological conditions, such as chronic inflammation in Crohn's disease (Pedica et al. 2008), psoriasis (Henno et al. 2009), renal (Kerjaschki et al. 2004) and corneal graft rejection (Dietrich et al. 2010).

In contrast to Angiogenesis, the growth of blood vessels, lymphangiogenesis has received trivial attention over the past few decades. However, our knowledge of the molecular mechanisms controlling lymphangiogenesis has improved considerably over the past few years, mainly thanks to progress in the identification of regulatory molecules and markers specific to the lymphatic endothelium. The genetic programs that determine lymphatic endothelial cell (LEC) differentiation and growth, and make them distinct from blood vessels, involve a number of newly described signal transduction pathways (Tammela et al. 2010).

Several markers have been used to identify the lymphatic endothelium. Since the late 1990s, lymphatic vessel endothelial hyaluronan receptor-1 (LYVE-1), a CD44 homologue protein involved in hyaluronan and immune cell transport, has been used to identify lymphatics vessels subtypes (Prevo et al. 2001). Podoplanin is a mucin-type transmembrane glycoprotein (Shayan et al. 2006) that was originally identified as a podocyte membrane protein in the renal corpuscle and was found to be specific for the lymphatic endothelium. Its expression is found specifically in the lymphatic endothelium in many organs, including the skin, kidney, and lung of normal individuals (Gu et al. 2008, Britto et al. 2009). D2-40 is a relative new marker to detect lymphatic vessels (Britto et al. 2009). It is a monoclonal antibody to a Mr 40,000 O-linked sialoglycoprotein expressed in normal lymphatic endothelium, and is reported to be highly sensitive for lymphatic endothelium, compared with other lymphatic endothelial specific antibodies, such as LYVE-1, podoplanin, and the homeobox transcription factor Prox1 (Lee et al. 2010; Hong et al. 2002). All these markers can be tested by immunohistochemistry. VEGFR-3 is another marker that was used to characterize lymphatic vessels, however, it was shown to be expressed also on blood vessels in tumors and wound granulation tissue (Shayan et al. 2006). There are other several proteins studied to identify lymphatic channels summarized in Tab. 12.1, but it is beyond the scope to this chapter to describe all of them.

The molecular mechanisms related to lymphangiogenesis are complex and the VEGF family seems to be the most important mediator to lymphangiogenesis. The

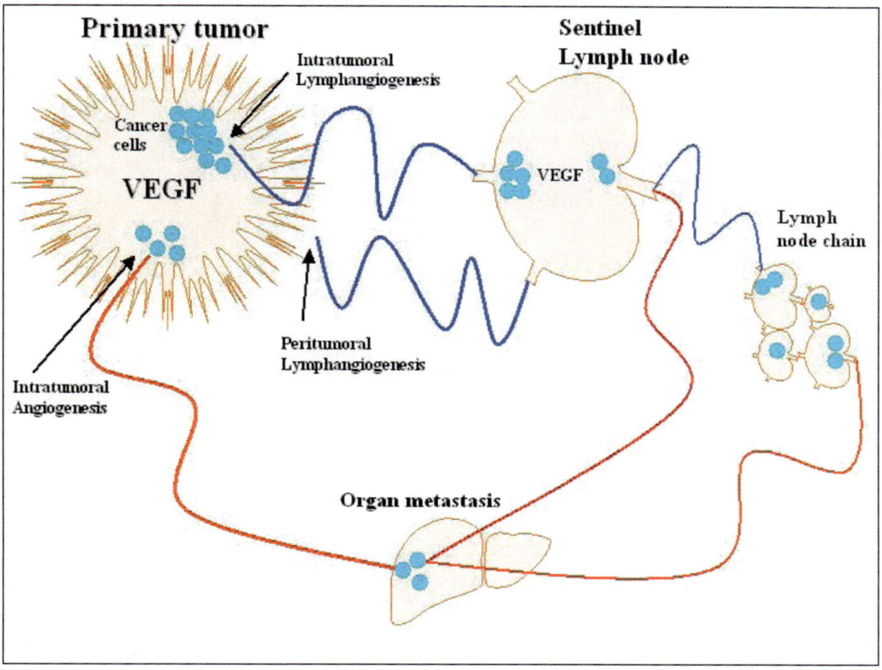

Fig. 12.2 Tumoral cells produce VEGF that induce lymphangiogenesis at the primary tumor. Once the tumoral cells have spread to sentinel lymph node, VEGF continues to be produced at the new site therefore maintaining the lymphangiogenic activity, facilitating the cells to spread to distant lymph nodes as well as to distant organs. (Cueni and Detmar 2008 #1)

best studied lymphangiogenic signaling system in cancer is the VEGF-C/VEGF-D/VEGFR-3 signaling axis in which the secreted lymphangiogenic growth factors VEGF-C or VEGF-D activate VEGFR-3, a cell surface receptor tyrosine kinase expressed on lymphatic endothelium, leading to proliferation of LECs, growth of lymphatic vessels and, potentially effects expression of molecules by LECs (Achen and Stacker 2006). In fact, the VEGF-C/VEGFR-3 signaling has been suggested to play a role in maintenance of the lymphatic endothelium or lymphangiogenesis (Scavelli et al. 2004). Therefore, this group of enzymes is very important to the tumorigenicity of cancers which secrete these growth factors (Shayan et al. 2006). In These lymphangiogenic factors are commonly expressed in malignant, tumor-infiltrating and stromal cells, creating a favorable environment for generation of new lymphatic vessels (Ran et al. 2009) (Fig. 12.2).

In gastric carcinoma, for example, VEGF-C expression was significantly higher in patients with positive lymph nodes (Amioka et al. 2002; Aurello et al. 2009; Kitadai et al. 2010). Also, VEGFR-3 expression has been associated with poor prognosis in colorectal carcinoma (Witte et al. 2002), non-small cell lung carcinoma (Donnem et al. 2009b, 2010), breast carcinoma (Gu et al. 2008) as well as with different stages of cervical carcinoma (Van Trappen et al. 2003). However, a meta-analysis showed no correlation of expression of VEGFC and VEGFR-3 with survival in patients with non-small cell lung carcinoma (Zhan et al. 2009).

Although VEGF-A is more related to angiogenesis, VEGF-A expression has also been correlated with lymph node metastasis in non-small cell lung carcinoma (Donnem et al. 2009a). VEGF-A induces active proliferation of VEGFR-2-expressing tumor-associated lymphatic vessels as well as metastastic dissemination to lymph nodes in transgenic mice (Hirakawa et al. 2005). Furthermore, primary tumors that overexpress VEGF-A induce lymphangiogenesis in the SLN prior to the actual nodal metastasis (Donnem et al. 2009a).

Nitric oxide (NO) is a diatomic free radical molecule synthesized from L-arginine by NO synthases that plays a critical role in various physiological and pathological processes, including tumor growth (Massi et al. 2009). It upregulates VEGF and Basic Fibroblastic Growth Factor being an important mediator of tumor angiogenesis (Ohhashi et al. 2005) NO is also produced and released by LECs and physiologically regulates lymphatic permeability and flow by modulating active lymph pump activity (Ohhashi et al. 2005). It has been demonstrated that NO mediates VEGF-C induced lymphangiogenesis and, consequently, plays a critical role in lymphatic metastasis (Lahdenranta et al. 2009). In squamous cell carcinoma of the head and neck, VEGF-C has been correlated to lymphangiogenesis and lymph node metastasis (Franchi et al. 2006). Also, it may play a hole in lymphangiogenesis in melanoma (Massi et al. 2009).

Recent studies have provided evidence that stromal cells are also important for lymphangiogenesis, as they are capable of secreting many potential lymphangiogenic factors, like hyaluronan, that possibly lead to *de novo* formation of lymphatic vessels. Therefore, lymphangiogenesis would be governed by interactions between tumor cells and stromal components (Koyama et al. 2008). Albeit interesting and promising, more studies are necessary to precisely determine this interaction.

Garmy-Susini et al. (2010) showed that integrin α4β1 and the signals it transduces regulate the adhesion, migration, invasion, and survival of proliferating LEC. Moreover, suppression of α4β1expression, signal transduction, or function in tumor lymphatic endothelium inhibits tumor lymphangiogenesis and further prevents metastatic disease. These results show that integrin α4β1-mediated tumor lymphangiogenesis promotes metastasis and is a useful target for the suppression of metastatic disease.

Also recently, the identification of genes selectively expressed in tumor lymphatics represents a major step toward identifying biomarkers for metastasis and for elucidating the mechanisms by which tumors invade the microvasculature and spread to lymph nodes (Clasper et al. 2008). Interesting, in tumoral LEC, there are approximately 800 genes are up or downregulated by a factor of twofold or greater in tumor as compared with normal LEC, and several of these have functions related to extracellular matrix and cell adhesion. Considerable changes in tumor LEC gene expression may therefore be induced either by the tumor environment or by growth-factor-induced proliferation, and the potential consequences of these changes for tumor invasion are truly fascinating (Witte et al. 2006).

It has been proposed that lymphangiogenesis in the lymph node may play a role in augmenting the metastatic spread of tumors in cancer patients. Metastatic tumors that overexpress VEGF-A or VEGF-C also induced new lymphatic vessel growth within the regional lymph nodes, probably contributing to enhanced distant lymph node metastasis. Moreover, primary tumors in the skin induced lymph node lymphangiogenesis even before they metastasized, thereby preparing the "lymphvascular niche", a tumor-conditioned microenvironment that serves as a future metastatic site within the regional lymph node (Hirakawa et al. 2009).

12.5 Summary

Lymphatic metastasis is an early and common event in most types of cancer, especially in carcinomas. Lymphatic vessels were seldom studied till the establishment of markers specific to lymphatic vessels some years ago. Lymphangiogenesis seems to be an important mechanism involving several signaling pathways that enable or enhances lymphatic metastases.

References

Achen MG, Stacker SA (2006) Tumor lymphangiogenesis and metastatic spread-new players begin to emerge. Int J Cancer 119:1755–1760

Achen MG, Stacker SA (2008) Molecular control of lymphatic metastasis. Ann N Y Acad Sci 1131:225–234

Amioka T et al (2002) Vascular endothelial growth factor-C expression predicts lymph node metastasis of human gastric carcinomas invading the submucosa. Eur J Cancer 38:1413–1419

Aurello P et al (2009) Vascular endothelial growth factor C and microvessel density in gastric carcinoma: Correlation with clinicopathological factors. Our experience and review of the literature. Oncol Res 17:405–411

Azzali G (2006) On the transendothelial passage of tumor cell from extravasal matrix into the lumen of absorbing lymphatic vessel. Microvasc Res 72:74–85

Balch CM et al (2001) Final version of the American Joint Committee on Cancer staging system for cutaneous melanoma. J Clin Oncol 19:3635–3648

Bolenz C et al (2009) The role of lymphangiogenesis in lymphatic tumour spread of urological cancers. BJU Int 104:592–597

Britto AV et al (2009) Immunostaining with D2–40 improves evaluation of lymphovascular invasion, but may not predict sentinel lymph node status in early breast cancer. BMC Cancer 9:109

Clasper S et al (2008) A novel gene expression profile in lymphatics associated with tumor growth and nodal metastasis. Cancer Res 68:7293–7303

Compton C, Fenoglio-Preiser CM, Pettigrew N, Fielding LP (2000) American Joint Committee on Cancer Prognostic Factors Consensus Conference: Colorectal Working Group. Cancer 88:1739–1757

Cueni LN, Detmar M (2008) The lymphatic system in health and disease. Lymphat Res Biol 6:109–122

Dadras SS et al (2003) Tumor lymphangiogenesis: A novel prognostic indicator for cutaneous melanoma metastasis and survival. Am J Pathol 162:1951–1960 de Boer M, van Dijck JA, Bult P, Borm GF, Tjan-Heijnen VC (2010) Breast cancer prognosis and occult lymph node metastases, isolated tumor cells, and micrometastases. J Natl Cancer Inst 102:410–425

De Giorgi V et al (2007) Outcome of patients with melanoma and histologically negative sentinel lymph nodes: one institution's experience. Oncology 73:401–406

Dietrich T et al (2010) Cutting edge: Lymphatic vessels, not blood vessels, primarily mediate immune rejections after transplantation. J Immunol 184:535–539

Donnem T et al (2009a) VEGF-A and VEGFR-3 correlate with nodal status in operable non-small cell lung cancer: inverse correlation between expression in tumor and stromal cells. Lung Cancer 63:277–283

Donnem T, Al-Shibli K, Al-Saad S, Busund LT, Bremnes RM (2009b) Prognostic impact of fibroblast growth factor 2 in non-small cell lung cancer: Coexpression with VEGFR-3 and PDGF-B predicts poor survival. J Thorac Oncol 4:578–585

Donnem T, Al-Saad S, Al-Shibli K, Busund LT, Bremnes RM (2010) Co-expression of PDGF-B and VEGFR-3 strongly correlates with lymph node metastasis and poor survival in non-small-cell lung cancer. Ann Oncol 21:223–231

Franchi A et al (2006) Inducible nitric oxide synthase activity correlates with lymphangiogenesis and vascular endothelial growth factor-C expression in head and neck squamous cell carcinoma. J Pathol 208:439–445

Franchi A, Gallo O, Massi D, Baroni G, Santucci M (2004) Tumor lymphangiogenesis in head and neck squamous cell carcinoma: a morphometric study with clinical correlations. Cancer 101:973–978

Garmy-Susini B et al (2010) Integrin {alpha}4{beta}1 Signaling Is Required for Lymphangiogenesis and Tumor Metastasis. Cancer Res

Govindarajan A, Ghazarian DM, McCready DR, Leong WL (2007) Histological features of melanoma sentinel lymph node metastases associated with status of the completion lymphadenectomy and rate of subsequent relapse. Ann Surg Oncol 14:906–912

Gu Y, Qi X, Guo S (2008) Lymphangiogenesis induced by VEGF-C and VEGF-D promotes metastasis and a poor outcome in breast carcinoma: A retrospective study of 61 cases. Clin Exp Metastasis 25:717–725

Harris JR, Lippman ME, Veronesi U, Willett W (1992) Breast cancer (3). N Engl J Med 327:473–480

Heindl LM et al (2009) Intraocular lymphangiogenesis in malignant melanomas of the ciliary body with extraocular extension. Invest Ophthalmol Vis Sci 50:1988–1995

Heindl LM et al (2010) Intraocular tumor-associated lymphangiogenesis a novel prognostic factor for ciliary body melanomas with extraocular extension? Ophthalmology 117:334–342

Henno A et al (2009) Altered expression of angiogenesis and lymphangiogenesis markers in the uninvolved skin of plaque-type psoriasis. Br J Dermatol 160:581–590

Hirakawa S et al (2005) VEGF-A induces tumor and sentinel lymph node lymphangiogenesis and promotes lymphatic metastasis. J Exp Med 201:1089–1099

Hirakawa S et al (2009) Nodal lymphangiogenesis and metastasis: Role of tumor-induced lymphatic vessel activation in extramammary Paget's disease. Am J Pathol 175:2235–2248

Hong YK et al (2002) Prox1 is a master control gene in the program specifying lymphatic endothelial cell fate. Dev Dyn 225:351–357

Iwase H, Yamamoto Y, Kawasoe T, Ibusuki M (2009) Advantage of sentinel lymph node biopsy before neoadjuvant chemotherapy in breast cancer treatment. Surg Today 39:374–380

Kerjaschki D et al (2004) Lymphatic neoangiogenesis in human kidney transplants is associated with immunologically active lymphocytic infiltrates. J Am Soc Nephrol 15:603–612

Kitadai Y et al (2005) Quantitative analysis of lymphangiogenic markers for predicting metastasis of human gastric carcinoma to lymph nodes. Int J Cancer 115:388–392

Kitadai Y (2010) Angiogenesis and lymphangiogenesis of gastric cancer. J Oncol 2010:468725

Koyama H et al (2008) Significance of tumor-associated stroma in promotion of intratumoral lymphangiogenesis: pivotal role of a hyaluronan-rich tumor microenvironment. Am J Pathol 172:179–193

Kyzas PA, Geleff S, Batistatou A, Agnantis NJ, Stefanou D (2005) Evidence for lymphangiogenesis and its prognostic implications in head and neck squamous cell carcinoma. J Pathol 206:170–177

Lahdenranta J et al (2009) Endothelial nitric oxide synthase mediates lymphangiogenesis and lymphatic metastasis. Cancer Res 69:2801–2808

Laurent TC, Fraser JR (1992) Hyaluronan. FASEB J 6:2397–2404

Lee K et al (2010) Increased intratumoral lymphatic vessel density correlates with lymph node metastasis in early gastric carcinoma. Ann Surg Oncol 17:73–80

Leong SP et al (2006) Clinical patterns of metastasis. Cancer Metastasis Rev 25:221–232

Mandriota SJ et al (2001) Vascular endothelial growth factor-C-mediated lymphangiogenesis promotes tumour metastasis. EMBO J 20:672–682

Massi D et al (2009) Inducible nitric oxide synthase expression in melanoma: implications in lymphangiogenesis. Mod Pathol 22:21–30

Matsumoto K et al (2007) Lymphatic microvessel density is an independent prognostic factor in colorectal cancer. Dis Colon Rectum 50:308–314

Maula SM et al (2003) Intratumoral lymphatics are essential for the metastatic spread and prognosis in squamous cell carcinomas of the head and neck region. Cancer Res 63:1920–1926

Moroi Y (2009) Significance of sentinel lymph node biopsy in malignant melanoma: Overview of international data. Int J Clin Oncol 14:485–489

Munoz-Guerra MF, Marazuela EG, Martin-Villar E, Quintanilla M, Gamallo C (2004) Prognostic significance of intratumoral lymphangiogenesis in squamous cell carcinoma of the oral cavity. Cancer 100:553–560

Murali R et al (2009) Interobserver reproducibility of histologic parameters of melanoma deposits in sentinel lymph nodes: implications for management of patients with melanoma. Cancer 115:5026–5037

Ohhashi T, Mizuno R, Ikomi F, Kawai Y (2005) Current topics of physiology and pharmacology in the lymphatic system. Pharmacol Ther 105:165–188

Padera TP et al (2002) Lymphatic metastasis in the absence of functional intratumor lymphatics. Science 296:1883–1886

Pasquali S et al (2010) Early (sentinel lymph node biopsy-guided) versus delayed lymphadenectomy in melanoma patients with lymph node metastases: Personal experience and literature meta-analysis. Cancer 116:1201–1209

Pedica F, Ligorio C, Tonelli P, Bartolini S, Baccarini P (2008) Lymphangiogenesis in Crohn's disease: an immunohistochemical study using monoclonal antibody D2–Virchows Arch 452:57–63

Pepper MS (2001) Lymphangiogenesis and tumor metastasis: Myth or reality? Clin Cancer Res 7:462-468

Prevo R, Banerji S, Ferguson DJ, Clasper S, Jackson DG (2001) Mouse LYVE-1 is an endocytic receptor for hyaluronan in lymphatic endothelium. J Biol Chem 276:19420–19430

Ran S, Volk L, Hall K, Flister MJ (2009) Lymphangiogenesis and lymphatic metastasis in breast cancer. Pathophysiology

Renyi-Vamos F et al (2005) Lymphangiogenesis correlates with lymph node metastasis, prognosis, and angiogenic phenotype in human non-small cell lung cancer. Clin Cancer Res 11:7344–7353

Rescigno J, Zampell JC, Axelrod D (2009) Patterns of axillary surgical care for breast cancer in the era of sentinel lymph node biopsy. Ann Surg Oncol 16:687–696

Rinderknecht M, Detmar M (2008) Tumor lymphangiogenesis and melanoma metastasis. J Cell Physiol 216:347–354

Salem A (2009) Sentinel lymph node biopsy in breast cancer: A comprehensive literature review. J Surg Educ 66:267–275

Scavelli C, Vacca A, Di Pietro G, Dammacco F, Ribatti D (2004) Crosstalk between angiogenesis and lymphangiogenesis in tumor progression. Leukemia 18:1054–1058

Schoppmann SF et al (2004) Prognostic value of lymphangiogenesis and lymphovascular invasion in invasive breast cancer. Ann Surg 240:306–312

Sedivy R, Beck-Mannagetta J, Haverkampf C, Battistutti W, Honigschnabl S (2003) Expression of vascular endothelial growth factor-C correlates with the lymphatic microvessel density and the nodal status in oral squamous cell cancer. J Oral Pathol Med 32:455–460

Shayan R, Achen MG, Stacker SA (2006) Lymphatic vessels in cancer metastasis: bridging the gaps. Carcinogenesis 27:1729–1738

Sleeman J, Schmid A, Thiele W (2009) Tumor lymphatics. Semin Cancer Biol 19:285–297

Sleeman JP, Thiele W (2009) Tumor metastasis and the lymphatic vasculature. Int J Cancer 125:2747–2756

Starz H, Balda BR, Kramer KU, Buchels H, Wang H (2001) A micromorphometry-based concept for routine classification of sentinel lymph node metastases and its clinical relevance for patients with melanoma. Cancer 91:2110–2121

Swartz MA, Skobe M (2001) Lymphatic function, lymphangiogenesis, and cancer metastasis. Microsc Res Tech 55:92–99

Tammela T, Alitalo K (2010) Lymphangiogenesis: Molecular mechanisms and future promise. Cell 140:460–476

Uhara H, Takata M, Saida T (2009) Sentinel lymph node biopsy in Japan. Int J Clin Oncol 14:490–496

Valencak J et al (2004) Selective immunohistochemical staining shows significant prognostic influence of lymphatic and blood vessels in patients with malignant melanoma. Eur J Cancer 40:358–364

van Akkooi AC, Spatz A, Eggermont AM, Mihm M, Cook MG (2009) Expert opinion in melanoma: the sentinel node; EORTC Melanoma Group recommendations on practical methodology of the measurement of the microanatomic location of metastases and metastatic tumour burden. Eur J Cancer 45:2736–2742

Van Trappen PO et al (2003) Expression of vascular endothelial growth factor (VEGF)-C and VEGF-D, and their receptor VEGFR-3, during different stages of cervical carcinogenesis. J Pathol 201:544–554

Wang TB, Huang YH, Lan P, Song XM, Wang JP (2005) [Correlation of lymphangiogenesis to progression of colorectal cancer]. Ai Zheng 24:1276–1279

Witte D, Thomas A, Ali N, Carlson N, Younes M (2002) Expression of the vascular endothelial growth factor receptor-3 (VEGFR-3) and its ligand VEGF-C in human colorectal adenocarcinoma. Anticancer Res 22:1463–1466

Witte MH et al (2006) Structure function relationships in the lymphatic system and implications for cancer biology. Cancer Metastasis Rev 25:159–184

Yarbro JW, Page DL, Fielding LP, Partridge EE, Murphy GP (1999) American Joint Committee on Cancer prognostic factors consensus conference. Cancer 86:2436–2446

Zeng Y, Opeskin K, Horvath LG, Sutherland RL, Williams ED (2005) Lymphatic vessel density and lymph node metastasis in prostate cancer. Prostate 65:222–230

Zhan P et al (2009) Prognostic value of vascular endothelial growth factor expression in patients with lung cancer: a systematic review with meta-analysis. J Thorac Oncol 4:1094–1103

Chapter 13
Hematogenous Dissemination

Bruno F. Fernandes

The changes in the ECM composition induced by the invading tumor cells have been discussed in previous chapters. We now focus on the following step of the metastatic cascade, the access of malignant cells to the host's bloodstream. The importance of understanding this early step of disease progression is crucial because most cancer patients die from metastases rather than from their primary tumors.

Even though cancers can be defined as lesions having the ability to cause distant metastases, the potential to spread varies greatly. For example, non-melanoma skin cancers are capable of invading deep tissues and adjacent structures, albeit rarely get access to the circulation. (American Cancer Society 2009) Fortunately, despite an annual incidence of 1 million cases in the United States, less than 1000 deaths are reported, and even fewer of those are due to distant metastases (American Cancer Society 2009).

We are now going to detail each aspect of the hematogenous dissemination of tumor cells.

13.1 Angiogenesis

Angiogenesis is defined by the development of new vessels from preexistent ones, which should be distinguished from vasculogenesis that derives from primordial endothelial cells during embryogenesis (Paku 1998). Understanding the importance of vascular biology to tumor development have led to important insights on the pathophysiology and treatment of malignancies. Tumors have high metabolic rates and a consequent higher need of nutrients and oxygen. It is believed that a tumor mass can not be greater than 2 mm in diameter without inducing angiogenesis. Beyond that, passive diffusion can no longer provide adequate nutrients in or allow waste products out of the tumoral tissue (Sutherland 1988). The inability of a tumor to promote

B. F. Fernandes (✉)
Department of Ophthalmology & Pathology, Henry C. Witelson Ocular Pathology Laboratory, McGill University, Montreal, Canada
e-mail: bruno.mtl@gmail.com

J. V. Burnier, M. N. Burnier, Jr. (eds.), *Experimental and Clinical Metastasis*,
DOI 10.1007/978-1-4614-3685-0_13,

neovascularization has even been linked to the dormant state of micrometastases (Folkman 1985; Blood and Zetter 1990). Thus, any tumor mass needs to induce the formation of new blood vessels that will supply an appropriate blood flow to sustain growth.

Judah Folkman is considered by some the father of angiogenesis (Cohen and Judah Folkman 2009). According to Folkman et al. (Folkman and Kalluri 2004), there are two critical phases in cancer development, the first being a somatic mutation resulting in a malignant cell. The second phase is the conversion into an angiogenic phenotype, in which the tumor recruits its own blood supply. A set of genes responsible for the activities of cell motility, epithelial-mesenchymal transition, extracellular matrix degradation and angiogenesis have been recently called metastases initiating genes (Nguyen et al. 2009).

As with other steps of the metastatic cascade, angiogenesis also depends on the interaction between the neoplasm and the host. Therefore, tumor progression depends on the balance between the release of antiogenic factors by the tumor and the individual's endogenous angiogenic inhibitors. Angiogenic output includes FGF2, VEGF, IL8, and PDGF while endogenous angiogenic inhibitors include thromboplastin, tumstatin, canstatin, endostatin, angiostatin, and interferon [alpha]/[beta]. Tumor cells and blood vessels constitutes a highly integrated system, where endothelial cells can be switched from a resting state to one of rapid growth by diffusible signals from tumor or associated inflammatory cells (Folkman 1971).

The process of angiogenesis related to tumor (or otherwise) can be summarized in the following steps (Paku 1998):

1. Dilatation of postcapillary venules situated around the tumor;
2. Local degradation of the basement membrane;
3. Weakened intercellular contacts between endothelial and emigration into the connective tissue towards the angiogenic stimulus
4. Formation of a solid cord of endothelial cells
5. Organization of a lumen, either by fusing of intracellular vacuoles or curving of single endothelial cells;
6. Loop formation by fusion of the sprouts;
7. Appearance of pericytes and synthesis of a basement membrane.

Tumor-induced angiogenesis not only provide the means for tumor growth, but it also grants an easier access to the blood stream. During angiogenesis, endothelial cell at the tip of invading capillaries release important paracrine growth factors for tumor cells such as basic fibroblast growth factor (bFGF), insulin growth factor-2, platelet-derived growth factor, and colony-stimulating factor (Hamada et al. 1992; Nicosia et al. 1986; Rak et al. 1994). Additionally, collagenases and other degradative enzymes secreted by endothelial cells facilitate the spread of tumor cells through the surrounding extracellular matrix (Fox et al. 1993; Gross et al. 1982). Not surprisingly, several reports have associated the tumoral microvessel density with aggressiveness and poor prognosis (Weidner et al. 1991; Weidner 1995; Bono et al. 2002; Thelen et al. 2008; Yildiz et al. 2008).

13.2 Intravasation

As stated previously, the original malignant clone needs to convert into a phenotype capable of initiating the metastatic processes. The genes responsible for the activities of cell motility, epithelial-mesenchymal transition, extracellular matrix degradation and angiogenesis.

Intravasation is the term used for the entry of any kind of foreign material into a blood or lymph vessels. As part of the process of metastasis, intravasation refers to the invasion of the systemic circulation by the malignant cells. Newly formed vessels lack the normal architectural support of a basement membrane and pericytes, which allows leakage of fluids into the extravascular space. Tumor-related angiogenesis however, has some particularities that make the angiogenic vasculature even more susceptible to the penetration of malignant cells.

Ultrastructural reports have shown that, under normal circumstances, angiogenic vessels are not permeable for molecules larger than 20kD (Rizzo and DeFouw 1996). On the other hand, tumor vasculature allows the passage of molecules larger than 70–150kD (Dvorak et al. 1988). Pericytes are usually absent and the basement membrane of tumor vessels is frequently fragmented or even completely absent (Paku et al. 1990). The lumen of the vessel itself is covered by thin endothelial cells with open intercellular junctions. Some areas even show vascular spaces delineated by malignant cells in direct contact with the tumor mass (Paku 1998). Those changes are explained by the invasive activities of tumor cells and the consequent changes in the composition of the extracellular matrix caused by malignant tumors, but not their benign counterparts (Skinner et al. 1995).

The actual process of intravasation has not completely elucidated. It might well be a passive process in which cells are sloughed off from the tumor into the lumen of a vessel. The other possibility is an active migration of cells through the capillary wall (Condeelis and Segall 2003). Cell motility is a principal requirement for the spreading of cancer cells (Stracke et al. 1991). The invasive cells often follow a gradient of extracellular compounds (often growth factors) that are detected by intracellular signal processing pathways, which in turn coordinate cell movement (Maghazachi 2000). At last, cell motility relies on the actin-based cytoskeleton for both generating protrusions and retracting the rear of the cell that results in the characteristic ameboid form of movement (Condeelis and Segall 2003). Studies using in vivo intravital microscopy showed that metastatic cells polarize towards blood vessels while nonmetastatic cells do not (Wyckoff et al. 2000). Moreover, nonmetastatic cells fragment upon crossing endothelial junctions.

Intravital imaging also demonstrated that macrophages are crucial in the processes of intravasation (Fig. 13.1). Cancer cells and macrophages are linked together in a paracrine loop using EGF and colony-stimulated factor 1 (CSF-1). Expression analysis showed that macrophages express CSF-1 receptor and secrete EGF, whereas carcinoma cells express EGF receptor and secrete CSF-1. Thus, these two cell types reciprocally induce each other to migrate (Wyckoff et al. 2004). Macrophages that are located in the vicinity of blood vessels help to direct cancer cells to the vessels. The outcome of this communication is the accumulation of cancer cells near blood vessels, which eventually leads to intravasation. Indeed, the presence of tumor-

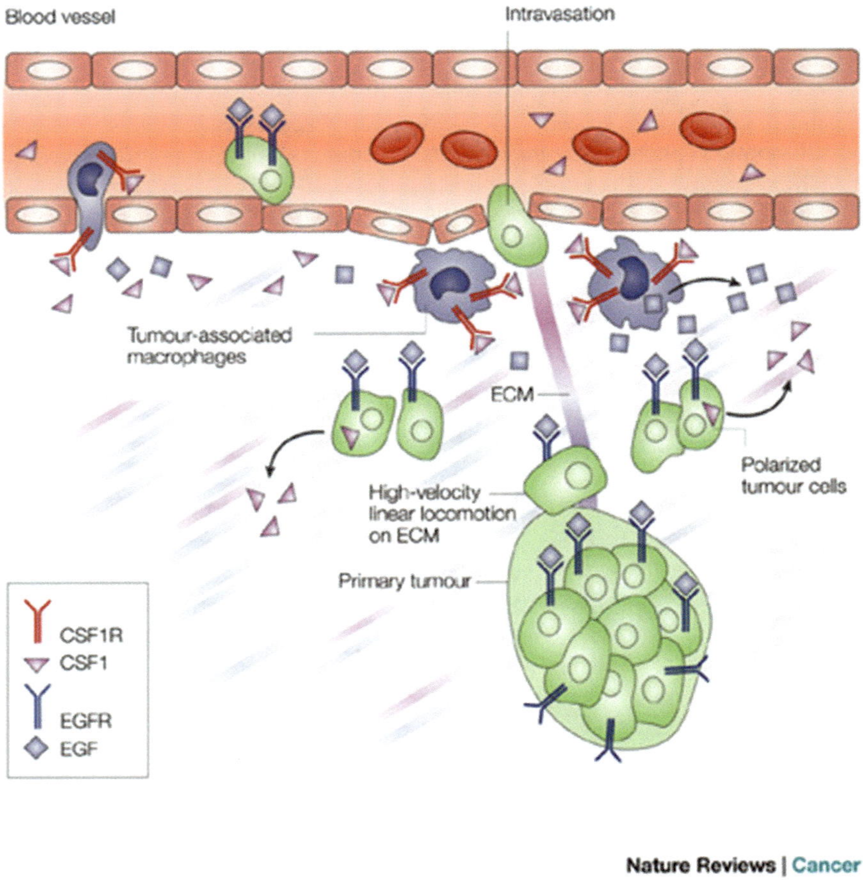

Fig. 13.1 An illustration that summarizes the interactions of carcinoma cells with blood vessels as seen by multiphoton-based intravital imaging. Carcinoma cells (*green*) of metastatic tumours collect near blood vessels as a polarized cell layer, which is a result of chemotaxis to the blood vessel in response to chemoattractants such as epidermal growth factor (*EGF*). Cancer cells express the EGF receptor (*EGFR*). Macrophages (*purple*) collect near the vessel in response to colony-stimulating factor-1 (*CSF1*), which is produced by tumour cells. Macrophages express the CSF1 receptor (*CSF1R*) and might be the source of EGF. The polarity of carcinoma cells is correlated with increased intravasation and metastasis. (Hernandez et al. 1992)

infiltrating macrophages in the primary tumor has been correlated with metastasis in several malignancies (Siveen and Kuttan 2009).

13.3 Tumor Cell Shedding and Survival in the Circulation

The well-know inefficiency of the metastatic process is compensated by the large numbers of cells that are constantly released by the primary tumor. An attempt to quantify tumor cell shedding estimated that the efferent blood from a tumor mass contains approximately 16,000 cells/ml. In a day, each gram of tumor sheds more than 3 million cells into the systemic circulation (Butler and Gullino 1975). Luckily, the blood is not an ideal place for malignant cells and most of them do not remain viable for long. After 24 h in circulation, only 1 % of the initial load survives (Fidler 1970). Cells die as a consequence of the process of anoikis (programmed cell death associated with loss of cellular contact), immune recognition and the sheer physical stress of the circulatory system (Mendoza and Khanna 2009). Some of the currently available data indicates that only 0.1 % of those injected tumor cells could form gross metastatic foci (Tsubura et al. 1983).

Metastatic cells can leave the primary site individually or in clumps, also called tumor emboli. Those tumor clumps represent approximately 10 % of circulating tumor cells and contains between 2 and 30 cells. It is believed that clumps actually liberated as such into the circulation during the natural course of the pathological process, instead of aggregating after dissemination (Liotta et al. 1974). Even though secondary growths can originate from the clonal expansion of a single cell, circulating multicell tumor emboli are more likely to successfully form metastases (Fidler and Talmadge 1986). It appears that aggregates of cells tend to survive longer in circulation compared to individual cells. Under light microscopy, isolated circulating cells from clumps are larger and better preserved than single ones. One possible explanation is that cells at the center of the clump would not be in direct contact with the blood itself and would also be protected from immune surveillance (Liotta et al. 1974). Then, centrally located cells would remain viable until the clumps arrest at the capillary network of the target organ.

It is recognized that platelets and coagulation factors are involved in hematogenous metastasis, more specifically in regards to cell survival in the bloodstream and adhesion to the vasculature of distant sites (Erpenbeck and Schon 2010). Trombocytosis, as a paraneoplastic unspecific phenomenon in the metabolism of the host triggered by the cancer, facilitates metastatic spread (Estrov et al. 1995). Elevated platelet counts have been associated with advanced stages of cancer and poor prognosis for a variety of malignancies, including endometrial carcinoma (Scholz et al. 2000), cervical (Hernandez et al. 1992), ovarian (Zeimet et al. 1994), gastric (Ikeda et al. 2002) or esophageal cancer (Shimada et al. 2004). Those clinical observations are supported by experimental data demonstrating that the ability of tumor cells to aggregate platelets in vitro is correlated with the metastatic potential of cancer cells in vivo. The process of tumor-cell induced platelet aggregation (TCIPA) appears to involve most known platelet receptors engaged in adhesion and aggregation of platelets, which in turn are attractive target of cancer therapies. Glycoprotein Ib-IX-V complex, GpIV, intergrins, ADP receptors, P-selectin and thrombin receptors are some of the targets being used for the development of potential treatments because of their implication in the metastatic process (Erpenbeck and Schon 2010). One of the explanations why TCIPA increase cell survival in circulation is that a protective thrombus may shield tumor cells from recognition by the immune system. Platelets also limit the ability of natural killer (NK) cells to lyse tumor cells in vitro and in vivo (Fig. 13.2, Palumbo et al. 2005).

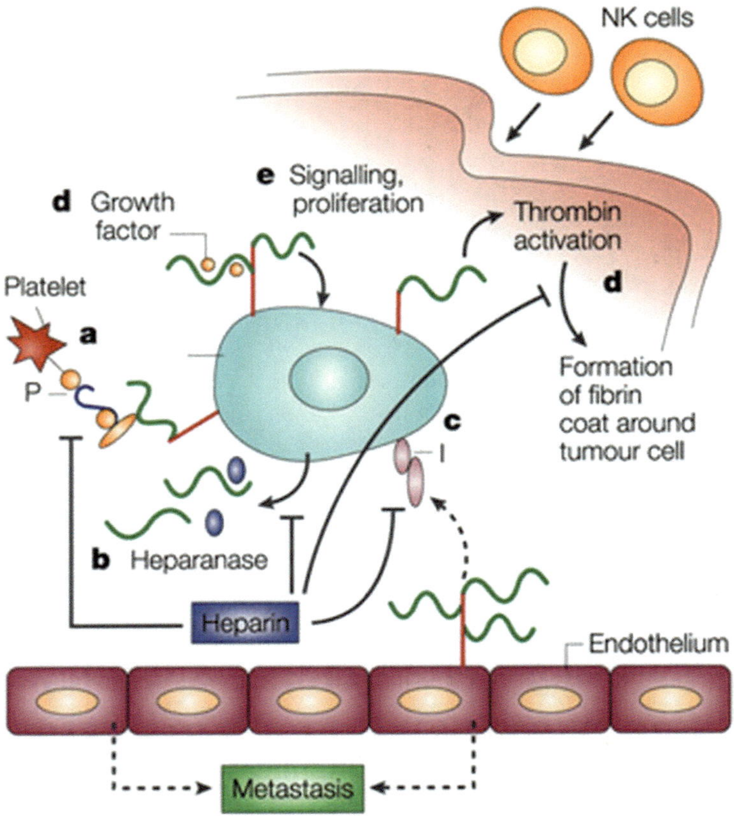

Fig. 13.2 Heparan-sulphate glycosaminoglycans (HSGAGs; *green lines*) function at the tumour-cell surface to mediate metastasis. **(a)** Cancer-cell-surface HSGAGs can act as ligands for P-selectin (*P*), which mediates adhesion either to platelets or to the endothelial lining of the capillary system. This allows cancer cells both to extravasate and enter the bloodstream, as well as to metastasize to other organs. Addition of exogenous heparin competes with P-selectin binding, inhibiting tumour-cell adhesion processes. **(b)** Heparanase cleaves HSGAGs, releasing growth-promoting factors and promoting tumour metastasis. Pharmacological doses of heparin are thought to inhibit heparanase action. **(c)** Cell-surface HSGAGs also act as coreceptors for integrins (*I*), mediating cancer-cell adhesion to blood vessels to promote extravasion. Pharmacological doses of heparin are also believed to interfere with these processes by competing with cancer-cell-surface HSGAG binding to integrins. **(d)** Cancer-cell-surface HSGAGs also contain sequences that modulate local coagulation, specifically by modulating the activity of coagulation serine proteases such as thrombin (*Factor IIa*). Tumour procoagulants promote the formation of a protective layer of fibrin around the tumour, and are also inhibited by heparin. This coat prevents attack by natural killer (*NK*) cells of the immune system. **(e)** Finally, HSGAGs at the tumour-cell surface interact with growth factors (*circles*), such as fibroblast growth factor and vascular endothelial growth factor, to regulate the proliferation and migration of cancer cells through autocrine signalling loops

Table 13.1 Organ-specific colonization

Tumour type	Principal sites of metastasis
Breast	Bone, lungs, liver and brain
Lung adenocarcinoma	Brain, bones, adrenal gland and liver
Skin melanoma	Lungs, brain, skin and liver
Colorectal	Liver and lungs
Pancreatic	Liver and lungs
Prostate	Bones
Sarcoma	Lungs
Uveal melanoma	Liver

Host immune defense against CTC can be immunologic specific or non-specific. Specific immunity against clumps of cells in circulation is attributable to (NK) cell activity. NK cells are able to destroy tumor emboli, albeit having a limited role in inhibiting growth after implantation (Tsubura et al. 1983). Experimental evidence supporting such theory shows that NK deficicient animals have a higher incidence of metastasis. On the other hand, metastasis is markedly inhibited in mice treated with interferon inducers (Hanna 1982). In the case of uveal melanoma, it was showed that intraocular tumors are able to inhibit NK activity and tumor cells are able to promote growth and maintain the immune privilege (Apte et al. 1997). Human uveal melanoma cells produce macrophage migration-inhibitory factor to prevent lysis by NK cells (Repp et al. 2000). The cells of the monocyte-macrophage series are responsible for the non-specific host defense. Activated macrophages can destroy a wide range of CTCs from different origins, regardless of their phenotypic diversity, antigenicity, chemosensitivity or metastatic potential. Tumoricidal macrophages are also able to control the progression of established micrometastasis in vivo. Furthermore, the effectiveness of agents such as BCG, levamisole and others are likely linked to the non-specific activation of monocyte-macrophages (Proctor et al. 1977).

13.4 Cell Arrest

After entering the circulation, individual or clumps of metastatic cells eventually reach the capillary bed of distant organs. The fact that some organs are more prone to suffer from metastatic colonization than others (Table 13.1) has puzzled scientists for decades. An old theory proposed by Virchow was that metastasis could be explained by the simple lodgment of emboli of disseminated cells in the vasculature of the affected organ (Virchow 1858). Other scientists supported such idea, like James Ewing that proposed that colonization of a distant organ would be ruled by mechanical factors determined by the anatomical structure of its vascular system (Ewing 1928). However, it was the "seed and soil" theory (Paget 1889) proposed by Stephen Paget in 1889 that survived until the present day. Its key findings after reviewing the autopsy records of 735 women with breast cancer are summarized below (Fidler and Poste 2008):

- The pattern of metastasis is not random;
- Some organs are more prone to be the seat of secondary neoplastic growth;

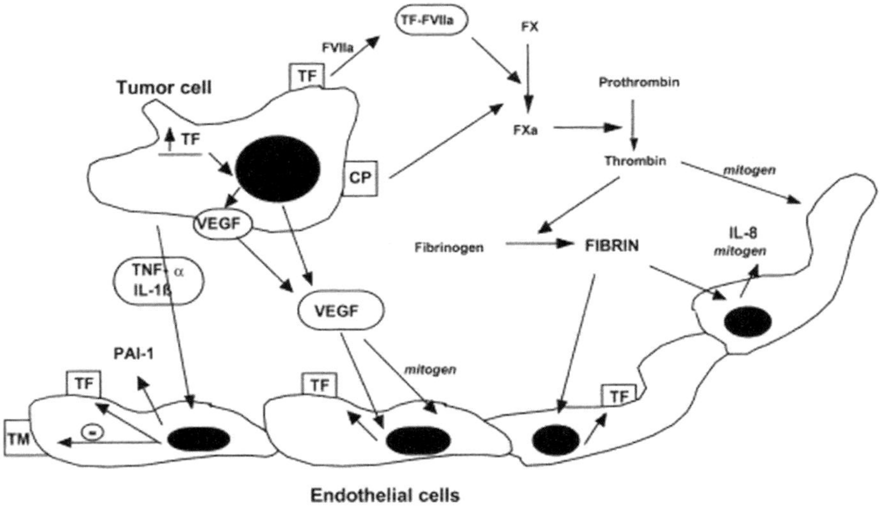

Fig. 13.3 Regulation of tumor cell and endothelial cell procoagulant functions in the pathogenesis of thrombosis in cancer. TF and CP expression are synthesized and expressed on the surface of tumor cells. The effect of these tumor cell procoagulants are enhanced by the local production of the important proangiogenic cytokines IL-8 (from the endothelial cell) and VEGF and the inflammatory cytokines TNF-α and IL-1β from tumor cells. These cytokines convert the normal anticoagulant endothelium to a procoagulant endothelium as follows: (1) down-regulation of TM expression and (2) increased synthesis of TF and PAI-1. Fibrin, produced in response to activation of clotting by TF and CP, increases both TF and IL-8 production by the endothelium, further enhancing thrombogenesis and angiogenesis. TF also increases angiogenesis by the tumor cell by increasing the synthesis of VEGF

- In breast cancer, the incidence of metastasis to the ovaries is higher than to the spleen and kidney combined;
- Bone metastasis cannot be explained by the theory of embolism alone;
- There is a high incidence of bone metastasis from thyroid cancer, and some bones have more metastases than others

To a certain degree, nonspecific entrapment and arrest of circulating tumor cells in the circulation are undoubtedly influenced by mechanical factors such as the size and deformability of tumor cells, and the diameter and distensibility of capillaries. Changes in microcirculatory hemodynamics such as slowing, flowback, sludge, and plasma-skimming phenomena occur after intravasation of tumor cells (Liotta et al. 1974). The interaction of tumor cells with one another in aggregating, and/or with host cells such as platelets and lymphocytes, may also influence and facilitate tumor cell arrest (Rickles and Falanga 2001). Interestingly, experimental models demonstrate that metastatic cell lines arrest in capillary beds at a significantly higher rate than cells of low metastatic potential of the same origin (Tsubura et al. 1983). Tissue Factor (TF) and cancer procoagulant (CP) are some of the procoagulant molecules that have been characterized in the process of tumor cell arrest (Fig. 13.3). Moreover, manipulation of cells can increase their ability to arrest and subsequently form metastasis (Poste and Nicolson 1980).

13.5 Extravasation

Even though this last step of hematogenous dissemination is one of the most intensively studied, the exact mechanism of extravasation is still debated. Most observations are inferred from ultrastructural studies of liver and lung metastasis and 4 possible mechanisms have been proposed:

1. Penetration of the endothelium and basement membrane by cancer cells in a leukocyte-like fashion (Kawaguchi and Nakamura 1986);
2. Destruction of the capillary wall caused by extension of the tumor cell to the subendothelial matrix followed by dissolution of the basement membrane (Crissman et al. 1988);
3. Migration of endothelial cells covering the intravascular tumor emboli before penetration of the basement membrane (Lapis et al. 1988);
4. Intracapillary proliferation leading to the mechanical destruction of the vessel (Machado et al. 1982).

Regardless of minor differences in these theories, tumor cells have 2 barriers to cross in order to get access to the organ parenchyma after the cell/clump arrives at the capillary and interacts with an intact endothelium. The first step is accomplished by either the endothelialization of cancer cells or retraction of endothelial cells. 12(S)-hydroxy-eicosatetraenoic and tumor derived retraction factor were both seen to cause reversible endothelial retraction in vitro (Honn et al. 1994; Kusama et al. 1995). The basement membrane is then degraded granting the invading cells a direct contact with the stroma of the target organ (Paku et al. 2000).

The particularities of the extravasation step of the metastatic cascade can offer interesting insights on the preferential colonization of specific organs. The endothelium of the capillary of different organ shows differences in ultrastructure and cell surface molecules (Fig. 13.4, Ruoslahti and Rajotte 2000). Moreover, in the liver, the penetration of the basement membrane is not necessary since it is not so well-defined as in other organs. As a consequence of those and possible other factors, tumor cells reach an extraluminal position more rapidly in organs that are more susceptible to metastasis (i.e. liver vs. brain) (Fig. 13.5, Paku et al. 2000).

As the disseminated cells progress towards the establishment of an established metastasis, cells need to readapt their genetic expression and molecular machinery to accomplish subsequent tasks. To date, several mediators of extravasation have been identified (Nguyen et al. 2009). Taking breast cancer as an example, pulmonary extravasation is related to the upregulation of mediators in the primary tumor. Epiregulin, COX2, matrix metalloproteinase 1 and 2 support not only vascular remodeling in the primary site but also distant extravasation (Gupta et al. 2007). Cytokine angiopoietin-like 4(ANGPTL4) does not confer any advantage for the primary tumor but specifically enhances extravasation by inducing the dissociation of endothelial cell-to-cell junctions (Padua et al. 2008). Last but not least, systemic secretion of LOX accumulates in the lung, where it could act on extracellular matrix proteins creating a more permissive niche for extravasating cells (Nguyen et al. 2009).

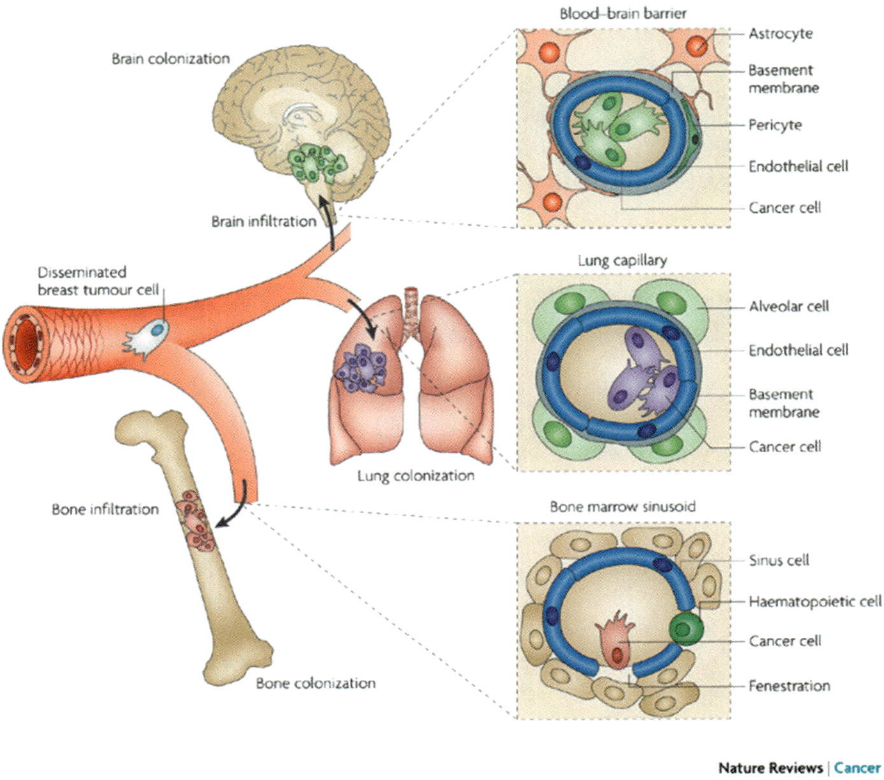

Fig. 13.4 The potential barriers to metastasis in different sites are exemplified by the case of breast cancer and the anatomy of capillary walls in different target tissues. Breast cancer cells entering the circulation can infiltrate a distant organ if they carry the necessary functions for extravasation. The fenestrated structure of bone marrow sinusoid capillaries is more permissive to cancer cell infiltration than the contiguous structure of lung capillary walls. Brain capillaries are more difficult to penetrate, owing to the unique nature of the haematoencephalic barrier. Infiltration through these barriers selects for tumour cells that express the necessary extravasation functions. These functions can be provided by genes for which expression in primary tumours independently provides a selective growth advantage (such as vascular remodelling) or by genes for which expression in primary tumours provides no benefit but is a consequence of tumour microenvironment signals

13.6 Summary

We detailed in this chapter the distinctiveness of each step of the hematogenous dissemination of tumor cells (Fig. 13.5). As demonstrated, there is a continuous interaction of the metastatic cells with the host, in agreement with the so called “seed and soil” theory originally proposed by Paget. Different cancer cells (seeds) show different potential to perform each step of the metastatic cascade. At the same time, certain characteristics of the host facilitate one or more steps of disease progression allowing the distant growth of disseminated cells in specific organs (host). Knowing

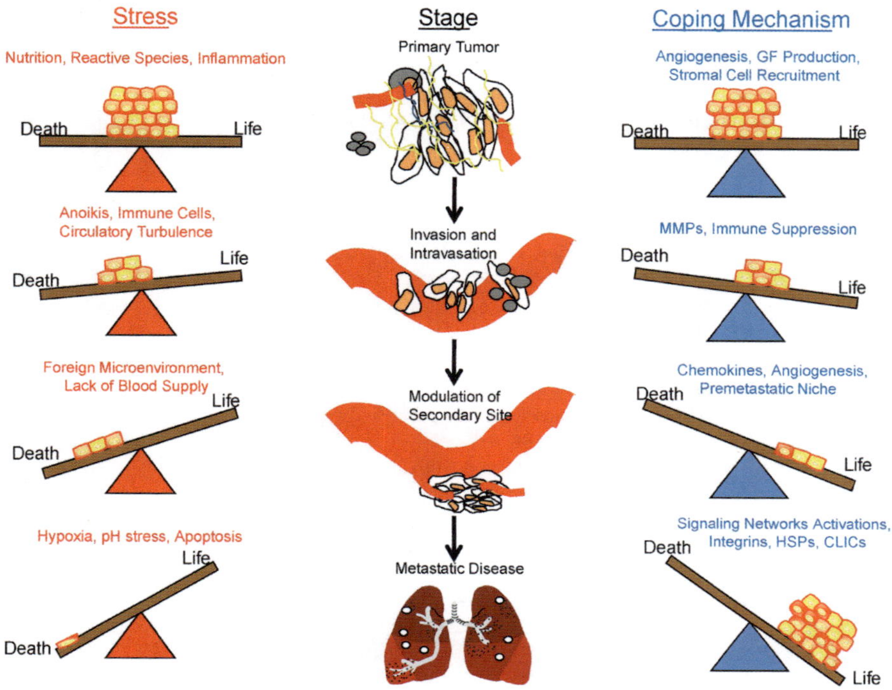

Fig. 13.5 Tumor cells must resist stress in order to metastasize. Metastasis is thought to be a very inefficient process, in part, due to the number of stresses tumor cells must overcome in order to reach secondary sites and develop into gross metastatic lesions. Throughout each stage, tumor cells are confronted with various stresses, any of which may kill the cell. This results in a fragile balance between life and death for the cell. Only those tumor cells which can successfully manage the stress will survive. Depicted are examples of the various stresses tumor cells face during each stage of the metastatic process and some of the mechanisms the cell may use to deal with those stresses. Note that each stress and coping mechanism listed above are not exclusive to a particular stage of metastasis and likely apply to more than one of the stages. Cancer stem cells, those cells which are thought most able to resist the stresses of the metastatic cascade, are depicted in yellow. GF = growth factor; MMPs = matrix metalloproteinases; HSPs = heat shock proteins; CLICs = chloride intracellular ion channels

that metastasis is the most common cause of death in cancer patients, research in the area will certainly enlightenour understanding of the whole process and translate into improved therapies and survival rates.

References

American Cancer Society (2009) Atlanta, GA

Apte RS, Mayhew E, Niederkorn JY (1997) Local inhibition of natural killer cell activity promotes the progressive growth of intraocular tumors. Invest Ophthalmol Vis Sci 38:1277–1282

Blood CH, Zetter BR (1990) Tumor interactions with the vasculature: angiogenesis and tumor metastasis. Biochim Biophys Acta 1032:89–118

Bono AV et al (2002) Microvessel density in prostate carcinoma. Prostate Cancer Prostatic Dis 5:123–127
Butler TP, Gullino PM (1975) Quantitation of cell shedding into efferent blood of mammary adenocarcinoma. Cancer Res 35:512–516
Cohen MM Jr, Judah Folkman MD (2009) 1933–2008: father of angiogenesis. J Craniofac Surg 20(Suppl 1):590–591
Condeelis J, Segall JE (2003) Intravital imaging of cell movement in tumours. Nat Rev Cancer 3:921–930
Crissman JD, Hatfield JS, Menter DG, Sloane B, Honn KV (1988) Morphological study of the interaction of intravascular tumor cells with endothelial cells and subendothelial matrix. Cancer Res 48:4065–4072
Dvorak HF, Nagy JA, Dvorak JT, Dvorak AM (1988) Identification and characterization of the blood vessels of solid tumors that are leaky to circulating macromolecules. Am J Pathol 133:95–109
Erpenbeck L, Schon MP (2010) Deadly allies: the fatal interplay between platelets and metastasizing cancer cells. Blood 115:3427–3436
Estrov Z et al (1995) Elevated plasma thrombopoietic activity in patients with metastatic cancer-related thrombocytosis. Am J Med 98:551–558
Ewing J (1928) Neoplastic Diseases. Saunders, Philadelphia
Fidler IJ (1970) Metastasis: guantitative analysis of distribution and fate of tumor embolilabeled with 125 I-5-iodo-2'-deoxyuridine. J Natl Cancer Inst 45:773–782
Fidler IJ, Poste G (2008) The "seed and soil" hypothesis revisited. Lancet Oncol 9:808
Fidler IJ, Talmadge JE (1986) Evidence that intravenously derived murine pulmonary melanoma metastases can originate from the expansion of a single tumor cell. Cancer Res 46:5167–5171
Folkman J (1971) Tumor angiogenesis: therapeutic implications. N Engl J Med 285:1182–1186
Folkman J (1985) Tumor angiogenesis. Adv Cancer Res 43:175–203
Folkman J, Kalluri R (2004) Cancer without disease. Nature 427:787
Fox RI, Luppi M, Kang HI, Ablshi D, Josephs S (1993) Detection of high levels of human herpes virus-6 DNA in a lymphoma of a patient with Sjogren's syndrome. J Rheumatol 20:764–765
Gross JL, Moscatelli D, Jaffe EA, Rifkin DB (1982) Plasminogen activator and collagenase production by cultured capillary endothelial cells. J Cell Biol 95:974–981
Gupta GP et al (2007) Mediators of vascular remodelling co-opted for sequential steps in lung metastasis. Nature 446:765–770
Hamada J, Cavanaugh PG, Lotan O, Nicolson GL (1992) Separable growth and migration factors for large-cell lymphoma cells secreted by microvascular endothelial cells derived from target organs for metastasis. Br J Cancer 66:349–354
Hanna N (1982) Inhibition of experimental tumor metastasis by selective activation of natural killer cells. Cancer Res 42:1337–1342
Hernandez E, Lavine M, Dunton CJ, Gracely E, Parker J (1992) Poor prognosis associated with thrombocytosis in patients with cervical cancer. Cancer 69:2975–2977
Honn KV et al (1994) Tumor cell-derived 12(S)-hydroxyeicosatetraenoic acid induces microvascular endothelial cell retraction. Cancer Res 54:565–574
Ikeda M et al (2002) Poor prognosis associated with thrombocytosis in patients with gastric cancer. Ann Surg Oncol 9:287–291
Kawaguchi T, Nakamura K (1986) Analysis of the lodgement and extravasation of tumor cells in experimental models of hematogenous metastasis. Cancer Metastasis Rev 5:77–94
Kusama T et al (1995) Enhancement of in vitro tumor-cell transcellular migration by tumor-cell-secreted endothelial-cell-retraction factor. Int J Cancer 63:112–118
Lapis K, Paku S, Liotta LA (1988) Endothelialization of embolized tumor cells during metastasis formation. Clin Exp Metastasis 6:73–89
Liotta LA, Kleinerman J, Saidel GM (1974) Quantitative relationships of intravascular tumor cells, tumor vessels, and pulmonary metastases following tumor implantation. Cancer Res 34:997–1004

Machado EA, Gerard DA, Mitchell JR, Lozzio BB, Lozzio CB (1982) Arrest and extravasation of neoplastic cells. An electron microscopy study of serial sections at sequential stages. Virchows Arch A Pathol Anat Histol 396:73–89

Maghazachi AA (2000) Intracellular signaling events at the leading edge of migrating cells. Int J Biochem Cell Biol 32:931–943

Mendoza M, Khanna C (2009) Revisiting the seed and soil in cancer metastasis. Int J Biochem Cell Biol 41:1452–1462

Nguyen DX, Bos PD, Massague J (2009) Metastasis: from dissemination to organ-specific colonization. Nat Rev Cancer 9:274–284

Nicosia RF, Tchao R, Leighton J (1986) Interactions between newly formed endothelial channels and carcinoma cells in plasma clot culture. Clin Exp Metastasis 4:91–104

Padua D et al (2008) TGFbeta primes breast tumors for lung metastasis seeding through angiopoietin-like 4. Cell 133:66–77

Paget S (1889) The distribution of secondary growths in cancer of the breast. Lancet 133:571–573

Paku S (1998) Current concepts of tumor-induced angiogenesis. Pathol Oncol Res 4:62–75

Paku S, Timar J, Lapis K (1990) Ultrastructure of invasion in different tissue types by Lewis lung tumour variants. Virchows Arch A Pathol Anat Histopathol 417:435–442

Paku S, Dome B, Toth R, Timar J (2000) Organ-specificity of the extravasation process: an ultrastructural study. Clin Exp Metastasis 18:481–492

Palumbo JS et al (2005) Platelets and fibrin(ogen) increase metastatic potential by impeding natural killer cell-mediated elimination of tumor cells. Blood 105:178–185

Poste G, Nicolson GL (1980) Arrest and metastasis of blood-borne tumor cells are modified by fusion of plasma membrane vesicles from highly metastatic cells. Proc Natl Acad Sci U S A 77:399–403

Proctor JW, Auclair BG, Stokowski L, Mansell WA, Shibata H (1977) Comparison of effect of BCG, glucan and levamisole on B16 melanoma metastases. Eur J Cancer 13:115–122

Rak JW, Hegmann EJ, Lu C, Kerbel RS (1994) Progressive loss of sensitivity to endothelium-derived growth inhibitors expressed by human melanoma cells during disease progression. J Cell Physiol 159:245–255

Repp AC, Mayhew ES, Apte S, Niederkorn JY (2000) Human uveal melanoma cells produce macrophage migration-inhibitory factor to prevent lysis by NK cells. J Immunol 165:710–715

Rickles FR, Falanga A (2001) Molecular basis for the relationship between thrombosis and cancer. Thromb Res 102:V215–224

Rizzo V, DeFouw DO (1996) Capillary sprouts restrict macromolecular extravasation during normal angiogenesis in the chick chorioallantoic membrane. Microvasc Res 52:47–57

Ruoslahti E, Rajotte D (2000) An address system in the vasculature of normal tissues and tumors. Annu Rev Immunol 18:813–827

Scholz HS et al (2000) Preoperative thrombocytosis is an independent prognostic factor in stage III and IV endometrial cancer. Anticancer Res 20:3983–3985

Shimada H et al (2004) Thrombocytosis associated with poor prognosis in patients with esophageal carcinoma. J Am Coll Surg 198:737–741

Siveen KS, Kuttan G (2009) Role of macrophages in tumour progression. Immunol Lett 123:97–102

Skinner SA, Frydman GM, O'Brien PE (1995) Microvascular structure of benign and malignant tumors of the colon in humans. Dig Dis Sci 40:373–384

Stracke ML, Aznavoorian SA, Beckner ME, Liotta LA, Schiffmann E (1991) Cell motility, a principal requirement for metastasis. EXS 59:147–162

Sutherland RM (1988) Cell and environment interactions in tumor microregions: the multicell spheroid model. Science 240:177–184

Thelen A et al (2008) Microvessel density correlates with lymph node metastases and prognosis in hilar cholangiocarcinoma. J Gastroenterol 43:959–966

Tsubura E, Yamashita T, Sone S (1983) Inhibition of the arrest of hematogenously disseminated tumor cells. Cancer Metastasis Rev 2:223–237

Virchow R (1858) Cellularpathologie. Hirschwald, Berlin

Weidner N (1995) Intratumor microvessel density as a prognostic factor in cancer. Am J Pathol 147:9–19

Weidner N, Semple JP, Welch WR, Folkman J (1991) Tumor angiogenesis and metastasis–correlation in invasive breast carcinoma. N Engl J Med 324:1–8

Wyckoff J et al (2004) A paracrine loop between tumor cells and macrophages is required for tumor cell migration in mammary tumors. Cancer Res 64:7022–7029

Wyckoff JB, Jones JG, Condeelis JS, Segall JE (2000) A critical step in metastasis: in vivo analysis of intravasation at the primary tumor. Cancer Res 60:2504–2511

Yildiz E, Ayan S, Goze F, Gokce G, Gultekin EY (2008) Relation of microvessel density with microvascular invasion, metastasis and prognosis in renal cell carcinoma. BJU Int 101:758–764

Zeimet AG, Marth C, Muller-Holzner E, Daxenbichler G, Dapunt O (1994) Significance of thrombocytosis in patients with epithelial ovarian cancer. Am J Obstet Gynecol 170:549–554

Chapter 14
Other Methods of Tumor Dissemination

Abelardo A. Rodríguez-Reyes

14.1 Introduction

Methods of cancer dissemination other than lymphatic and hematogenous spread are direct seeding of body cavities or surfaces and perineural spread (Robbins et al. 1994; Laerum 2005). Seeding of body cavities and surfaces may occur whenever a malignant tumor penetrates into a natural "open field". The peritoneum is the most often involved cavity, but other cavities such as pleura, pericardium, subarachnoid space and the eye globe may be affected.

14.2 Peritoneal Cavity

Seeding is particularly characteristic of carcinoma arising in organs such as ovaries, in which all peritoneal surfaces frequently become coated with a heavy layer of cancerous glaze. The tumor cells may remain confined to the surface of the coated abdominal viscera without penetrating into the substance (Robbins et al. 1994).

Peritoneal carcinomatosis is a common event that develops in the natural history of many neoplastic diseases, representing a major problem encountered in cancer management. Peritoneal tumor dissemination arising from colorectal cancer, appendiceal cancer, gastric cancer, gynecologic malignancies or peritoneal mesothelioma is a common sign of advanced tumor stage or disease recurrence, and mostly associated with poor prognosis (Glockzin et al. 2009). The peritoneal cavity may be involved by all types of metastatic tumors. The most common sites of the primary tumors are the ovary followed by large bowel and pancreas (Chu et al. 1989; Sadeghi et al. 2000).

A. A. Rodríguez-Reyes (✉)
Asociación Para Evitar la Ceguera en México,
Hospital "Dr. Luis Sánchez Bulnes", Faculty of Medicine,
Universidad Nacional Autónoma de Mexico (UNAM),
Ciudad de México, México
e-mail: bruno.mtl@gmail.com

J. V. Burnier, M. N. Burnier, Jr. (eds.), *Experimental and Clinical Metastasis*,
DOI 10.1007/978-1-4614-3685-0_14,

Tumors of the ovary and uterus resulting in peritoneal carcinomatosis are commonly of the serous type (Soslow et al. 2000). The gross pattern varies from single, well-defined nodules to a diffuse peritoneal thickening. The consistency varies depending on cellularity, amount of connective tissue and other elements such as mucin, calcium, etc.

Metastatic carcinoma may mimic the gross and microscopic appearance of malignant mesothelioma. This is particularly the case with papillary serous carcinoma of the lung, in conjunction with pleural spread (Shah et al. 1999). Sometimes the peritoneal cavity contain large amounts of mucinous or gelatinous material, a distinctive form of tumor implant referred to as *pseudomyxoma peritonei* (Kahn and Demopoulos 1992; Smith et al. 1992). The bowel is relatively spared, but polypoid mucinous masses can develop on the peritoneal surface of the small bowel (Sugarbaker et al. 2001). Mucinous cysts can also seen in the substance of the spleen (Du Plessis et al. 1999). For those cases, it has been stated that the primary lesion may be a borderline or malignant mucinous neoplasm of the appendix, ovary, or pancreas (Lee and Scully 2000). The appendix is the primary site of origin of pseudomyxoma in the vast majority of the cases in both men and women (Young et al. 1991; Prayson et al. 1994; Ronnett et al. 1995). The associated mucinous ovarian tumors—when present—are most likely additional implants from appendiceal lesions rather than independent synchronous tumors (Young et al. 1991; Prayson et al. 1994; Ronnett et al. 1995).Microscopically,large amounts of mucinous material are seen accompanied by congestive vessels and chronic inflammatory cells. Mucus intermingled with viable epithelial glandular cells must be identified to diagnose *pseudomyxoma peritonei*. These cells have bland appearance both on histologic and cytologic preparations and show no infiltrative properties (Shin and Sneige 2000; Jackson et al. 2001). This process has been designated as adenomucinosis in order to distinguish it from peritoneal mucinous carcinomatosis accompanied by cytologic atypia and resulting from an invasive mucinous adenocarcinoma usually located in the gastrointestinal tract (Ronnett et al. 2001). By immunohistochemistry, the cells of pseudomyxoma characteristically show expression of MUC2, a mucin possessing the physicochemical property of being gel forming (Lee and Scully 2000). *Pseudomyxoma peritonei* is characterized by a slow but relentless clinical course, with recurrent ascites that eventually reaches massive proportions ("jelly-belly syndrome").

Wide surgical resection is the treatment currently recommended, with most patients requiring multiple laparotomies, and in some including a total gastrectomy (Sugarbaker and Chang 1999; Sugarbaker 2002). Mucinous cystadenomas of the ovary and appendix can rupture and discharge their content into the peritoneal cavity. The resulting condition, which is self-limited and microscopically lacks tumor cells, should not be designated as *pseudomyxoma peritonei* (Cariker and Dockerty 1954; Higa et al. 1973). Pseudomyxoma-like changes have also been described in other sites such as the stroma of prostatic adenocarcinoma following neoadjuvant androgen ablation therapy (Tran et al. 1998).

Another form of tumor implantation is the *gliomatosis peritonei* resulting from the selective growth of glial tissue from ovarian teratoma (Harms et al. 1989), which in rare circumstances may undergo malignant transformation (Dadmanesh et al. 1997); The implants appear grossly as miliary grayish white nodules in the peritoneal surface or omentum and may be accompanied by fibrosis and chronic inflammation. This is a benign process, as long as the glial tissue is entirely mature and unaccompanied by other teratomatous elements (Fortt and Mathie 1969; Truong et al. 1982; Nielsen et al. 1985).

A pathogenetically related conditions is peritoneal "melanosis", which can also follow the rupture of a cystic teratoma (Jaworski et al. 2001). Metastatic carcinoma or peritoneal seedings in the peritoneal cavity tends to be accompanied by recurrent ascites resulting in a source of significant discomfort to the patient. This is sometimes treated by peritoneovenous shunting, by which the effusion is returned to the general circulation; this technique has not resulted in an increase in the number of extra-abdominal metastases (Tarin et al. 1984).

The diagnosis of metastatic carcinoma in the peritoneal cavity is possible in about 75 % of cases on the basis of cytologic examination of the ascitic fluid (Cardozo 1966). This also applies to *pseudomyxoma peritonei* (Jackson et al. 2001). With malignant lymphoma and leukemia, the overall yield is approximately 60 %, these figures being slightly better for large cell lymphoma (Melamed 1963).

The most difficult problems in cytology of ascitic fluid are the distinction between reactive and neoplastic mesothelium and that between malignant mesothelioma and metastatic carcinoma. False-positive diagnoses have been caused by disorders associated with mesothelial hyperplasia; confusion occurs because reactive cells may form pseudoacini resembling the true acini of adenocarcinoma, have multiple nuclei or a "signet ring" appearance, or undergo mitotic division. Evaluation of the nuclei-cytoplasmic ratio and of nuclear features is essential in this differential diagnosis.

Considered in the past as a terminal condition, peritoneal carcinomatosis was approached during the last 2 decades as a curable disease. The introduction of cytoreductive surgery or peritonectomy in the treatment of peritoneal neoplastic diseases drastically changed the natural history of peritoneal carcinomatosis. Another technique that showed an important impact on disease control is intraperitoneal hyperthermic perfusion, one of the most successful treatments of peritoneal carcinomatosis that results in an impressive increase in overall survival and quality of life in treated patients with low morbidity. A review published by Deraco et al. illustrates the modality of dissemination of peritoneal carcinomatosis in relation to the primary tumor site and grade of malignancy. Peritoneal carcinomatosis is a term used to define an advanced stage of many abdominal neoplastic diseases that differ in biologic aggressiveness and prognosis. The different presentation of peritoneal carcinomatosis in relation to a different primary tumor and different grade of malignancy strongly influences the potentially radical therapeutic approaches using new and advanced modalities, like cytoreductive surgery and intraperitoneal hyperthermic perfusion (Deraco et al. 1999).

14.3 Pleural Cavity

A malignant pleural effusion may be the first evidence of cancer. About 75 % of metastatic tumors in the pleura are of carcinomatous nature, metastatic carcinoma being the most common malignant tumor in the pleura. Dyspnea, cough, and chest pain are the most common presenting symptoms. Usually malignant pleural effusions are greater than 500 ml, most serous to sanguineous. The most common sites for the primary tumors are lung (33 %), breast (21 %), and stomach (73 %) (Chernow and Sahn 1977). The lung, breast, and ovarian malignant effusion are ipsilateral to the primary tumors in approximately 90 % of the cases. If pleural effusion is present, cytologic examination of the fluid has been found to be more effective in detecting malignancy than pleural biopsy (Nance et al. 1991). When the possibility of malignancy is considered in the presence of pleural effusion, a cytologic examination of the pleural fluid is mandatory, regardless of the gross appearance of the fluid.

14.4 Pericardium

Metastatic carcinoma to the pericardium usually arises in the lung in the form of direct extension or lymphatic permeation. The constrictive "pericarditis" is the result of the associated intense desmoplastic reaction. Other tumors that commonly give rise to pericardial metastases are breast carcinoma, malignant melanoma, and malignant lymphoma (Adenle and Edwards 1982; Mambo 1981). Cytology is the most important technique for the evaluation of malignant pericardial effusions.

14.5 Cerebrospinal Fluid

The high incidence of vertebral and paravertebral metastases in cancer developing patients developing diffuse leptomeningeal carcinomatosis, usually derived from the lung and breast adenocarcinomas (Kokkoris 1983). This diagnosis is commonly established by the demonstration of malignant cells on cytologic inspection of the CSF.

Metastasis of intraventricular meningiomas through CSF pathways is a rarity and only four cases have been reported in world literature describing meningiomas which were intraventricular and malignant (Ramakrishnamurthy et al. 2002).

14.6 Intraocular Dissemination

In some intraocular tumors of neuroepithelial origin such as medulloepithelioma, the proliferating medullary epithelium is characteristically arranged in cords and sheets separated by cystic spaces that contain hyaluronic acid. In some instances, spheric cysts containing hyaluronic acid and lined by a single layer of epithelium are present on the surface of the tumor and may break of and become free floating in the vitreous and the posterior and anterior chambers (Broughton and Zimmerman 1978; Gifford 1966; Zimmerman 1971).

Endophytic retinoblastoma is composed of friable tumor masses that grow and seed the vitreous body. Vitreous seeds grow into separate, small, spheroidal masses, which on clinical examination appear as cotton balls. Such tumors seedings may grow along the inner surface of the retina and invade the retina away from the site of the main mass. Even though the seedings are often difficult to distinguish from a retinoblastoma with multicentric origin (McLean et al. 1994), they are mostly seen on the inner surface of the retina rather than within it. They are also usually seen in association with tumor cell cluster within the vitreous body (McLean et al. 1994). The neoplastic seeds in the vitreous body may spread into the posterior and the anterior chamber and deposit on the lens, zonular fibers, ciliary epithelium, iris, corneal endothelium, and trabecular meshwork. Through the meshwork, the tumor cells gain access to the aqueous outflow pathways to reach an extraocular site.

Diffuse infiltrating retinoblastomas are the least common and often are the most difficult to diagnose clinically (Mansour et al. 1989; Nicholson and Norton 1980; Shields et al. 1988). These tumors grow diffusely within the retina without greatly thickening it. Tumors cells are discharged into the vitreous, often with seeding of the anterior chamber, thereby producing a pseudohypopion. These tumors, which occur in older children, can be devoid of calcium deposits. Occasionally, diffuse retinoblastoma arise from the anterior retina, and seed the vitreous body and anterior chamber (Grossniklaus et al. 1998).

14.7 Perineural Tumor Spread

Perineural tumor spread (PNS) of head and neck malignancies is a well-known form of metastatic disease in which a tumor can migrate away from the primary site along the endoneurium or perineurium, its overall incidence ranges from 2.5–5 %. This pattern of spread is potentially devastating complication of head and neck cancer, has a high impact on the therapeutical management and may create a poor prognosis. PNS is more frequently associated with carcinoma arising from minor or major salivary glands (more often adenoid cystic carcinoma), lacrimal glands, mucosal or cutaneous squamous cell carcinoma, basal cell carcinoma, melanoma, lymphoma, and sarcoma (Ojiri 2006; Maroldi et al. 2008; Nemec et al. 2007). Although PNS can be insidious, often is a delaying diagnosis and in the past was previously associated with worsening prognosis, increasing evidence shows that cure is possible. Knowledge of anatomy of the nerves is crucial in the imaging diagnosis of PNS, to detect early curable disease. The facial nerve and the maxillary and mandibular divisions of the trigeminal nerve are most commonly affected (Ojiri 2006). Magnetic resonance imaging is the modality of choice in the assessment of PNS because of its multiplanar capability and its superior soft-tissue contrast (Maroldi et al. 2008; Nemec et al. 2007). Perineural and to a lesser extent, intraneural invasion is a common and frequently conspicuous feature of adenoid cystic carcinoma and oncocytic carcinoma of the salivary and lacrimal glands. Tumors can extend along nerves for a considerable distance beyond the clinically apparent boundaries of the tumor.

14.8 Summary

This chapter presents less common pathways of cancer dissemination such as direct seeding of body cavities or surfaces and perineural spread.

In presence of any type of fluid in a cavity such as pleura, pericardium, subarachnoid or the globe, a cytologic examination is mandatory, regardless of its gross appearance to rule out malignancy.

Perineural tumor spread in the course of head and neck tumors is a form of metastatic disease in which the tumor disseminates centrifugally or centripetally along the nerve to contiguous regions.

References

Adenle AD, Edwards JE (1982) Clinical and pathologic features of metastatic neoplasms of the pericardium. Chest 81:166–169

Broughton WL, Zimmerman LE (1978) A clinicopathologic study of 56 cases of intraocular medulloepitheliomas. Am J Ophthalmol 85:407–418

Cariker M, Dockerty M (1954) Mucinous cystadenomas and mucinous cystadenocarcinomas of the ovary; a clinical and pathological study of 355 cases. Cancer 7:302–310

Cardozo PL (1966) A critical evaluation of 3000 cytologic analyses of pleural fluid ascitic fluid and pericardial fluid. Acta Cytologica 10:455

Chernow B, Sahn SA (1977) Carcinomatous involvement of the pleura: An analysis of 96 patients. Am J Med 63:695–702

Chu DZ, Lang NP, Thompson C, Osteen PK, Westbrook KC (1989) Peritoneal carcinomatosis in nongynecologic malignancy. A prospective study of prognostic factors. Cancer 63:364–367

Dadmanesh F, Miller DM, Swenerton KD, Clement PB (1997) Gliomatosis peritonei with malignant transformation. Mod Pathol 10:597–601

Deraco M et al (1999) Peritoneal carcinomatosis: feature of dissemination. A review. Tumori 85:1–5

Du Plessis DG, Louw JA, Wranz PA (1999) Mucinous epithelial cysts of the spleen associated with pseudomyxoma peritonei. Histopathology 35:551–557

Fortt RW, Mathie IK (1969) Gliomatosis peritonei caused by ovarian teratoma. J Clin Pathol 22: 348–353

Gifford H (1966) A cystic diktyoma. Surv Ophthalmol 11:557–561

Glockzin G, Schlitt HJ, Piso P (2009) Peritoneal carcinomatosis: patients selection, perioperative complications and quality of life related to cytoreductive surgery and hyperthermic intraperitoneal chemotherapy. World J Surg Oncol 7:5

Grossniklaus HE, Dhaliwal RS, Martin DF (1998) Diffuse anterior retinoblastoma. Retina 18: 238–241

Harms D, Janig U, Gobel U (1989) Gliomatosis peritonei in childhood and adolescence. Clinicopathological study of 13 cases including immunohistochemical findings. Pathol Res Pract 184:422–430

Higa E, Rosai J, Pizzimbono CA, Wise L (1973) Mucosal hyperplasia, mucinous cystadenoma, and mucinous cystadenocarcinoma of the appendix. A re-evaluation of appendiceal "mucocele". Cancer 32:1525–1541

Jackson SL, Fleming RA, Loggie BW, Geisinger KR (2001) Gelatinous ascites: A cytohistologic study of pseudomyxoma peritonei in 67 patients. Mod Pathol 14:664–671

Jaworski RC, Boadle R, Greg J, Cocks P (2001) Peritoneal "melanosis" associated with a ruptured ovarian dermoid cyst: Report of a case with electron-probe energy dispersive X-ray analysis. Int J Gynecol Pathol 20:386–389

Kahn MA, Demopoulos RI (1992) Mucinous ovarian tumors with pseudomyxoma peritonei: A clinicopathological study. Int J Gynecol Pathol 11:15–23

Kokkoris CP (1983) Leptomeningeal carcinomatosis. How does cancer reach the pia-arachnoid? Cancer 51:154–160

Laerum OD (2005) Tumour spread in serosal cavities: What have we learned? Montebello Conference–PSC, Lillehammer, Norway, June 18–22 2004. Diagn Cytopathol 33:292–293

Lee KR, Scully RE (2000) Mucinous tumors of the ovary: A clinicopathologic study of 196 borderline tumors (of intestinal type) and carcinomas, including an evaluation of 11 cases with 'pseudomyxoma peritonei'. Am J Surg Pathol 24:1447–1464

Mambo NC (1981) Diseases of the pericardium: Morphologic study of surgical specimens from 35 patients. Hum Pathol 12:978–987

Mansour AM, Greenwald MJ, O'Grady R (1989) Diffuse infiltrating retinoblastoma. J Pediatr Ophthalmol Strabismus 26:152–154

Maroldi R, Farina D, Borghesi A, Marconi A, Gatti E (2008) Perineural tumor spread. Neuroimaging Clin N Am 18:413–429 (xi)

McLean IW, Burnier MN, Zimmerman LE, Jakobiec FA (1994) In tumors of the eye and ocular adnexa. Armed Forces Institute of Pathology, Washington DC pp 97–151

Melamed MR (1963) The cytological presentation of malignant lymphomas and related diseases in effusions. Cancer 16:413–431

Nance KV, Shermer RW, Askin FB (1991) Diagnostic efficacy of pleural biopsy as compared with that of pleural fluid examination. Mod Pathol 4:320–324

Nemec SF, Herneth AM, Czerny C (2007) Perineural tumor spread in malignant head and neck tumors. Top Magn Reson Imaging 18:467–471

Nicholson DH, Norton EW (1980) Diffuse infiltrating retinoblastoma. Trans Am Ophthalmol Soc 78:265–289

Nielsen SN, Scheithauer BW, Gaffey TA (1985) Gliomatosis peritonei. Cancer 56:2499–2503

Ojiri H (2006) Perineural spread in head and neck malignancies. Radiat Med 24:1–8

Prayson RA, Hart WR, Petras RE (1994) Pseudomyxoma peritonei. A clinicopathologic study of 19 cases with emphasis on site of origin and nature of associated ovarian tumors. Am J Surg Pathol 18:591–603

Ramakrishnamurthy TV, Murty AV, Purohit AK, Sundaram C (2002) Benign meningioma metastasizing through CSF pathways: A case report and review of literature. Neurol India 50:326–329

Robbins SL, Cotran RS, Kumar V (eds) (1994) Pathologic basis of disease. Saunders, Philadelphia

Ronnett BM et al (1995) Pseudomyxoma peritonei in women: a clinicopathologic analysis of 30 cases with emphasis on site of origin, prognosis, and relationship to ovarian mucinous tumors of low malignant potential. Hum Pathol 26:509–524

Ronnett BM et al (2001) Patients with pseudomyxoma peritonei associated with disseminated peritoneal adenomucinosis have a significantly more favorable prognosis than patients with peritoneal mucinous carcinomatosis. Cancer 92:85–91

Sadeghi B et al (2000) Peritoneal carcinomatosis from non-gynecologic malignancies: Results of the EVOCAPE 1 multicentric prospective study. Cancer 88:358–363

Shah IA, Salvatore JR, Kummet T, Gani OS, Wheeler LA (1999) Pseudomesotheliomatous carcinoma involving pleura and peritoneum: A clinicopathologic and immunohistochemical study of three cases. Ann Diagn Pathol 3:148–159

Shields JA, Shields CL, Eagle RC, Blair CJ (1988) Spontaneous pseudohypopyon secondary to diffuse infiltrating retinoblastoma. Arch Ophthalmol 106:1301–1302

Shin HJ, Sneige N (2000) Epithelial cells and other cytologic features of pseudomyxoma peritonei in patients with ovarian and/or appendiceal mucinous neoplasms: A study of 12 patients including 5 men. Cancer 90:17–23

Smith JW et al (1992) Pseudomyxoma peritonei of appendiceal origin. The memorial sloan-kettering cancer center experience. Cancer 70:396–401

Soslow RA, Pirog E, Isacson C (2000) Endometrial intraepithelial carcinoma with associated peritoneal carcinomatosis. Am J Surg Pathol 24:726–732

Sugarbaker PH (2002) Cytoreduction including total gastrectomy for pseudomyxoma peritonei. Br J Surg 89:208–212

Sugarbaker PH, Chang D (1999) Results of treatment of 385 patients with peritoneal surface spread of appendiceal malignancy. Ann Surg Oncol 6:727–731

Sugarbaker PH, Yan H, Shmookler B (2001) Pedunculated peritoneal surface polyps in pseudomyxoma peritonei syndrome. Histopathology 39:525–528

Tarin D et al (1984) Mechanisms of human tumor metastasis studied in patients with peritoneovenous shunts. Cancer Res 44:3584–3592

Tran TA, Jennings TA, Ross JS, Nazeer T (1998) Pseudomyxoma ovariilike posttherapeutic alteration in prostatic adenocarcinoma: A distinctive pattern in patients receiving neoadjuvant androgen ablation therapy. Am J Surg Pathol 22:347–354

Truong LD, Jurco S 3rd, McGavran MH (1982) Gliomatosis peritonei. Report of two cases and review of literature. Am J Surg Pathol 6:443–449

Young RH, Gilks CB, Scully RE (1991) Mucinous tumors of the appendix associated with mucinous tumors of the ovary and pseudomyxoma peritonei. A clinicopathological analysis of 22 cases supporting an origin in the appendix. Am J Surg Pathol 15:415–429

Zimmerman LE (1971) Verhoeff's "terato-neuroma". A critical reappraisal in light of new observations and current concepts of embryonic tumors. The fourth Frederick H. Verhoeff lecture. Am J Ophthalmol 72:1039–1057

Part V
Animal Models of Metastasis

Editor:
Patrick Logan

Chapter 15
Haematogenous Models of Metastases

Patrick T. Logan

15.1 Animal Models of Metastasis

Animal models of cancer and of metastasis in particular, provide a critical link between *in vitro* studies and the treatment of human disease. Animal models allow scientists to understand and interpret disease pathogenesis in an environment in which metastatic cells are constantly bombarded by autocrine, paracrine, and endocrine signals from a multitude of sources. Disease pathogenesis can only be elucidated through observation of organs, organ systems, and, ultimately, whole organisms. In addition to contributing to our knowledge of disease pathogenesis, animal models also provide an avenue for testing both the safety and efficacy of various anti-metastatic drugs and biological compounds. Animal models allow interpretation of the physiological effects of administrating a drug or biological compound in a complex organism. In this respect, animal models are critical to the drug development process and are a required element of the drug approval process. Within the umbrella term 'animal models', there are various types of models that present unique advantages and disadvantages to understanding metastasis and the ability to test anti-metastatic compounds. Ideally, animal models that closely mimic human cancers, with respect to disease duration, progression, mode of dissemination, and metastatic location, are desirable. However, due to the often inefficiency that is inherent in the metastatic process, animal models in which metastasis takes many years to develop are impractical. To overcome this innate obstacle, several different types of animal models have been developed to expedite the metastatic process: there are ectopic models, in which malignant cells are explanted into foreign locations on the animal, and there are haematogenous models of metastasis, in which cells are dispersed into circulation with the intention of simulating a natural course of dissemination. Occasionally, metastatic locations differ between human and their animal counterparts and thus, metastatic cells can be transplanted directly into a desired organ. Finally, there are spontaneous models of metastasis chemically induced, and

P. T. Logan (✉)
McGill University, Montreal, QC, Canada
e-mail: patrick.logan@mail.mcgill.ca

J. V. Burnier, M. N. Burnier, Jr. (eds.), *Experimental and Clinical Metastasis*,
DOI 10.1007/978-1-4614-3685-0_15,

transgenic models, in which a primary tumour is borne either in a normal host or in a host that has been predisposed to developing a desired tumour and subsequent metastatic development. This chapter will serve to introduce the reader to the various types of models, including the types of animals that are typically used. It will also present the advantages and disadvantages of the different models with respect to furthering our understanding of disease pathogenesis and the treatment of metastatic disease.

15.2 Haematogenous models

While spontaneous or comparative models of metastasis might be considered the gold standard for studying the natural history of metastasis they are not without several inherent disadvantages. The natural history of uveal melanoma in canines, for instance, may be different in terms of metastasis location, aggressiveness, and lethality when compared to the human disease (Wilcock and Peiffer 1986). However, the major detriment to these models is that they are rare and often take many years in order to develop metastasis. Thus, other 'high-throughput' models have been developed. Some of these models, such as the intravenous (IV) injection of tumor cells, omit the development and maturation of a primary tumour by injecting cells directly into an animal's circulation. In these models, cells are exposed to the stresses of being in circulation (such as pH, turmoil, anoikis) prior to metastatic organ seeding. As opposed to spontaneous models of metastases, a variety of different cell types, from metastatic to primary tumors, can be injected. Cells can also be selected for their affinity to metastasize to a particular organ and cells can be modified to express or suppress different genes in order to determine the effects of these on the development of metastases. Intravenous models of metastasis also allow for the use of human cells in these models which is not an option in spontaneous models of metastasis. Although, it must be noted, these models require immunosuppression of the animal and thus the natural history or metastatic profile may be affected. By injecting cells into the circulation, there is tremendous flexibility in the types of animals that can be used. Perhaps the most common animal used in these studies of intravenous injection of malignant cells leading to metastases, is the nude mouse. The nude mouse lacks a thymus gland and thus is inherently immunocompromised, lacking the ability to produce T-cells. Thus, the relatively inexpensive nude mouse that does not require immunosuppression is a prime candidate for the production and evaluation of intravenous models of metastasis. In addition to nude mice, other types of mice that have native malignant cell lines can be used without the risk of graft-host rejection. B-16 mice in combination with mouse melanoma cell lines are commonly used in intravenous models of metastasis. Although not as common as mouse models, intravenous injections of malignant cells in rats is also an approved method of metatasis development (Shingu et al. 2003). Despite the popularity of the mouse and rat, several models also use guinea pigs, gerbils, and hamsters to study the development of metastases (Perk et al. 1974; Shimizu et al. 1999; Uchida et al.

2008). Not unpredictably, each type of animal offers its own benefits and drawbacks; however, mice are the most common animals due to the ease of handling them, as well as their relatively inexpensive nature.

Haematogenous models of metastasis, whether the injection method is intravenous, intracardiac, or intraportal, all suffer from the same drawback—they do not allow for the investigation or observation of the cells' ability to extravasate into the blood from the primary tumor. As a result, all cells that are injected have the opportunity to colonize and metastasize in other organs while, in reality, the cells that are unable to enter into the blood stream from the primary tumor would never gain this opportunity. Another drawback of these models is that the majority of cells injected into circulation are cells that have been through several cell culture passages. Cultured cells are grown in an artificial environment that likely alters their phenotype: cells are not exposed to competitive situations, do not experience hypoxia, and are typically provided with a supra-physiological source of nourishment.

In order to study human cells in an animal model, the animal must be immunocompromised in order to ensure that implantation does not fail due to host-graft rejection. Thus, there is an inherent trade-off: researchers get the benefit of observing the behaviour of human cancer cells in an animal system, yet the system is incomplete as the important role of the immune system in metastasis development has been eliminated.

However, despite their drawbacks, these models provide excellent insight into many of the steps in the metastatic process and allow for the testing of therapeutics that would not otherwise be possible.

15.2.1 Intravenous Models

Typcically, **intravenous animal models** involve the injection of malignant cells into the dorsal tail-vein of either a rat or mouse. Although there are many variants on this procedure, the most common method involves either restraining or anesthetizing the rodent and warming the tail vein with a heat lamp or immersing in warm water. The visible tail-vein can now be injected with volumes of solution of around 100 μL.

Intravenous (IV) animal models, in particular mouse models, have been used to study a wide variety of cancers ranging from breast, colon, prostate, and melanoma. One particular advantage of intravenous models is that they must be injected as either single cells or in clumps of only a few cells. Thus, the development of subsequent metastases can be attributed to the clonal expansion of either one or a few cells. This is more comparable to human cancer, as cells that leave the primary site via hematogenous dissemination would do so in the same linear fashion. Other types of animal models, such as models which involve injection a large bolus of cells directly into the organ of interest, may induce large changes to the microenvironment that are superficial in nature. However, IV models of metastasis also pose their own unique set of disadvantages; cells are not required to invade locally or extravasate into the bloodstream. If human cells are used, the animal must be immunosuppressed and this eliminates the influence of the innate immune system on metastasis development. By utilizing cultured cell lines, further unwanted variables can be introduced including genetic drift due to prolonged culturing, mycoplasma infections, and artificial cell selection could lessen the impact of any discoveries or advances acquired during the metastatic animal model.

Often the location of metastasis formation following intravenous injection varies between the murine and human counterpart. This is further compounded by the formation of several metastatic colonies in the same animal at various locations (Ji et al. 2009). While these locations do not always correspond to the natural history of metastasis in humans, some locations are common, and by harvesting the metastatic cells from these locations, serial injections in subsequent animals can lend to an organ specific cell line. This has proven to be an invaluable tool to study the genetic characteristic of cells that metastasize to one particular organ. The aforementioned artificial selection technique has also been used to select for a more metastatic cell type from the heterogeneous cell culture population. Fidler et al., increased the ability of B16 mouse melanoma cells to metastasize roughly five fold through a series of selections in which intravenously injected cells that developed into lung metastases were recultured and reinjected into a host mouse (Fidler and Nicolson 1977). This process has since been successfully replicated for murine mammary, osteosarcoma, rhabdomyosarcoma, lung, and colon tumors (Aslakson and Miller 1992; Rusciano et al. 1994; Khanna et al. 2000; Yu et al. 2004; Sacchi et al. 1981). Minn et al. (2005), used this serial selection process in order to isolate a lung metasatasis specific cohort of the human, MDA-MB-231 breast cell line. Development of this lung-specific metastatic cohort facilitated the identification of genes that may be implicated in lung metastasis development. This information may prove valuable in identifying those patients who's primary tumors express the lung metastasis signature which include specific genes such as MMP1, VCAM1, CXCR4, and CXCL1 amongst others (Minn et al. 2005).

The validity and usefulness of an animal model of metastasis and cancer in general is often evaluated based on the similarities with the human disease; including, but not limited to, metastasis location and development. Thus, when considering hematogenous models of metastsis, the three most common introduction routes include intravenous (IV), intrasplenic or portal vein injection, or intracardiac injection. Typically, IV injections result in lung metastases, portal vein injections result in liver metastases, and intracardiac injections result in bone metastasis (Khanna and Hunter 2005). Although not a steadfast rule, it is generally accepted that the consistent development of metastasis in organs depending on injection route is attributed to the fact that these organs typically correspond with a high degree of vascularity that is first encountered. However, the ability to image single cells *in vivo* immediately post-injection suggests broad organ seeding of cells in various organs and that survival in these organs may be the limiting factor (Logan et al. 2008; Holleran et al. 2002). This is apparent when the frequency of bone metastasis developing post-intracardiac injection of malignant cells. Holleran et al., used a lacZ tagged prostate cancer cell line and injected a single cell suspension in the tail-vein of nude mice and determined that micrometastasis were present immediately following injection in the lung, bone, kidney, brain and liver of the animals. Logan et al., using GFP labelled uveal melanoma cells, found similar broad-organ seeding following tail-vein injection in nude mice, and observations revealed that the presence of micrometastasis in non-native metastatic or hostile organs are quickly destroyed or eliminated (Logan et al. 2008; Holleran et al. 2002). This should not be suprising though, as the seed and soil theory that metastatic development is contingent upon interactions between tumor cells and the organ microenvironment was proposed more than a century ago (Fidler and Poste 2008).

15.2.2 Intracardiac Injections

Intracardiac injections of malignant cells is another popular method for developing metastases. This technique involves inserting a needle in the second intercostal space aimed in the direction of the anatomical location of the heart of an anesthetized mouse. Advancing the needle should be accompanied by frequent aspirations and the presence of fresh blood indicates that the correct injection location has been achieved. The malignant cells should be injected slowly over a period of roughly thirty seconds.

As previously mentioned, this method is preferable if the development of bone metastases is desired. In humans, breast, prostate, and lung primary malignancies often metastasize to the bone (Yoneda 1998). In fact, breast cancer and prostate cancer metastasize preferentially to bone in 70 % of cases of metastasis (Lelekakis et al. 1999; Chiarodo 1991). Unlike portal vein and intravenous method of inoculation, the rationality regarding the development of metastases in the first capillary rich bed that is encountered, intracardiac animal models and subsequent bone metatases do not follow this pattern. It has been suggested that the development of bone metastases in these animal models may be a result of complex host-tumor interactions that are not completely understood (Khanna and Hunter 2005). One suggestion is that the bones of young animals are growing and remodelling which requires a high degree of blood flow. The blood flow in these growing bones are highly convoluted which could be conducive to the lodging of injection malignant cells and subsequent metastasis development (Rosol et al. 2003; Yoneda 1997). Whatever the reason, intracardiac injections of metastatic cells have proven invaluable in increasing our understanding of bone. In rat model of metastasis, the intracardiac injection of Mat-LyLu rat Dunning carcinoma cells resulted in 100 % bone metastasis that caused paralysis and death within five days (Haq et al. 1992). However, injecting the same Mat-LyLu cells either intravenously or subcutaneously resulted in lung or lymph metastases but failed to develop any bone metastases (Haq et al. 1992). Human bone metastases are typically either osteolytic (breast) or osteoblastic (prostate) and occasionally tumors express both osteolytic and osteoblastic properties (Rose and Siegel 2006). Although there are other methods of developing bone metastases, mainly, injecting malignant cells directly into the bone, cardiac injections avoid the additional complication of bone remodelling that can occur as a direct result of the

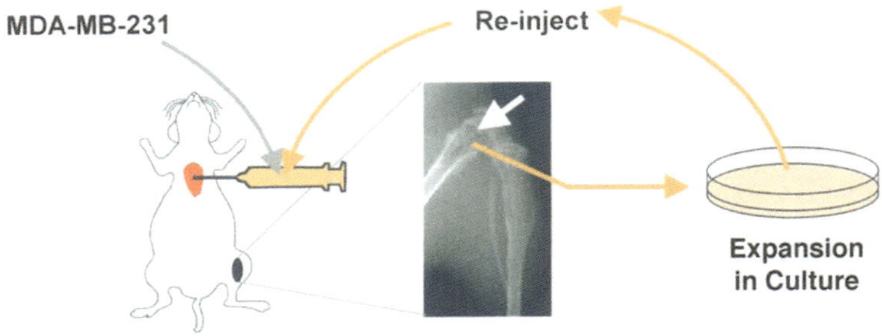

Fig. 15.1 Example of the selection process for a highly bone metastatic phenotype derived from intracardiac injections of a human breast cancer cell line. (From Kang et al. 2003)

Table 15.1 A list of select mouse models of breast cancer metastasis established by either tail vein or intracardiac injection. (Adapted from Kim and Baek 2010)

Injection site	Cell number	Metastasis location	Latency (weeks)	Reference
Tail vein	2×10^5	Lung	8–15	Minn et al. (2005)
Intracardiac	1×10^4–1×10^5	Brain, bone	4	Bos et al. (2009)
Intracardiac	1×10^5	Bone	4	Charafe-Jauffret et al. (2009)
Tail vein	2×10^6	Lung	8	Kuperwasser et al. (2005)
Intracardiac	1×10^6	Bone	4	Lu et al. (2009)

injection (Rose and Siegel 2006). Kang et al. (2003) injected a human breast cancer cell line intracardially in nude mice which resulted in bone and adrenal metastases and through selection and reinjection, was able to select a highly bone metastatic subpopulation of cells (Fig. 15.1, Table 15.1).

Transcriptional profiling of the original breast cancer cell line, the highly bone metastatic selected group, and the adrenal metastasis group revealed a unique expression profile (Kang et al. 2003). When compared to the original cell line, using a cut-off of a four fold increase in gene expression in the highly bone metastasis subpopulation, a variety of cell membrane or secretory proteins were identified (Fig. 15.2).

Perhaps not surprisingly, several of these have been implicated, including, most prominently, CXCR4 in the 'homing' of malignant cells to a particular organ for the purpose of metastatic formation. In fact, the CXCR4 and its receptor SD-1 has been implicated in the ability of tumor cells to migrate, adhere, invade (facilitated by secretion of proteolytic enzymes such as MMPs), proliferation, and tumor angiogenesis (Libura et al. 2002; Di Cesare et al. 2007; Ding et al. 2003; Majka et al. 2000; Wang et al. 2005). Perhaps the most critical role in bone metastasis development is the gradient of SD-1 produced by the host/receptive tissue. This gradient draws tumor cells expressing the CXCR4 to that organ for preferential metastasis formation (Fig. 15.3, Kucia et al. 2005).

Although more factors than the CXCR4/SD-1 axis are likely involved in the specificity for bone metastases, as many other organs such as the lung and liver produce

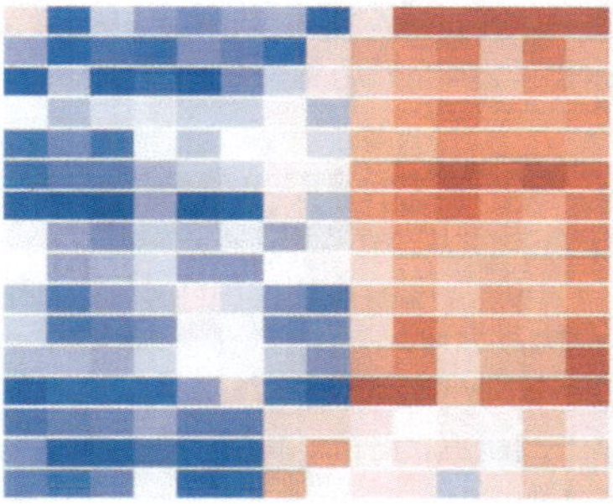

Probe set	Fold	Gene Symbol, Gene Name
222162_s_at	18.46	*ADAMTS1*
210310_s_at	12.29	*FGF5, Fibroblast growth factor 5*
208378_x_at	15.51	*FGF5, Fibroblast growth factor 5*
209101_at	4.32	*CTGF, Connective tissue growth factor*
201859_at	6.68	*PRG1, Proteoglycan 1, secretory granule*
201858_s_at	12.99	*PRG1, Proteoglycan 1, secretory granule*
204749_at	51.09	*NAP1L3, Nucleosome assembly protein 1-like 3*
209949_at	4.34	*NCF2, Neutrophil cytosolic factor 2*
201041_s_at	4.23	*DUSP1, Dual specificity phosphatase 1*
207345_at	4.64	*FST, Follistatin*
204948_s_at	5.99	*FST, Follistatin*
211919_s_at	4.06	*CXCR4, Chemokine (C-X-C motif), receptor 4*
209201_x_at	21.72	*CXCR4, Chemokine (C-X-C motif), receptor 4*
206926_s_at	4.06	*IL11, Interleukin 11*
206924_at	10.06	*IL11, Interleukin 11*
204475_at	5.28	*MMP1, Matrix metalloproteinase 1*

Fig. 15.2 List of genes that are upregulated in a bone metastasis enriched subpopulation derived from a human breast cancer cell line. (From Kang et al. 2003)

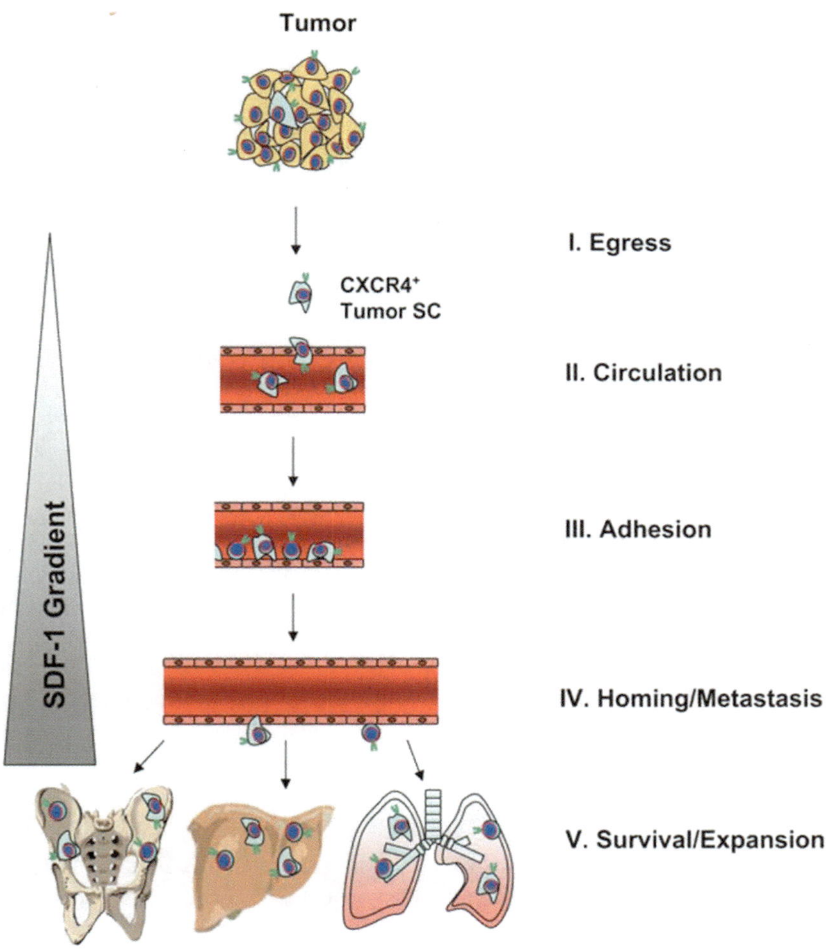

Fig. 15.3 An example of the proposed role of the CXCR4/SD-1 axis in the development of metastatic disease. (Adapted from Kucia et al. 2005)

large quantities of SD-1, its role has been well documented in a variety of cancers. Indeed, the combination of upregulating CXCR4, IL11, and osteopontin resulted in increased frequency and aggressiveness of bone metastases compared to upregulation of CXCR4 alone (Kang et al. 2003).

In addition to forming bone metastases, a study of 2050 cases of breast cancer revealed that roughly 20 % of patients develop brain metastases (Jonkers and Derksen 2007). Yoneda et al., developed a preferential brain and bone metastasis strains of the breast cancer cell line MDA-231 through repeated inoculations as described above (Fig. 15.1, Yoneda et al. 2001). After seven such passages, the MDA-231BR cell line was established with properties that resulted in 100 % brain metastases development following intracardiac injection with no alternative metastasis sites in these animals. Similarly, after 11 passages, a bone exclusive strain, MDA-231BO was generated. By developing these clones using the same methods and derived from the same original cell line, it was possible to identify several genetic differences that may play a key role in the site-specific metastasis development. Insulin-like growth factor 1 (IGF-1) had a significantly greater effect on colony growth in culture of MDA-231BO compared to MDA-231BR (Yoneda et al. 2001). Another protein implicated in the development of bone metastases is parathryroid hormone-related protein (PTHrP). PTHrP is produced by tumor cells and is responsible for bone osteoclastic resorption and umors that produce PTHrP are more likely to metastasize to bone in patients (Abou-Samra et al. 1992; Juppner et al. 1991; Bundred et al. 1991, 1996). Mice that were inoculated with PTHrP anti-bodies prior to ventricle injection of breast cancer cells had a significantly lower tumor bone metastasis burden than those without the PTHrP antibodies (Guise et al. 1996). Considering that TGF-B is the most common growth factor in the bone matrix, it comes as no surprise that it is capable of inducing the production of PTHrP by metastatic tumor cells (Yin et al. 1999). When comparing the MDA-231BO (bone) and MDA-231BR (brain) selected cell lines, the bone metastasis population expresses greater basal levels of PTHrP than the brain population (Yoneda et al. 2001). Additionally, stimulating of these cultured cell lines with TGF-B causes a greater increase in the bone metastasis cells compared to the brain metastasis cells (Yoneda et al. 2001). Thus, utilizing established intracardiac injection murine metastasis models discovered the importance of PTHrP in the development of breast cancer bone metastases. This information may be critical in determining primary lesions of patients that are capable of metastasizing preferentially to a particular site and could be used to tailor patient-specific therapies.

15.2.3 Intraportal Injections

Considering that liver metastases are common and frequently inoperable in many human cancers, including melanoma, breast cancer, colorectal cancer, lung cancer, esophageal cancer, pancreatice cancer, and stomach cancer, it is critical that animal models of liver metastasis are developed in order to study this disease. While intravenous injections tend to give rise to lung metastases and intracardiac injections give rise to bone metastases, intraportal injections almost excusively give rise to liver metastases. **Intraportal animal model** injection surgeries typically involve making an incision in the abdomen of the mouse from the zyphoid process to above the bladder and inserting a cannula in the portal vein just after the bifurcation (Stapfer et al. 2003). By slowly injecting a single celled suspension of tumor cells (ranging from 10,000–1,000,000 cells depending on the aggressiveness of the cells) the most likely location for the development of metastases is the liver (Stapfer et al. 2003; Hamada et al. 2008). Stapfer et al. (2003), repeated this process with pancreatic, breast, and colon cancer cell lines and successfully developed a liver metastasis nude mouse model of each of the aforementioned cancers. Hamada et al. (2008), injected eleven different human colon cancer cell lines into the portal vein of immunosuppressed mice and determined that six were capable of forming liver metastases and the other cell lines did not form any metastases. Intraportal injection models of liver metastases have also revealed information about the host inflammatory response to tumor cell invasion that would have otherwise likely remained unknown. E-selectin is a vascular endothelial cell receptor which is induced by the production of the cytokine TNF-α (Dejana et al. 1992; Tozeren et al. 1995; Brodt et al. 1997). The use of intrasplenic animal models have revealed that colon cancer cells express the ligand for E-selectin and that malignant cells exploit this ligand to bind to vascular endothelial cells. Abolishment of this expression through the use of antibody therapy inhibited the formation of liver metastases (Brodt et al. 1997). Furthermore, additional animal studies confirmed that the tumor cells themselves were capable and perhaps culpable for the upregulation of TNF-α and other cytokines that have been shown to upregulate E-selectin (Khatib et al. 1999). Thus, the ability of tumor cells to manipulate the microenvironment of organs in animal models likely contributes to the organ specificity of metastasis.

15.2.4 Animals of Haematogenous Models

There are several different species and strains of animals that are used to study metastases. Traditionally, if the malignant cells to be used are of mouse origin, then selection is usually predetermined; malignant mouse cells are almost exclusively injected in the mouse species of origin. Multiple inbreeding sessions result in no host-graft rejection and thus immunosuppression is not required. The most popular mouse used in animal models of metastasis that does not require immunosuppression is the **Black 6 mouse (C57BL/6)** a heavily inbred strain that demonstrates robust breeding characteristics. Black 6 mice are typically paired with B16 mouse melanoma cell lines in order to study metastatic development. For instance, Yang et al. (1999) used intravenous injections of B16 mouse melanoma cells in the Black 6 mouse to generate skeletal and visceral metastases.

In order to study metastases from human derived cell lines, mice must be immunosuppressed. There are several strains of immunodeficient mice, the most popular of

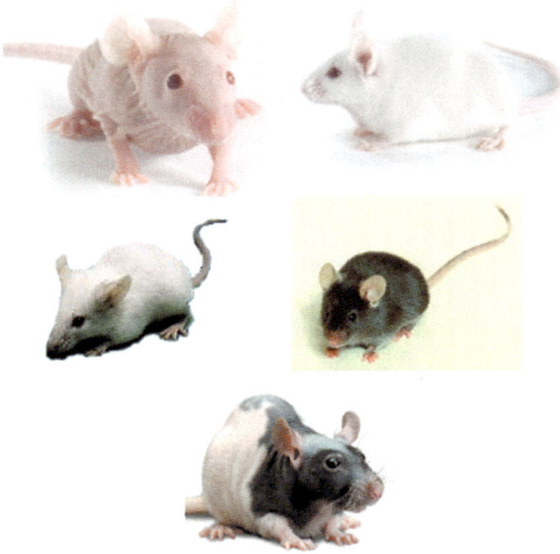

Fig. 15.4 Images of some of the typical rodents used in animal models. Clockwise from *top right*—BALB/c nude mouse (image from Charles River), SCID mouse (Charles River), NOG mouse (CIEA), Black 6 mouse (Jackson Labs Archive), RNU nude rat (Charles River)

which is likely the **nude mouse (BALB/c)** which lacks a thymus gland and thus is incapable of producing T-cells but produces both B-cells and NK cells. The nude mouse derives its name from the fact that a side-effect of the lack of thymus results in a hairless appearance. Logan et al. (2008), used nude mice to study the broad organ seeding of metastatic uveal melanoma cells following tail-vein injections. A similar mouse is the **SCID mouse** (severe combined immonudeficiency) that lacks both B-cell and T-cell production but produces a normal NK cell count. The latest iteration of immunodeficient mice is the NOD/Shi-*scid*/IL-2Rγ^{null} **(NOG) mouse**. This mouse lacks T-cell, B-cell, and NK cell function in addition to having dysfunctional macrophages and dendritic cells. NOG mice were created by the Central Institute for Experimental Animals in Japan and is considered one of the most immunologically inept mouse for consideration in animal models of disease (Nomura et al. 2008). An athymic rat (RNU rat) was also created by Charles River Labs and has the same general properties as the nude mouse; mainly, the lack of thymus generated lymphocytes (Fig. 15.4). Successful brain metastases have been developed as a result of intracardiac injections of breast cancer lines in these animals and the larger animal size can be desirable for some studies (Song et al. 2009).

15.2.5 Drug Development and Discovery

While the importance of basic scientific studies and cell cultures should not be overlooked, animal models play a paramount role in the discovery and evaluation of new drugs or treatment compounds. In fact, prior to entering into the clinical trial phases of drug approval, scientists must first provide sufficient evidence of a compounds' biological activity. This step includes a variety of *in vitro* tests in order to determine the potential benefits and risks of a compound or drug. The compound is then tested in a variety of animal models (*in vivo*) to provide further evidence of desired biological activity (Health, U.S.N.I.o. 2006). Thus, almost every drug, including those that are approved for the treatment of metastastases, that has been FDA or Health Canada approved for human use has also been tested in at least one animal model.

In 2004, the most prescribed treatment for breast cancer, in particular estrogen receptor positive (ER+) tumors was tamoxifen. Tomixifen is a Selective Estrogen Receptor Modulator (SERM): tamoxifen binds to the estrogen receptor preventing the binding of estrogen and subsequent growth signal induction (Nowak-Markwitz et al. 2010). Tamoxifen is used for treatment of both early and late, metastastic, stages of breast cancer.

Tamoxifen has also been shown to inhibit the growth of experimental colorectal liver metastases. Karuppu et al. (1998), injected mice intrasplenicly with a colon cancer cell line that generates liver metastases within 10 days. Daily sub-coetaneous injections of 1 mg/kg dose of tamosifen citrate caused a significant delay in the growth of liver metastasis nodules. Tumor burden was significantly less between days 16–22 in the tamoxifen treated and control, untreated groups. Interestingly, the colon cancer cell line used in this study does not express the estrogen receptor, suggesting additional roles to tamoxifen treatment aside from estrogen receptor modulation (Kuruppu et al. 1998). It has been proposed that tamoxifen's benefit in ER− tumors arises from its anti-angiogenic properties (Blackwell et al. 2000). Current studies are evaluating the benefits of combining tamoxifen and other drugs, such as the anti-angiogenic bevacizumab, in order to treat cancer metastases in both ER+ and ER− tumors (Mittal et al. 2005).

Melanoma metastases have a poor prognosis with a mean survival time of roughly 6 months (Klimek et al. 2000). The current treatment for melanoma metastases typically includes the alkalating agent dacarbazine (DCIT) the mechanism of action of which has not been fully elucidated (Eggermont and Kirkwood 2004). However, the response rate to DCIT is estimated at around only 15 % with rapidly induced resistance (Chapman et al. 1999). Thus, alternative methods of treatment for metastatic melanoma are under investigation. In 2010, Valera et al., investigated the use of a new compound Dimethylfumarate (DMF) alone and in combination with DCIT. SCID mice received intradermal injections of the human M24met melanoma cell lines. Both DMF and DCIT treatment alone caused a marked reduction in the number of lymph node metastases. However, treatment with both DMF and DCIT resulted in further, statistically significant reduction in the total volume of lymph node metastases compared to the control group (Valero et al. 2010, Fig. 15.5). Additional studies are evaluating the effectiveness of DMF and DCIT in combination to treat metastatic melanoma.

Ocular melanoma has a metastasis rate of roughly 40 % almost all of which are incurable and result in death in six months (Diener-West et al. 2004). As a similar, yet more rare counterpart to coetaneous melanoma, ocular melanoma treatments often arise secondary to their discovery for the treatment of coetaneous

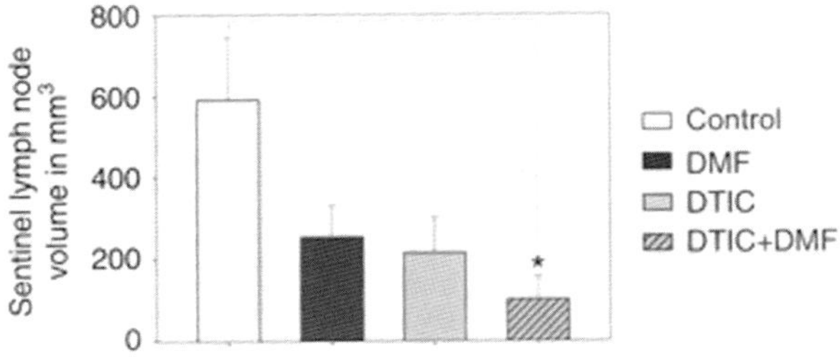

Fig. 15.5 Reduction in metastases post treatment with Dimethylfumarate (DMT), dacarbazine (DCIT), or a combination of both in a SCID mouse model of melanoma lymph node metastases. (From Valero et al. 2010)

melanoma. Never-the-less, animal studies evaluating the effectiveness in treating metastatic ocular melanoma are often conducted. For instance, intraocular inoculation of B16 melanoma cells into the eye of Black 6 mice results in the formation of numerous lung metastases (Sanborn et al. 1992). High doses of DCIT bolus injections caused a dramatic decrease in the incidence of metastases in these animals (Sanborn et al. 1992).

Bevacizumab is a monoclonal antibody raised against the powerful angiogenic factor Vascular Endothelial Growth Factor (VEGF). The antiangiogenic effects of bevacizumab have been tested in many animal models for many different types of cancer metastases. The FDA approved bevacizumab in 2004 for treatment of metastatic colon cancer. Since approval, bevacizumb's effectiveness in treating metastasis has been tested in breast, lung, ocular melanoma, and gastric cancer animal models (Bauerle et al. 2008; Yang et al. 2010; Otsuka et al. 2009; Ninomiya et al. 2009). Countless studies have also been performed in a variety of animal models of metastasis using bevacizumab in conjunction with other therapies in order to increase efficacy (Gerber and Ferrara 2005).

Bauerle et al. (2008), injected the MDA-MB-231 human breast cancer cell line into the superficial epigastric artery of nude rats. Thirty-five days post inoculation, rats were injected with a10 mg/kg weekly, intravenous dose of bevacizumab. Treated rats saw a 63 % reduction in bone metastases compared to the control group (Bauerle et al. 2008). In a similar model using lung cancer cell lines, bevacizumab showed efficacy in reducing the overall number of metastases in an immunodeficient mouse model of bone metastases (Otsuka et al. 2009).

In 2010, Yang et al. assessed the efficacy of bevacizumab in preventing metastasis formation following an intraocular injection of the human uveal melanoma cell line Mel290 into nude mice or B16LS9 mouse melanoma cell line in immunocompetent Black 6 mice. In both cases, the formation of micrometastases were reduced in a dose dependant manner following intraperitoneal doses of 50 or 250 μg/100 μL (Yang et al. 2010). Intraperitoneal injection of bevacizumab following inoculation of human gastric cancer cell lines into nude mice resulted in a reduction of the number of metastatic tumors in addition to a reduction in the overall mass of the tumors (Ninomiya et al. 2009). Additional animal models studying the effects of bevacizumab treatment on metastasis formation can be seen in Table 15.2.

All of these animal studies provide the footwork and background necessary to establish clinical trials for the use of bevacizumab in a wide variety of human cancers, as well as providing support for the off-label use of this compound.

Table 15.2 The effects of bevacizumab on metastasis formation in various animal models. (Adapted from Gerber and Ferrara 2005)

Tumor type	Graft location	Dosing regimen (twice weekly) (μg i.p.)	Species	Results	Reference
Prostate carcinoma	Sub-cutaneous	10 + 100	Mouse/CB-17 SCID/SCID	Suppression of primary tumor growth (82 %) and lung metastases	Melnyk et al. (1999)
Colon adenocarcinoma	Splenic portal injections	10–200	Mouse/athymic	90 % reduction in tumor size of primary tumor; reduction in liver metastases	Warren et al. (1995)
Wilms' tumor	Intrarenal	100	Mouse/nude	Significant > 95 % reduction in tumor weight and > 40 % in lung metastases	Rowe et al. (2000)
Wilms' tumor	Intrarenal	100	Mouse/athymic	Significant reduction in tumor growth, vascularity, and lung metastases	Soffer et al. (2001)
Pancreatic cancer	Sub-cutaneous	100	Mouse/nude mice	Single treatment reduced primary tumor size, metastasis, angiogenesis, and increased survival	Hotz et al. (2003)

15.3 Key Terms

Intravenous Animal Models These models typically involve the injection of a malignant cell suspension into the tail-vein of rodents. This type of model allows for the study of circulating malignant cells, extravasation out of the blood, and organ seeding and proliferation. It does not permit the observation of the initial escape of malignant cells from the primary tumor. The most common site of metastases in these models is the lung.

Intracardiac Animal Models Malignant cells are injected into the left ventricle of anaesthetized rodents in these models. Similar to intravenous models, intracardiac animal models allow the observation of the stages of metastases development post-intravasation from the primary tumor. Metastases typically develop in the bone and thus these animal models are a useful tool to study breast and prostate cancer metastases.

Intraportal Animal Models This type of model is ideal for studying liver seeding of metastatic cells and overt metastatic development in the liver. Classically, an intraportal model is developed by injecting malignant cells into the portal vein of rodents following an abdominal incision. Subsequent metastatic development occurs almost exclusively in the liver of these animals.

Black 6 (C57BL/6) Mouse This heavily inbred animal is used in animal models of metastases that involve the injection of malignant mouse cells. As an immunocompetent animal, studies using this model allow for the observation of the effects of the immune system on metastatic development yet preclude the ability to study human malignant cells due to host-graft rejection. The most common cancer studied in models that use the Black 6 mouse are those involving the B16 mouse melanoma cell line.

Nude Mouse (BALB/c) The nude mouse does not have a thymus and thus does not produce T-cells. This mutation generates a hairless phenotype and hence the name nude mouse. This naturally immunosuppressed rodent permits the study of human malignant cells. The nude mouse produces normal B-cells and NK cells.

SCID (severe combined immunodeficient) Mouse The SCID mouse developed as a result of a mutation in a DNA repair enzyme. This mutation inhibits proper somatic recombination of immunoglobulin heavy chains which renders SCID mice incapable of producing T-cells or B-cells. SCID mice produce normal NK cells.

NOG Mouse Generated through multiple backcrosses of SCID and Black 6 mouse variants, this mouse is almost completely immunodefficient; the NOG mouse is incapable of producing T-cells, B-cells, or NK cells. This mouse also has diminished macrophage and dendritic cell production. As a result of such extensive immunosuppression, these animals are ideal for addressing specific questions regarding metastases in which the immune system is not a consideration.

References

Abou-Samra AB et al (1992) Expression cloning of a common receptor for parathyroid hormone and parathyroid hormone-related peptide from rat osteoblast-like cells: a single receptor stimulates intracellular accumulation of both cAMP and inositol trisphosphates and increases intracellular free calcium. Proc Natl Acad Sci U S A 89:2732–2736

Aslakson CJ, Miller FR (1992) Selective events in the metastatic process defined by analysis of the sequential dissemination of subpopulations of a mouse mammary tumor. Cancer Res 52:1399–1405

Bauerle T et al (2008) Bevacizumab inhibits breast cancer-induced osteolysis, surrounding soft tissue metastasis, and angiogenesis in rats as visualized by VCT and MRI. Neoplasia 10:511–520

Blackwell KL et al (2000) Tamoxifen inhibits angiogenesis in estrogen receptor-negative animal models. Clin Cancer Res 6:4359–4364

Bos PD et al (2009) Genes that mediate breast cancer metastasis to the brain. Nature 459:1005–1009

Brodt P et al (1997) Liver endothelial E-selectin mediates carcinoma cell adhesion and promotes liver metastasis. Int J Cancer 71:612–619

Bundred NJ et al (1991) Parathyroid hormone related protein and hypercalcaemia in breast cancer. Bmj 303:1506–1509

Bundred NJ, Walls J, Ratcliffe WA (1996) Parathyroid hormone-related protein, bone metastases and hypercalcaemia of malignancy. Ann R Coll Surg Engl 78:354–358

Chapman PB et al (1999) Phase III multicenter randomized trial of the Dartmouth regimen versus dacarbazine in patients with metastatic melanoma. J Clin Oncol 17:2745–2751

Charafe-Jauffret E et al (2009) Breast cancer cell lines contain functional cancer stem cells with metastatic capacity and a distinct molecular signature. Cancer Res 69:1302–1313

Chiarodo A (1991) National Cancer Institute roundtable on prostate cancer: future research directions. Cancer Res 51:2498–2505

Dejana E et al (1992) Endothelial leukocyte adhesion molecule-1-dependent adhesion of colon carcinoma cells to vascular endothelium is inhibited by an antibody to Lewis fucosylated type I carbohydrate chain. Lab Invest 66:324–330

Di Cesare S et al (2007) In vitro characterization and inhibition of the CXCR4/CXCL12 chemokine axis in human uveal melanoma cell lines. Cancer Cell Int 7:17

Diener-West M et al (2004) Screening for metastasis from choroidal melanoma: the collaborative ocular melanoma study group report 23. J Clin Oncol 22:2438–2444

Ding Z, Issekutz TB, Downey GP, Waddell TK (2003) L-selectin stimulation enhances functional expression of surface CXCR4 in lymphocytes: implications for cellular activation during adhesion and migration. Blood 101:4245–4252

Eggermont AM, Kirkwood JM (2004) Re-evaluating the role of dacarbazine in metastatic melanoma: what have we learned in 30 years? Eur J Cancer 40:1825–1836

Fidler IJ, Nicolson GL (1977) Fate of recirculating B16 melanoma metastatic variant cells in parabiotic syngeneic recipients. J Natl Cancer Inst 58:1867–1872

Fidler IJ, Poste G (2008) The "seed and soil" hypothesis revisited. Lancet Oncol 9:808

Gerber HP, Ferrara N (2005) Pharmacology and pharmacodynamics of bevacizumab as monotherapy or in combination with cytotoxic therapy in preclinical studies. Cancer Res 65:671–680

Guise TA et al (1996) Evidence for a causal role of parathyroid hormone-related protein in the pathogenesis of human breast cancer-mediated osteolysis. J Clin Invest 98:1544–1549

Hamada K et al (2008) Liver metastasis models of colon cancer for evaluation of drug efficacy using NOD/Shi-scid IL2Rgammanull (NOG) mice. Int J Oncol 32:153–159

Haq M, Goltzman D, Tremblay G, Brodt P (1992) Rat prostate adenocarcinoma cells disseminate to bone and adhere preferentially to bone marrow-derived endothelial cells. Cancer Res 52:4613–4619

Holleran JL, Miller CJ, Edgehouse NL, Pretlow TP, Culp LA (2002) Differential experimental micrometastasis to lung, liver, and bone with lacZ-tagged CWR22R prostate carcinoma cells. Clin Exp Metastasis 19:17–24

Hotz HG et al (2003) Evaluation of vascular endothelial growth factor blockade and matrix metalloproteinase inhibition as a combination therapy for experimental human pancreatic cancer. J Gastrointest Surg 7:220–227 (discussion 227–228)
Ji X et al (2009) Noninvasive visualization of retinoblastoma growth and metastasis via bioluminescence imaging. Invest Ophthalmol Vis Sci 50:5544–5551
Jonkers J, Derksen PW (2007) Modeling metastatic breast cancer in mice. J Mammary Gland Biol Neoplasia 12:191–203
Juppner H et al (1991) A G protein-linked receptor for parathyroid hormone and parathyroid hormone-related peptide. Science 254:1024–1026
Kang Y et al (2003) A multigenic program mediating breast cancer metastasis to bone. Cancer Cell 3:537–549
Khanna C et al (2000) An orthotopic model of murine osteosarcoma with clonally related variants differing in pulmonary metastatic potential. Clin Exp Metastasis 18:261–271
Khanna C, Hunter K (2005) Modeling metastasis in vivo. Carcinogenesis 26:513–523
Khatib AM et al (1999) Rapid induction of cytokine and E-selectin expression in the liver in response to metastatic tumor cells. Cancer Res 59:1356–1361
Kim IS, Baek SH (2010) Mouse models for breast cancer metastasis. Biochem Biophys Res Commun 394:443–447
Klimek VM, Wolchok JD, Chapman PB, Houghton AN, Hwu WJ (2000) Systemic chemotherapy. Clin Plast Surg 27:451–461 (ix–x)
Kucia M et al (2005) Trafficking of normal stem cells and metastasis of cancer stem cells involve similar mechanisms: pivotal role of the SDF-1-CXCR4 axis. Stem Cells 23:879–894
Kuperwasser C et al (2005) A mouse model of human breast cancer metastasis to human bone. Cancer Res 65:6130–6138
Kuruppu D, Christophi C, Bertram JF, O'Brien PE (1998) Tamoxifen inhibits colorectal cancer metastases in the liver: a study in a murine model. J Gastroenterol Hepatol 13:521–527
Lelekakis M et al (1999) A novel orthotopic model of breast cancer metastasis to bone. Clin Exp Metastasis 17:163–170
Libura J et al (2002) CXCR4-SDF-1 signaling is active in rhabdomyosarcoma cells and regulates locomotion, chemotaxis, and adhesion. Blood 100:2597–2606
Logan PT et al (2008) Single-cell tumor dormancy model of uveal melanoma. Clin Exp Metastasis 25:509–516
Lu X et al (2009) ADAMTS1 and MMP1 proteolytically engage EGF-like ligands in an osteolytic signaling cascade for bone metastasis. Genes Dev 23:1882–1894
Majka M et al (2000) Stromal-derived factor 1 and thrombopoietin regulate distinct aspects of human megakaryopoiesis. Blood 96:4142–4151
Melnyk O, Zimmerman M, Kim KJ, Shuman M (1999) Neutralizing anti-vascular endothelial growth factor antibody inhibits further growth of established prostate cancer and metastases in a pre-clinical model. J Urol 161:960–963
Minn AJ et al (2005) Genes that mediate breast cancer metastasis to lung. Nature 436:518–524
Mittal A, Maxuitenko Y, Rinehart J, Waud WR, Thottassery J, Frost AR, Grizzle W, Li R, Qu Z (2005) A preclinical study of tamoxifen in combination with bevacizumab (Avastin) for the treatment of ER-positive breast cancer. AACR Meeting Abstracts: 254-b
Ninomiya S et al (2009) Effect of bevacizumab, a humanized monoclonal antibody to vascular endothelial growth factor, on peritoneal metastasis of MNK-45P human gastric cancer in mice. J Surg Res 154:196–202
Nomura T, Tamaoki N, Takakura A, Suemizu H (2008) Basic concept of development and practical application of animal models for human diseases. Curr Top Microbiol Immunol 324:1–24
Nowak-Markwitz E et al (2010) Influence of tamoxifen on cisplatin-sensitivity and estrogen receptors expression in ovarian carcinoma cell lines. Ginekol Pol 81:183–187
Otsuka S et al (2009) A bone metastasis model with osteolytic and osteoblastic properties of human lung cancer ACC-LC-319/bone2 in natural killer cell-depleted severe combined immunodeficient mice. Oncol Res 17:581–591

Perk K, Pearson JW, Torgersen JA, Chirigos MA (1974) An animal model for meningeal leukemia. Int J Cancer 13:863–866

Rose AA, Siegel PM (2006) Breast cancer-derived factors facilitate osteolytic bone metastasis. Bull Cancer 93:931–943

Rosol TJ, Tannehill-Gregg SH, LeRoy BE, Mandl S, Contag CH (2003) Animal models of bone metastasis. Cancer 97:748–757

Rowe DH et al (2000) Anti-VEGF antibody suppresses primary tumor growth and metastasis in an experimental model of Wilms' tumor. J Pediatr Surg 35:30–32 (discussion 32–33)

Rusciano D, Lorenzoni P, Burger M (1994) Murine models of liver metastasis. Invas Metast 14:349–361

Sacchi A, Calabresi F, Greco C, Zupi G (1981) Different metastatic potential of in vitro and in vivo lines selected from Lewis lung carcinoma: correlation with response to different bleomycin schedulings. Invas Metast 1:227–238

Sanborn GE, Niederkorn JY, Gamel JW (1992) Efficacy of dacarbazine (DTIC) in preventing metastases arising from intraocular melanomas in mice. Graefes Arch Clin Exp Ophthalmol 230:192–196

Shimizu N et al (1999) New animal model of glandular stomach carcinogenesis in Mongolian gerbils infected with Helicobacter pylori and treated with a chemical carcinogen. J Gastroenterol 34(Suppl 11):61–66

Shingu K et al (2003) Intratracheal macrophage-activating lipopeptide-2 reduces metastasis in the rat lung. Am J Respir Cell Mol Biol 28:316–321

Soffer SZ et al (2001) Combination antiangiogenic therapy: increased efficacy in a murine model of Wilms tumor. J Pediatr Surg 36:1177–1181

Song HT et al (2009) Rat model of metastatic breast cancer monitored by MRI at 3 T and bioluminescence imaging with histological correlation. J Transl Med 7:88

Stapfer M, Hu J, Wei D, Groshen S, Beart RW Jr (2003) Establishment of a nude mouse model of hepatic metastasis for evaluation of targeted retroviral gene delivery. J Surg Oncol 82:121–130 (discussion 131)

Tozeren A et al (1995) E-selectin-mediated dynamic interactions of breast- and colon-cancer cells with endothelial-cell monolayers. Int J Cancer 60:426–431

Uchida E et al (2008) Experimental pancreatic cancer model using PGHAM-1 cells: characteristics and experimental therapeutic trials. J Nippon Med Sch 75:325–331

United States National Institute of Health Year (2006) http://www.cancer.gov/cancertopics/factsheet/information/clinical-trials. Accessed July 2010

Valero T et al (2010) Combination of dacarbazine and dimethylfumarate efficiently reduces melanoma lymph node metastasis. J Invest Dermatol 130:1087–1094

Wang J et al (2005) Diverse signaling pathways through the SDF-1/CXCR4 chemokine axis in prostate cancer cell lines leads to altered patterns of cytokine secretion and angiogenesis. Cell Signal 17:1578–1592

Warren RS, Yuan H, Matli MR, Gillett NA, Ferrara N (1995) Regulation by vascular endothelial growth factor of human colon cancer tumorigenesis in a mouse model of experimental liver metastasis. J Clin Invest 95:1789–1797

Wilcock BP, Peiffer RL Jr (1986) Morphology and behavior of primary ocular melanomas in 91 dogs. Vet Pathol 23:418–424

Yang H, Jager MJ, Grossniklaus HE (2010) Bevacizumab suppression of establishment of micrometastases in experimental ocular melanoma. Invest Ophthalmol Vis Sci 51:2835–2842

Yang M et al (1999) Genetically fluorescent melanoma bone and organ metastasis models. Clin Cancer Res 5:3549–3559

Yin JJ et al (1999) TGF-beta signaling blockade inhibits PTHrP secretion by breast cancer cells and bone metastases development. J Clin Invest 103:197–206

Yoneda T (1997) Arterial microvascularization and breast cancer colonization in bone. Histol Histopathol 12:1145–1149

Yoneda T (1998) Cellular and molecular mechanisms of breast and prostate cancer metastasis to bone. Eur J Cancer 34:240–245

Yoneda T, Williams PJ, Hiraga T, Niewolna M, Nishimura R (2001) A bone-seeking clone exhibits different biological properties from the MDA-MB-231 parental human breast cancer cells and a brain-seeking clone in vivo and in vitro. J Bone Miner Res 16:1486–1495

Yu Y et al (2004) Expression profiling identifies the cytoskeletal organizer ezrin and the developmental homeoprotein Six-1 as key metastatic regulators. Nat Med 10:175–181

Chapter 16
Spontaneous, Induced, and Transgenic Models of Metastasis

Patrick T. Logan

Spontaneous, chemically induced, and transgenic models of metastases provide a unique framework for studying disease progression; in most cases, they allow the observation of the full spectrum of metastasic development including intravasation, survival in the blood, extravasation, organ seeding, and proliferation, in one immunocompetent animal. This is an advantage over haematogenous and ectopic counterparts that only offer the ability to observe specific fragments of the metastatic cascade. However, observing the intricate processes of metastasis, in particular those such as extravasation and intravasation, which involve single cells, in a spontaneous or induced model is challenging. With respect to chemically and radiation induced models, the methods needed to initiate tumor formation poses potential health risks to the practitioner. Spontaneous and induced models also do not permit the study of human malignant cells; due to the nature of these models, observations made regarding the behaviour and development of metastasis must be prefaced by mentioning that these cells are of animal origin.

However, spontaneous, induced, and transgenic models offer a unique background for the testing of pharmaceutical compounds in an immunocompetent animal that represents all stages of malignant development.

16.1 Spontaneous Models

Spontaneous models of metastases in animals, that is, naturally occurring malignancies, are rare. Also, by definition, they randomly appear in the animal population and this makes them difficult to study. That being said, canines, felines, rodents, and primates are susceptible to developing several types of cancer including prostate and mammary tumors. Unlike breast cancer in humans in which 30 % of patients develop metastases, 50 % of the mammary tumors that develop in canines result in lymph node metastases (O'Shaughnessy 2005). However, it must be noted that the

P. T. Logan (✉)
McGill University, Montreal, QC, Canada
e-mail: patrick.logan@mail.mcgill.ca

J. V. Burnier, M. N. Burnier, Jr. (eds.), *Experimental and Clinical Metastasis*,
DOI 10.1007/978-1-4614-3685-0_16, © Springer Science+Business Media New York 2013

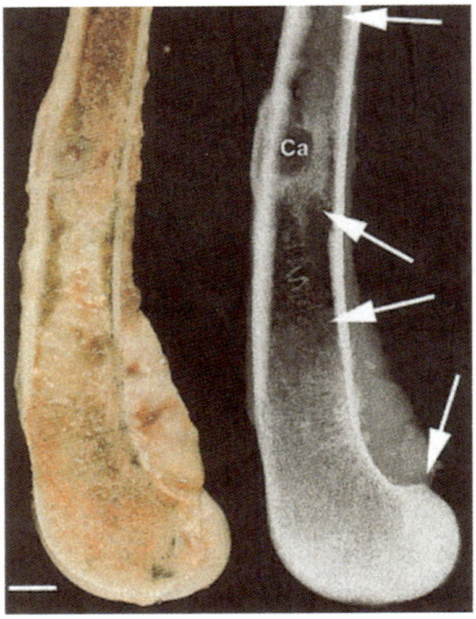

Fig. 16.1 Example of bone metastasis in a spontaneous occurrence of prostate cancer in a dog. The *arrows* indicate osteolytic, osteoblastic, and new bone trabeculae; features that are consistent with the human disease. (From Rosol et al. 2003)

treatment methods for breast cancer in humans are more elaborate and established than those for canines or other animals, which likely contributes to the differential rate of metastasis.

Feline mammary tumors share a striking resemblance to its human counterpart with respect to incidence and metastasis (MacEwen 1990). There is also evidence that hormones may be involved in the development of mammary tumors in cats owing to the attenuated reduction in incidence from ovariohysterectomized animals (Overley et al. 2005). It has been estimated that as many as 90 % of feline mammary tumors are malignant and these tumors typically metastasize to the lung (Burrai et al. 2010). Recent studies by Burrai et al. 2010, identified that intra-epithelial lesions from felines closely resemble those from humans, including the frequency of loss of hormonal receptors, and thus should be investigated further to increase our understanding of breast cancer.

Canines and rats are also susceptible to developing prostate cancer. It is estimated that 90 % of Lobund Wistar rats will develop prostate cancer by one year and these tumors occasionally metastasize to the lungs (Pollard et al. 1989). Prostate cancer in dogs can metastasize to a wide variety of organs including bone which, similar to human bone metastases, can possess both osteolytic and osteoblastic qualities (Fig. 16.1).

Although the benefit of these models is limited due to their rare and unpredictable nature, these models provide a unique advantage; these tumors must undergo all of the steps of the metastatic process that occur in humans and offer unparalleled insight into the natural history of these metastases. Additionally, these models serve to produce a reservoir of naturally occurring malignant cells that can be used in more controlled situations; for instance, several cell lines have been isolated from Wistar rats and canine prostate cancers that can be used in xenograft studies (Koutsilieris 1992; Anidjar et al. 2001).

16.2 Chemically and Radiation Induced Models

Chemically induced animal models of metastases are similar to spontaneous models in the sense that they allow for the study of the entire development of cancer from transformation to metastases. However, unlike spontaneous models, a carcinogenic agent must be used to induce these tumors. Considering that roughly 80 % of all human cancers are a result of carcinogens or are preventable, it seems appropriate to study these reasonable facsimiles (Higginson 1997). In addition, there is no requirement for the animal to be immunosuppressed and thus the effects of the immune system on the development of metastases can be assessed and extrapolated to human cancers. For instance, 1, 2-dimethylhydrazine (DMH) induced colorectal carcinomas express very similar immunological antigens to the human disease (Sjogren and Steele 1975). Future studies using the same DMH induced model revealed that if the tumors would metastasize if they were left to grow large enough (Belnap et al. 1979).

In other models, repeated applications of either benzo[a]pyrene or N-methyl-N'-nitro-N-nitrosogaunidine to the skin of mice will result in a high percentage of metastases to the lymph nodes, adrenal glands, and kidneys (Patskan et al. 1987).

Similar to chemically induced animal models, there are, albeit more rare, radiation induced models of metastases. Cobb (1970) discovered that implanting discs containing the radioactive isotope of phosphorous (^{32}P) in the femoral metaphysis of rats could induce the formation of osteaosarcomas. The rate of metastasis in these models, primarily to the lung, was almost 85 % and the disease was pathologically similar to osteosarcomas in humans.

Chemical and radiation induced animal models of metastases are desirable because they emulate all of the stages development that occurs in humans. However, the potential dangers to research by using these modalities, the relative difficulty in obtaining consistent results, and the advent of more reliable transgenic models renders these models all but obsolete.

16.3 Transgenic Models

One of the first, and likely the most infamous, transgenic mouse was created by Leder and Stewart in 1980 and involved the generation of a cancer prone mouse by genetically implanting the Myc oncogene (Hanahan et al. 2007). This mouse, aptly named the Harvard Oncomouse, a reflection of the university in which it was created, showed a high propensity to develop a variety of tumors throughout its body. Many other mice have been created that follow in the Harvard Mouse's footsteps, including genetic knockouts of popular tumor suppression genes such as Rb and p53. Recently, new types of knockout models specific for a particular malignancy and metastatic location have been developed and are discussed below.

The predictability of the development of both tumors and metastases in **genetically modified mice** (GMM) provide the framework for understanding disease progression. For instance, by cloning the mammary oncogene PyMT under the control of

Table 16.1 An overview of popular GMM models of breast cancer and metastasis progression, attenuation, and suppression. (Adapted from Kim and Baek 2010)

	Primary tumor	Metastasis		
	Incidence (%)	Incidence	Organ	Reference
Tumor progression				
MMTV-PyMT	100	85–100	Lung, lymph nodes	Maglione et al. 2001
MMTV-Neu	100	75	Lung	Bouchard et al. 1989
MMTV-Neu^{NDL}	60	75	Lung	Siegel et al. 1994
WAP-Ras	100	14	Lung	Jonkers and Derksen 2007
Tumor attenuating				
MMTV-Neu; PTP1B-/-	40	0		Julien et al. 2007
MMTV-PyMT; AKT-/-	100	37		Maroulakou et al. 2007
MMTV-PyMT; CD44-/-	100	66		Lopez et al. 2005
Tumor suppressor				
MMTV-cre; MMTV-p53$^{flox/flox}$	100	50		Lin et al. 2004

the mouse mammary tumor virus (MMTV) into a susceptible mouse host, 100 % of mice will development primary tumors confined to the mammary glad within 8 weeks and predictable lung metastases will occur by week 14 (Yang et al. 2004). Substituting PyMT for other oncogenes, such as Erb2 or Ras will also result in the development of predictable metastatic models (Table 16.1).

Due to the predictability of metastatic development, GMM can be crossed with other GMM that have specific genes of interest knocked out. The offspring of these mice will thus have the same mutation that results in the development of the tumor as the parent GMM, however, will also provide a model to explore the effects of the gene of interest on primary and metastatic tumor development. Julien et al., backcrossed an *Erbb2* negative mouse strain (see Table 16.1) with a *Ptpn1-/-* mouse. The *Ptpn1* gene encodes the PTB1 tyrosine phosphatase protein that is upregulated in the vast majority of human breast carcinomas, however, the exact role in cancer development had not been completely elucidated (Wiener et al. 1994). The *Erbb2/Ptpn-/-* resultant mouse strain had a marked delay in the development of primary tumors and subsequent lung metastases. Further exploration revealed that PTB1 overexpression in these animals caused spontaneous breast cancer development and that PTB1 induced carcinogenesis was fuelled by the upregulation of the MAPK/Ras pathway (Wiener et al. 1994). As a result of this and other supporting studies, the importance of PTB1 expression in breast cancer has been identified and is currently the target of the development of several inhibiting, pharmaceutical compounds.

In a similar study using a cross of two GMM, Lopez investigated the role of CD44, a transmembrane protein that binds to the secreted hyaluronin, on metastatic development. Crossing a spontaneously metastasizing MMTV-PyV mouse with a CD44$^{-/-}$ mouse generated a spontaneous tumor model lacking CD44 expression. This new GMM resulted in a reduction in the overall incidence of metastasis and a

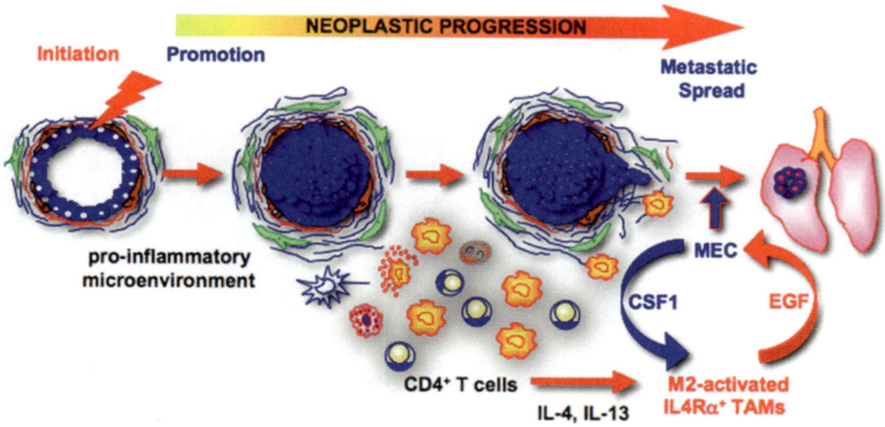

Fig. 16.2 Pictorial of the influence of pro-inflammatory cytokines induced by CD4$^+$ as determined by several iterations of CD4$^+$ knockouts in transgenic mice. (From DeNardo et al. 2009)

lower tumor burden in the experimental mice that did develop metastases compared to the control, MMTV-PyV mice (Lopez et al. 2005). It has been postulated that the binding of CD44 to hyaluronin may prevent invasion of metastatic cells and thus high levels of hyaluronin as an indicator of poor prognosis may be a result of lack of CD44 expression and subsequent CD44-hyaluronin binding (Lopez et al. 2005; Auvinen et al. 2000).

Like spontaneous models of metastases, transgenic models also permit the study of the effects of the immune system on metastatic development. Knockout of CD4$^+$ T-cell production through genetic modifications and crosses with MMTV-PyMT mice resulted in a reduction of lung cancer metastases in these animals (DeNardo et al. 2009). Subsequent crosses and experiments involving blocking IL-4 production and EGF signalling determined that the pro-inflammatory environment produced by the CD4$^+$ T-cells is conducive to the development of metastases (Fig. 16.2) (DeNardo et al. 2009). It was only through the use of these knockout mice that the rationale behind how the presence of CD4$^+$ T-cells potentiates the development of lung metastases.

Transgenic models of metastasis have also served to clarify some of the more puzzling aspects of tumor spread and invasion; traditional logic suggests that metastasis is a late stage process. Thus, it reasons that circulating malignant cells or disseminated tumor cells found in the bone marrow would increase over time and only after subsequent mutations and acquisitions of metastatic phenotypes would they be capable of populating distant organs. However, recent studies indicate that circulating or disseminated cell numbers are irrespective of primary disease progression (Husemann et al. 2008; Callejo et al. 2007). Husseman et al., discovered that in both MMTV-Her2 and MMTV-PyMT transgenic models, malignant cells were capable of leaving the primary site during the premalignant stage of development and were detected in metastatic locations prior to clinical manifestation of the primary tumors (Husemann and Klein 2009).

In general, tumors of host origin in immunocompetent animals can contribute to our body of knowledge regarding malignancies and compliment the observations from haematogenous and ectopic models of metastases. Transgenic models in particular allow for investigations regarding the effects of paradoxical role of immune cells in metastases development. Like all animal models of metastasis, they also offer a mechanism to test pharmaceutical agents and can be useful in identifying and evaluating promising treatment modalities.

16.4 Key Terms

Spontaneous Models Cancer and subsequent metastases occur in canines, felines, and rodents. The most common location of malignancy in these animals is the breast or prostate and theese tumors are capable of metastasizing both locally and to distant organs. Due to their rarity and unpredictability their usefulness is limited. However, these models' utility is derived from their ability to generate cell lines that can subsequently be used in more controlled models of metastases.

Chemically Induced Animal Models Chemical induction of primary tumors involves the application of carcinogens to a susceptible host animal. Considering the prevalence of carcinogen-induced malignancies in the human population, these models have the potential to emulate human disease progression. Radiation models follow the same principals. However, developing these models poses potential risk to the individuals applying the carcinogen.

Genetically Modified Mice Genetic models of metastasis are created by means of knocking-out specific genes (tumor suppressor genes) or by knocking-in tumor inducing genes (oncogenes) which results in the development of primary tumors. Both primary and metastatic tumor development occurs in a predictable and reproducible manner in these models. Additional genes can be knocked out of these animals and the effects on the predictable tumor development can be observed. This is a major advantage of these models as it allows the characterization of particular genes in the development and progression of metastases.

References

Anidjar M et al (2001) In vivo model mimicking natural history of dog prostate cancer using DPC-1, a new canine prostate carcinoma cell line. Prostate 46:2–10

Auvinen P et al (2000) Hyaluronan in peritumoral stroma and malignant cells associates with breast cancer spreading and predicts survival. Am J Pathol 156:529–536

Belnap LP, Cleveland PH, Colmerauer ME, Barone RM, Pilch YH (1979) Immunogenicity of chemically induced murine colon cancers. Cancer Res 39:1174–1179

Bouchard L, Lamarre L, Tremblay PJ, Jolicoeur P (1989) Stochastic appearance of mammary tumors in transgenic mice carrying the MMTV/c-neu oncogene. Cell 57:931–936

Burrai GP et al (2010) Spontaneous feline mammary intraepithelial lesions as a model for human estrogen receptor- and progesterone receptor-negative breast lesions. BMC Cancer 10:156

Callejo SA, Antecka E, Blanco PL, Edelstein C, Burnier MN Jr (2007) Identification of circulating malignant cells and its correlation with prognostic factors and treatment in uveal melanoma. A prospective longitudinal study. Eye (Lond) 21:752–759

Cobb LM (1970) Radiation-induced osteosarcoma in the rat as a model for osteosarcoma in man. Br J Cancer 24:294–299

DeNardo DG et al (2009) CD4(+) T cells regulate pulmonary metastasis of mammary carcinomas by enhancing protumor properties of macrophages. Cancer Cell 16:91–102

Hanahan D, Wagner EF, Palmiter RD (2007) The origins of oncomice: a history of the first transgenic mice genetically engineered to develop cancer. Genes Dev 21:2258–2270

Higginson J (1997) From geographical pathology to environmental carcinogenesis: a historical reminiscence. Cancer Lett 117:133–142

Husemann Y et al (2008) Systemic spread is an early step in breast cancer. Cancer Cell 13:58–68

Husemann Y, Klein CA (2009) The analysis of metastasis in transgenic mouse models. Transgenic Res 18:1–5

Jonkers J, Derksen PW (2007) Modeling metastatic breast cancer in mice. J Mammary Gland Biol Neoplasia 12:191–203

Julien SG et al (2007) Protein tyrosine phosphatase 1B deficiency or inhibition delays ErbB2-induced mammary tumorigenesis and protects from lung metastasis. Nat Genet 39:338–346

Kim IS, Baek SH (2010) Mouse models for breast cancer metastasis. Biochem Biophys Res Commun 394:443–447

Koutsilieris M (1992) PA-III rat prostate adenocarcinoma cells (review). In Vivo 6:199–203

Lin SC et al (2004) Somatic mutation of p53 leads to estrogen receptor alpha-positive and -negative mouse mammary tumors with high frequency of metastasis. Cancer Res 64:3525–3532

Lopez JI et al (2005) CD44 attenuates metastatic invasion during breast cancer progression. Cancer Res 65:6755–6763

MacEwen EG (1990) Spontaneous tumors in dogs and cats: models for the study of cancer biology and treatment. Cancer Metast Rev 9:125–136

Maglione JE et al (2001) Transgenic Polyoma middle-T mice model premalignant mammary disease. Cancer Res 61:8298–8305

Maroulakou IG, Oemler W, Naber SP, Tsichlis PN (2007) Akt1 ablation inhibits, whereas Akt2 ablation accelerates, the development of mammary adenocarcinomas in mouse mammary tumor virus (MMTV)-ErbB2/neu and MMTV-polyoma middle T transgenic mice. Cancer Res 67:167–177

O'Shaughnessy J (2005) Extending survival with chemotherapy in metastatic breast cancer. Oncologist 10(Suppl 3):20–29

Overley B, Shofer FS, Goldschmidt MH, Sherer D, Sorenmo KU (2005) Association between ovarihysterectomy and feline mammary carcinoma. J Vet Intern Med 19:560–563

Patskan GJ, Klein-Szanto AJ, Phillips JL, Slaga TJ (1987) Metastasis from squamous cell carcinomas of SENCAR mouse skin produced by complete carcinogenesis. Cancer Lett 34:121–127

Pollard M, Luckert PH, Snyder DL (1989) The promotional effect of testosterone on induction of prostate-cancer in MNU-sensitized L-W rats. Cancer Lett 45:209–212

Rosol TJ et al (2003) Animal models of bone metastasis. Cancer 97:748–757

Siegel PM, Dankort DL, Hardy WR, Muller WJ (1994) Novel activating mutations in the neu proto-oncogene involved in induction of mammary tumors. Mol Cell Biol 14:7068–7077

Sjogren HO, Steele G Jr (1975) Colon carcinoma antigens in the rat. Ann N Y Acad Sci 259:404–411

Yang J et al (2004) Twist, a master regulator of morphogenesis, plays an essential role in tumor metastasis. Cell 117:927–939

Wiener JR et al (1994) Overexpression of the protein tyrosine phosphatase PTP1B in human breast cancer: association with p185c-erbB-2 protein expression. J Natl Cancer Inst 86:372–378

Chapter 17
Orthotopic and Ectopic Models of Metastasis

William J. Muller and Ian Swanson

The implantation of syngeneic or xenogeneic tissue into living models allows cancer researchers to follow primary tumor growth and the development of secondary metastases in an *in vivo* host microenvironment. Host animals are constantly releasing stimuli (autocrine, endocrine, and paracrine factors), which influences the progression and pathogenesis of the primary tumor and secondary metastatases. Animal models allow researchers to observe the complex interactions of these physiological factors with the metastatic cascade *in vivo*, a process that is not possible to replicate *in vitro*. Successful models allow for the observation and elucidation of the pathways implicated in the development of metastatic disease. These models are used to delineate the critical factors influencing the success and failure at each step in metastatic disease progression. Furthermore, these models allow for the opportunity to examine the effects of pharmacological and anti-cancer therapies on both the primary tumor and the secondary metastases in order to develop better therapies for treating human disease.

17.1 Limitations of Intravenous (Experimental) Models of Metastasis

Experimental metastases models of metastases offer several advantages over other techniques used to study cancer; mainly, they exhibit consistent and reproducible metastasis biologies, mature rapidly, and give the user control over the number and type of cell used. Injection site specificity allows the user to generally target a specific organ in which they would like the metastases to grow, as most common injection locations result in the development of metastases at the first capillary bed encountered. As previously described, a popular model is the injection in the lateral tail vein of mice, which primarily results in the development of pulmonary metastases.

W. J. Muller (✉) · I. Swanson
Department of Biochemistry and Medicine, McGill University,
Montreal, QC, Canada
e-mail: william.muller@mcgill.ca

J. V. Burnier, M. N. Burnier, Jr. (eds.), *Experimental and Clinical Metastasis*,
DOI 10.1007/978-1-4614-3685-0_17, © Springer Science+Business Media New York 2013

Although the ability to generate metastases in a particular organ of interest is desirable, injecting cells directly into circulation eliminates several crucial steps of the metastatic cascade; growth and survival in the primary tumor site, migration and degradation of the basement membrane, and intravasation into the circulatory system. All of the aforementioned steps are critical selection barriers that human cancer cells must overcome in order to develop into overt metastases. Finally, experimental metastases generated by these models use cells that have been pre-selected for their metastatic potential and rapid tumor development and thus these models have the tendency to ignore important attributes of metastatic biology such as metastatic dormancy. While experimental metastases models offer several advantages, including the ease in which they can provide answers to specific questions regarding metastases, their limitations preclude them from use in many studies.

17.2 Ectopic and Orthotopic Models of Metastasis

Orthotopic models of metastasis involve the injection of malignant cells or the transplantation of tumors into the same anatomical location in which they were derived. Conversely, **ectopic models** involve injections into incorrect anatomical locations. The most popular ectopic model involves a subcutaneous injection and was originally developed as a simple and rapid method to grow primary tumors. Subcutaneous injections represent a simple and reproducible model that is used in the pre-clinical setting to examine the effectiveness of anticancer agents to limit primary tumor growth. Another advantage of subcutaneous models is that they allow for the ability of the primary tumor to be resected in order to lengthen the time for metastases formation and to examine the effect of primary tumor removal on metastatic development. While primary tumor resection is possible in some orthotopic models, the vast majority of animals used in these studies do not survive primary tumor resection. Subcutaneous injections have the advantage over intravenous metastasis models as they recreate the host-tumor interaction leading to a more realistic tumor and metastasis model. However, the growth of subcutaneous tumors has been criticized as an unrealistic growth location for the majority of human tumors. Furthermore, subcutaneous models rarely metastasize, a characteristic that can be attributed to the lack of normal (organ specific) host-tumor interactions, the famous “seed and soil” hypothesis.

In order to overcome the limitations of subcutaneous models, orthotopic animal models were developed. Implantation into their normal environment allows for the complete recapitulation of the metastatic cascade and for the cancer to develop in its natural milieu. Jessani et al. showed that breast cancer cells which had been implanted in the mammary fat pad displayed different proteomic profiles than cultured cells. Upon reinjection, the orthotopically-derived cells developed more metastases and primary tumors grew more quickly. Taken together, these results suggest that the tumor microenvironment selects for cell variants with metastatic and tumorigenic properties (Jessani et al. 2004). In another study by Lee et al., human breast cancer cells were implanted in the mammary fat pad and the resulting lymph and thoracic cavity metastases were isolated for gene expression profiling. When compared to the parental cells, the metastases derived cells showed overexpression of the transmembrane protein CD73. Thus, in addition to being a regulator of normal lymphocyte homing, CD73, was also revealed to be an important factor in metastasizing to the lymph node (Lee et al. 2003). These studies demonstrate the ability of orthotopic models to recapitulate metastatic pathogenesis and identify key regulators of that process which may in turn become important clinical targets for intervention and screening.

The strength of orthotopic models lies in their ability to recapitulate the metastatic cascade from a primary tumor grown in its normal environment. When compared to experimental metastases systems, orthotopic models represent a more realistic physiological system to select relevant metastatic phenotypes due to their inclusion of primary tumor growth and basement membrane degradation and intravasation into the circulatory system. There are two main types of orthotopic models; orthotopic injection of cellular suspensions, and surgical orthotopic implantation of intact tumor tissue. Orthotopic injection using suspensions of xenograph or syngeneic tissues represents the next logical step in model development from subcutaneous and intravenous injections. Cells from tissue culture or tumor tissue are disaggregated and injected as a cell suspension into the relevant organ from which primary tumors develop and seed secondary metastases. One of the limitations in regards to orthotopic injection is that injection directly into the organ of choice requires a skilled technician and the need to anesthetize the mouse prior to injection. While injections into sites such as the mammary fat pad are relatively simple procedures, internal organs pose a more difficult and time consuming task, which increases the risk of animal mortality. Instead of suspensions of disaggregated cells, surgical orthotopic implantation uses small pieces of intact tumors for implantation into the organ of choice. Using this method circumvents the cell disaggregation step and instead retains the intact three dimensional tumor architecture for direct implantation. The obvious limitation of surgical implantation is that it requires even greater surgical skill for implantation of the tumor tissue into the host animal. While this is a valid concern, surgical implantation of tissue into immunocompromised or humanized host animals allows for the implantation of human tumor fragments from patients in the clinic. Both orthotopic injection of cell suspensions and surgical implantation of tumor fragments offer advantages over intravenous and subcutaneous injections; however, they require increasing technical skill and the implantation process itself may influence physiological changes in the host animal. Nevertheless, orthotopic injections represent relatively rapid, and reproducible models useful for dissection of the metastatic cascade and as models for pre-clinical therapeutic screening.

17.3 Differences Between Intravenous, Ectopic, Orthotopic and Surgical Orthotopic Implantation Models

The importance and advantageous of orthotopic models has been validated through experimental differences observed between experimental metastases and spontaneous metastases models. Yamamoto et al. developed a system of two identical human fibrosarcoma HT-1080 cell lines individually tagged with either GFP or RFP. A mixture of the two differentially labeled cell lines were injected either orthotopically or intravenously, and resultant metastases were scored as monoclonal for green or red metastases, while yellow metastases were considered polyclonal. Orthotopic injections led to a predominance of monoclonal metastases, while intravenous injection developed almost purely as polyclonal metastases (Yamamoto et al. 2003). Hall and Thompson observed similar results when they compared orthotopic injection with experimental metastases using prostate tumor and lung metastasis explants cell lines. Their results indicated that while only the metastasis derived cell lines were able to create new lung metastases in the orthotopic model all cell lines were able to develop lung metastases in the experimental assay (Hall and Thompson 1997). These results demonstrate that spontaneous models have a more stringent selection criterion in order for metastases to form when compared with experimental metastases models. A study by Xue et al. demonstrates the limited utility of intravenous models due to their inability to recapitulate the complete metastatic cascade. They established that epidermal growth factor receptor (EGFR) overexpression in human breast cancer cells did not affect the growth of the primary tumor, or the ability to form lung metastases through intravenous injections. However, they determined that overexpression increased intravasation and subsequent lung metastases from orthotopic injections in the mammary fat pad (Xue et al. 2006). This study highlights the limited ability of intravenous models to act as models for preclinical therapy due to their inability to fully emulate human metastatic progression. However the rapidity, ease of use, and reproducibility of experimental metastasis models represent an important initial tool useful in the study of metastasis.

Due to their ease of use, subcutaneous injection became the prevalent method for which to model primary tumor growth, and later to model spontaneous metastases. Studies have demonstrated that, when compared to orthotopic models, the differences in the injection site location lead to differences in chemosensitivity and metastatic propensity. Kubota showed that even when using identical cell lines there are differences in chemosensitivity of small-lung carcinoma cells injected either subcutaneously or othotopically (Kubota 1994). Similarly, Troiani et al. showed that ectopic and orthotopic injections responded differently to chemotherapeutics for epidermal growth factor driven cancer cells (Troiani et al. 2008). Another study by Bao et al. looked at whether the addition of extracellular matrix components (matrigel) co-injected into either ectopic or orthotopic sites would influence the metastatic phenotype of MDA-MB-435 breast cancer cells. Their results showed that the subcutaneously injected cells with matrigel did slightly increase metastasis, but that the cells injected orthotopically with matrigel resulted in a much higher metastatic phenotype. The authors concluded that while matrigel could recapitulate part of the orthotopic microenvironment they showed that the diversity of the orthotopic site microenvironment could not be completely recapitulated (Bao et al. 1994). The technical ease and simplicity of subcutaneous injection models will enable their continued use as early stage preclinical models, but more complex orthotopic models are able to more closely emulate human metastatic pathogenesis and may therefore be more appropriate models for preclinical screening.

Injection of cellular suspensions into orthotopic sites increases the metastatic efficiency of cell lines when compared to subcutaneous injection. The metastatic efficiency is further increased when surgical orthotopic implantation was used instead of orthotopic injection of cell suspensions. Surgical orthotopic implantation improves on cell suspension injection due to the ability to retain tumor architecture. While all methods of metastatic modeling allow for the use of cultured and human tumor cells, surgical implantation offers the unique ability to implant primary tumor fragments directly from biopsied human tumor samples into immunocompromised mice. By combining injections of cell suspensions into subcutaneous sites to allow for the growth of primary tumors, followed by the surgical orthotopic implantation of intact tumor fragments there is an increase the metastatic efficiency compared to cell suspensions. Furthermore, surgically implanted tumor fragments lead to primary tumors that more closely resemble the histological and phenotypic properties of the tumors from which they were derived compared to cell suspensions. Morioka et al. demonstrated that a pancreatic cancer cell line grown subcutaneously before surgical implantation of intact tumor in increased invasiveness and metastases better mimicked the human disease when compared to an injection of a simple cell suspension (Morioka et al. 2000). Similarly, models of breast cancer metastases which used cell suspensions of MDA-MB-435 cells injected orthotopically did not display liver metastatses (Schmidt 1999). However, Li et al. found that MDA-MB-435 cells injected via surgical implantation were able to metastasize to the liver whereas cell suspensions were not (Li et al. 2002). Surgical orthotopic implantation represents the continuous development of improved metastatic models from years of cancer research. However this method has not reached a broad audience due to the limitations imposed by the necessary technical skill associated with the surgeries necessary for implantation. As more people become increasingly these techniques and become more skilled at carrying them out, the popularity of orthotopic implantation models are likely to continue to grow in popularity owing to their accurate modeling of human malignancies.

17.4 Continued Development of Orthotopic Models

Orthotopic models continue to increase in sophistication in order to better mimic metastatic disease progression and serve as more accurate preclinical models. These models have greatly benefited from the advances in *in vivo* imaging through the use of fluorescent and bioluminescently labeled syngeneic and xenographic human tumor lines. Coupled with advanced imaging devices such as CT, PET, and MRI the metastatic progression of orthotopic models can be followed through living animals, saving unnecessary sacrifices thereby lowering the number of animals needed to complete a study. Gros et al. combined fluorescent imaging for rapid imaging of the primary tumor and secondary metastases coupled with MRI to provide highly sensitive anatomical data on the metastasis location. Together these technologies were able to characterize the spread of metastases in a model of aggressive esophageal cancer in order to develop an effective model for preclinical drug screening (Gros et al. 2010). Temporal control of gene activation and gene silencing through inducible promoter systems allows for key proteins to be activated and deactivated at different stages in the metastatic progression. Le Dévédec et al. combined inducible oncogene expression with dual fluorescently labeled cells with intravital imaging in order to better dissect the metastatic behavior of breast cancer cells *in vivo* (Le Dévédec et al. 2011). Combining these tools with further refinement and development of new more sophisticated models will allow researchers to create animal models which better recapitulate the human metastatic pathogenesis and create more effective treatments in order to combat it.

17.5 The Role of Orthotopic Models in Breast Cancer Metastasis

Breast cancer will affect 1 in 9 women in the western world and will ultimately affect the lives of thousands of Canadians each year (Society et al. 2010). Improvements in breast cancer screening and new therapies have resulted in a 30 % drop in breast cancer mortality since 1986 and this downward trend is estimated to continue. Orthotopic animal models have helped breast cancer researchers understand disease progression, identify new therapeutic targets and biomarkers while serving as preclinical models for new anticancer agents. Orthotopic animal models allowed Hendrix et al. to relate *in vitro* data suggesting that Rab27 proteins promoted proliferation and invasive growth in tissue culture with increased invasiveness and metastatic burden using *in vivo* orthotopic models. Their research exemplifies the scientific progression from *in vitro* cell culture through to *in vivo* models to confirm the role of a previously unknown agent in breast cancer. Finally, their *in vivo* information regarding the role of Rab27s role in human breast cancer combined with clinical samples showed a correlation with poor patient prognosis (Hendrix et al. 2010). Orthotopic models have allowed breast cancer researchers to derive cell lines with increased tumorigenic and metastatic properties through *in vivo* selection through orthotopic injection. Jessani et al. compared the proteomic profile of parental MDA-MB-231 cells with that of MDA-MB-231 explants to identify key differences in tissue plasminogen activator (tPA) and urokinase plasminogen activator (uPA) (Jessani et al. 2004). Jessani's work revealed key differences in the production of proteins of cells while in culture compared to those *in vivo* and thus emphasizes that animal models should emulate the human disease as accurately as possible in order to ensure the validity of findings and discoveries.

While 5 year survival rates have been increasing for breast cancer patients, once the disease spreads to distant organs, there are no effective treatments available. Human breast cancers are known to develop secondary bone metastases, however, in order to model bone metastases, previous models have required the injection of malignant breast cancer cells into an animals heart. Lelekakis et al. developed an orthotopic model of breast cancer using explanted bone metastasis cells to select for preferential bone metastasis formation from the primary tumor. This model accurately recapitulates the metastatic spread seen in human breast cancers. Studies

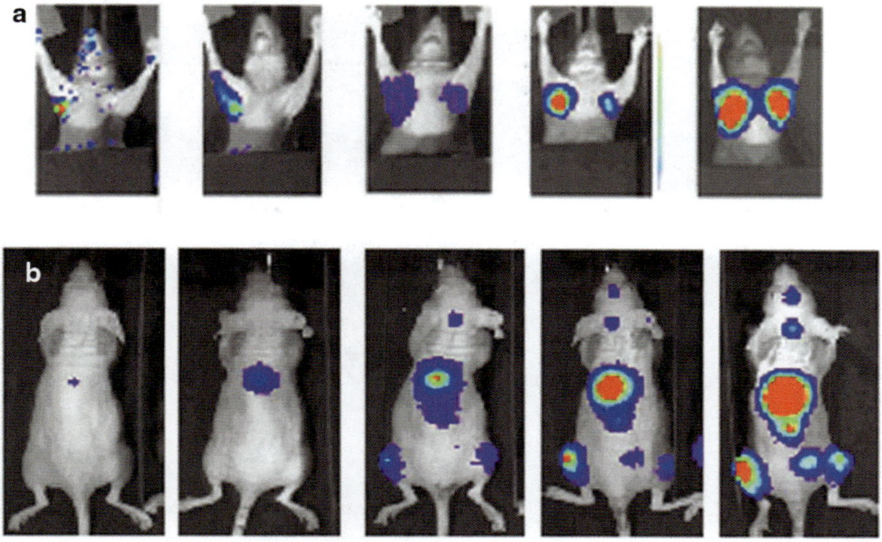

Fig. 17.1 Differential location of metastasis depending on injection location. Metastasis to the lymphnodes **a** following orthotpic injection into the abdominal fat pad, metastasis to rib cage and lung **b** following intracardiac injection of the same cell line. (Adapted from Jenkins et al. 2005)

using this model of breast cancer bone metastases revealed the important role of the parathyroid hormone-related protein in this process (Lelekakis et al. 1999). In an effort to improve bone metastasis models and overcome the interspecies limitations, Kuperwasser et al. used a novel model where normal human bone was implanted into NOD/SCID mice, followed by human breast cancer SUM1315 cell line injected into the mammary fat pad. Interestingly, metastases from the breast cancer cell line formed exclusively within the implanted human bone, which is highly suggestive of specific osteotroprism selection (Kuperwasser 2005). Further study of this model will help to elucidate osteotropism associated genes and provide a model to study therapeutic intervention of bone metastases. Finally, to demonstrate the utility of orthotopic animal models as tools for preclinical screening of therapeutics, Bandyopadhyay et al. showed that a common chemotherapeutic agent, doxorubicin, activated epithelial-mesenchymal transition through TGFβ signaling, leading to resistant cell populations. It was discovered that by combining doxorubicin with a TGFβ inhibitor, they could achieve synergistic inhibition of the resistant cell population, while decreasing the required effective dose of doxorubicin (Bandyopadhyay et al. 2010). This model helps to identify the cause of therapeutic resistance while helping to develop a treatment regime to overcome it.

The ultimate goal of cancer research remains to delineate the mechanisms through which cancer develops, metastasizes, and resists anticancer agents in order to develop more effective therapeutic treatments. Continuing improvements and innovation of orthotopic animal models will increase the similarities with their human counterparts and will thereby maintain its important role in the fight against cancer (Fig. 17.1, Table 17.1).

Table 17.1 Primary tumors and their resultant location of metastases in orthotpic animal models

Primary tumor injection site	Metastatic sites	References
Bladder	Lymph nodes Liver Lung Pancreas Spleen Diaphragm	Chan et al. (2009a, b)
Breast	Lymph nodes Liver Lung Bone	Li et al. (2002), Fu et al. (1993)
Colon	Lymph nodes Liver Lung Brain	Rashidi et al. (2000a, b)
Kidney	Lymph nodes Liver Lung	Chang et al. (1999)
Liver	Lymph nodes Liver Lung Peritoneum	Sun et al. (1996)
Melanoma	Lymph nodes Lung Bone Brain Adrenal Glands	Yang et al. (1999)
Ovarian	Colon Lymph nodes Liver Stomach Diaphragm	Fu and Hoffman (1993)
Pancreas	Lymph nodes Liver Lung Kidney Spleen	Lee et al. (2000)
Prostate	Lymph nodes Liver Lung Bone	Yang et al. (1999)
Stomach	Lymph nodes Liver Lung Pancreas Kidney	Furukawa et al. (1993)

17.6 Key Terms

Orthotopic Models These models are developed by injecting malignant cells or by grafting intact tumor sections into the correct anatomical location of an animal. The major advantage of these types of models lies in their ability to provide information regarding the entire gamut of malignant development from primary tumor proliferation to distant metastases. However, metastatic development in these animals does not always occur in the same locations as the human disease that they are intended to model.

Ectopic Models These models are similar to orthotopic models of metastases, however, cells or graft material is delivered to a location that differs from the origin of the original tumor. Sub-cutaneous injections are the most common location for these models and they are used extensively in breast cancer research.

References

Astoul P, Colt HG, Wang X, Hoffman RM (1994) A "patient-like" nude mouse model of parietal pleural human lung adenocarcinoma. Anticancer Res 14:85–91

Bandyopadhyay A et al (2010) Doxorubicin in combination with a small TGFβ inhibitor: A potential novel therapy for metastatic breast cancer in mouse models. PLoS ONE 5:e10365

Bao L, Matsumura Y, Baban D, Sun Y, Tarin D (1994) Effects of inoculation site and matrigel on growth and metastasis of human breast cancer cells. Br J Cancer 70:228–232

Chan E, Patel A, Heston W, Larchian W (2009a) Mouse orthotopic models for bladder cancer research. BJU Int 104:1286–1291

Chan ES et al (2009b) Optimizing orthotopic bladder tumor implantation in a syngeneic mouse model. J Urol 182:2926–2931

Chang XH et al (1999) Improved metastatic animal model of human prostate carcinoma using surgical orthotopic implantation (SOI). Anticancer Res 19:4199–4202

Fu X, Hoffman RM (1993) Human ovarian carcinoma metastatic models constructed in nude mice by orthotopic transplantation of histologically-intact patient specimens. Anticancer Res 13:283–286

Fu X, Le P, Hoffman RM (1993) A metastatic orthotopic-transplant nude-mouse model of human patient breast cancer. Anticancer Res 13:901–904

Furukawa T et al (1993) Nude mouse metastatic models of human stomach cancer constructed using orthotopic implantation of histologically intact tissue. Cancer Res 53:1204–1208

Gros SJ et al (2010) Complementary use of fluorescence and magnetic resonance imaging of metastatic esophageal cancer in a novel orthotopic mouse model. Int J Cancer 126:2671–2681

Hall SJ, Thompson TC (1997) Spontaneous but not experimental metastatic activities differentiate primary tumor-derived vs metastasis-derived mouse prostate cancer cell lines. Clin Exp Metastasis 15:630–638

Hendrix A et al (2010) Effect of the secretory small GTPase Rab27B on breast cancer growth, invasion, and metastasis. J Natl Cancer Inst 102(12):866–880

Jenkins D, Hornig Y, Oei Y, Dusich J, Purchio T (2005) Bioluminescent human breast cancer cell lines that permit rapid and sensitive in vivo detection of mammary tumors and multiple metastases in immune deficient mice. Breast Cancer Res 7:R444–R454

Jessani N et al (2004) Carcinoma and stromal enzyme activity profiles associated with breast tumor growth in vivo. Proc Natl Acad Sci U S A 101:13756–13761

Kubota T (1994) Metastatic models of human cancer xenografted in the nude mouse: the importance of orthotopic transplantation. J Cell Biochem 56:4–8
Kuperwasser C et al (2005) A Mouse model of human breast cancer metastasis to human bone. Cancer Res 65:6130–6138
Le Dévédec SE, Lalai R, Pont C, de Bont H, van de Water B (2011) Two-photon intravital multicolor imaging combined with inducible gene expression to distinguish metastatic behavior of breast cancer cells in vivo. Mol Imaging Biol 13(1):67–77
Lee H, Lin ECK, Liu L, Smith JW (2003) Gene expression profiling of tumor xenografts: In vivo analysis of organ-specific metastasis. Int J Cancer 107:528–534
Lee NC et al (2000) Antimetastatic efficacy of adjuvant gemcitabine in a pancreatic cancer orthotopic model. Clin Exp Metastasis 18:379–384
Lelekakis M et al (1999) A novel orthotopic model of breast cancer metastasis to bone. Clinical and Experimental Metastasis 17:163–170
Li X et al (2002) Optically imageable metastatic model of human breast cancer. Clin Exp Metastasis 19:347–350
Morioka CY, Saito S, Ohzawa K, Watanabe A (2000) Homologous orthotopic implantation models of pancreatic ductal cancer in Syrian golden hamsters: which is better for metastasis research–cell implantation or tissue implantation? Pancreas 20:152–157
Rashidi B et al (2000a) A nude mouse model of massive liver and lymph node metastasis of human colon cancer. Anticancer Res 20:715–722
Rashidi B et al (2000b) An orthotopic mouse model of remetastasis of human colon cancer liver metastasis. Clin Cancer Res 6:2556–2561
Schmidt CM et al (1999) Characterization of spontaneous metastasis in an aggressive breast carcinoma model using flow cytometry. Clin Exp Metastasis 17:537–544
Society CC (ed) Canadian Cancer Statistics 2010 (Toronto, Canada, 2010)
Sun FX et al (1996) Metastatic models of human liver cancer in nude mice orthotopically constructed by using histologically intact patient specimens. J Cancer Res Clin Oncol 122:397–402
Troiani T et al (2008) The use of xenograft models for the selection of cancer treatments with the EGFR as an example. Crit Rev Oncol Hematol 65:200–211
Xue C et al (2006) Epidermal growth factor receptor overexpression results in increased tumor cell motility in vivo coordinately with enhanced intravasation and metastasis. Cancer Res 66:192–197
Yamamoto N et al (2003) Determination of clonality of metastasis by cell-specific color-coded fluorescent-protein imaging. Cancer Res 63:7785–7790
Yang M et al (1999) A fluorescent orthotopic bone metastasis model of human prostate cancer. Cancer Res 59:781–786

Chapter 18
Animal Model Imaging Techniques

Patrick T. Logan

In recent years, the advent of new imaging technologies has enabled researchers to portray the development of metastases in animal models in a new light. Previously, observing the behaviour of metastatic cells required the sacrifice of the animal and thus the progress of development or treatment is often incomplete and necessarily elucidated from sequential sacrifices of inbred animals. Considering the technical difficulties in visualizing individual metastatic cells by traditional immunohistochemical or staining methods, understanding the critical first steps of micrometastatic development was difficult and often impractical. New technologies, in particular the ability to force cells of interest to fluoresce amongst a dull background, have enabled researchers to visualize the behaviour of individual metastatic cells in host organisms. These methods, in conjunction with new, non-lethal intravital imaging methods, have contributed greatly to the body of knowledge regarding malignant cells and the development of metastases. This chapter will discuss several of the more popular imaging methods such as luciferase, green fluorescent protein, MRI, CT, PET, and will analyze the advantages and limitations of each method.

18.1 Luciferase Imaging

Several organisms possess the ability to bioluminesce as a means of either communicating, or as an offensive or defensive reaction (Haddock and Moline 2010). Organisms possible of such light-emmitting reactions include bacteria, fireflies, vargulin, oplophorus, renilla, and aequorin and is typically achieved through the enzyme-substrate reaction Luciferase-luciferin (Greer and Szalay 2002). In the presence of oxygen and the substrate luciferin, the luciferase enzyme will produce light. The luciferase enzyme has since been isolated and sequenced from these organisms, the firefly in particular, as early as 1975 (Gates and Luca 1975). Since this time, more than 14 different luciferase genes have been identified and sequenced (Greer

P. T. Logan (✉)
McGill University, Montreal, QC, Canada
e-mail: patrick.logan@mail.mcgill.ca

J. V. Burnier, M. N. Burnier, Jr. (eds.), *Experimental and Clinical Metastasis*, 237
DOI 10.1007/978-1-4614-3685-0_18, © Springer Science+Business Media New York 2013

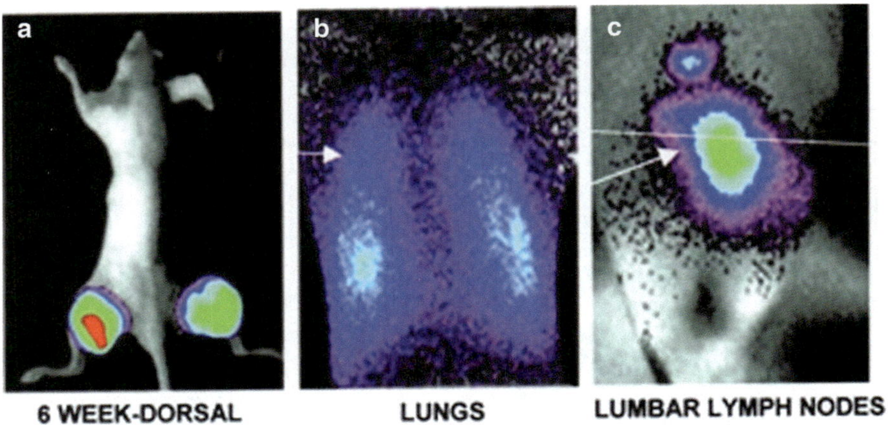

Fig. 18.1 Whole body imaging of luciferase labeled human prostate cancer cells in a nude mouse (**a**) and subsequent metastases in the lung (**b**) and thoracic lymphnodes (**c**) following intramuscular injection in the thigh. (Adapted from El Hilali et al. 2002)

and Szalay 2002). In 1985, the firefly luciferase gene was cloned and inserted into E. coli for visualization (Wet et al. 1985). Expression of the luciferase enzyme in mammalian cells is obtained by cloning the gene into either a constitutive or inducible expression vector. Subsequent exposure to luciferin will generate a bioluminescent signal which can then be detected using a charge-coupled device (CCD) specific for the visualization of bioluminescent cells (Hooper et al. 1990). For a comprehensive list of luciferase-reporter gene constructs please see Greer and Szalay (2002).

The luciferase reporter gene constructs have gained tremendous popularity in metastatic imaging studies in animal models; transfection of malignant cells with the reporter gene prior to implantation allows for a non-invasive method of visualizing malignant cells in an entire animal. This method clearly allows for the visualization of tumors that would not otherwise be visible. For instance, Nadia et al. used transfected human prostate cancer cells injected into the thigh of nude mice in order to visualize metastases (El Hilali et al. 2002). Two-weeks post-injection, luciferase emissions were visible from the primary tumors in the thigh in addition to multiple pelvic and lymph node metastases (Fig. 18.1).

Luciferase imaging permits the identification of metastastic lesions in early stages of development when they are smaller than the size required for angiogenesis (Wetterwald et al. 2002). Luciferase labelled breast cancer cell line injected intracardiacly can be clearly identified ten minutes post-injection via whole body imaging (Fig. 18.2). Twenty-four hours post injection, the total bioluminescence produced by the same animal drastically declined indicating destruction of the majority of breast cancer cells that were injected. Forty-eight hours post injection, clear, defined signals, later confirmed via traditional methods, representing bone and brain metastases were identified. Such studies have been used to confirm the inefficiency of the metastatic process (Wetterwald et al. 2002). In fact, Heyn et al. (2006) estimate the

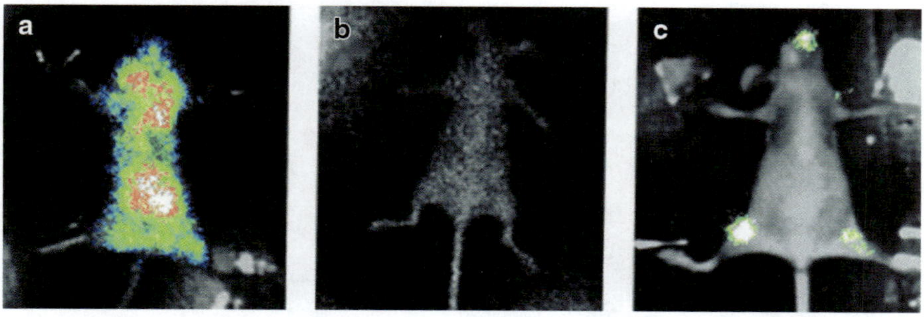

Fig. 18.2 Formation of micrometastatic bone metastases following intracardiac injection of human breast cancer cell line labeled with the luciferase reporter gene at (**a**) 10 min, (**b**) 24 h, and (**c**) 48 h post injection. (Adapted from Wetterwalt et al. 2002)

metastatic efficiency at less than 5 %; thus it can be extrapolated that, as a result of the high proportion of metastatic development in human cancers, that shedding of malignant cells from the primary tumor must be an almost constant process (Heyn et al. 2006) Furthermore, Shakman et al, report that there is a high degree of correlation between the intensity of the bioluminesce produced by colorectal liver metastases *in vivo* when compared to traditional measures of tumor burden (Smakman et al. 2004).

The benefits of the luciferase reporter gene system include the ability to observe metastatic development in a non-invasive manner. The high degree of correlation between emitted light and tumor burden has permitted the testing of pharmacological compounds in treating prostatic bone metastases in a non-invasive manner that would otherwise have not been possible (24th Congress of the International Association for Breast Cancer Research 2003). However, despite its advantages, luciferase imaging in animal models is not without its drawbacks; requirements for visualizing cells includes a minimum of 1000 cells which prevents the imaging of single-celled or small cluster of cells that comprise micrometastases (Contag et al. 2000). Further limitations of the luciferase system is the requirement of injecting the exogenous luciferin substrate; differential tissue absorption and distribution can confound calculating accurate tumor burden in certain organs (El Hilali et al. 2002). Assessing tumor burden can be further complicated as a result of the requirement of oxygen to complete the luciferase reaction in addition to technical complications owing to the differing optical densities of body tissues (El Hilali et al. 2002).

18.2 Green Fluorescent Protein (GFP)

Green Fluorescent Protein is, as the name suggests, a protein that emits green light when excited by a particular wavelength. Originally isolated from the *A. victoria* jellyfish, the GFP fluorophore is excited by blue light with a wavelength of roughly 488 nm and a peak emission wavelength of roughly 507 nm (Tsien 1998). For imaging purposes, the GFP protein gene is cloned with a constitutive promoter gene into a

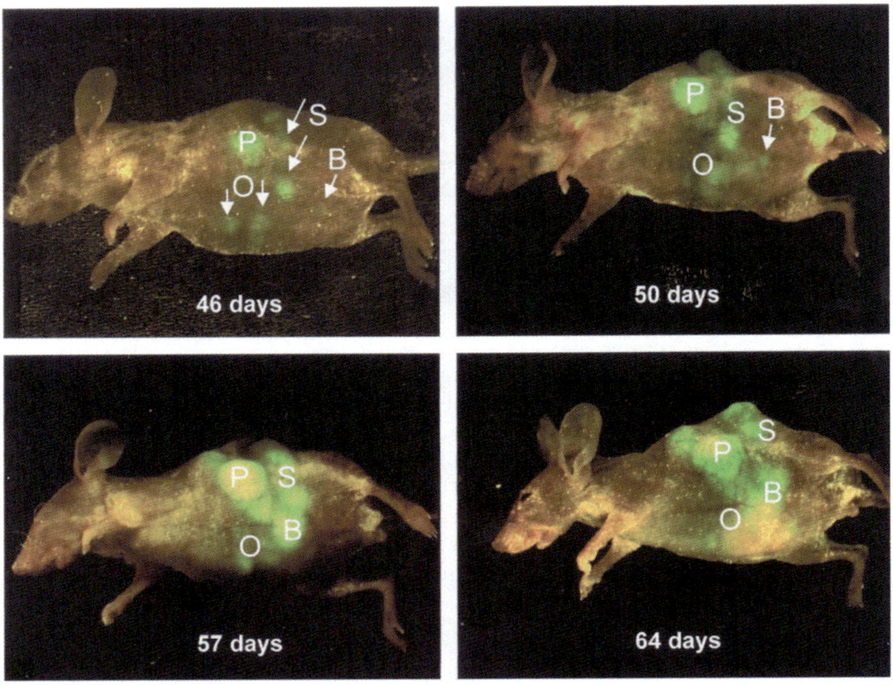

Fig. 18.3 External images of pancreas (*P*), spleen (*S*), omental (*O*), and bowel (*B*) metastases using GFP-labeled pancreatic cancer cells. (From Bouvet et al. 2002)

plasmid. This plasmid is then transfected into mammalian cells using a variety of techniques including electroporation, lipofection, or sonication. Since its inaugural use to detect gene expression in *C. elegans*, GFP has since gained rapid popularity in the field of *in vivo* imaging in cancer and metastases (Chalfie et al. 1994). Imaging of cancer cells *in vivo* using animal models is typically done in one of two ways: external observation of internal metastases or through **intravital videomicroscopy (IVVM)** (Hoffman 2002a). Pioneered by Robert Hoffman, successful GFP whole body-imaging a multitude of tumors ranging from brain to lymphnodes has been achieved (Hoffman 2002b). In one of the first animal models using GFP whole-body imaging, Hoffman et al, injected GFP-labeled human pancreatic cell line into the portal vein of nude mice (Bouvet et al. 2002). Consecutive whole-body imaging of the mice revealed pancreas, spleen, omental, and bowel metastases (Fig. 18.3).

While whole-body imaging offers the ability to visualize metastatic nodules *in vivo*, the brilliance and specificity of GFP expression by transfected cancer cells offers additional benefits. By utilizing skin-flap imaging methods, it is possible to visualize individual GFP-labeled malignant cells circulate in a live animal. In essence, IVVM involves creating a small skin-flap in the abdomen of a live, anesthetized animal, (typically a mouse) which is placed on a cover slip and illuminated and recorded with a conventional camera. Ann Chambers et al, used this technique and

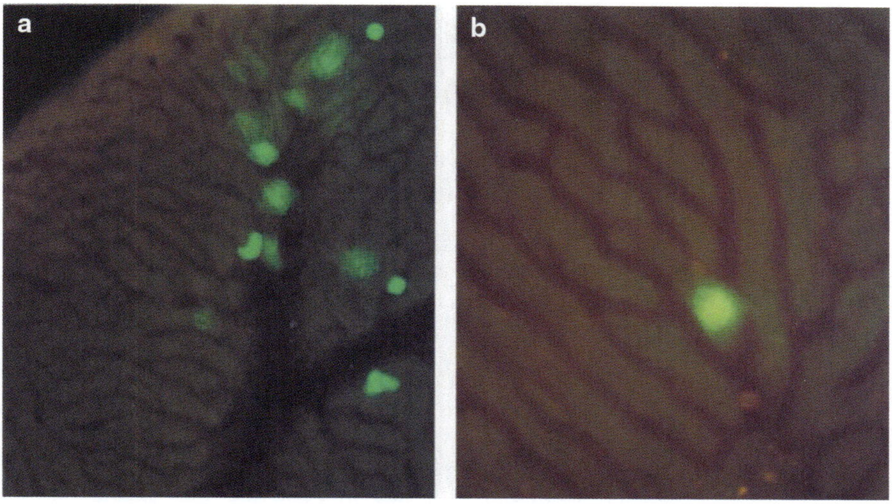

Fig. 18.4 IVVM of individual metastatic cells in the capillaries of the liver 1 h post injection (**a**) and a single cell that has extravasated into the liver parenchyma 24 h post injection (**b**). (From Naumov et al. 1999)

illuminated organs with blue light in order to visualize individual cells in circulation (Chambers et al. 1995). Building on these studies, Naumov used IVVM and GFP Chinese hamster ovary cells to visualize individual malignant cells pre and post-extravasation from blood vessels into the liver parenchyma (Fig. 18.4, Naumov et al. 1999). In fact, the GFP imaging was sensitive enough to discern and visualize the formation of new blood vessels (Naumov et al. 1999).

IVVM and GFP imaging has provided invaluable information regarding the steps of intravasation; the exit of malignant cells from the bloodstream and into organ parenchyma. Studies observing uveal melanoma cell lines in circulation indicate that perhaps the initial cause of arrest in the blood vessel is related to mechanical constraints involving large cells and small capillaries.

The single celled sensitivity of GFP imaging allows the testing of pharmacological agents on single cells and dormant micrometastases which, as a result of their lack of divisions, are typically difficult to target via traditional therapies (Naumov et al. 2003).

Recently, genetic mutations and engineering have produced a wide gamut of fluorescent proteins ranging from blue to yellow, all of which maintain the same basic properties of GFP. These new fluorophores have encouraged dual imaging techniques in which subtly different cell lines can be distinguished in the same animal *in vivo*. Yamamoto et al. (2003), used a co-injection of RFP and GFP human fibrosarcoma cells in order to determine that the majority of resultant metastases in a SCID mouse were the result of clonal expansion of individual cells.

Despite not needing the addition of an exogenous substrate like luciferase systems, GFP models are confounded by the fact that native tissue has a tendency to autofluoresce, which can occasionally render identification of GFP labelled cells difficult.

Nevertheless, GFP whole body and IVVM imaging offers researchers a valuable tool of identifying malignant cells *in vivo* and thus increasing our knowledge of dormancy and micrometastases in animal models.

18.3 Magnetic Resonance Imaging (MRI)

A recent technology, the first MRI image was produced in 1973, and its advent use for imaging metastases in animal models occurred in the twenty-first century (Lauterbur 1989). A traditional MRI uses a magnetic field to align hydrogen molecules in the water present in tissues, which are then rotated using a radiofrequency, and a composite image based on the differing hydration of tissues in the body is developed (Novelline 2004). MRI offers a non-invasive method of imaging metastases with resolutions capable of discerning individual cells. Simoes et al. (2008), injected the 439-Br1 breast cancer cell line intracardiacly in nude mice and then imaged the brain metastases produced by these cells with an MRI 20 days post injection. The resolution of malignant cells via **MRI imaging** contrast can be further improved by introducing micron-sized iron oxide particles (MPIO) into the cell lines (Bulte and Kraitchman 2004). Heyn et al. (2006), pre-incubated a human breast cancer, brain metastatic specific cell line, MDA-231BR, with MPIOs and subsequently injected these labeled cells into the left ventricle of nude mice. Subsequent MRI images of the mouse brain allowed tracking the fate of individual cells. Such studies revealed that, although the vast majority of malignant cells lodged in the brain do not survive and only a small number of the remaining cells developed into overt metastases, cells that enter and lodge in the brain may constitute a reservoir of dormant cells (Fig. 18.5, Heyn et al. 2006). These dormant cells remained present and viable even in the presence and proximity of growing, overt metastatic lesions.

MRI in animal models of metastases is perhaps the gold standard for non-lethal imaging with respect to sensitivity. However, the cost of imaging many animals is prohibitive and the imaging itself can be toxic to the animals that are being observed (Simoes et al. 2008).

18.4 Computerized Tomography (CT) and Positron Emission Tomography (PET)

Like MRI, **CT imaging** allows for non-invasive imaging of metastatic cells *in vivo*. Three-dimensional (3D) CT images are reconstructed from composites of X-ray images obtained from one axis (Harman 1980). These 3D reconstructions provide a backdrop for the visualization of GFP or luciferase labelled malignant cells. CT scans increase the sensitivity of these more traditional imaging modalities in addition to offering a non-invasive method of determining the depth of tumor growth. Strube et al. (2010), implemented CT scan as part of a mutli-modal animal model of renal

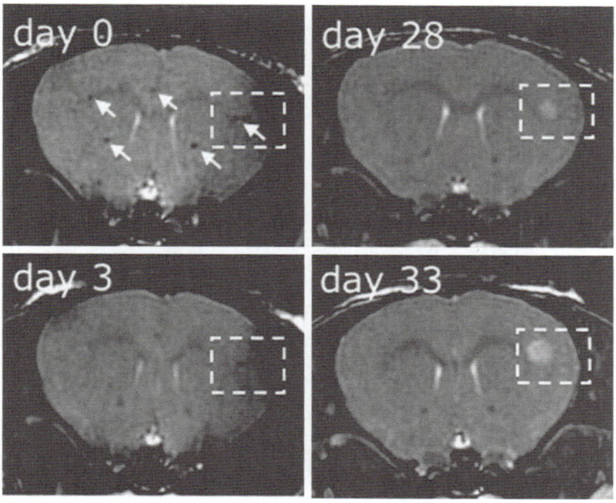

Fig. 18.5 MRI of mouse brain post injection of MPIO labeled breast cancer cells. The *arrows* indicate areas of signal void which is indicative of MPIO labeled cells. Subsequent images reveal that the majority of the cells visible in the first pane are no longer viable. The hyperintensive areas in panes 3 and 4 represent an overt metastases. (From Heyn et al. 2006)

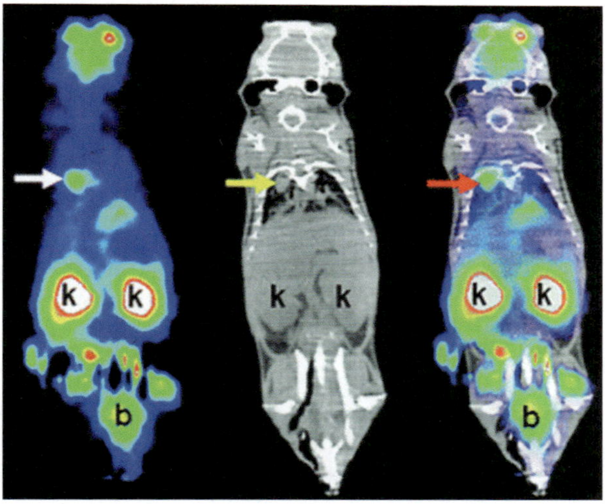

Fig. 18.6 PET, CT and combined PET/CT scan of lung metastasis (denoted by the *arrow*) in a SCID mouse. Physiological tracer uptake kidney (*k*) and bladder (*b*) is noted. (From Deroose et al. 2007)

cell carcinoma bone metastases in nude mice CT scans of the osteolytic damage from hind leg metastases correlated well with traditional luciferase images (Strube et al. 2010).

PET scans are developed with the aid of a radionucleotide; a radiolabeled tag (typically a glucose molecule) is transfected into a cell line and the PET scanner detects its degradation in the live animal. A three dimensional image is then reconstructed using CT technology. In a SCID mouse model of malignant melanoma, cells were tagged with both a radiolabelled glucose molecule and a luciferase reporter gene (Deroose et al. 2007). Metastases were then imaged by PET and CT (Deroose et al. 2007). Although the PET scan provided excellent resolution, the images obtained by this method were limited to visualization of the malignant cells

Table 18.1 Overview of various methods of visualizing metastases in animal models

Imaging method	Substrate required	Invasive	Single-Cell resolution	Toxic	Cost
Luciferase	Yes	No	No	No	Low
GFP	No	No (except IVVM)	No (except IVVM)	No	Low
MRI	No	No	Yes	Yes	High
CT	No	No	No	No	High
PET	Yes	No	Yes	No	High

in the absence of anatomical landmarks. However, by combining the PET and CT scans, metastatic cells were identified and located within the anatomy of the SCID mouse (Fig. 18.6). Together, PET/CT scans were capable of providing non-invasive, quantitative measurements of metastases.

In vivo imaging of metastases, whether it be of individual cells or full-blown metastases, is critical to our understanding of the metastatic disease. The ability to visualize the growth or recession of metastatic cells in an animal is also paramount in evaluating the promise of pharmaceutical agents. Each of the imaging modalities discussed in this chapter has their advantages and disadvantages, some of which are described in Table 18.1. For instance, CT and MRI scans provide anatomical relevance to observations but lack the specificity of PET or GFP models. Selecting the correct imaging technique, or combination of techniques, is critical for visualizing the developing metastases as required for the model.

18.5 Summary

Animal models, in all of their iterations, are critical contributors to our ambition to understand, treat, and ultimately eliminate metastasis as a clinical burden. The knowledge gained from observing the behaviour of malignant cells amidst the plethora of factors experienced *in vivo* would not be possible without animal models. They have allowed the visualization of all the steps of the metastatic cascade ranging from escaping the primary tumor to proliferation within a metastatic lesion. The advent of new, transgenic models has allowed us to isolate and characterize the implications of individual genes on the development of metastases. The exploitation of natural phenomena, such as green fluorescent protein and luciferase enzyme, has facilitated the visualization and characterisation of micrometastases and dormant cells. Technological advances, such as MRI and CT/PET imaging, now permits the non-lethal visualization of these cells *in vivo*.

Animal models of metastases continue to initiate the development of new therapies, including combination therapies, to destroy existing metastases and prevent metastatic development. They are critical in providing the *in vivo* evidence necessary for clinical trial approval by both Health Canada and the Food and Drug Administration in the United States.

Considering the deadly encumbrance of metastases, it is imperative that the research community continues to improve current animal models and develop new models that recapitulate human disease progression. Considering all of the recent advancements in animal models, it is foreseeable that a new model that combines all of the advantages without any of the disadvantages of the animal models described in this chapter will emerge as the gold standard for understanding and treating metastases.

18.6 Key Terms

Luciferase Imaging This technique involves forcing malignant cells to express the luciferase enzyme. Following injection of these cells into and metastases development, luciferin is injected in to the animal where it is catalyzed by luciferase and light is emitted. This emission can be detected non-invasively through the animal's skin and thus semi-quantitative analysis of tumor growth can be conducted. The minimum number of cells required to emit a visible signal is 1000 and thus this method is not ideal for observing micrometastases or dormant cells.

Green Fluorescent Protein (GFP) Malignant cells can be forced to express GFP, a protein that can be excited by a specific wavelength of light, which results in the emission of a vibrant green light. This technique can be used to identify individual malignant cells in animals through invasive, non-lethal surgery. Tissue auto-fluorescence is one of the complications of this imaging method as it can render identification of cells difficult.

Intravital Videomicroscopy (IVVM) Typically coupled with GFP labelled malignant cell imaging, IVVM involves making either a temporary or permanent window in the animal via abdominal incision. Malignant cells can then be videotaped over time as they circulate in the animal's blood or develop into metastatic lesions.

Magnetic Resonance Imaging (MRI) MRI uses a magnetic field to align water molecules in a tissue of interest. Metastatic lesions produce aberrations in these images and thus can be identified. Further resolution, including the ability to identify individual cells, can be acquired by using malignant cells that contain micron-sized iron oxide particles. One of the disadvantages to MRI is that the imaging process itself can be toxic to the animals.

Computerized Tomography (CT) and Positron Emission Tomography (PET) Scans CT scans are 3-D images produced through the computerized reconstruction of multiple X-rays. PET scans involve the injection of radiolabelled glucose molecules into the animal. The high metabolic activity of the metatatic lesions result in a large uptake of the labelled glucose molecules, which can then be detected as radiation is emitted from the cells. CT and PET scans are often used together as while the CT scan provides anatomical orientation, the sensitive PET image is used to identify metastatic lesions.

References

Bouvet M et al (2002) Real-time optical imaging of primary tumor growth and multiple metastatic events in a pancreatic cancer orthotopic model. Cancer Res 62:1534–1540

Bulte JW, Kraitchman DL (2004) Iron oxide MR contrast agents for molecular and cellular imaging. NMR Biomed 17:484–499

Chalfie M, Tu Y, Euskirchen G, Ward WW, Prasher DC (1994) Green fluorescent protein as a marker for gene expression. Science 263:802–805

Chambers AF et al (1995) Steps in tumor metastasis: new concepts from intravital videomicroscopy. Cancer Metastasis Rev 14:279–301

24th Congress of the International Association for Breast Cancer Research (2003) Advances in human breast cancer research: preclinical models. Sacramento, USA. 1–5 Nov 2003. Abstracts. Breast Cancer Res 5(Suppl 1):S1–18

Contag CH, Jenkins D, Contag PR, Negrin RS (2000) Use of reporter genes for optical measurements of neoplastic disease in vivo. Neoplasia 2:41–52

de Wet JR, Wood KV, Helinski DR, DeLuca M (1985) Cloning of firefly luciferase cDNA and the expression of active luciferase in Escherichia coli. Proc Natl Acad Sci U S A 82:7870–7873

Deroose CM et al (2007) Multimodality imaging of tumor xenografts and metastases in mice with combined small-animal PET, small-animal CT, and bioluminescence imaging. J Nucl Med 48:295–303

El Hilali N, Rubio N, Martinez-Villacampa M, Blanco J (2002) Combined noninvasive imaging and luminometric quantification of luciferase-labeled human prostate tumors and metastases. Lab Invest 82:1563–71

Gates BJ, DeLuca M (1975) The production of oxyluciferin during the firefly luciferase light reaction. Arch Biochem Biophys 169:616–621

Greer LF 3rd, Szalay AA (2002) Imaging of light emission from the expression of luciferases in living cells and organisms: a review. Luminescence 17:43–74

Haddock S, Moline M (2010) Case J Bioluminescence in the Sea. Annu Rev Marine Sci 2:443–493

Harman G (1980) Fundamentals of computerized tomography. Academic, New York

Heyn C et al (2006) In vivo MRI of cancer cell fate at the single-cell level in a mouse model of breast cancer metastasis to the brain. Magn Reson Med 56:1001–1010

Hoffman RM (2002a) In vivo imaging of metastatic cancer with fluorescent proteins. Cell Death Differ 9:786–789

Hoffman RM (2002b) Green fluorescent protein imaging of tumour growth, metastasis, and angiogenesis in mouse models. Lancet Oncol 3:546–556

Hooper CE, Ansorge RE, Browne HM, Tomkins P (1990) CCD imaging of luciferase gene expression in single mammalian cells. J Biolumin Chemilumin 5:123–130

Lauterbur PC (1989) Image formation by induced local interactions. Examples employing nuclear magnetic resonance. 1973. Clin Orthop Relat Res 224:3–6

Naumov GN et al (1999) Cellular expression of green fluorescent protein, coupled with high-resolution in vivo videomicroscopy, to monitor steps in tumor metastasis. J Cell Sci 112 (Pt 12):1835–1842

Naumov GN et al (2003) Ineffectiveness of doxorubicin treatment on solitary dormant mammary carcinoma cells or late-developing metastases. Breast Cancer Res Treat 82:199–206

Novelline R (2004) Squire's Fundamentals of Radiology, 6th edn. Harvard University Press, Cambridge

Simoes RV et al (2008) Preliminary characterization of an experimental breast cancer cells brain metastasis mouse model by MRI/MRS. Magma 21:237–249

Smakman N, Martens A, Kranenburg O, Borel Rinkes IH (2004) Validation of bioluminescence imaging of colorectal liver metastases in the mouse. J Surg Res 122:225–230

Strube A et al (2010) Characterization of a new renal cell carcinoma bone metastasis mouse model. Clin Exp Metastasis 27:319–330

Tsien RY (1998) The green fluorescent protein. Annu Rev Biochem 67:509–544

Wetterwald A et al (2002) Optical imaging of cancer metastasis to bone marrow: a mouse model of minimal residual disease. Am J Pathol 160:1143–1153

Yamamoto N et al (2003) Determination of clonality of metastasis by cell-specific color-coded fluorescent-protein imaging. Cancer Res 63:7785–7790

Part VI
Diagnosis and Treatment of Metastatic Disease

Editors:
Silvin Bakalian and Dana Faingold

Chapter 19
Diagnosis of Metastasis

Dawn Russell-Hermanns

19.1 Introduction

The process of metastasis is characterized by the propagation of a primary tumour to other organ sites. This is an unfortunate and often terrifying progression in the already arduous course of a patient with cancer. In some cases, patients may in actuality have metastasis at diagnosis and the primary site may either be known or the patient may be given a diagnosis of "unknown primary cancer" (Khoor 2010). It cannot be sufficiently emphasized that a careful and detailed approach to the overall management of metastatic disease is essential.

Metastasis results from a stepwise process (Chambers et al. 2002). The stages resulting in the formation of metastatic lesions initially include intravasation and survival of the tumour cells in circulation. Arrest in the secondary site then occurs, with subsequent extravasation, survival of the tumour cells, growth and formation of pre-angiogenic micro metastasis (Winnard et al. 2008). The tumour cells can either enter a stage of dormancy or apoptosis. In order to have the end result of metastasis, each of these stages must occur to completion (Fig. 19.1).

Overall, the metastatic process has been found to be largely inefficient (Fig. 19.2). Efficiency with regard to metastasis is generally defined as the ability of cells from the primary tumour to successfully form lesions at a distant or secondary site. In most cases, few cells are able to achieve this and are deemed inefficient (Luzzi et al. 1998). Inefficiency has been observed clinically where patients have a seemingly large quantity of cancer cells detected in the peripheral circulation, while only a small number of resulting metastatic lesions. This hypothesis of inefficiency of the metastatic process was later confirmed using video microscopy on an *in vivo* murine model (Chambers et al. 2000). Animal studies such as these have revealed that some stages in the process of metastasis are actually efficient while others are not (Chambers et al. 2002). It was found that the overall survival of tumour cells in

D. Russell-Hermanns (✉)
McGill University, Montreal, QC, Canada
e-mail: dr.russell@sympatico.ca

J. V. Burnier, M. N. Burnier, Jr. (eds.), *Experimental and Clinical Metastasis*, 251
DOI 10.1007/978-1-4614-3685-0_19, © Springer Science+Business Media New York 2013

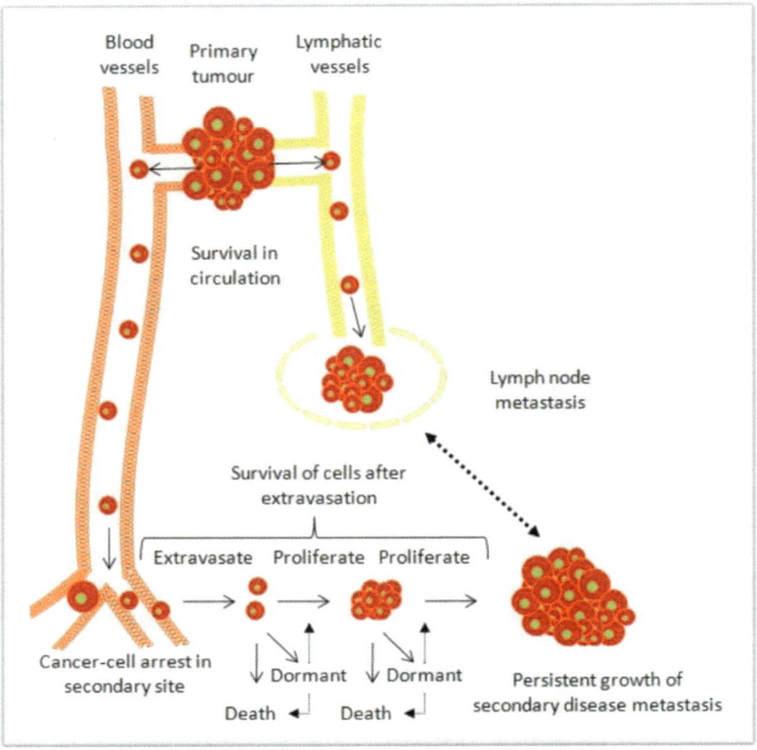

Fig. 19.1 Summary of the metastatic process. Cancer cells break from primary tumour and disseminate either hematogenously or via the lymphatic system. (Courtesy of J. Isenberg, McGill University school of medicine)

circulation, their arrest and subsequent extravasation were the more efficient stages in metastasis whereas tumour cell intravasation, post-extravasation cell survival and distal secondary tumour growth were actually found to be inefficient (Chambers et al. 2000). These early investigations were successful in revealing the fact that the presence of tumour cells or tissue at distant sites is not predictive of progression to clinically relevant metastatic disease. Furthermore, both mechanical and seed-soil (cancer cell-secondary organ) compatibility factors are involved in the propensity for certain cancers to metastasize to specific organs (Chambers et al. 2002).

An important aspect of the management of patients diagnosed with cancer is the early identification of metastases. It has been shown that early detection of the primary tumour itself will lead to more successful treatment outcomes (Chambers et al. 2002).

This chapter will address the various aspects involved in the diagnosis of metastatic disease and will also provide a comprehensive review of traditional and novel modalities of therapy for metastatic disease.

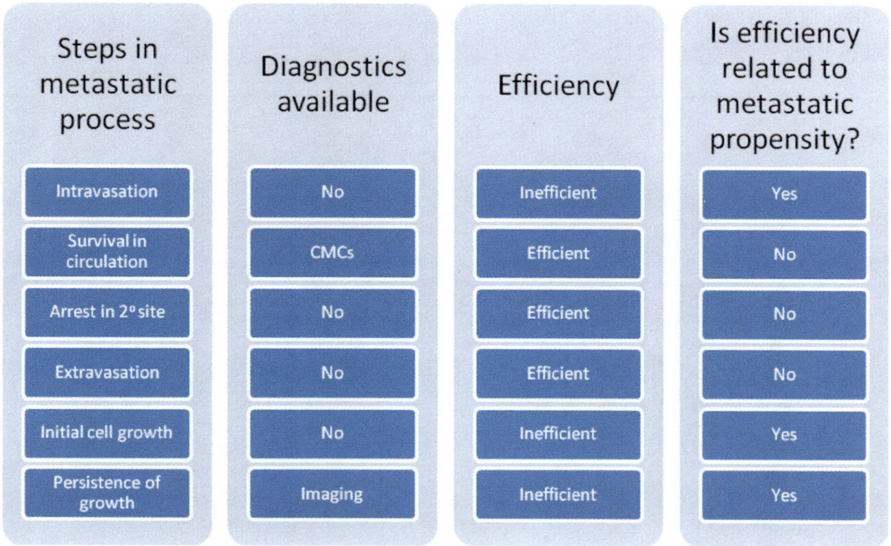

Fig. 19.2 Summary of observations regarding diagnosis of major metastatic processes and efficiencies of the major steps in metastasis with regards to their propensity for metastatic disease. (CMC = circulating malignant cells). (Courtesy of J. Isenberg, McGill University school of medicine)

19.2 Screening Tests

A screening test is a tool used to identify healthy members of the population who possibly have a disease from those that possibly do not have the disease. It has a role not only in determining of the presence of a primary cancer but there is also a role in metastatic disease. Specifically there are patients who present with a constellation of signs and symptoms with an unclear diagnosis of primary cancer and in whom screening tests are advantageous. There are three main types of screening tests based on the targeted stage of malignancy:

1. Tests to screen for pre-invasive lesions e.g. Papanicolaou test (PAP).
2. Tests to screen for "organ-confined" invasive cancer e.g. serum Prostatic specific antigen (PSA); mammography in breast cancer.
3. Screening tests for genetic predispositions to certain cancer types e.g. BRCA1 for breast cancer (Sharon 2007).

The goal of a screening test is naturally achievement of 100 % specificity and 100 % sensitivity. Sensitivity is defined as the number of individuals that actually have the disease that the screening test correctly identifies as positive. Specificity is the number of individuals that do not have disease that are correctly identified by the screening test as negative. In most cases, the sensitivity and specificity may have an inverse relationship. That is, a screening test may be highly sensitive in identifying truly positive individuals but may also have a large number of falsely positive results, which decreases the sensitivity of the test (Sharon 2007) (Table 19.1).

Table 19.1 A list of basic terms, definitions and calculations relevant for diagnostic assays. (Adapted from Sharon 2007)

Terms	Disease	No disease
Screening test positive	True positive (TP)	False positive (FP)
Screening test negative	False negative (FN)	True negative (TN)
	Definition	*Calculation*
Sensitivity	Percentage of diseased individuals who are correctly identified by the test	TP/(TP + FN) × 100
Specificity	Percentage of disease-free individuals who are correctly identified by the test	TN/(TN + FP) × 100

It is unfortunate that there are really only a small number of cancers for which screening tests have proven their efficacy with regard to decreasing cancer-associated mortality.

Key Points

- Metastasis is the spread of a primary tumour to a secondary site
- It is the end result of a sequence of events
- Stages of metastasis include:
  - Intravasation
  - Arrest in the secondary site
  - Extravasation
  - Growth
  - Angiogenesis
- Efficiency is the ability to successfully achieve metastasis
- Early detection of cancer is essential to improve treatment outcomes
- There may be circulating tumour cells in patients who do not develop metastatic disease

19.3 Clinical Diagnosis of Metastasis

Seventy percent of patients with cancer may have occult metastasis at the time of diagnosis (Liotta and Kohn 1990). It is crucial to approach the care of these patients systematically in order to arrive at a specific diagnoses with appropriate testing and investigations (Marchevsky et al. 2010). A study done evaluating follow up of breast cancer patients emphasizes the importance of history taking and applicable investigations (Kindler and Steinhoff 1989). Therefore a thorough work up starting with a detailed medical history and physical examination play a key role in the diagnosis of metastatic disease.

The clinical signs and symptoms exhibited by the patient can elude to the specific organ system affected by metastasis. In metastasis affecting the central nervous system, symptoms can include headaches, seizures, impairment of speech, visual disturbances, weakness, dizziness and vertigo. Pulmonary metastatic disease can

Table 19.2 Summary of organ specific clinical signs and symptoms of metastases

Tumour site	Symptoms
Central nervous system (CNS)	Headaches, seizures, speech impairment, visual disturbance, weakness, dizziness, vertigo
Pulmonary system	Cough, haemoptysis, chest pain, pneumonia, dyspnoea
Hepatic system	Jaundice, hepatomegaly
Hematopoietic system	Anaemia, leucopenia, thrombocytopenia
Skeletal system	Bone pain, pathological fractures, hypercalcemia, spinal cord compression
Generalized signs/symptoms	Weight loss, anorexia, aphagia, nausea, lymphadenopathy

present with multiple symptoms including cough, haemoptysis, chest pain or discomfort, as well as difficulty breathing and pneumonia. Hepatic involvement may be manifested by jaundice or yellow discolouration of the skin, anorexia, and hepatomegaly. If there is involvement of the hematopoietic system, this can result in leucopenia, anaemia and thrombocytopenia. Other nonspecific clinical signs of metastasis include ascites (fluid collection in the abdomen), lymphedema, weight loss, and lymphadenopathy. In metastasis to the bone, patients may present with bone pain, pathological fractures, spinal cord compression, and decreased mobility which can result in poor quality of life (Vassiliou et al. 2007). There are a wide variety as well as a paucity of symptoms that can occur in metastatic disease as there can be involvement of almost any organ system, be it the renal system, genitourinary and/or skeletal systems. There was one case reported in the literature of a patient who presented with monoarthritis of the hip who was subsequently found to have metastatic adenocarcinoma (Ruparelia et al. 2006). There are many other rare manifestations of metastatic disease that have been reported. These cases emphasize the importance of a complete and thorough physical examination in patients with confirmed or suspected malignancy (Table 19.2).

There are some primary malignancies however where the clinician can almost predict the most likely site of metastasis and this can guide the history, physical examination and investigations toward a particular target. This propensity for certain primary tumours to metastasize to specific organs is explained by the seed and soil theory. A recent study of the metastatic potential of cancers revealed quantitative reports of how different cancers had different metastatic targets and varying frequencies (Disibio and French 2008) (Table 19.3).

19.4 Diagnosis of Metastasis: Blood Testing

The management of a patient with metastatic disease or any malignancy goes beyond the history and physical to involve blood investigations, inclusive of tumour markers as well as routine lab tests. Routine lab tests will include a complete blood count

Table 19.3 Table showing frequent metastatic sites of various primary tumors

Primary tumour	Frequent sites of metastasis
Breast cancer	Lymph nodes, lungs, bones, brain
Lung cancer	Brain, bones
Prostate cancer	Regional lymph nodes, bone, distant lymph nodes, lung, liver
Colon cancer	Liver
Testicular cancer	Distant lymph nodes, liver, lung, kidney, bone

to rule out anaemia, neutropenia, and thrombocytopenia. A serum chemistry panel is also included in the work-up to evaluate renal function and assess calcium levels, urinalysis, and faeces for occult blood.

Tumour markers are substances that can be isolated from bodily fluids such as blood, urine, pleural and ascitic fluid as well as tissue and can be indicative of a particular type of cancer. They can be produced either by the tumour itself or by normal surrounding tissue as a result of the tumour (Schrohl et al. 2003). Tumour markers can be proteins, surface antigens, foetal antigens, oncogenic products, enzymes or hormones (Schrohl et al. 2003). It must be understood however that although they may be elevated in the presence of cancer, there are other non-cancerous conditions where they may be elevated as well.

There are a number of instances where the measurement of tumour markers is indicated. Screening for the presence of cancer in high risk and healthy populations as well as confirmation of the diagnosis of a particular type of cancer are two main indications for the use of tumour markers. They are also used in monitoring the efficacy of therapeutic interventions such as chemotherapy, radiation therapy or surgery, while also playing a role in the prognosis of a patient with cancer, and hence important in the management of metastatic disease. The varying role of tumour markers can thus be separated into diagnostic, predictive, prognostic, and monitoring markers. All of the available cancer markers fail at having both significant sensitivity and specificity and hence no solitary marker has met all the criteria of the ideal screening tool for a population. The two main protein specific markers that have been approved as screening tools as they met most of the criteria are prostatic specific antigen (PSA) and hem-occult blood testing (Schrohl et al. 2003).

Tumour markers can be cancer specific markers or tissue specific markers. Tissue specific markers are not directly related to malignancy and can be at high levels in the absence of cancer, as previously mentioned. Examples of tissue specific markers include alpha-fetoprotein (AFP), human chorionic gonadotropin (beta-HCG), prostatic specific antigen (PSA), thyroglobulin and a lectin-reactive AFP (AFP-L3). Cancer specific markers are elevated predominantly in the presence of malignancy, and examples include carcinoembryonic antigen (CEA), CA 19-9, and CA 125 (Schrohl et al. 2003).

19.4.1 Alpha Fetoprotein

This marker is a glycoprotein that is a significant constituent of foetal plasma, reaching a peak at twelve weeks gestation with a rapid decline after birth. In the foetus, it is made by the yolk sac, the gastrointestinal tract and the liver. Elevated levels have been associated with hepatocellular and germ cell carcinoma, typically greater than 500 ng/ml. The normal level in a healthy adult is less than 10 μg/ml. AFP is a tissue specific marker and hence can also be elevated in cirrhosis, hepatitis, and normal pregnancy (Schrohl et al. 2003). It is however still thought to be a suitable marker in detecting hepatocellular carcinoma in liver cirrhosis (Leandro et al. 1989).

19.4.2 Tissue Polypeptide Antigen (TPA)

Tissue polypeptide antigen is a protein antigen that was originally developed by Bjorklund and Bjorklund in 1957 (Weber et al. 1984). Initial studies revealed this antigen to be strongly associated with epithelial tissues as opposed to nonepithelial tissues (Nathrath et al. 1985). TPA may in certain settings be useful in determining the presence of hepatocellular carcimoma (Leandro et al. 1989). It was also found to be of use in patients with bladder cancer as a means of evaluating recurrence as well as in being a prognostic indicator (Maulard-Durdux et al. 1997).

19.4.3 Prostatic Specific Antigen (PSA)

This tissue specific antigen is also a glycoprotein that has very low levels in normal adult males, with a range from 0 to 4 ng/ml. It is used as a screening tool for prostate cancer, however its level can be affected by prostatitis as well as benign prostatic hypertrophy. Additionally, the PSA levels can vary according to age and race. Asians have been found to have lower PSA levels whereas African Americans have been found to have higher levels. Generally, there is an associated increase in the normal range of PSA with age. For these reasons, measurement of PSA levels may not be a very ideal screening tool however with regard to prognosis it has been found to be of great benefit. Patients with very high PSA levels prior to surgical intervention have a greater likelihood of recurrent prostate cancer than those with lower pre-operative levels (Schrohl et al. 2003).

19.4.4 Human Chorionic Gonadotropin

This is a hormone that is normally made by the syncytiotrophoblastic cells of the placenta and its elevation is a normal and expected feature of pregnancy. HCG is however also grossly elevated in gestational trophoblastic tumours, in most cases correlating well with tumour mass. There have been reported cases of breast, gastrointestinal, and lung cancer where the level of HCG has been elevated, however its use as a tumour marker has been restricted to trophoblastic tumours. It has been beneficial in monitoring for recurrence (Schrohl et al. 2003).

19.4.5 Carcinoembryonic Antigen (CEA)

This is a tumour marker produced in colon cancer, however can also be produced by a number of other cell types as well as the developing foetus. Its normal range in blood is less than 2.5 ng/ml. The normal level in smokers is doubled to 5 ng/ml. CEA has been used as a tool to monitor for recurrence of colon cancer with specific criteria for surgical intervention based on level of rise from baseline (Schrohl et al. 2003). It has been shown to be elevated in other conditions such as pancreatitis, inflammatory bowel disease and cirrhosis.

19.4.6 CA 125

This marker is mainly elevated in ovarian cancer although it can also be elevated in colon cancer, breast cancer, lung cancer and endometrial cancer. Other conditions such as endometriosis, menstruation and pregnancy can also have elevated CA 125 levels. CA 125 is a monoclonal antibody (OC 125) and has been reported to be present in 80 % of nonmucinous ovarian carcinomas. This marker can also be used to monitor for disease recurrence (Schrohl et al. 2003).

19.4.7 CA 19-9

This marker is also a monoclonal antibody and its clinical use has been predominantly in gastrointestinal adenocarcinoma. It has also been shown to be elevated in cases of gastric cancer and can be used to monitor for early disease recurrence after therapy (Schrohl et al. 2003). CA 19–9 is also elevated in pancreatic cancer. In a study of patients with metastatic pancreatic cancer, decline in the level of serum CA 19–9 was found to be comparable to radiographic response as a good predictor of overall outcome and time to progression. These findings reveal a promising role for CA 19–9 in metastatic pancreatic cancer (Wong et al. 2008).

19.4.8 CA 15-3

This is a monoclonal antibody that is derived from mucin (MUCI). It has been shown to be of some prognostic value in breast cancer and when compared with CEA, it is more sensitive and specific (Bartsch et al. 2006). It is a more useful tumour marker for breast cancer follow up than TPA or CEA given its higher sensitivity (Given et al. 2000). One study in particular however, revealed no significant prognostic benefit of this marker in monitoring disease progression in patients on fulvestrant therapy (Bartsch et al. 2006).

Table 19.4 Summary of common tumour specific markers

Malignancy	Tumour marker
Colorectal cancer	CEA
Germ cell tumours	AFP, β-HCG
Hepatoma	AFP, TPA
Ovarian cancer	CA 125
Choriocarcinoma	β-HCG
Prostate cancer	PSA
Breast cancer	CA 15-3, HER2/neu

19.4.9 Human Epidermal Growth Factor Receptor 2 (HER2/neu)

Testing for human epidermal growth factor receptor 2 gene is indicated at the time of diagnosis of primary breast cancer and also for monitoring patients with metastatic breast cancer (Hanna et al. 2007). This gene is not inherited and has been associated with aging and some have postulated a possible link with environmental factors. The HER2/neu gene is responsible for signalling cells during division, growth and repair. Healthy breast cells possess two copies of the gene however in some forms of breast cancer, approximately 18–20 %, the gene is over amplified (Hanna et al. 2007).

Decreasing levels of serum HER2/neu can be interpreted as favourable response to therapy and increasing levels are indicative of progression of disease (Table 19.4).

19.5 Diagnosis of Metastasis: Imaging Studies

The purpose of imaging in the management of the patient with metastatic disease goes far beyond merely screening for the presence of metastatic disease but also involves staging, monitoring progress of disease before and after therapy, as well as in gaining volumetric data in instances where surgical resection may be a therapeutic option (Choi 2006). Additionally, the age and sex of the patient along with the location of the metastasis confirmed by imaging can be predictive of the likely origin of the primary tumour (Khoor 2010).

There are various imaging modalities available and their specific role will obviously be dictated by the type of metastatic disease involved. In general, imaging modalities used in this arena must be of course be highly sensitive and specific, reproducible, consistent and provide all of these features while being tolerable to the patient (Choi 2006).

The response evaluation criteria in solid tumours (RECIST) was originally published in 2000 and has since been revised (RECIST 1.1) and provides criteria to be used in assessing tumour response to therapy in clinical trials (Choi 2006). With respect to imaging, RECIST has provided guidelines for the use and interpretation of specific imaging techniques allowing for a more accurate evaluation of tumour response in clinical trials (Eisenhauer et al. 2009). The purpose of RECIST however, is specifically for clinical trials and not to provide general imaging recommendations for oncologists in their daily practice (Eisenhauer et al. 2009).

The following sections will review the various imaging modalities available with specific examples of the various conditions where they are most commonly indicated.

19.5.1 Radiographic Modalities

There are some areas in medicine where plain radiography is no longer of significant benefit, however in the evaluation of certain forms of metastatic disease it still plays a role. Plain X-rays are of particular benefit in the evaluation of bone metastasis. After the liver and the lung, the bone follows as the third most frequent site of distant metastasis (Vassiliou et al. 2007).

Thirty to seventy percent of patients with cancer have bone metastasis (Salvo et al. 2009; Byun et al. 2002), usually occurring late in the disease process (King 2006). The way in which a metastatic lesion appears on plain radiography is dependent on the amount of bone that is resorbed or deposited (Lipton et al. 2004), with the radiographic appearance being either osteolytic or sclerotic. Osteolytic lesions are usually more frequently observed. Plain X-rays allow for the detailed assessment and classification of these lesions.

The use of plain films in bone metastasis is as an adjunct to bone scintigraphy scanning, which will be discussed in detail in the upcoming sections. In clinical practice, bone scanning is often followed by further evaluation with plain X-rays of the particular lesions found on scintiscan (Salvo et al. 2009). This is due to the fact that the appearance of the mestastatic bone lesions on plain film can be indicative of the primary cancer. Carcinomas of the thyroid, renal system (Lipton et al. 2004), and lung are typically associated with osteolytic bone lesions whereas carcinomas of the prostate, colon or bladder may be sclerotic. Some cancers such as that of breast may have a mixed appearance having both osteolytic and osteoblastic features on radiography (Vassiliou et al. 2007).

Plain radiography also plays a role in evaluating the response to therapy along with clinical, laboratory and bone scan findings (Coleman et al. 1988). Healing of an osteolytic lesion is manifested radiographically by the presence of a sclerotic rim of bone that progressively migrates from the edges toward the center of the lesion throughout the healing process with subsequent decrease in size and resolution. Radiographic evidence of decreased size and disappearance of a sclerotic metastatic bone lesion indicates therapeutic response and is often difficult to assess. Mixed lesions either show generalized sclerotic changes as response to therapy or increased osteolytic changes indicating disease progression. These findings may not be evident on plain radiographs at less than 6 months into therapy and so additional modalities for assessing response to therapy must be employed as well (Coleman et al. 1988).

Plain films are limited overall as a single imaging modality as they can only detect lesions that are 1–2 cm in size and where there has been greater than 50 % loss of the bone mineral content (Salvo et al. 2009).

Plain chest X-rays may also be of some benefit in the evaluation for metastatic lung disease, and in various instances may in fact be the first test performed to detect pulmonary metastasis. In some cases metastatic lesions may be an incidental finding on routine chest X-ray. Its overall role however is becoming less significant, as computed tomography (CT) scanning has better resolution and is a more accurate modality for detecting small metastatic lung lesions.

One of the many example of the declining significance of plain X-rays in the work up of metastatic disease is its use in the preoperative evaluation of patients with primary melanoma. One particular study found no additional benefit in the use of chest X-ray in this setting (Vermeeren et al. 2009b). Another example is in a subset of patients with disseminated non-seminomatous testicular cancer (marker positive patients in complete remission), one study found no benefit in doing routine chest X-rays for surveillance for relapse post chemotherapy (Gietema 2002). These are just a few of numerous examples where plain chest films no longer have a significant role in the work up of metastasis.

19.5.2 Ultrasonography

By evaluating and recording the sound waves that are reflected by tissues, an ultrasound scan (US) can detect abnormalities in various organs of the body. Its still remains relevant as a part of the evaluation of metastatic disease in certain settings.

Ultrasound scanning becomes important particularly in investigating for liver metastasis. Liver metastasis is unfortunately a common pathway for a number of malignancies, for example colorectal cancer and uveal melanoma. In colorectal cancer, it has been reported that approximately 70 % patients eventually advance to hepatic metastasis (Bipat et al. 2005). Discovery of liver metastasis in a patient with known malignancy can have a grave impact on the overall prognosis and hence early and accurate detection is essential (Liu and Francis 2010).

As an imaging modality for hepatic metastasis, US was thought by some to be a great tool for screening purposes (Bipat et al. 2005). This is because US is widely available, cost effective and non-invasive, hence tolerable to the patient. US can detect those patients with large numbers of metastatic liver lesions and who are therefore not appropriate for surgical resection versus other patients who may have few or no lesions at all (Bipat et al. 2005).

Others however, have found less utility of US as a screening tool given its low sensitivity and specificity and operator dependent efficacy (Choi 2006). Another limitation of the use of US in hepatic metastasis is that in some cases portions of the liver may not be accessible by US (Bipat et al. 2005). US is believed to be of greater benefit in the setting of indeterminate lesions found on other imaging modalities that require additional investigation (Choi 2006).

The appearance of the metastatic lesions of the liver on an US can be hypoechoic or hyperechoic. Features highly suggestive of hepatic metastasis on US are the presence of many solid lesions or one lesion surrounded by a hypoechoic halo (Choi 2006).

Recent advancements in US, namely Power Doppler and Contrast Harmonic Imaging (CHI) have been successful in providing a more accurate evaluation of solid hepatic lesions (Choi 2006; Robinson 2000).

Contrast Harmonic Imaging (CHI) uses contrast agents that improve the quality of US in various ways. When the contrast agent is introduced intravenously into the patient, it functions by increasing the back-shadowed echoes from regions that need to be visualized and the oral agent works by decreasing unwanted reflectivity from certain tissues. The various enhancement patterns produced allows for improved characterization of different hepatic tumours (Choi 2006).

Power Doppler is a newer form of assessing blood flow that is reported to be about 5 times more sensitive than color Doppler. It makes use of a color map and is able to demonstrate the Doppler signal power while eliminating information regarding flow or velocity, hence providing an improved report of the flow characteristics (Choi 2006).

Endoscopic US is another method of evaluating liver metastasis. It has also been shown in some studies to be superior to computed tomography (CT) scanning with regard to the accuracy of the number of lesions (Singh et al. 2009). With endoscopic US, fine needle aspiration biopsy can also be carried out which has been beneficial in the characterization of lesions that were not visualized on CT scan.

US can also be used to investigate the lymphatic system and lymph nodes for diagnosis of metastasis. In most cases, lymph node metastasis may actually occur before metastasis occurs hematogenously. Features of malignancy of the lymph nodes on gray scale US includes deformity of the normal echogenic hilus and the overall shape of the lymph node as opposed to features of benign reactive nodes where the shape and echogenic hilar structure may appear normal (Sohn et al. 2010).

19.5.3 Computed Tomography (CT)

A CT scan is a diagnostic modality created in 1972 by Godfrey Hounsfield (Choi 2006) that uses X-rays to generate detailed three dimensional (3D) images of structures within the body. The X-rays are taken at different angles and processed through a computer giving rise to the final 3D image called a tomogram. Advances in this technology have lead to the multi-detector helical CT which has improved the accuracy, resolution and detail of the images created in comparison to the original CT scans. CT scan has been a key imaging modality in evaluating various forms of metastatic disease.

Multi-detector helical CT is the standard imaging modality in suspected liver metastasis. Its role in hepatic metastatic disease involves being part of the initial work up, monitoring and surveillance pre- and post-treatment as well as in preoperative planning (Choi 2006). With helical CT, the vascularity of the liver can be evaluated by dual phase studies during the hepatic arterial and portal venous phases with the use of intravenous contrast. Dual phase helical CT has been reported to have a specificity of 86–91 % and sensitivity of 69–71 % in hepatic lesions that were confirmed surgically (Choi 2006).

In hepatic metastasis, evaluating the vascularity of the lesion in comparison to the normal surrounding tissue is important as it may dictate how the lesion appears on CT scan. Primary tumours that can produce very vascular metastatic lesions in the liver include melanoma, sarcoma, neuro-endocrine tumours and renal cell carcinoma. On CT scan, these highly vascular lesions will appear more enhanced than the normal surrounding liver especially during the arterial phase of liver enhancement. Colorectal adenocarcinoma typically produces metastatic lesions in the liver that have minimal vascularity and so can be seen better during venous phase in dual phase helical CT studies (Choi 2006).

In certain instances where liver resection may be an option, the use of CT scan during arterial portography has proven to be of some benefit. Unfortunately, given that this procedure is more invasive as well as expensive, it has not gained much popularity when compared to helical CT or MRI (Choi 2006).

In skeletal or bone metastasis, CT scan has several roles. It been useful in providing more detailed evaluation of lesions seen on bone scintiscan that were not confirmed on plain radiography. Additionally, CT scan is used as a confirmatory test in symptomatic patients whose initial plain films are negative for any obvious metastatic lesions.

In the detection of bone metastasis, CT scan has been shown to be more sensitive than plain films. It is better at identifying small sclerotic areas than plain radiographs and has no anatomical limitations with respect to the bones being studied as is the case with plain films (Lipton et al. 2004).

CT scan is also used to determine the presence of metastasis to the brain. It has been shown that in brain metastasis, several factors are key to obtaining accuracy on CT scan. These include not only the dose of contrast agent used but also the timing with which the image is obtained after administration of the contrast agent. The result can be an altered image of the metastatic lesions. As such, the choice of imaging technique for evaluation of brain metastasis or metastatic disease in general is essential to overall management of the patient, in particular surgical planning (Sidhu et al. 2004).

CT scan is also useful in the evaluation of metastatic lesions of the lungs, lymph nodes and other systems in the body and has been shown to be an integral part of the work up in the metastatic patient (Fig. 19.3, 19.4 and 19.5).

19.5.4 Magnetic Resonance Imaging (MRI)

MRI is an imaging modality that uses a magnetic field and the principle of magnetic resonance. The hydrogen ions in the human body are magnetized in the MRI machine and they emit signals that are processed through a computer to produce an image. Like CT scan, MRI plays an integral role in the evaluation of patients with metastatic disease and is more sensitive in detection of soft tissue abnormalities than CT scan. Advances in MRI technology have included T1-weighted spoiled gradient echo and T2-weighted fast spin echo which has resulted in faster acquisition of images (Choi 2006). This has been particularly useful in the evaluation of hepatic metastasis.

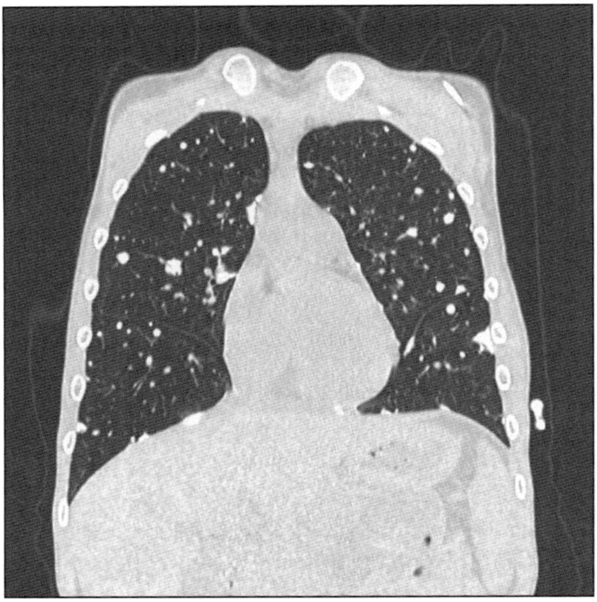

Fig. 19.3 CT scan chest in the coronal plane demonstrating multiple metastatic lesions in the lungs bilaterally in a patient with metastatic osteosarcoma. (Courtesy of Dr. R. Faingold)

Whole body MRI is a concept that has been extensively explored for both screening and staging in the management of the patient with known malignancy. It was found by some to be an excellent screening method for detecting bone metastasis, especially of the vertebral bodies (Nakanishi et al. 2005). Whole body MRI initially failed due to limitations in data acquisition time and accuracy. VIBE (volumetric interpolated breath-hold examination) was introduced to overcome the limitations initially faced with whole body MRI (Lauenstein et al. 2004). VIBE imaging involves T1-weighted, 3D gradient echo sequence used with integrated fat saturation and near isotropic spatial resolution. The data acquisition time is reported to be around 20 s and occurs during breath holding. With the use of gadolinium contrast, detection of metastasis in parenchymal organs has been markedly improved (Lauenstein et al. 2004). Other studies of this technique have reported promising results as well with regard to staging (Thomson et al. 2008; Barkhausen et al. 2001).

There has been recent work with regard to liver specific contrast agents for MRI in hepatic metastasis. MRI for liver metastasis is done routinely with contrast enhancement and newer agents specific to the liver have been introduced to increase accuracy of detection of metastatic lesions. Contrast enhanced MRI for investigation of hepatic metastasis is said to be the most accurate imaging technique for this purpose (Kim et al. 2008). An example of a hepatic specific agent is Mangafodipir trisodium (MnDPDP, Telescan) (Choi 2006). There have been studies comparing the efficacy of other new contrast agents such as gadoacetic acid (Zech 2007) and ferucarbotran-enhanced MRI (Kim et al. 2010). Another study comparing MnDPDP and ferucarbotran-enhanced MRI in hepatic metastasis revealed comparable efficacy between these two agents (Choi et al. 2006).

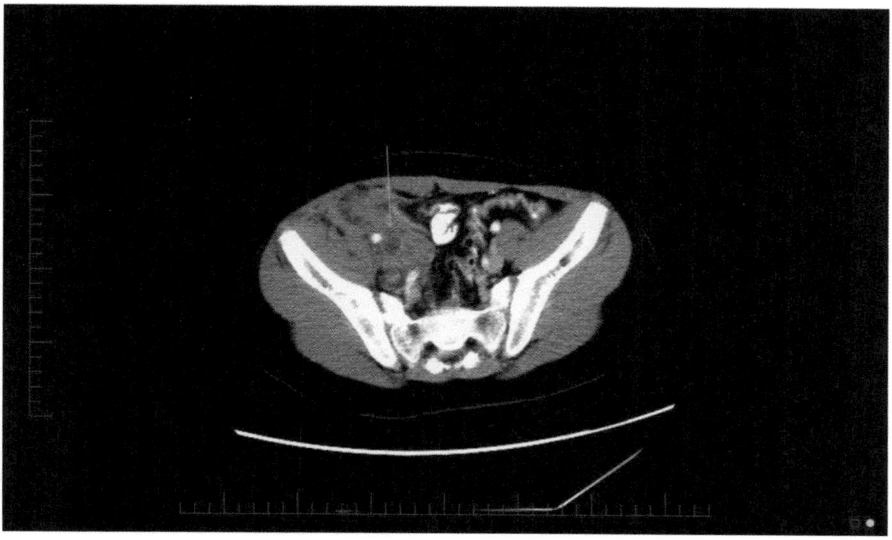

Fig. 19.4 CT scan pelvis in the axial plane demonstrating a metastatic lesion (*arrow*) involving the right iliopsoas muscle in a patient with metastatic rhabdomyosarcoma. (Courtesy of Dr. R. Faingold)

Fig. 19.5 CT Scan abdomen, axial plane demonstrating multiple hypodense metastatic liver lesions. (Courtesy of Dr. R. Faingold)

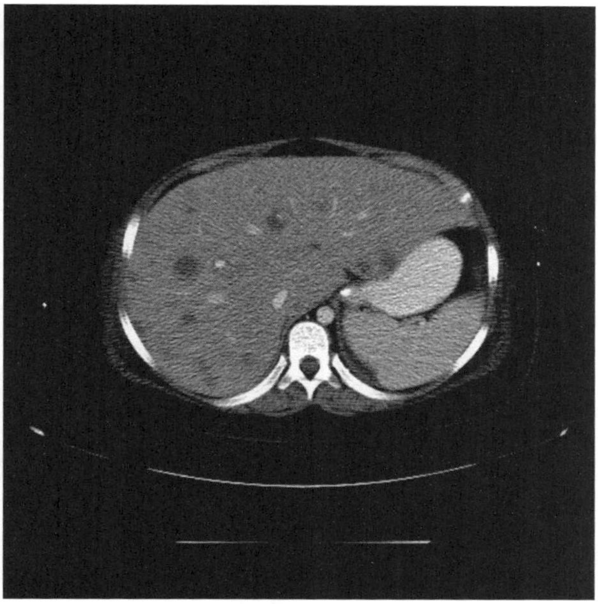

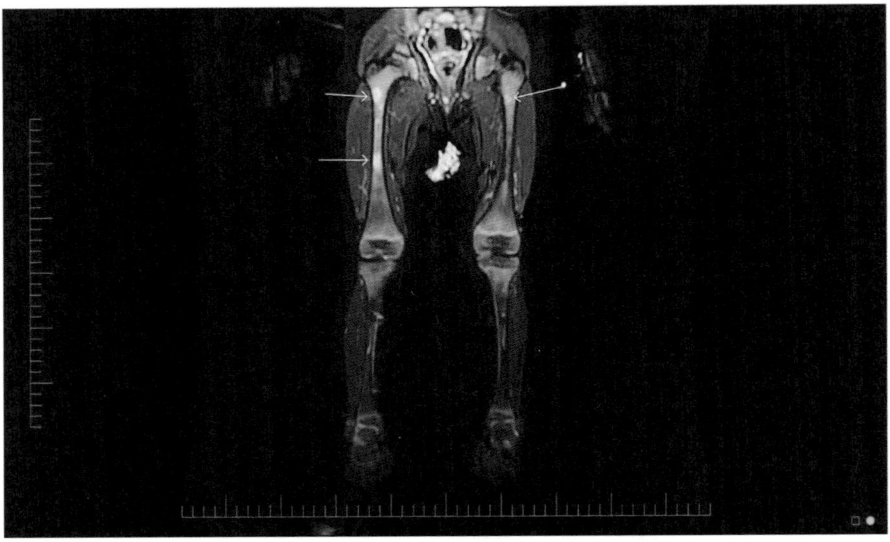

Fig. 19.6 Coronal view of MRI (STIR (short T1 inversion recovery) weighted sequence) showing bilateral bone marrow metastases involving femur and tibia bilaterally in a patient with metastatic neuroblastoma. (Courtesy of Dr. R. Faingold)

Fig. 19.7 T1 weighted MRI with gadolinium and fat suppression (*coronal view*) showing metastatic osteosarcoma involving distal left femur and contralateral proximal right femur. (Courtesy of Dr. R. Faingold)

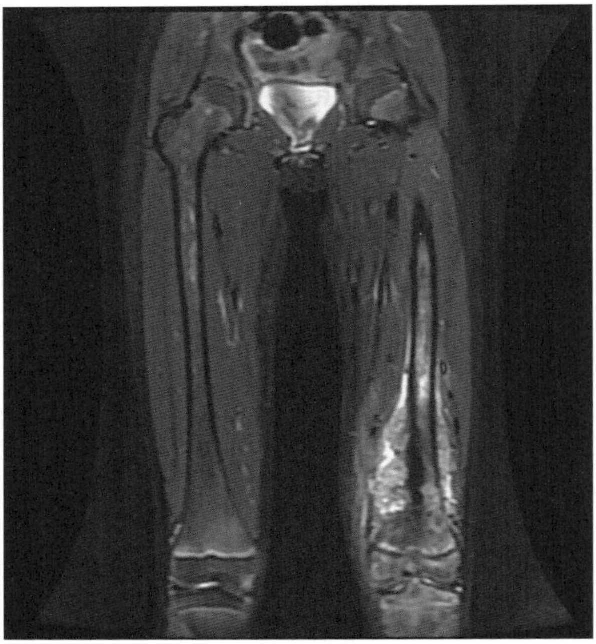

In the evaluation of lymph node metastases, gadolinium enhanced MRI has been shown to be of some benefit. The results of a systematic review and meta analysis of the gadolinium enhanced MRI in lymph node staging revealed moderate accuracy with regard to detection of lymph node metastases (Klerkx et al. 2010) (Fig. 19.6 and Fig. 19.7).

19.5.5 Nuclear Imaging

This is a diagnostic modality whereby images are produced by detection of radiation from various parts of the body following administration of a radioactive tracer agent either intravenously in most cases or in some instances orally. Technetium-99m bone scintigraphy, positron emission tomography (PET) and single photon emission computed tomography (SPECT) are examples of nuclear imaging that can be used in the evaluation of metastatic disease.

Bone scintigraphy, also known as radionuclide bone scanning, is an imaging modality that can be used for whole body screening in the evaluation of bone metastasis. It has the advantage of being more widely available and cost effective than other imaging studies for bone metastasis. It is usually the first imaging study for investigating bone metastasis in asymptomatic breast cancer patients (Costelloe et al. 2009). On a bone scan, metastasis can be seen as multiple, irregular, randomly distributed areas of increased tracer uptake. Tracer uptake is increased because when bone metastasis form there is an associated increase in blood flow and reactive new bone formation (Jackson et al. 1975). Advances in the accuracy and sensitivity of other nuclear imaging techniques such as PET scans may eventually lead to a decreased role for bone scan in evaluation of osseous metastasis in some cases (Cheran et al. 2004) (Fig. 19.8).

PET scans have many indications in the evaluation of metastatic disease. With the use of 2-deoxy-2-[18 F] fluoro-D-glucose (FDG-PET), glucose metabolism can be imaged. This has allowed for the detection of metabolic changes prior to anatomical changes leading to earlier identification of tumours and discovery of lesions in previously unknown locations. This information is also useful for staging of malignancies, monitoring for recurrence and response to therapy (Choi 2006). FDG-PET is indicated in the evaluation of hepatic, colorectal and skeletal metastases as well as many others. In lung metastasis, although spiral CT is still the superior imaging modality, given its high specificity, a positive FDG-PET can be used as a confirmatory test for suspected metastatic lesions found on thoracic CT (Franzius et al. 2001).

There are limitations with the use of conventional PET scans and a major one is the inability to accurately identify the corresponding anatomical site with the abnormal area that is detected on the scan. This has lead to the integration of CT scan with PET for more accurate anatomical localization (Choi 2006). A comparative study by Dandrup-Link et al. of imaging modalities revealed sensitivities of 90 % for FDG-PET, 82 % for whole body MRI, and 71 % for Technetium bone scan (Daldrup-Link et al. 2001) (Fig. 19.9).

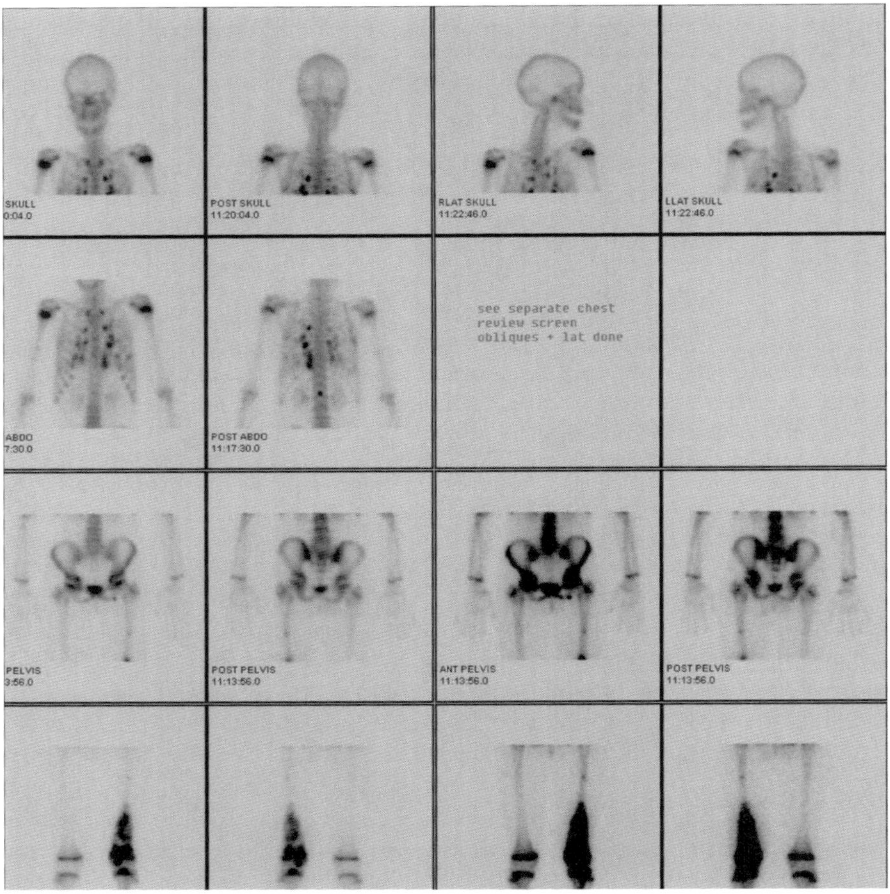

Fig. 19.8 Bone scan of a patient with primary osteosarcoma, involving the distal left femur and extending into proximal tibia. Metastatic lesions of the lumbar vertebrae, ribs and multiple mediastinal and lung lymph nodes. (Courtesy of Dr. R. Faingold)

SPECT is another imaging modality whereby molecules labelled with a radionuclide emit gamma ray photons. It differs from PET in that during this process, only a single photon is detected and emitted directly from the radioactive atom. SPECT has multiple roles in evaluating metastatic disease. Bone SPECT has been found to be better at detecting osseous abnormalities than planar bone scan. In breast cancer, bone SPECT was found to be superior to FDG-PET (Uematsu et al. 2005).

The integration of SPECT with CT was found to have additional benefit in localization of more sentinel lymph nodes when compared with planar imaging in prostate cancer (Vermeeren et al. 2009a).

It can thus be seen that the application of these nuclear imaging modalities has made quite an impact on the management of metastatic disease.

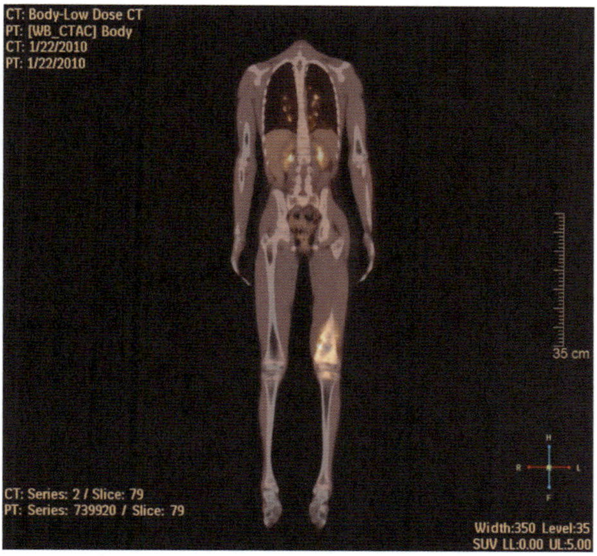

Fig. 19.9 PET/CT fused, coronal plane demonstrating osteosarcoma involving the left distal femur with metastatic lung disease. (Courtesy of Dr. R. Faingold)

Table 19.5 Table showing the site of metastases and the indicated imaging modality

Sites of metastasis	Common imaging modalities
Liver	Ultrasound scan, power doppler, contrast harmonic imaging (CHI), endoscopic ultrasound, CT scan, CT scan with arterial portography, FDG-PET, MRI (with liver specific contrast)
Lung	Plain chest X-ray, CT scan, FDG-PET
Bone	Plain X-ray, planar bone scintigraphy, CT scan, bone-SPECT
Brain	CT scan, MRI
Lymph nodes	USS, CT scan, MRI, SPECT

19.5.6 Molecular Imaging

Molecular imaging is a new technology that incorporates molecular biology with *in vivo* imaging. Molecular events within living organisms can be studied in detail with the use of tracers (Gambhir 2002). One of its many uses in medicine is to capture the metastatic potential and status of a tumour through imaging. This should allow for earlier detection and an improvement in the overall management of metastatic patients (Apolo et al. 2008).

In this field, MRI has been used as a tool to study metastatic potential by various methods. Firstly, there are *in vivo* studies of animals with metastatic tumour xenografts and secondly, it has been studied with chamber type assays in evaluating cancer cellular invasive characteristics. Another method has been investigations delineating the targets of labelled metastatic cancer cells (Winnard et al. 2008). Most of these techniques have been used in animal models of metastases, however there are some examples of other MRI techniques that are currently used in clinical practice. We previously mentioned the technique of screening using whole body MRI. Another technique is applied in detection of axillary lymph nodes in breast cancer patients. Yet another current clinically relevant technique that makes use of this technology is the detection of occult lymph nodes metastasis in prostate cancer. This is done noninvasively with extremely lymphotrophic super-magnetic iron oxide nanoparticles (Winnard et al. 2008). A recent study evaluated the large number of tracers now available for study in prostate cancer, inclusive of metabolic, angiogenic, and apoptotic pathways as well as others (Apolo et al. 2008).

PET technology has also been used along with radiopharmaceuticals in imaging tumour glucose metabolism and hypoxia with the goal of studying metastatic potential. Currently, major work is being done with angiogenesis-specific radiopharmaceuticals for imaging metastatic potential (Winnard et al. 2008).

19.5.7 Angiography

In the current era where there are so many new imaging modalities for metastatic disease, angiography plays a limited role. In liver metastasis, catheter angiography has been useful for preoperative planning as well as detection of metastatic hepatic lesions (Choi 2006). In skeletal metastasis, it may be useful in the assessment of pain palliation in cases where there are multiple, non-resectable lesions. Additionally, in surgical cases, it can be useful preoperatively in displaying devascularisation of vascular metastasis (Jonsson and Johnell 1982) (Table 19.5).

Key Points

- At initial diagnosis, 70 % of patients with cancer may have undetectable metastasis.
- A detailed history, physical examination, blood work (complete blood count, chemistry panel, tumor markers) are initial steps in the work up of metastatic disease.
- Imaging plays multiple roles in metastatic disease that include:
  - Screening
  - Staging
  - Monitoring response to therapy

References

Apolo AB, Pandit-Taskar N, Morris MJ (2008) Novel tracers and their development for the imaging of metastatic prostate cancer. J Nucl Med 49:2031–2041

Barkhausen J et al (2001) Whole-body MR imaging in 30 sec with real-time true FISP and a continuously rolling table platform: feasibility study. Radiology 220:252–256

Bartsch R et al (2006) Prognostic value of monitoring tumour markers CA 15-3 and CEA during fulvestrant treatment. BMC Cancer 6:81

Bipat S et al (2005) Colorectal liver metastases: CT, MR imaging, and PET for diagnosis–meta-analysis. Radiology 237:123–131

Byun WM et al (2002) Diffusion-weighted MR imaging of metastatic disease of the spine: assessment of response to therapy. AJNR Am J Neuroradiol 23:906–912

Chambers AF, Naumov GN, Vantyghem SA, Tuck AB (2000) Molecular biology of breast cancer metastasis. Clinical implications of experimental studies on metastatic inefficiency. Breast Cancer Res 2:400–407

Chambers AF, Groom AC, MacDonald IC (2002) Dissemination and growth of cancer cells in metastatic sites. Nat Rev Cancer 2:563–572

Cheran SK, Herndon JE 2nd, Patz EF Jr (2004) Comparison of whole-body FDG-PET to bone scan for detection of bone metastases in patients with a new diagnosis of lung cancer. Lung Cancer 44:317–325

Choi J (2006) Imaging of hepatic metastases. Cancer Control 13:6–12

Choi JY et al (2006) Detection of hepatic metastasis: manganese—and ferucarbotran-enhanced MR imaging. Eur J Radiol 60:84–90

Coleman RE et al (1988) Bone scan flare predicts successful systemic therapy for bone metastases. J Nucl Med 29:1354–1359

Costelloe CM et al (2009) Imaging bone metastases in breast cancer: techniques and recommendations for diagnosis. Lancet Oncol 10:606–614

Daldrup-Link HE et al (2001) Whole-body MR imaging for detection of bone metastases in children and young adults: comparison with skeletal scintigraphy and FDG PET. AJR Am J Roentgenol 177:229–236

Disibio G, French SW (2008) Metastatic patterns of cancers: results from a large autopsy study. Arch Pathol Lab Med 132:931–939

Eisenhauer EA et al (2009) New response evaluation criteria in solid tumours: revised RECIST guideline (version 1.1). Eur J Cancer 45: 228–247

Franzius C et al (2001) FDG-PET for detection of pulmonary metastases from malignant primary bone tumors: comparison with spiral CT. Ann Oncol 12:479–486

Gambhir SS (2002) Molecular imaging of cancer with positron emission tomography. Nat Rev Cancer 2:683–693

Gietema JA, Meinardi MT, Sleijfer DT, Hoekstra HJ, Van Der Graaf WT (2002) Routine chest X-rays have no additional value in the detection of relapse during routine follow-up of patients treated with chemotherapy for disseminated non-seminomatous testicular cancer. Ann Oncol 13:1616–1620

Given M, Scott M, Mc Grath JP, Given HF (2000) The predictive of tumour markers CA 15-3, TPS and CEA in breast cancer recurrence. Breast 9:277–280

Hanna W et al (2007) Updated recommendations from the Canadian National Consensus Meeting on HER2/neu testing in breast cancer. Curr Oncol 14:149–153

Jackson FI, Lentle BC (1975) Scintiscan methods in cancer diagnosis. Can Fam Physician 21:79–83

Jonsson K, Johnell O (1982) Preoperative angiography in patients with bone metastases. Acta Radiol Diagn (Stockh) 23:485–489

Khoor A (2010) Diagnosis of metastatic neoplasms: an overview. Arch Pathol Lab Med 134:192–193

Kim YK, Lee YH, Kwak HS, Kim CS, Han YM (2008) Small malignant hepatic tumor detection in gadolinium- and ferucarbotran-enhanced magnetic resonance imaging: does combining ferucarbotran-enhanced T2*-weighted gradient echo and T2-weighted turbo spin echo images have additive efficacy? Korean J Radiol 9:510–519

Kim YK, Lee YH, Kwak HS, Kim CS, Han YM (2010) Detection of liver metastases: gadoxetic acid-enhanced three-dimensional MR imaging versus ferucarbotran-enhanced MR imaging. Eur J Radiol 73:131–136

Kindler M, Steinhoff G (1989) Follow-up of breast cancer patients. Oncology 46:360–365

King DM (2006) Imaging of metastatic melanoma. Cancer Imaging 6:204–208

Klerkx WM et al (2010) Detection of lymph node metastases by gadolinium-enhanced magnetic resonance imaging: systematic review and meta-analysis. J Natl Cancer Inst 102:244–253

Lauenstein TC et al (2004) Whole-body MR imaging: evaluation of patients for metastases. Radiology 233:139–148
Leandro G et al (1989) Do CA 19-9 and TPA play a minor role as compared to AFP in diagnosing primary hepatocellular carcinoma? Oncology 46:381–385
Liotta LA, Kohn E (1990) Cancer invasion and metastases. JAMA 263:1123–1126
Lipton A et al (2004) Skeletal complications in patients with bone metastases from renal cell carcinoma and therapeutic benefits of zoledronic acid. Clin Cancer Res 10:6397S–6403S
Liu PS, Francis IR (2010) Hepatic imaging for metastatic disease. Cancer J 16:93–102
Luzzi KJ et al (1998) Multistep nature of metastatic inefficiency: dormancy of solitary cells after successful extravasation and limited survival of early micrometastases. Am J Pathol 153:865–873
Marchevsky AM, Gupta R, Balzer B (2010) Diagnosis of metastatic neoplasms: a clinicopathologic and morphologic approach. Arch Pathol Lab Med 134:194–206
Maulard-Durdux C, Toubert ME, Hennequin C, Housset M (1997) Serum tissue polypeptide antigen in bladder cancer as a tumor marker: a prospective study. J Clin Oncol 15:3446–3450
Nakanishi K et al (2005) Whole body MRI for detecting metastatic bone tumor: comparison with bone scintigrams. Magn Reson Med Sci 4:11–17
Nathrath WB, Heidenkummer P, Bjorklund V, Bjorklund B (1985) Distribution of tissue polypeptide antigen (TPA) in normal human tissues: Immunohistochemical study on unfixed, methanol-, ethanol-, and formalin-fixed tissues. J Histochem Cytochem 33:99–109
Robinson PJ (2000) Imaging liver metastases: current limitations and future prospects. Br J Radiol 73:234–241
Ruparelia N, Ahmadi H, Cobiella C (2006) Metastatic adenocarcinoma of the colon presenting as a monarthritis of the hip in a young patient. World J Surg Oncol 4:95
Salvo N et al (2009) The role of plain radiographs in management of bone metastases. J Palliat Med 12:195–198
Schrohl AS et al (2003) Tumor markers: from laboratory to clinical utility. Mol Cell Proteomics 2:378–387
Sharon Poltis Wilczynski (ed) (2007) Introduction to the diagnosis of cancer. Wiley, Etobicoke
Sidhu K et al (2004) Delineation of brain metastases on CT images for planning radiosurgery: concerns regarding accuracy. Br J Radiol 77:39–42
Singh P et al (2009) Endoscopic ultrasound versus CT scan for detection of the metastases to the liver: results of a prospective comparative study. J Clin Gastroenterol 43:367–373
Sohn YM et al (2010) Diagnostic approach for evaluation of lymph node metastasis from thyroid cancer using ultrasound and fine-needle aspiration biopsy. AJR Am J Roentgenol 194:38–43
Thomson V et al (2008) Whole-body MRI for metastases screening: a preliminary study using 3D VIBE sequences with automatic subtraction between noncontrast and contrast enhanced images. Am J Clin Oncol 31:285–292
Uematsu T et al (2005) Comparison of FDG PET and SPECT for detection of bone metastases in breast cancer. AJR Am J Roentgenol 184:1266–1273
Vassiliou V, Kalogeropoulou C, Petsas T, Leotsinidis M, Kardamakis D (2007) Clinical and radiological evaluation of patients with lytic, mixed and sclerotic bone metastases from solid tumors: is there a correlation between clinical status of patients and type of bone metastases? Clin Exp Metastasis 24:49–56
Vermeeren L et al (2009a) Value of SPECT/CT for detection and anatomic localization of sentinel lymph nodes before laparoscopic sentinel node lymphadenectomy in prostate carcinoma. J Nucl Med 50:865–870
Vermeeren L, Van Der Ent FW, Hulsewe KW (2009b) Is there an indication for routine chest X-Ray in initial staging of melanoma? J Surg Res 166:114
Weber K, Osborn M, Moll R, Wiklund B, Luning B (1984) Tissue polypeptide antigen (TPA) is related to the non-epidermal keratins 8, 18 and 19 typical of simple and non-squamous epithelia: re-evaluation of a human tumor marker. EMBO J 3:2707–2714
Winnard PT Jr et al (2008) Molecular imaging of metastatic potential. J Nucl Med 49(Suppl 2):96S–112S

Wong D et al (2008) Serum CA19-9 decline compared to radiographic response as a surrogate for clinical outcomes in patients with metastatic pancreatic cancer receiving chemotherapy. Pancreas 37:269–274

Zech CJ, Herrmann KA, Reiser MF, Schoenberg SO (2007) MR imaging in patients with suspected liver metastases: value of liver-specific contrast agent Gd-EOB-DTPA. Magn Reson Med Sci 6:43–52

Chapter 20
Cancer Staging

Alexandre Nakao Odashiro

Cancer staging (CS) describes the extent and/or severity of a malignant neoplasia by the time of diagnosis (Edge and Compton 2010). It helps to stratify patients into groups that are prognostically and therapeutically similar (Greene and Sobin 2009). CS is based on knowledge of how cancer develops and spreads, as well as on prognostic factors. It is one of the most important tools used for planning treatment, determining prognosis, evaluating treatment outcomes and exchanging information between clinicians and centres around the world (Allen and MyiLibrary 2006).

There are currently a few staging systems used around world. TNM (tumor-node-metastasis) system (Edge and American Joint Committee on Cancer 2010; Fleming 1997; Greene et al. 2002) is one of the main CS systems used worldwide. It is maintained by the American Joint Committee on Cancer (AJCC) and the International Union for Cancer Control (UICC). The AJCC published the 1st edition of the Cancer Staging Manual in 1977 and began using the TNM as an organized staging scheme to express the extent of disease. This provides physicians and others with a useful tool to plan treatment, project prognosis, and measure outcomes (Yarbro et al. 1999).

TNM is updated periodically based on advances in the understanding of cancer prognosis in order to remain current and relevant to clinical practice. The latest revision of TNM, presented in the 7th edition of the AJCC Cancer Staging Manual, takes effect for cases diagnosed on or after January 1, 2010 (Edge and Compton 2010; Greene et al. 2002).

The TNM system is used for CS of most cancer types, with exceptions including brain and spinal cord, and blood/ bone marrow cancers. These exceptions are staged according to the cell type and grade, and the Ann Arbour classification system, respectively (Allen and MyiLibrary 2006).

TNM codes the extent of the primary tumor (T), regional lymph nodes (N), and distant metastases (M) and provides a "stage grouping" based on these T, N, and M

A. N. Odashiro (✉)
Département de Pathologie & Cytologie du Centre Hospitalier Affilié universitaire de Québec (CHA), Hôpital l'Enfant-Jésus, local C-1210 1401, 18e rue, Québec, Canada
e-mail: alexandre.odashiro.cha@ssss.gouv.qc.ca

J. V. Burnier, M. N. Burnier, Jr. (eds.), *Experimental and Clinical Metastasis*, DOI 10.1007/978-1-4614-3685-0_20, © Springer Science+Business Media New York 2013

Table 20.1 TNM staging categories for cutaneous melanoma. (Balch et al. 2009)

Classification	Thickness (mm)	Ulceration Status/Mitoses
Tis	NA	NA
T1	≤ 1.00	Without ulceration and mitosis $< 1/mm^2$
		With ulceration or mitoses $\geq 1/mm^2$
T2	1.01–2.00	Without ulceration
		With ulceration
T3	2.01–4.00	Without ulceration
		With ulceration
T4	>4.00	Without ulceration
		With ulceration
N	*No. of Metastatic Nodes*	*Nodal Metastatic Burden*
N0	0	NA
N1	1	Micrometastasis[a]
		Macrometastasis[b]
N2	2–3	Micrometastasis[a]
		Macrometastasis[b]
		In transit metastases/satellites without metastatic nodes
N3	4+ metastatic nodes, or matted nodes, or in transit metastases/satellites with metastatic nodes	
M	*Site*	*Serum LDH*
M0	No distant metastases	NA
M1a	Distant skin, subcutaneous, or nodal metastases	Normal
M1b	Lung metastases	Normal
M1c	All other visceral metastases	Normal
	Any distant metastasis	Elevated

NA not applicable, *LDH* lactate dehydrogenase
[a]Micrometastases are diagnosed after sentinel lymph node biopsy
[b]Macrometastases are defined as clinically detectable nodal metastases confirmed pathologically

factors (Edge and Compton 2010), using a combination of clinical and pathological data. This classification system is based on the anatomy and biological progression of tumor growth. Generally speaking, a solid tumor first grows locally in overall size and extent (T classification); metastases to regional lymph nodes may then occur (N classification); and finally metastases occur past these nodal basins either into non-regional lymph nodes or into a variety of solid organs (M classification) (Greene and Sobin 2009). Each primary tumor site has a different classification according to the anatomy of the site (Edge and American Joint Committee on Cancer 2010; Fleming 1997; Greene et al. 2002), and oncologists, radiologists and pathologists play an important role in determining the TNM of each patient.

To assess the TNM, there is a two-step process: first, the clinician estimates the tumor's extent as a basis for determining the therapeutic strategy; secondly, the pathologist describes the tumor's extent based on gross and microscopic features of a resected specimen (Greene and Sobin 2009). The post-surgical pathological classification of TNM is designated as pTNM and is based on pre-treatment, surgical and pathological information (Allen and MyiLibrary 2006) and is designated as follows:

- pT: requires resection of the primary tumor or a biopsy to evaluate the highest pT category or the extent of local tumor spread.
- pN: requires removal of lymph nodes. It is sufficient to evaluate the presence or absence of regional node metastasis and also the highest pN category.
- pM: requires microscopic examination of distant metastases which is often not available to the pathologist and therefore designated on clinical and/or radiological grounds.

In some tumors, TNM classification uses parameters other than pure anatomy. For example, in cutaneous melanoma staging, since 2002, the serum levels of LDH is incorporated in the classification as shown in the above table (Table 20.1).

After determining the stage of the tumor, treatment options are discussed with the patients according to the stage. For example, the European-consensus based interdisciplinary guideline recommends that sentinel lymph node dissection be routinely offered as a staging procedure in patients with tumours more than 1 mm in thickness, although there is no resultant survival benefit. Interferon-α treatment can be offered to patients with more than 1.5 mm in thickness and stage II to III melanoma as an adjuvant therapy, as this treatment increases the relapse-free survival (Garbe et al. 2010). Anatomy continues to be a key prognostic factor for cancer, and anatomic-based staging will remain critically important. However, the rapidly increasing specific knowledge of cancer biology provides prognostic information that complements and in some cases is more relevant than anatomic extent (Edge and Compton 2010). Recently, new technology has lead to the development of new molecular biomarkers (eg. HER2, c-Kit, EGF-Kras, etc.) that either predict the therapeutic benefit of target-specific drug treatment or improve the forecasting of disease natural history over that based on anatomic criteria alone (Epstein 2009). Because the main importance of CS is for treatment and prognosis, it is expected that the staging system may become less anatomical and more biological in the future, or more likely, a combination and integration of both.

References

Allen DC, MyiLibrary (2006) Histopathology reporting guidelines for surgical cancer. Springer, London

Balch CM et al (2009) Final version of 2009 AJCC melanoma staging and classification. J Clin Oncol 27:6199–6206

Edge SB, American Joint Committee On Cancer (2010) AJCC cancer staging manual. Springer, New York

Edge SB, Compton CC (2010) The American joint committee on cancer: the 7th edition of the AJCC cancer staging manual and the future of TNM. Ann Surg Oncol 17:1471–1474

Epstein RJ (2009) TNM: therapeutically not mandatory. Eur J Cancer 45:1111–1116

Fleming ID, American Joint Committee on Cancer, American Cancer Society, American College of Surgeons (1997) AJCC cancer staging manual. Lippincott-Raven, Philadelphia

Garbe C et al (2010) Diagnosis and treatment of melanoma: European consensus-based interdisciplinary guideline. Eur J Cancer 46:270–283

Greene FL, Sobin LH (2009) A worldwide approach to the TNM staging system: collaborative efforts of the AJCC and UICC. J Surg Oncol 99:269–272

Greene FL, American Joint Committee on Cancer, American Cancer Society (2002) AJCC cancer staging manual. Springer, New York

Yarbro JW, Page DL, Fielding LP, Partridge EE, Murphy GP (1999) American joint committee on cancer prognostic factors consensus conference. Cancer 86:2436–2446

Chapter 21
Diagnostic Immunohistochemistry in Tumor Metastasis

Mohib Wadie Morcos

Immunohistochemistry (IHC) refers to the process of localizing antigens (e.g. proteins) in cells of a tissue section using antibodies that bind specifically to these antigens in bisological tissues (Ramos-Vara 2005). Immunohistochemical staining is widely used in the diagnosis of abnormal cells such as those found in cancerous tumors and in metastasis (Webster et al. 2009).

Specific molecular markers are often characteristic of particular cellular events such as proliferation or cell death (apoptosis). Immunohistochemistry is a tool that recognizes an antigen antibody reaction. This process comprises the antigen which is present in the tumor tissues and the antibody represented by a glycoprotein.

Visualization of an antibody-antigen interaction can be, accomplished in a number of ways. Most commonly, an antibody is conjugated to an enzyme, such as a peroxydase, that can catalyze a color producing reaction (Sternberger et al. 1970; Sternberger and Sternberger 1986).

Antibodies may be of either *monoclonal* or *polyclonal* types (Colcher et al. 1981). A monoclonal antibody is an antibody that is produced artificially from a single cell clone and therefore consists of a single type of immunoglobulin exhibiting more specificity. (Buchwalow and Böcker 2010; Colcher et al. 1981). Polyclonal antibodies are multiple antibodies produced by different types of immune cells and are useful in detecting proteins which have lower expression levels (Buchwalow and Böcker 2010).

There are two strategies used for the immunohistochemical detection of antigens in tissues: the *direct* and *indirect* methods. In direct method, a labeled antibody reacts directly with an antigen in tissue. In indirect method, an *unlabelled primary antibody* reacts with an antigen in tissue, and a *labeled secondary antibody* reacts with the primary antibody (Fig. 21.1). The direct method is quick, but the indirect method is more sensitive (Buchwalow and Böcker 2010).

M. W. Morcos (✉)
Department of Pathology, Centre Hospitalier Affilié Universitaire de Québec,
Hôpital l'Enfant-Jésus, Faculty of Medicine,
Laval University, Quebec, QC, Canada
e-mail: mohib-w.morcos.cha@ssss.gouv.qc.ca

J. V. Burnier, M. N. Burnier, Jr. (eds.), *Experimental and Clinical Metastasis*, 279
DOI 10.1007/978-1-4614-3685-0_21, © Springer Science+Business Media New York 2013

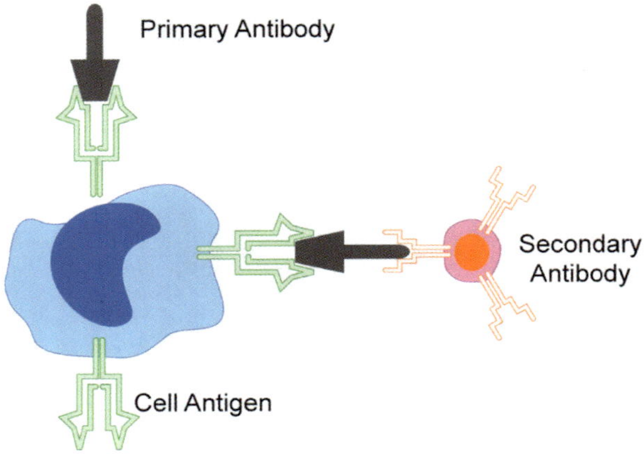

Fig. 21.1 Schematic diagram of an antigen-antibody reaction. The antigen is depicted in *green*, *primary antibody* in *black* and *secondary antibody* in *orange*

21.1 Diagnostic IHC markers

IHC is an excellent detection technique and has the advantage of being able to show exactly where a given protein is located within the tissue examined. The technique is widely used in diagnostic surgical pathology for typing tumors, and hence their metastases (Schlom 1986).

Many antibodies can be used in cancer diagnosis, for example the E-Cadherin antibody is used in breast surgical pathology. This antibody stains positive in ductal carcinomas whether invasive or in-situ, whereas it stains negative in lobular carcinomas, whether invasive or in-situ (lobular neoplasia). Table 21.1 shows various antibodies used for the diagnosis of tumors, and/or their metastases, in surgical pathology.

Tumor cell histology, morphology, and biological behavior are similar in the original tumor site as well as in the metastatic site (Scartozzi et al. 2004). Moreover, the same antigen-antibody reactions would take place in both primary tumor, or after spreading at a distance. It is here where IHC plays an essential and efficient role in the diagnosis of metastatic disease. The immune profile (antigens expressed) in a metastatic tumor can direct a surgical pathologist to identify a primary site.

For example, if a lung nodule is found in a heavy-smoking male patient, and the same patient has had a past history of colon cancer, this nodule could clinically be either a primary lung lesion, or a metastasis of his already known colon cancer. Besides histological morphology, IHC can help the surgical pathologist in identifying and underlining whether this nodule is a primary or secondary (metastatic) lesion. If the tumor cells express cytokeratin-7 and antigen TTF-1, then the lesion is a primary lung tumor as cytokeratin-7 is expressed in lung cancers together with antigen TTF-1 (Rossi et al. 2004). However, if these markers were negative, whereas the Cytokeratin-20 was positive, then a pathologist could concluded that the nodule is a metastasis of the already known colon cancer, since Cytokeratin-20 is expressed in the colorectal cancers (Ikeda et al. 2006). The same principle can be used with various antibodies, in various types of lesions, to identify if a specific lesion is a primitive or secondary (metastatic) lesion.

Table 21.1 Antibodies directed against antigens in specific tumor tissue cells

Antibody	Antigens targeted in specific tumor tissue cells
Carcinoembryonic antigen (CEA)	Adenocarcinoma (Hansen et al. 1974)
Cytokeratins (Fig. 21.3)	Carcinomas, and some sarcomas (Leader et al. 1986)
CD15 and CD 30	Hodgkin's Lymphoma (Siebert et al. 1995)
Alpha Feto-protein (AFP)	Yolk sac tumors (Dällenbach et al. 2006) & hepatocellular carcinoma (Guzman et al. 2005)
CD117 (C-KIT) (Fig. 21.3)	Gastrointestinal stromal tumors (GIST) (Miettinen and Lasota 2006)
CD10	Renal cell carcinoma (Martignoni et al. 2004) & acute lymphoblastic leukemia (Gleissner et al. 2005)
Prostate specific antigen (PSA)	Prostate adnenocarcinoma (Israeli et al. 1994)
CD20	B-Cell Lymphoma (Hans et al. 2004)
CD3	T-Cell Lymphoma, or reaction lymphocytes (Sigel and Hsi 2000)
Estrogen (Fig. 21.2a) & Progesterone receptors (ER & PR)	Breast (Molino et al.1995), and gynaecological (ovary, uterus) tumors (van Doorn et al. 2000)
Her2/neu (Fig. 21.2b)	Breast cancer (Ridolfi et al. 2000)
HMB45 & MART-1	Malignant Melanoma (Zubovits et al. 2004)
Protein S100	Nerve origin Tumors & Malignant Melanoma (Fernando et al. 1994)
Antigen TTF-1	Thyroid adenocarcinoma and adenocarcinoma of lung origin (Ordóez 2000)
CD31 & CD34	Tumors of vascular origin (Yilmazer et al. 2007)
Smooth actin muscle & desmin	Tumors of muscle origin (Riddle et al. 2010)

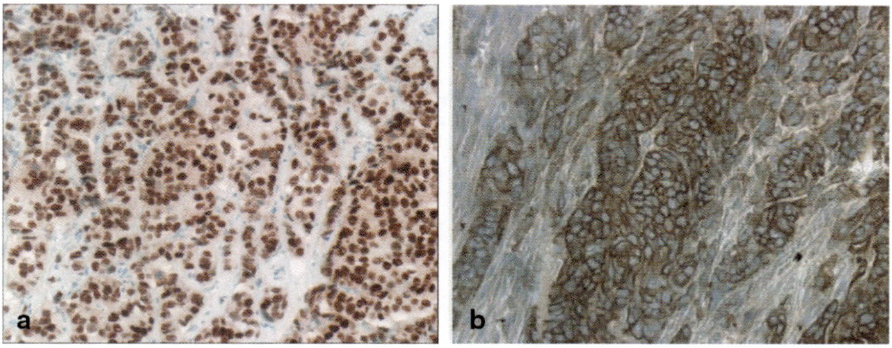

Fig. 21.2 **(a)** Positive estrogen receptors in invasive ductal carcinoma of breast. **(b)** Her2/neu expression in same invasive ductal carcinoma of breast

21.2 IHC & Directing (Targeted) Therapy

A variety of molecular pathways are altered in cancers and some of these alterations can be targeted in cancer therapy. Immunohistochemistry can be used to assess which tumors are likely to respond to therapy, by detecting the presence or elevated levels of specific molecular targets.

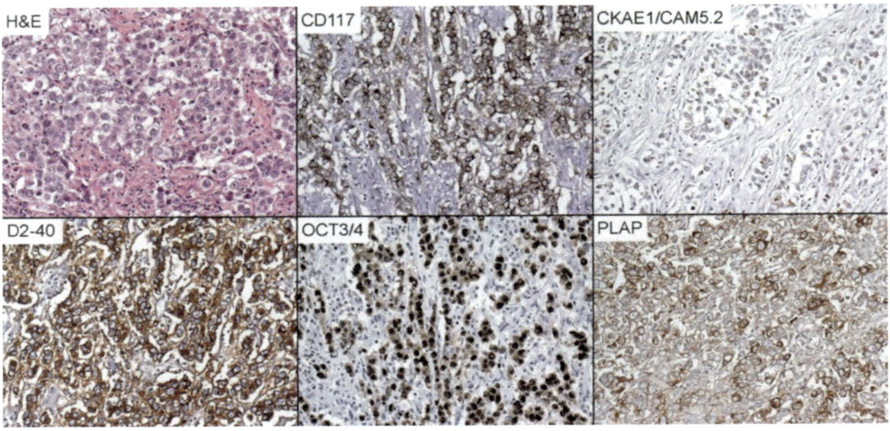

Fig. 21.3 Various IHC antibodies being expressed in an ovarian tumor called dysgerminoma

21.3 Chemical Inhibitors

Tumors contain a number of potential intracellular targets. Many tumors are hormone dependant. The presence of hormone receptors can be used to determine if a tumor is potentially responsive to anti-hormonal therapy. One of the first such therapies was the anti-estrogen receptor, *Tamoxifen*, used to treat breast cancer. Such hormone receptors can be detected by immunohistochemistry (Jorgensen et al. 2007). *Imatinib*, an intracellular tyrosine kinase inhibitor, was developed to treat chronic myelogenous leukemia, a disease characterized by the formation of a specific abnormal tyrosine kinase. Imatinib also has proven effective in tumors that express other tyrosine kinases, most notably KIT. Most gastrointestinal stromal tumors (GIST) express KIT (CD117), which can be detected by immunohistochemistry (Gold and Dematteo 2006).

21.4 Monoclonal Antibodies

Many proteins known to be highly up-regulated in pathological states and detectable by IHC can be potential targets for therapies utilizing *monoclonal antibodies*. For example, the *epidermal growth factor receptor* (EGFR) family, of transmembrane proteins. Of these, *HER2/neu* (also known as Erb-B2) was the first to be developed. The molecule is highly expressed in a variety of cancer cell types, most notably breast cancer. As such, antibodies against HER2/neu have been approved for clinical treatment of breast cancer under the name *Herceptin* (Harari 2004). Similarly, EGFR (HER-1) is over-expressed in a variety of cancers including head & neck (Rastushny et al. 2009) and colorectal cancer (Bibeau et al. 2006). In this respect the detection of EGFR expression performed in primary tumors for treatment with

EGFR-targeted monoclonal antibodies is used to determine patients who may benefit from therapeutic antibodies such as *Erbitux* (cetuximab) (Scartozzi et al. 2004).

In conclusion, IHC is an important and efficient technique that can be used by clinicians and surgical pathologists to diagnose the type of tumor, and assess whether it is a primary or a metastatic tumor. Additionaly it can be utilized in targeted therapy leading to a better prognosis in cancer therapy.

References

Bibeau F et al (2006) Assessment of epidermal growth factor receptor (EGFR) expression in primary colorectal carcinomas and their related metastases on tissue sections and tissue microarray. Virchows Arch 449:281–287

Buchwalow IB, Böcker W (ed) (2010) Antibodies for immunohistochemistry. SpringerLink, p 153

Colcher D, Hand PH, Nuti M, Schlom J (1981) A spectrum of monoclonal antibodies reactive with human mammary tumor cells. Proc Natl Acad Sci U S A 78:3199–3203

Dällenbach P, Bonnefoi H, Pelte MF, Vlastos G (2006) Yolk sac tumours of the ovary: an update. Eur J Surg Oncol 32:1063–1075

Fernando SS, Johnson S, Bate J (1994) Immunohistochemical analysis of cutaneous malignant melanoma: comparison of S-100 protein, HMB-45 monoclonal antibody and NKI/C3 monoclonal antibody. Pathology 26:16–19

Gleissner B et al (2005) CD10- pre-B acute lymphoblastic leukemia (ALL) is a distinct high-risk subgroup of adult ALL associated with a high frequency of MLL aberrations: results of the German Multicenter Trials for Adult ALL (GMALL). Blood 106:4054–4056

Gold JS, Dematteo RP (2006) Combined surgical and molecular therapy: the gastrointestinal stromal tumor model. Ann Surg 244:176–184

Guzman G et al (2005) p53, Ki-67, and serum alpha feto-protein as predictors of hepatocellular carcinoma recurrence in liver transplant patients. Mod Pathol 18:1498–1503

Hans CP et al (2004) Confirmation of the molecular classification of diffuse large B-cell lymphoma by immunohistochemistry using a tissue microarray. Blood 103:275–282

Hansen HJ et al (1974) Carcinoembryonic antigen (CEA) assay. A laboratory adjunct in the diagnosis and management of cancer. Hum Pathol 5:139–147

Harari PM (2004) Epidermal growth factor receptor inhibition strategies in oncology. Endocr Relat Cancer 11:689–708

Ikeda S et al (2006) Combined immunohistochemistry of beta-catenin, cytokeratin 7, and cytokeratin 20 is useful in discriminating primary lung adenocarcinomas from metastatic colorectal cancer. BMC Cancer 6:31

Israeli RS, Powell CT, Corr JG, Fair WR, Heston WDW (1994) Expression of the prostate-specific membrane antigen. Cancer Res 54:1807–1811

Jorgensen JT, Nielsen KV, Ejlertsen B (2007) Pharmacodiagnostics and targeted therapies—a rational approach for individualizing medical anticancer therapy in breast cancer. Oncologist 12:397–405

Leader M, Patel J, Makin C, Henry K (1986) An analysis of the sensitivity and specificity of the cytokeratin marker CAM 5.2 for epithelial tumours. Results of a study of 203 sarcomas, 50 carcinomas and 28 malignant melanomas. Histopathology 10:1315–1324

Martignoni G et al (2004) CD10 is expressed in a subset of chromophobe renal cell carcinomas. Mod Pathol 17:1455–1463

Miettinen M, Lasota J (2006) Gastrointestinal stromal tumors: review on morphology, molecular pathology, prognosis, and differential diagnosis. Arch Pathol Lab Med 130:1466–1478

Molino A. et al (1995) Estrogen receptors in 699 primary breast cancers: a comparison of immunohistochemical and biochemical methods. Breast Cancer Res Treat 34:221–228

Ordóez NG (2000) Thyroid Transcription Factor-1 is a Marker of Lung and Thyroid Carcinomas. Adv Anat Pathol 7:123–127

Ramos-Vara JA (2005) Technical aspects of immunohistochemistry. Vet Pathol 42:405–426

Ratushny V, Astsaturov I, Burtness BA, Golemis EA, Silverman JS (2009) Targeting EGFR resistance networks in head and neck cancer. Cell Signal 21:1255–1268

Riddle ND, Quigley BC, Browarsky I, Bui MM (2010) Leiomyosarcoma arising in the pancreatic duct: a case report and review of the current literature. Case Report Med 2010:252–364

Ridolfi RL, Jamehdor MR, Arber JM (2000) HER-2/neu testing in breast carcinoma: a combined immunohistochemical and fluorescence in situ hybridization approach. Mod Pathol 13:866–873

Rossi G et al (2004) TTF-1, Cytokeratin 7, 34βE12, and CD56/NCAM Immunostaining in the subclassification of large cell carcinomas of the lung. Am J Clin Pathol 122:884–893

Scartozzi M et al (2004) Epidermal Growth Factor Receptor (EGFR) Status in primary colorectal tumors does not correlate with egfr expression in related metastatic sites: implications for treatment with egfr-targeted monoclonal antibodies. J Clin Oncol 22:4772–4778

Schlom J (1986) Basic Principles and applications of monoclonal antibodies in the management of carcinomas: the Richard and Hinda Rosenthal Foundation award lecture. Cancer Res 46:3225–3238

Siebert JD, McClure SP, Banks PM, Gulley ML (1995) Hodgkin's disease, mixed cellularity type, with a B-cell immunophenotype. Report of a case and literature review. Arch Pathol Lab Med 119:474–479

Sigel JE, Hsi ED (2000) Immunohistochemical analysis of CD30-positive lymphoproliferative disorders for expression of CD95 and CD95L. Mod Pathol 13:446–451

Sternberger LA, Sternberger NH (1986) The unlabeled antibody method: comparison of peroxidase-antiperoxidase with avidin-biotin complex by a new method of quantification. J Histochem Cytochem 34:599–605

Sternberger LA, Hardy PH Jr, Cuculis JJ, Meyer HG (1970) The unlabeled antibody enzyme method of immunohistochemistry: preparation and properties of soluble antigen-antibody complex (horseradish peroxidase-antihorseradish peroxidase) and its use in identification of spirochetes. J Histochem Cytochem 18:315–333

van Doorn HC, Burger CW, van der Valk P, Bonfrér HMG (2000) Oestrogen, progesterone, and androgen receptors in ovarian neoplasia: correlation between immunohistochemical and biochemical receptor analyses. J Clin Pathol 53:201–205

Webster JD, Miller MA, Dusold D, Ramos-Vara J (2009) Effects of prolonged formalin fixation on diagnostic immunohistochemistry in domestic animals. J Histochem Cytochem 57:753–761

Yilmazer D, Han Ü, Önal B (2007) A comparison of the vascular density of VEGF expression with microvascular density determined with CD34 and CD31 staining and conventional prognostic markers in renal cell carcinoma. Int Urol Nephrol 39:691–698

Zubovits J, Buzney E, Yu L, Duncan LM (2004) HMB-45, S-100, NK1/C3, and MART-1 in metastatic melanoma. Hum Pathol 35:217–223

Chapter 22
Genomics and Proteomics

Dominique Fausto de Souza

22.1 Introduction

Understanding the specific changes that occur in the DNA, RNA, and proteins of cancerous cells may allow for the identification of markers for early cancer detection, prevention and in the development of molecular-targeted treatments. Gene expression profiling is a powerful tool that allows for the evaluation of thousands of genes simultaneously and can provide insight into the complex interactions between genes in biologic specimen (Fingleton 2007). Proteomic tools have enabled the analysis of thousands of proteins and the identification of disease-specific proteins (Hudler et al. 2010). These tools have the potential to lead to clinical applications such as improved diagnosis, an understanding of the specific tumor behavior, prognosis indicators and prediction of response to different treatment modalities.

Traditional diagnosis of disease relied on histopathologic characteristics and immunohistochemistry (IHC) analysis. These methods provide data that is broad and imprecise for the individual tumor or patient. Gene expression profiling and proteomics profiling hold great potential as new approaches to cancer diagnosis and prognosis. The combination of genomics and proteomics has provided clinicians with a unique opportunity to more precisely diagnose, classify, and detect malignant disease; to understand and define the behavior of specific tumors; and to develop direct and targeted therapy (Caprioli 2005).

Key Points Applications of Genomics and Proteomics

- Determination of the tissue-of-origin in metastatic tumors
- Knowledge of somatic mutations involved in the development and progression of cancer
- New ways of classifying tumors
- Development of targeted therapy
- Prediction of tumor response and choice of therapy
- Prediction of recurrence

D. F. de Souza (✉)
Department of Pathology, Henry C. Witelson Ocular Pathology Laboratory
and Department of Dermatology, McGill University, Montreal, QC, Canada
e-mail: dominique.faustodesouza@mail.mcgill.ca

J. V. Burnier, M. N. Burnier, Jr. (eds.), *Experimental and Clinical Metastasis*,
DOI 10.1007/978-1-4614-3685-0_22, © Springer Science+Business Media New York 2013

22.2 Genomics

Since the mid 1990s, DNA microarray technology has been successfully applied to the molecular profiling of tumors (Schena et al. 1995; DeRisi et al. 1996). This has resulted in a much more detailed classification scheme, as well as in the identification of the major genetic alterations and signaling pathways involved in cancer. Through the use of powerful genomic technologies, it is now possible to identify the genetic determinants that drive cancer formation and progression (Parikh et al. 2008; Jeffrey et al. 2005).

22.2.1 Gene Expression Microarray

Microarray technology evolved from Northern (RNA-DNA hybridization) and Southern (DNA-DNA hybridization) blotting, in which a small number of complementary DNA probes are used to detect RNA or DNA target sequences. Microarrays consist of a small solid support surface with a glass slide, silicon chip, or nylon membrane that has thousands of DNA probes imprinted directly to the support. RNA is extracted from a tissue of interest, the RNA is reverse transcribed and converted into complementary DNA (cDNA), labeled with a detectable fluorescent substance and allowed to bind to the chip where any specific sequences will hybridize to complementary DNA sequences (Fig. 22.1). Detection of a fluorescent signal in a specific location of the microarray indicates the presence of the transcript complementary to that probe, and the relative fluorescent intensity is indicative of the level of expression for that particular gene. After the data are analyzed by bioinformatics software that performs background correction and normalization, a gene expression profile is obtained. In general, the greater the degree of hybridization and the more intense the signal, a higher level of expression is implied (Chung et al 2007; Quackenbush 2006; Harris and McCromick 2010; Ramaswamy and Golub 2002).

Expression arrays have been applied to primary human samples to detect differences between normal tissues and cancers. The gene-expression profiling of breast cancer has dramatically altered its classification and has identified at least four major breast cancer phenotypes: luminal A, luminal B, HER 2 -like, and basal-like. The expression-based classification of a tumor has prognostic and therapeutic implications, and can provide information that enhances the prediction of clinical outcome. As an example, the luminal B subtype of breast cancer has an increase in expression of genes associated with cell proliferation and has a poorer overall outcome than the luminal A subtype (Ramaswamy and Perou 2003; Sorlie et al. 2003; Perou et al. 2000; Hu et al. 2006).

Obtaining adequate human RNA, typically from tissue, remains a limiting step in many studies. Fresh frozen biospecimens are usually of a limited number and size and once samples are fixed in formalin, the RNA is degraded and traditional methods for gene expression profiling are not suitable. The cDNA mediated annealing, selection, extension, and ligation (DASL) assay have been developed for gene

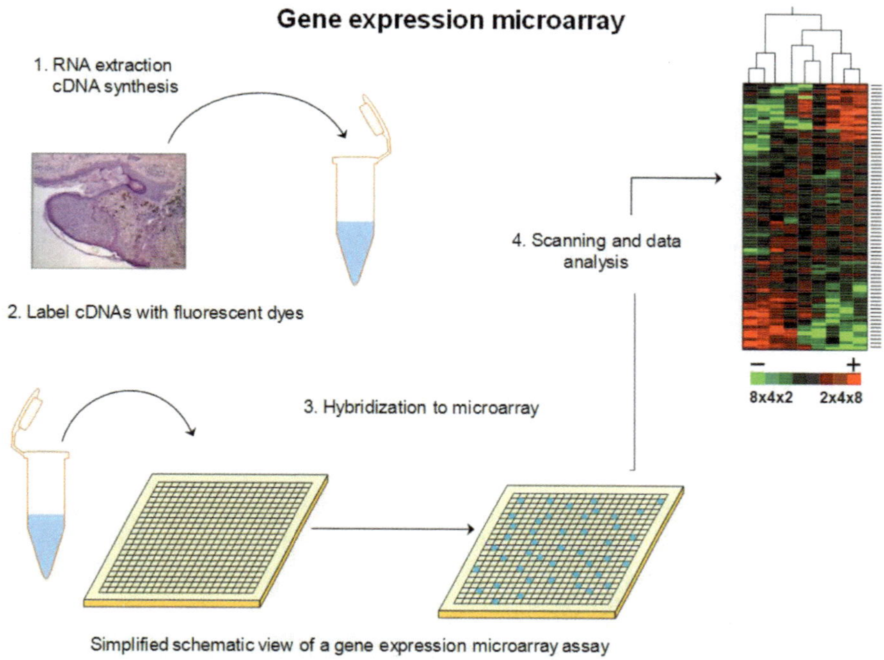

Fig. 22.1 Illustrates a gene expression microarray assay

expression profiling of this degraded RNA from formalin-fixed, paraffin-embedded blocks (FFPE) (Waddell et al. 2010; Conway et al. 2009).

22.2.2 Fluorescence In Situ Hybridization

As a combined molecular and cytological approach, Fluorescence in situ hybridization (FISH) detects nucleic acids sequences by a fluorescent probe that hybridizes specifically to its complementary target sequence within the intact cell. Hydrogen bonds are broken by heating, making the DNA single-stranded to allow the probes to bind (hybridize) to the sequences to which they are homologous. This technique allows specific genome regions to be visualized using a light microscope. It was often used in methaphase spreads (M phase) and it is now used in interphase chromossomes (I phase) as well. The fact that FISH can evaluate nondividing (interphase) nuclei, makes it unnecessary to evaluate the neoplastic cells in culture and allows retrospective analysis of formalin-fixed, paraffin embedded tissue (Sugimura et al. 2010; Volpi and Bridger 2008; Van Prooijen-Knegt et al. 1982; Bayani and Squire 2004). One of the applications of FISH in cancer is to distinguish between entities with similar histologic appearances such as soft tissue neoplasms, which harbor consistent molecular alterations (Tanas and Goldblum 2009). One of the limitations in the use of FISH is that to detect a specific DNA sequence and structural aberrations, the underlying genetic abnormalities need to be identified as a possibility by the pathologist.

22.2.3 Quantitative Real-Time PCR

Polymerase chain reaction (PCR) methods are particularly valuable when amounts of RNA are low, since the amplification step results in a more sensitive method. Quantitative Real-Time PCR (qRT-PCR) technology represents an important genomic platform that has great sensitivity and specificity and that requires small amounts of cells or tissue from which to isolate RNA (Chung et al. 2007; Weksberg et al. 2005). This technique is used to amplify and simultaneously quantify a targeted DNA molecule. Relative quantification measures the fold difference in expression when normalized to a control gene. Absolute quantification requires the construction of a standard curve for each target; this standard curve is based on a serial dilution of a sample with a known copy number. qRT-PCR is useful when validating the results of microarrays or when measuring the expression of a particular set or family of genes (Quackenbush 2002; Goswami et al. 2010).

22.2.4 MicroRNAs

MicroRNAs (miRNAs) are short RNA molecules of between 19 and 24 nucleotides in length that have been linked with some types of cancer. miRNAs can regulate the translation of hundreds of genes through sequence specific binding to messenger RNA (mRNA) and can result in the inhibition of translation and/or degradation of target mRNA. Since Calin et al described abnormalities in the expression levels of miRNAs in B-cell chronic lymphocytic leukaemia (CLL) (Calin et al. 2002), abnormal miRNA expression has been identified in many different types of human cancers. MiRNAs can also be hybridized to microarrays, slides or chips to allow the assessment of cancer-specific expression levels of hundreds of miRNAs in a large number of samples; these assays are the most commonly used high-throughput technique for miRNAs profiling in cancer (Lu et al. 2005; Couzin 2008).

22.2.5 Validation

Once a gene expression pattern is discovered, the next step is to validate the results. Microarray data is difficult to exchange due to the lack of standardization in platform fabrication, assay protocols, and analysis methods. This presents an interoperability problem in bioinformatics. To facilitate comparisons between different studies, various methods for standardizing data have been developed (Papadopoulos et al. 2006). The Minimum Information About a Microarray Experiment (MIAME) (Quackenbush 2009; Brazma et al. 2001) is one such example. Other examples include the MicroArray Quality Control (MAQC) project (Shi et al. 2006) that is being conducted by the US Food and Drug Administration (FDA) and the MicroArray and Gene Expression group (Spellman et al. 2002).

22.2.6 Unknown Primary Cancer

Unknown primary cancer (UPC) accounts for 3–5 % of new cancer cases. Studies have suggested that metastatic tumors often retain gene expression patterns of their primary tumor (Ramaswamy et al. 2001; Tothill et al. 2005). Gene expression profiling may therefore enable an accurate identification of the cancer of origin in patients who have metastatic disease of an unknown primary tumor. Patient management has the potential to be improved through the use of molecular tests for the identification of the tissue-of-origin in metastatic tumors. Commercially available clinical tests for this purpose are offered clinically (Monzon and koen 2010). For example, the Pathwork Tissue of Origin Test (Monzon and koen 2010; Dumur et al. 2008) can be used to test frozen and formalin-fixed, paraffin-embedded (FFPE) tissues (http://www.accessdata.fda.gov/cdrh_docs/pdf9/K092967.pdf).

22.3 Technologies Driving Molecular Diagnosis

DNA sequencing is one of the technologies currently driving molecular diagnostics to identify changes in genes and their expression in tumors. The following methods use next-generation sequencing (Mardis 2008a; Mardis 2008b):

- Genome Analyzer™ by Illumina (San Diego, CA, USA),
- 454 Genome Sequencer™ FLX system from Roche (Branford, CT, USA),
- Life Technologies SOLiD™ (sequencing by oligonucleotide ligation and detection) platforms (Foster City, CA, USA).

Third-generation systems (Pushkarev et al. 2009) are being developed with clinical utility in mind, such as:

- HeliScope™ Platform (Helicos, Cambridge, MA, USA),
- SMRT™ DNA sequencing (Pacific Biosciences, Menlo Park, CA, USA),
- Sequencing from Complete Genomics (Mountain View, CA, USA) and
- Nanopore sequencing (Oxford Nanopore Technologies, Oxford, UK).

Selection systems for isolating different types of DNA for analysis, including exons, regions of genetic association, and different types of RNA, such as microRNAs (miRNAs), are available (Stratton 2008), including Agilent (Santa Clara, CA, USA) and Roche NimbleGen (Madison, WI, USA).

The Cancer Genome Atlas (TCGA) is a project established by The National Institutes of Health (NIH), to generate comprehensive multi-dimensional maps of the key genomic changes in major types and subtypes of cancer (Stratton et al. 2009). This catalog serves as a powerful resource for a new generation of research aimed at developing better strategies for diagnosing, treating and preventing each type of cancer. Following the success of a pilot phase initiated in 2006, the National Cancer Institute (NCI) and National Human Genome Research Institute (NHGRI) announced in September 2009 that TCGA will produce comprehensive genomic maps of at least 20 types of cancer over the next 5 years (http://cancergenome.nih.gov).

A central aim of cancer research has been to identify the mutated genes involved in cell proliferation, differentiation and death. So far, some 300 cancer genes have been reported, more than 1 % of all the genes in the human genome. Mutations that have been discovered so far are summarized in the Catalogue of Somatic Mutations In Cancer (COSMIC) (http://www.sanger.ac.uk/genetics/CGP/cosmic) (Pleasance et al. 2010). The Cancer Gene Census (Futreal et al. 2004) is an ongoing effort to catalogue those genes for which mutations have been causally implicated in cancer and this census is updated regularly (http://www.sanger.ac.uk/genetics/CGP/Census). The importance of this work can be exemplified with recent studies that were done with the protein kinase gene family. The protein kinase gene family is the most common domain that is encoded by cancer genes. Imatinib is a drug that inhibits several protein kinases, and has proved remarkably effective in treating certain types of cancers in which these genes are mutated and activated (Harris and McCromick 2010; Greenman et al. 2007).

Genome-Wide Association Studies (GWAS) is another technology driver that has led to novel insights into the biology of cancer and other diseases. This project compares most of the genes of different individuals to see how much the genes vary from individual to individual (Hirschhorn 2009). To conduct GWAS researchers analyze the DNA of two groups of participants: people with the disease being studied and similar people without the disease. Each person's complete set of DNA, or genome, is placed on tiny chips and scanned on automated laboratory machines, which quickly survey each participant's genome for strategically selected markers of genetic variation, which are called single nucleotide polymorphisms (SNPs) (Hirschhorn 2009; Manolio et al. 2008). The common alleles conferring low risk that have been identified by GWAS have not yet been linked to outcome (only susceptibility), and they do not account for all of the genetic risk of the cancers in question (Altshuler et al. 2008). The utility of screening at-risk individuals for mutations in genes known to confer a much higher increase in relative risk of cancer predisposition can be exemplified by measuring mutations in BRCA1 and BRCA2, which confer a considerable increase in the risk of breast and ovarian cancer in women. The potential to look for rare mutant alleles is alluring and will probably lead to the identification of genes that can be of diagnostic utility (Foulkes 2008; Turnbull et al. 2010).

22.4 Proteomics

Proteomics is defined as the simultaneous analysis of all the proteins expressed by the human genome, referred to as the human proteome. As proteins represent the vast majority of biologically active molecules responsible for cellular function, the

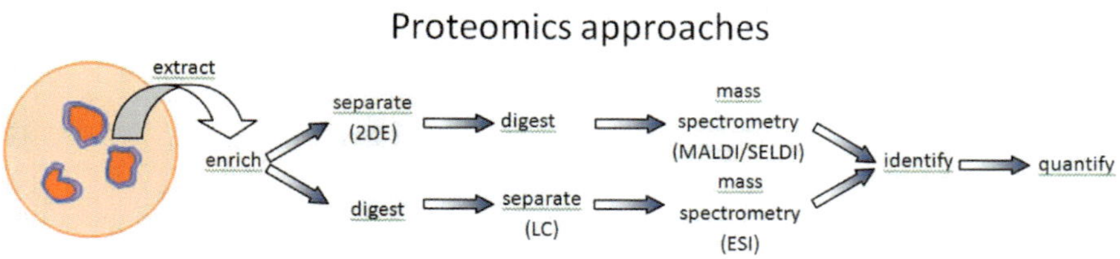

Fig. 22.2 Illustrates two different proteomics approaches

field of proteomics promises to expand our understanding of the molecular basis of diseases such as cancer (Alaiya et al. 2005). Proteomics platforms are often used for protein profiling, protein identification and protein quantification (Parikh et al. 2008). An important goal when studying the protein expression between samples is to establish specific proteomic signatures that discriminate between disease states, and that can perhaps differentiate metastatic from non-metastatic patients in a subclinical stage of the disease.

Proteomics usually begins with the separation of proteins from complex mixtures. The most commonly used proteomics approaches are: "top down" and "bottom up" ("shotgun") (Fig. 22.2). In top down proteomics intact protein molecules expressed by cells are detected by two-dimensional gel electrophoresis (2DE) and identified (Henzel et al. 1993). The isolated protein is then submitted to enzymatic (e.g. trypsin) digestion to generate peptides. Then matrix-assisted laser desorption/ionization-time-of-flight mass spectrometry (MALDI-TOF MS) may be used to produce peptide mass maps (Mann et al. 1993; Mann et al. 2001; Yates et al. 1993).

Shotgun proteomics refers to the use of bottom-up proteomics techniques in which the protein in a biological sample mixture is first digested to small peptides prior to separation by multidimensional liquid chromatography (LC) and mass spectrometry (MS) analysis with an electrospray ionization mass spectrometer (ESI-MS) (Motoyama and Yates 2008; Kubota et al. 2009).

22.4.1 Gel Electrophoresis

Gel electrophoresis has been used for many years as a protein-separation technique based on molecular weight (Fig. 22.3). Prior to the advent of serum proteomics, two-dimensional gel electrophoresis (2DE) coupled with mass spectrometric (MS) based protein identification was the classic tool of proteomic analysis. Although two-dimensional gel electrophoresis (2DE) has been used in protein research for decades, problems with quantification of protein expression differences as well as the need for protein characterization and identification have kept it from the forefront of biomarker discovery research even when combined with mass spectrometry (Iwadate 2008; Wong et al. 2009; Hanash 2003).

Difference in gel electrophoresis (DIGE) is a quantitative extension of 2DE and allows multiple variables to be quantitatively compared simultaneously. This

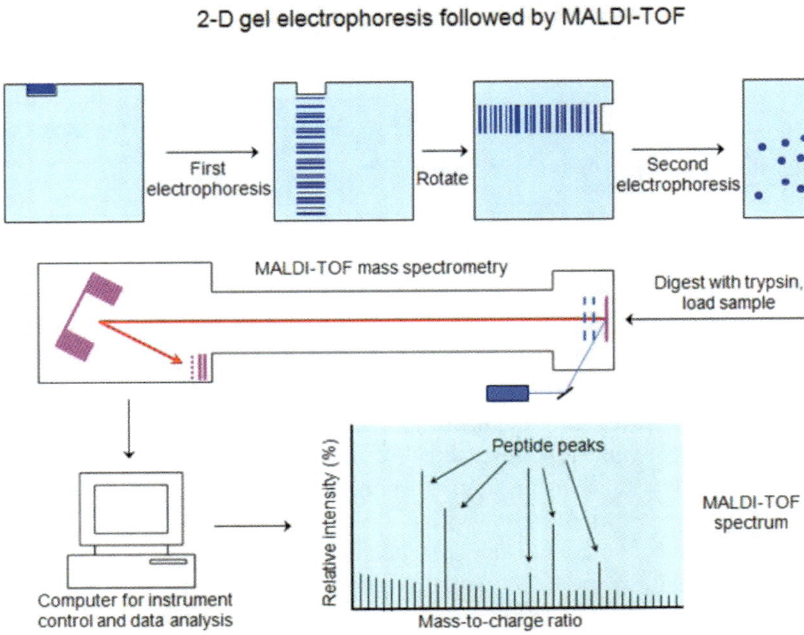

Fig. 22.3 Illustrates a proteomic platform composed of two-dimensional gel electrophoresis (2DE) coupled with matrix-assisted laser desorption/ionization (MALDI)

technology allows for separation of thousands of proteins first by charge using isoelectric focusing in one dimension and then by molecular mass in the other. To compare two cell types directly, protein extracts from two samples (e.g. cancer and healthy cells) can be labeled with fluorescent dyes. Differentially expressed proteins of interest can be identified by alterations in the ratios of signals. Proteins of interest then are excised from the gels and analyzed using mass spectrometry (MS) and protein databases to identify statistically significant candidate protein matches (Lilley and Friedman 2004; Minden et al. 2009).

22.4.2 Mass Spectrometry

MS has rapidly emerged as the technique of choice for the analysis of proteins and peptides. Mass spectrometers accurately measure the mass-to-charge (m/z) ratios of ionizable compounds. The ionization methods most commonly used for analysis of peptides and proteins are electrospray ionization (ESI), matrix-assisted laser desorption/ionization (MALDI) and surface-enhanced laser desorption/ionization (SELDI). These ionization sources are often coupled to time-of-flight (TOF) or quadrupole analyzers (Rossenbalt et al. 2004). The standardization of mass spectrometers across laboratories is essential for the reproducibility of diagnostic tests.

MALDI and SELDI are similar in that both involve the spotting of biological samples onto a solid surface, sometimes referred to as a probe, or for SELDI a chip (Roboz 2005). After the sample is applied to the probe or chip array, the surface is washed to remove unbound proteins and impurities. A matrix is then applied to the chip surface and subsequently irradiated, which results in the ionization and desorption of the proteins after a laser pulse (Fig. 22.3). This technique has been modified so that laser desorption can be carried out without the addition of a chemical matrix (Mann et al. 2001). The difference between SELDI and MALDI is that the SELDI probes employ selective surfaces to capture only a fraction of proteins from a complex mixture in biological samples (Merchant and Weinberger 2000). Surfaces with diverse affinities for different proteins of interest can be generated to carry out on-probe chromatography, including hydrophobicity, anionic or cationic charge, and metal affinity (Simpkins et al. 2005).

ESI-MS is used to analyze peptides directly from liquid samples. In this technique, a peptide solution is forced through a small channel and positively charged to create an ion gas cloud (spray). Varying the flow rate through the channel changes the size of the droplets that are created and, thus, the size of ions produced. The mass-to-charge ratio information then is obtained and the sample can be analyzed. The fact that ESI produces gas clouds from a liquid solution makes it highly compatible with LC (Fenn et al. 1989).

The ionized gaseous molecules then are accelerated through a voltage tunnel, the time-of-flight mass spectrometer (TOF-MS) region of the instrument, which measures the mass-to-charge (m/z) of each protein, based on the time requirement for the ions to travel down the vacuum tube towards an oppositely charged electrode called the detector (Cornish and Cotter 1993). Ions reach the detector at different times depending on their weight; heavier ones take longer (Fig. 22.4). Each ion that strikes the electrode is registered as a component of the data spectrum that emerges from the analysis. The output generated from the TOF-MS analysis is a series of peaks showing the relative abundance versus the molecular weights (MW) of the detected proteins. Advantages of this approach include simplicity of sample preparation and the small amount of sample needed for analysis of complex mixtures, such as serum and whole tissues (Jr et al. 1999).

Proteins secreted by cancer cells are attractive candidates for biomarkers. As an approach to serum biomarker discovery, detecting proteomic expression in cancer has been developed as a means to identify novel markers when comparing samples from patients with disease with those from healthy subjects (Simpkins et al. 2005; Chaerkady and Pandey 2008). It has emerged as a high-throughput tool for detection and differentiation of several cancer types (Abramovitz and Leyland-Jones 2006). Theoretically, such a method is well suited for biomarker discovery because of rapid analysis, and minimal sample requirement. Together with a suite of bioinformatics software, proteomics platforms are capable to identifying differences in protein expression profiles of two or more distinct samples (Rosenblatt et al. 2004).

However, the application of 2DE-MS and protein microarrays, as well as DNA microarray technology to clinical samples requires the direct acquisition of patient tissue for the extraction of proteins or nucleic acids. Proteomic pattern analysis

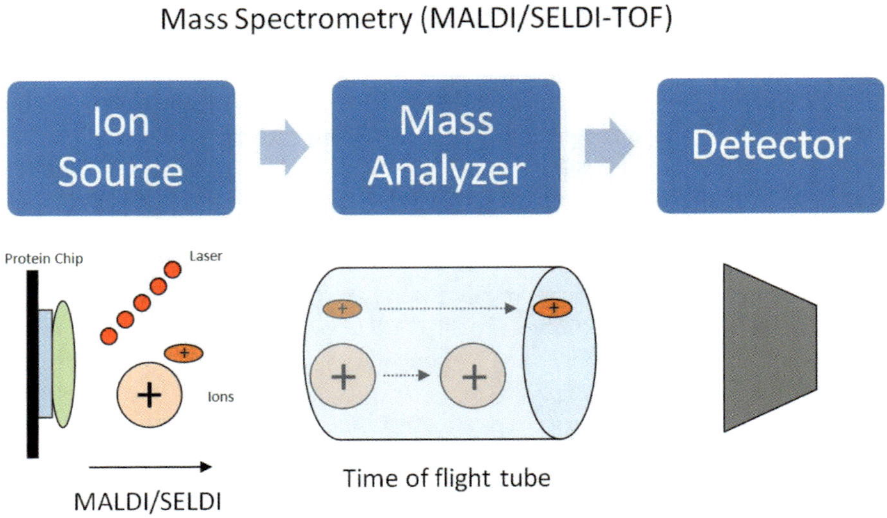

Fig. 22.4 Mass spectrometry technique coupled to time-of-flight (TOF) analyzer

requires only relatively small amounts of easily accessible serum and body fluids for protein detection. Because the procedures are simple, inexpensive, and minimally invasive, proteomic profiling is an emerging technology that is increasingly employed and its ease promises to translate into routine clinical practice. It can be applied to screen clinical samples for early detection of disease, for prognosis, measurement of therapeutic toxicity and therapeutic monitoring of cancers, and for the discovery of new drug targets for therapy (Petricoin et al. 2002a). For example, recent studies on prostate cancer using SELDI-MS and other techniques were able to detect the presence of cancer with excellent sensitivity (82–100 %) and specificity (67–88 %), potentially avoiding the need for prostate biopsies in a significant number of patients who have mildly elevated prostate-specific antigen (Ornstein et al. 2004; Wang et al. 2005; Adam et al. 2002; Petricoin et al. 2002b). Although these results are promising, additional studies are needed to confirm these results.

Finally, genomics and proteomics are advancing the goal of personalized medicine where each and every patient will receive individualized therapy based upon the key signaling pathways of their cancer cells (Harris and McCormick 2010; Gonzalez-Angulo et al. 2010).

References

Abramovitz M, Leyland-Jones B (2006) A systems approach to clinical oncology: focus on breast cancer. Proteome Sci 4:5

Adam BL et al (2002) Serum protein fingerprinting coupled with a pattern-matching algorithm distinguishes prostate cancer from benign prostate hyperplasia and healthy men. Cancer Res 62:3609–3614

Alaiya A, Al-Mohanna M, Linder S (2005) Clinical cancer proteomics: promises and pitfalls. J Proteome Res 4:1213–1222. doi:10.1021/pr050149f

Altshuler D, Daly MJ, Lander ES (2008) Genetic mapping in human disease. Science 322, 881–888. doi:322/5903/881 [pii] 10.1126/science.1156409

Bayani J, Squire JA (2004) Fluorescence in situ hybridization (FISH). Curr Protoc Cell Biol Chapter 22, Unit 22 24, doi:10.1002/0471143030.cb2204s23

Brazma A et al (2001) Minimum information about a microarray experiment (MIAME)-toward standards for microarray data. Nat Genet 29:365–371

Calin GA et al (2002) Frequent deletions and down-regulation of micro-RNA genes miR15 and miR16 at 13q14 in chronic lymphocytic leukemia. Proc Natl Acad Sci U S A 99:15524–15529. doi:10.1073/pnas.242606799 242606799 [pii]

Chaerkady R, Pandey A (2008) Applications of proteomics to lab diagnosis. Ann Rev Pathol 3:485–498

Caprioli RM (2005) Deciphering protein molecular signatures in cancer tissues to aid in diagnosis, prognosis, and therapy. Cancer Res 65:10642–10645. doi:65/23/10642 [pii] 10.1158/0008-5472.CAN-04–3581

Chung CH, Levy S, Chaurand P, Carbone DP (2007) Genomics and proteomics: emerging technologies in clinical cancer research. Crit Rev Oncol Hematol 61:1–25. doi:S1040–8428(06)00109–0 [pii] 10.1016/j.critrevonc.2006.06.005

Conway C et al (2009) Gene expression profiling of paraffin-embedded primary melanoma using the DASL assay identifies increased osteopontin expression as predictive of reduced relapse-free survival. Clin Cancer Res 15:6939–6946

Cornish TJ, Cotter RJ (1993) A curved-field reflectron for improved energy focusing of product ions in time-of-flight mass spectrometry. Rapid Commun Mass Spectrom 7:P1037–P1040. doi:10.1002/rcm.1290071114

Couzin J (2008) MicroRNAs make big impression in disease after disease. Science 319:1782–1784. doi:319/5871/1782 [pii] 10.1126/science.319.5871.1782

DeRisi J et al (1996) Use of a cDNA microarray to analyse gene expression patterns in human cancer. Nat Genet 14, 457–460. doi:10.1038/ng1296–457

Dumur CI et al (2008) Interlaboratory performance of a microarray-based gene expression test to determine tissue of origin in poorly differentiated and undifferentiated cancers. J Mol Diagn 10:67–77. doi:jmoldx.2008.070099 [pii] 10.2353/jmoldx.2008.070099

Fenn JB, Mann M, Meng CK, Wong SF, Whitehouse CM (1989) Electrospray ionization for mass spectrometry of large biomolecules. Science 246:64–71

Fingleton B (2007) Molecular targets in metastasis: lessons from genomic approaches. Cancer Genom Proteom 4:211–221

Foulkes WD (2008) Inherited susceptibility to common cancers. N Engl J Med 359:2143–2153. doi:359/20/2143 [pii] 10.1056/NEJMra0802968

Futreal PA et al (2004) A census of human cancer genes. Nat Rev Cancer 4:177–183. doi:10.1038/nrc1299 nrc1299 [pii]

Gonzalez-Angulo AM, Hennessy BT, Mills GB (2010) Future of personalized medicine in oncology: a systems biology approach. J Clin Oncol 28:2777–2783. doi:JCO.2009.27.0777 [pii] 10.1200/JCO.2009.27.0777

Goswami RS et al (2010) Optimization and analysis of a quantitative real-time PCR-based technique to determine microRNA expression in formalin-fixed paraffin-embedded samples. BMC Biotechnol 10:47. doi:1472–6750-10–47 [pii] 10.1186/1472–6750-10–47

Greenman C et al (2007) Patterns of somatic mutation in human cancer genomes. Nature 446:153–158. doi:nature05610 [pii] 10.1038/nature05610

Harris TJ, McCormick F (2010) The molecular pathology of cancer. Nature rev 7:251–265

Henzel WJ et al(1993) Identifying proteins from two-dimensional gels by molecular mass searching of peptide fragments in protein sequence databases. Proc Natl Acad Sci U S A 90:5011–5015

Hirschhorn JN (2009) Genomewide association studies–illuminating biologic pathways. N Engl J Med 360. 1699–1701. doi:NEJMp0808934 [pii] 10.1056/NEJMp0808934

Hu Z et al (2006) The molecular portraits of breast tumors are conserved across microarray platforms. BMC Genomics 7:96. doi:1471–2164-7–96 [pii] 10.1186/1471–2164-7–96

Hanash S (2003) Disease proteomics. Nature 422:226–232, doi:10.1038/nature01514 nature01514 [pii]

Hudler P, Gorsic M, Komel R (2010) Proteomic strategies and challenges in tumor metastasis research. Clin Exp Metastasis 27:441–451. doi:1007/s10585–010-9339–7

Iwadate Y (2008) Clinical proteomics in cancer research-promises and limitations of current two-dimensional gel electrophoresis. Curr Med Chem 15:2393–2400

Jeffrey SS, Lonning PE, Hillner BE (2005) Genomics-based prognosis and therapeutic prediction in breast cancer. J Natl Compr Canc Netw 3:291–300

Jr GW et al (1999) Proteinchip® surface enhanced laser desorption/ionization (SELDI) mass spectrometry: a novel protein biochip technology for detection of prostate cancer biomarkers in complex protein mixtures. Prostate Cancer Prostatic Dis 2:264–276.doi:10.1038/sj.pcan.4500384 4500384 [pii]

Kubota K, Kosaka T, Ichikawa K (2009) Shotgun protein analysis by liquid chromatography-tandem mass spectrometry. Methods Mol Biol Clifton NJ 519:483–494. doi:10.1007/978–1-59745–281-6_32

Lilley KS, Friedman DB (2004) All about DIGE: quantification technology for differential-display 2D-gel proteomics. Expert Rev Proteomics 1:401–409. doi:10.1586/14789450.1.4.401

Lu J et al (2005) MicroRNA expression profiles classify human cancers. Nature 435:834–838. doi:nature03702 [pii] 10.1038/nature03702

Mann M, Hojrup P, Roepstorff P (1993) Use of mass spectrometric molecular weight information to identify proteins in sequence databases. Biol Mass Spectrom 22:338–345. doi:10.1002/bms.1200220605

Mann M, Hendrickson RC, Pandey A (2001) Analysis of proteins and proteomes by mass spectrometry. Annu Rev Biochem 70:437–473. doi:70/1/437 [pii] 10.1146/annurev.biochem.70.1.437

Manolio TA, Brooks LD, Collins FS (2008) A HapMap harvest of insights into the genetics of common disease. J Clin Invest 118:1590–1605. doi:10.1172/JCI34772

Mardis ER (2008a) The impact of next-generation sequencing technology on genetics. Trends Genet 24:133–141

Mardis ER (2008b) Next-generation DNA sequencing methods. Annu Rev Genomics Hum Genet 9:387–402. doi:10.1146/annurev.genom.9.081307.164359

Merchant M, Weinberger SR (2000) Recent advancements in surface-enhanced laser desorption/ionization-time of flight-mass spectrometry. Electrophoresis 21:1164–1177. doi:10.1002/(SICI)1522–2683(20000401)21:6 < 1164::AID-ELPS1164 > 3.0.CO;2–0 [pii] 10.1002/(SICI)1522–2683(20000401)21:6 < 1164::AID-ELPS1164 > 3.0.CO;2–0

Minden JS, Dowd SR, Meyer HE, Stuhler K (2009) Difference gel electrophoresis. Electrophoresis 30 (Suppl 1):S156–161. doi:10.1002/elps.200900098

Monzon FA, Koen TJ (2010) Diagnosis of metastatic neoplasms: molecular approaches for identification of tissue of origin. Arch Pathol Lab Med 134:216–224

Motoyama A, Yates JR 3rd (2008) Multidimensional LC separations in shotgun proteomics. Anal Chem 80:7187–7193, doi:10.1021/ac8013669

Ornstein DK et al (2004) Serum proteomic profiling can discriminate prostate cancer from benign prostates in men with total prostate specific antigen levels between 2.5 and 15.0 ng/ml. J Urol 172:1302–1305. doi:00005392–200410000-00019 [pii]

Parikh AA, Johnson JC, Merchant NB (2008) Genomics and proteomics in predicting cancer outcomes. Surg Oncol Clin N Am 17:257–277 (vii)

Papadopoulos N, Kinzler KW, Vogelstein B (2006) The role of companion diagnostics in the development and use of mutation-targeted cancer therapies. Nat Biotechnol 24:985–995. doi:nbt1234 [pii] 10.1038/nbt1234

Perou CM et al (2000) Molecular portraits of human breast tumours. Nature 406:747–752. doi:10.1038/35021093

Petricoin EF, Zoon KC, Kohn EC, Barrett JC, Liotta LA (2002a) Clinical proteomics: translating benchside promise into bedside reality. Nat Rev Drug Discov 1:683–695. doi:10.1038/nrd891 nrd891 [pii]

Petricoin EF 3rd et al (2002b) Serum proteomic patterns for detection of prostate cancer. J Natl Cancer Inst 94:1576–1578

Pleasance ED et al (2010) A comprehensive catalogue of somatic mutations from a human cancer genome. Nature 463:191–196. doi:nature08658 [pii] 10.1038/nature08658

Pushkarev D, Neff NF, Quake SR (2009) Single-molecule sequencing of an individual human genome. Nat Biotechnol 27:847–852

Quackenbush J (2002) Microarray data normalization and transformation. Nat Genet 32 (Suppl):496–501, doi:10.1038/ng1032 ng1032 [pii]

Quackenbush J (2006) Microarray analysis and tumor classification. N Engl J Med 354:2463–2472. doi:354/23/2463 [pii] 10.1056/NEJMra042342

Quackenbush J (2009) Data reporting standards: making the things we use better. Genome Med 1:111. doi:gm111 [pii] 10.1186/gm111

Ramaswamy S et al (2001) Multiclass cancer diagnosis using tumor gene expression signatures. Proc Natl Acad Sci U S A 98:15149–15154. doi:10.1073/pnas.211566398 211566398 [pii]

Ramaswamy S, Golub TR (2002) DNA microarrays in clinical oncology. J Clin Oncol 20:1932–1941

Ramaswamy S, Perou CM (2003) DNA microarrays in breast cancer: the promise of personalised medicine. Lancet 361:1576–1577. doi:S0140–6736(03)13322–3 [pii] 10.1016/S0140–6736(03)13322–3

Roboz J (2005) Mass spectrometry in diagnostic oncoproteomics. Cancer Invest 23:465–478

Rosenblatt KP et al (2004) Serum proteomics in cancer diagnosis and management. Annu Rev Med 55:97–112

Schena M, Shalon D, Davis RW, Brown PO (1995) Quantitative monitoring of gene expression patterns with a complementary DNA microarray. Science 270:467–470

Shi L et al (2006) The Microarray quality control (MAQC) project shows inter- and intraplatform reproducibility of gene expression measurements. Nat Biotechnol 24:1151–1161

Simpkins F, Czechowicz JA, Liotta L, Kohn EC (2005) SELDI-TOF mass spectrometry for cancer biomarker discovery and serum proteomic diagnostics. Pharmacogenomics 6:647–653. doi:10.2217/14622416.6.6.647

Sorlie T et al (2003) Repeated observation of breast tumor subtypes in independent gene expression data sets. Proc Natl Acad Sci U S A 100:8418–8423. doi:10.1073/pnas.0932692100932692100 [pii]

Spellman PT et al (2002) Design and implementation of microarray gene expression markup language (MAGE-ML). Genome Biol 3:Research0046

Stratton M (2008) Genome resequencing and genetic variation. Nat Biotechnol 26:65–66. doi:nbt0108–65 [pii] 10.1038/nbt0108–65

Stratton MR, Campbell PJ, Futreal PA (2009) The cancer genome. Nature 458:719–724. doi:nature07943 [pii] 10.1038/nature07943

Sugimura H et al (2010) Fluorescence in situ hybridization analysis with a tissue microarray: 'FISH and chips' analysis of pathology archives. Pathol Int 60:543–550. doi:PIN2561 [pii] 10.1111/j.1440–1827.2010.02561.x

Tanas MR, Goldblum JR (2009) Fluorescence in situ hybridization in the diagnosis of soft tissue neoplasms: a review. Adv Anat Pathol 16:383–391. doi:10.1097/PAP.0b013e3181bb6b86 00125480–200911000-00002 [pii]

Tothill RW et al (2005) An expression-based site of origin diagnostic method designed for clinical application to cancer of unknown origin. Cancer Res 65:4031–4040

Turnbull C et al (2010) Genome-wide association study identifies five new breast cancer susceptibility loci. Nat Genet 42:504–507. doi:ng.586 [pii] 10.1038/ng.586

Van Prooijen-Knegt AC et al (1982) In situ hybridization of DNA sequences in human metaphase chromosomes visualized by an indirect fluorescent immunocytochemical procedure. Exp Cell Res 141:397–407

Volpi EV, Bridger JM (2008) FISH glossary: an overview of the fluorescence in situ hybridization technique. Biotechniques 45:385–386, 388, 390 passim. doi:000112811 [pii] 10.2144/000112811

Waddell N et al (2010) Gene expression profiling of formalin-fixed, paraffin-embedded familial breast tumours using the whole genome-DASL assay. J Pathol 221:452–461. doi:10.1002/path.2728

Wang X et al (2005) Autoantibody signatures in prostate cancer. N Engl J Med 353:1224–1235. doi:353/12/1224 [pii] 10.1056/NEJMoa051931

Weksberg R et al (2005) A method for accurate detection of genomic microdeletions using real-time quantitative PCR. BMC Genomics 6:180. doi:1471–2164-6–180 [pii] 10.1186/1471–2164-6–180

Wong SC et al (2009) Advanced proteomic technologies for cancer biomarker discovery. Expert Rev Proteomics 6:123–134. doi:10.1586/epr.09.1

Yates JR 3rd, Speicher S, Griffin PR, Hunkapiller T (1993) Peptide mass maps: a highly informative approach to protein identification. Anal Biochem 214:397–408. doi:S0003–2697(83)71514–9 [pii] 10.1006/abio.1993.1514

Chapter 23
The Role of Chemotherapy for Metastatic Disease

Catalin Mihalcioiu

23.1 Introduction

Advances in understanding the molecular and biochemical changes underlying the metastatic disease resulted in development of promising chemotherapeutic agents. Treatment of metastatic disease has improved significantly with the addition of drugs that affect specific processes like nucleotide bases, DNA (synthesis, degradation and repair) as well as microtubules.

A. Alkylating agents These agents have antitumor and mutagenic properties by interfering with DNA synthesis and ultimately with cell division. They act through formation of DNA adducts that lead to somatic point mutations or cell death. Several types of alkylating agents used in chemotherapy treatments are nitrogen mustards derivatives, ethyleneimine, alkyl sulfonates, nitrosoureas and the triazenes. Other agents in this category include platinum complexes such as cisplatin and carboplatin. Platinating agents act by a similar mechanism as the alkylating agents forming covalent adducts with DNA (Huitema et al. 2000) (Table 23.1).

B. Antimetabolites These agents are similar in structure with DNA base pairs. These compounds compete with the metabolites in RNA and DNA synthesis resulting in decreased cancer cell proliferation (Kaye 1998). Several agents in this class are currently in use for the treatment of colorectal, breast, head and neck and other cancers (Table 23.2).

C. Microtubule-targeting agents These agents function by disrupting microtubule polymerization or hyper-stabilizing of the microtubule polymers. They interfere with microtubular network and induce mitotic arrest in cancer cells (Jordan and Kamath 2007) (Table 23.3).

D. Topoisomerase inhibitors Topoisomerase inhibitors disrupt key enzymes, such as topoisomerases I and II which are involved in the control of replicative DNA

C. Mihalcioiu (✉)
Department of Medicine & Oncology, Royal Victoria Hospital,
McGill University Health Center, McGill University, Montreal, QC, Canada
e-mail: catalin.mihalcioiu@muhc.mcgill.ca

J. V. Burnier, M. N. Burnier, Jr. (eds.), *Experimental and Clinical Metastasis*,
DOI 10.1007/978-1-4614-3685-0_23,

Table 23.1 Alkylating agents

Alkylating agents	Names of the drugs
Mustard gas derivatives (Goodman et al. 1946)	Mechlorethamine, Cyclophosphamide, Chlorambucil, Melphalan, and Ifosfamide
Ethylenimines (Maanen et al. 2000)	Thiotepa and Hexamethylmelamine
Hydrazines and Triazines (Marchesi et al. 2007)	Altretamine, Procarbazine, Dacarbazine and Temozolomide
Nitrosureas (Hurley 2002)	Carmustine, Lomustine and Streptozocin
Platinum salts (Jakupec et al. 2003; Olszewski and Hamilton 2010)	Carboplatin, Cisplatin, and Oxaliplatin, Satraplatin, Picoplatin and Triplatin

Table 23.2 Antimetabolites

Antimetabolites	Name of the drugs
Folate antagonists (Matherly et al. 2007)	Methotrexate, Pemetrexed (Alimta®)
Purine antagonists (Szyf et al. 2005)	6-Mercaptopurine, Dacarbazine, Fludarabine
Pyrimidine antagonists (Maring et al. 2005)	5-fluorouracil or 5-FU, Arabinosylcytosine, Capecitabine (Xeloda), Gemcitabine

synthesis. These agents induce breaks in single and double strand DNA, disrupting DNA ligation and result in apoptosis and cell death (Denny 2004) (Table 23.4).

The following section aims to identify and disscuss the evidence of chemotherapeutic options in the biological context of metastatic melanoma and breast cancer metastatic disease.

23.2 Treatment of Metastatic Melanoma

At present the survival in metastatic melanoma is influenced by several tumor characteristics such as the extent and progression pace of the disease. Favourable tumor predictors include: good performance status (ECOG 0 or 1), normal LDH (marker of tumor burden) and absence of visceral disease (liver, bone and brain metastases) (Blach and Peters 1993) (Table 23.5).

The median survival of metastatic melanoma is ranging from 4–6 months for patients belonging to unfavourable prognostic group and from 10–12 months in patients with favourable tumor characteristics. Overall, the median survival is expected to be 6–9 months with a 5 year survival of 1–2 %, mainly from patients who achieved a complete response (CR) with treatment (Anderson et al. 1995).

In the last 40 years most of the chemotherapeutic agents that have been discovered have been tested for efficacy against melanoma *in vitro* and *in vivo* with few encouraging results. The relative lack of active treatment is explained by natural resistance mechanisms of this tumor. As a result there is no widely accepted standard of care for the treatment of metastatic melanoma. Chemotherapeutic options include: single agent cytotoxic chemotherapy, combination chemotherapy or biochemotherapy.

Table 23.3 Microtubule-targeting agents. (Carlson 2008; Harrison et al. 2009)

Microtubule-targeting agents	Name of the drugs
Vinca alkaloids	Vinblastine, Vincristine, Vinorelbine and Vindesine
Taxanes	Paclitaxel (Taxol), Docetaxel (Taxotere)
Epothilones	Ixabepilone (Ixempra)

23.2.1 *Single Agent Chemotherapy*

Accepted single chemotherapeutic agents that proved to have antitumor effect in melanoma include: dacarbazine (DTIC), temozolomide, nitrosourea, platinum analogs and tubular toxins (Table 23.6).

Dacarbazine remains the most widely tested single agent since its discovery in 1970. This is due in part to the perception that DTIC is considered one of the most active cytotoxic agent in metastatic melanoma. Dacarbazine (DTIC) is the only single-agent approved by FDA for treating metastatic melanoma. This drug yields 20 % objective response rate with median response duration of 5–6 months and complete response rates of 5 % with one forth of CR experiencing long term survival (Serrone et al. 2000). The patients who are proned to respond to DTIC are more likely to have the disease limited to soft tissue and lung. DTIC is administered intravenously, every 3–4 weeks, dose and schedule varies depending on personal preference, logistics and patient characteristics. The typical dose and schedule include 850–1000 mg/m^2 day 1 every 3 weeks, 200–250 mg/m^2 day 1–5 every 3 weeks, or 4.5 mg/kg/day on day 1–10 every 4 weeks. The main toxicity is nausea and vomiting. Bone marrow suppression is modest; fatigue is minimal allowing patients to enjoy relatively normal function during treatment.

Temozolomide is a novel oral alkylating agent of the imidazotetrazine series (Crosby et al. 2000). It is structurally related to DTIC; both agents require conversion to (monomethyl triazeno imidazole carboxamide) MTIC, for their clinical activity. Whereas DTIC is metabolically activated in the liver, temozolomide undergoes decarboxylation and ring opening to form MTIC which is additionally fragmented to the highly reactive methyldiazonium ion that alkylates DNA. It remains stable under acid conditions providing an important basis of targeted therapy directed towards tumors such as gliomas and melanoma. It has the advantage of good oral bioavailability and blood brain barrier penetration. The most utilized dose schedule for temozolomide is 200 mg/m^2/day $\times$ 5 days every 4 weeks or 150 mg/m^2/day $\times$ 5 days for elderly patients with poor bone marrow reserve or those who received prior radiotherapy or

Table 23.4 Topoisomerase inhibitors

Topoisomerase inhibitors	Name of the drugs
Topoisomerase I inhibitors (Ewesuedo and Ratain 1997)	Irinotecan, Topotecan, Camptothecine
Topoisomerase II inhibitors (Larsen et al. 2003)	Etoposide, Suramine
Anthracyclines (Sessa et al. 2007)	Doxorubicin, Nemorubicin

Table 23.5 Average survival in months with metastatic melanoma

	Site alone	Other sites
Skin, soft tissue, lymph nodes	7.2	5.0
Lung	11.4	4.0
Brain	5.0	1.4
Liver	2.4	2.0
Bone	6.0	4.0
Other	2.2	2.0
Widespread	2.4	2.4

chemotherapy. Other schedules include 75 mg/m^2 daily for 6–7 consecutive weeks or alternating weeks in an attempt to overcome resistance (circumvent the DNA repair process) (Hwu et al. 2002; Danson and Middleton 2001; Brock et al. 1998). The most significant side effects are headache, constipation, fatigue and decrease appetite during the 5 days of administration. Myelotoxicity is mild and mainly in the elderly or post radiotherapy.

A phase II clinical study, showed objective response in 21 % of patients with metastatic melanoma (brain metastases allowed), treated with temozolamide including 5 % CR (Bleehen et al. 1995). Clinical trial data showed no significant differences between the efficacy of the agent temozolomide and DTIC in patients with advanced metastatic melanoma(Middleton et al. 2000; Atkins 1997). A phase III study comparing temozolomide to DTIC, showed a progression free survival (PFS) of 1.9 months versus 1.5 months in favour of temozolomide, but no significant change in response rates (13.5 vs 12.1 %) or overall surviva (OS)l (7.7 vs 6.4 months). However, there was less incidence of brain metastases in temozolamide treated patients (Middleton et al. 2000). Because of lack of significant superiority to DTIC, temozolomide has not been approved by FDA in the treatment of metastatic melanoma.

Nitrosoureas agents are represented by carmustine (BCNU), lomustine (CCNU) and fotemustine. Both BCNU and CCNU showed response rates of 13–18 % in advanced cutaneous melanoma (Anderson et al. 1995; Ahmann et al. 1974). Toxicities are more severe specially fatigue, alopecia and thrombocytopenia. The proposed proposed mechanism of resistance is endogenous production of glutathione (Gajewski 2004).

Table 23.6 Single drug activity in metastatic melanoma

Drug	No. patients	Overall response %
Fotemustine (Jacquillat et al. 1990b)	153	24
Dacarbazine (Anderson et al. 1995; Hill et al. 1984)	1,936	20
Carmustine (Anderson et al. 1995; Wolchok et al. 2003)	122	18
Temozolomide (Su et al. 2004; Middleton et al. 2000)	200	17
Cisplatin (Al-Sarraf et al. 1982; Schilcher et al. 1984)	114	15
Paclitaxel (Wood et al. 1995)	34	15
Docetaxel (Aamdal et al. 1994; Bedikian et al. 1995)	43	14
Lomustine (Anderson et al. 1995; Ahmann et al. 1974)	270	13
Vinblastine (Atkins 1997)	62	13
Carboplatinum (Atkins 1997)	30	16

Fotemustine (FTMU) a novel chloroethyl nitrosourea, has shown consistent response rates of 20–24 %. Dose of administration as single agent is 100 mg/m^2 on day 1, 8 and 15. Mechanism of action is rapid alkylation of thioenzimes involved in DNA synthesis (Avril et al. 2004) and because of the ability to cross the blood brain barrier has activity on cerebral metastases (Jacquillat et al. 1990a). Fotemustine is well tolerated with myelosuppression as the main side-effect and modest extra-hematologic toxicity. When compared with DTIC fotemustine yielded RR in first-line treatment of disseminated melanoma (Avril et al. 2004)

Platinum analogs represented by cisplatin and carboplatin are used for the treatment of metastatic melanoma. Response rates range from 17–29 % for cisplatin when used as a single agent and the results for carboplatin appear to be similar. Carboplatin compared with cisplatin has shown tolerable renal, neural and ototoxic effects, and reversible myelosuppression (Balch and Peters 1993; Evans et al. 1987; Lens and Eisen 2003).

Microtubule toxins such as taxanes (paclitaxel and docetaxel) and vinca alkaloids (vinblastin) interfere with microtubule disassembly and have shown modest activity in metastatic melanoma. A phase II study using paclitaxel produced an overall response rate of 13 % (Einzig et al. 1991; Legha et al. 1990). Doses of 150 mg/m^2 weekly for 6 weeks out of 8 weeks were well tolerated. Similar results were demonstrated in phase II studies using docetaxel (Bedikian et al. 1995; Einzig et al. 1996). Vinca alkaloids have limited activity on their own and have been used in combination regimens (Bedikian et al. 2010).

New agents like epothilones, a nontaxane tubuline polymerization agent showed no clinical activity in newly diagnosed and pretreated metastatic melanoma (Ott et al. 2010).

23.2.2 Combination Chemotherapy

Retrospective analysis comparing chemotherapy to historical controls suggested a small benefit with 30–50 % response rates (RR). Subsequent prospective phase III studies were undertaken comparing combination chemotherapy to DTIC as a control arm. These studies showed a RR of 18–24 % for combination therapy and 10–11 % for DTIC alone with no significant difference in median survival (Lens and Eisen 2003; Chapman et al. 1999).

Some of the chemotherapeutic combinations frequently used are: Dartmouth regimen, CVD, FDV and BHD (Atallah and Flaherty 2005; Rixe et al. 1995) (Table 23.7).

Tamoxifen was used as part of combination therapy since 1985, based on suggestion from small phase II studies showing a 50 % RR (McClay et al. 1992). However, the lack of benefit from the addition of Tamoxifen to chemotherapy was proved by Rusthoven and Folkson in phase III studies. A recent meta-analysis including nine randomized controlled trials showed that chemotherapies with tamoxifen improved overall and partial response, but do not improve mortality in 1 year in advanced melanoma (Beguerie et al. 2010; Rusthoven 1998; Falkson et al. 1998).

Table 23.7 Chemotherapy combination regimens in metastatic malignant melanoma

Dartmouth regimen	Cisplatin 25 mg/m^2 day 1–3, Q3–4 week, DTIC 220 mg/m^2 day 1–3, Q3–4 week, BCNU 150 mg/m^2 day 1, Q6–8 week
CVD	Cisplatin 20 mg/m^2 day 1–4, Q3 week, Vinblastine 2 mg/m^2 day 1–4, Q3 week, DTIC 800 mg/m^2 day 1, Q3 week
FDV	Fotemustine, DTIC, Vindesine
BHD	BCNU 150 mg/m^2 day 1, Q8 weeks, Q4 weeks, Hydroxyurea 1500 mg/m^2 day 1–5, Q4 weeks DTIC 150 mg/m^2 day 1–5

Although combination chemotherapy showed higher RR than single agent chemotherapy no benefit in median survival rates was observed when compared to single agent DTIC (Chapman et al. 1999).

23.2.3 Biochemotherapy

Biochemotherapy is based on synergistic interaction between immunotherapy and combination chemotherapy (McDermott et al. 2000; Atkins et al. 2002; González Astorga et al. 2009).

Immunotherapeutic approaches that are currently evaluated in metastatic melanoma include interferon-alpha (IFN) and interleukin-2 (IL-2). The immune-modulating agent IFN-α is approved by the FDA for the adjuvant treatment of high-risk melanoma patients. Due to the lack of impact on overall survival OS and toxicity profile this type of treatment is not considered as a standard therapeutic option as a single agent (Seetharamu et al. 2009). With the exception of a small study (Pyrhonen et al. 1992), the combination of chemotherapy with INF-α resulted in similar RR and survival rates when compared to chemotherapy alone (Schultz et al. 1997; Feun et al. 1995). On the other hand, several phase III studies comparing DTIC single agent to the combination DTIC-IFN-α showed superiority for clinical response to DTIC alone (Falkson et al. 1998; González Astorga et al. 2009; Kirkwood et al. 1990; Young et al. 2001).

Interleukin-2 (IL-2) is a cytokine produced by CD4-positive T lymphocytes. Immunotherapy with high- dose IL-2 is associated with an objective response rate of 5–27 % with complete responses in 0–4 % of patients (Rosenberg et al. 1993; Sparano et al. 1993).

In an attempt to further improve response and survival, several investigators used combination chemotherapy concomitantly with combination immunotherapy (IFN-α and IL-2) (Garbe et al. 2011). Most of phase III clinical trials compared the efficacy of the combination chemotherapy with IFN-α and IL-2 as the experimental arm and a control arm varying from IFN-α/IL-2 to CVD alone or cisplatin-IL-2. Those studies showed significantly higher RR but no significant OS. However, these type of combinations were associated with hemodynamic and myelosuppressive toxic effects (Seetharamu et al. 2009; Rosenberg et al. 1999; Eton et al. 2002; Atkins et al. 2008). Moreover, several European studies showed similar results (Keilholz et al. 1997; Keilholz et al. 2005; Dorval et al. 1999). A meta-analysis comparing single-agent DTIC versus combination chemotherapy with or without immunotherapy revealed that biochemotherapy was not associated with a statistically significant survival benefit (Hofmann et al. 2007; Hamm et al. 2008). Due to the lack of durable response in terms of OS and a high toxicity profile, biochemotherapy cannot be considered as standard treatment for advanced metastatic melanoma.

Other approaches used for immunotherapy in cutaneous melanoma include cancer vaccines that stimulate the response of the immune system against tumor cells (Jain 2010). Tumor-derived vaccines are based on antigens expressed on a specific to the tumor. (MAGE)-A3 is tumor-antigen-based vaccine for melanoma. This vaccine was evaluated in phase II clinical trial and was shown to induce specific T-cell responses and clinical objective responses in metastatic melanoma (Kruit et al. 2008). In a randomized phase III clinical trial a peptide vaccine, gp100:209–217 (200M), in combination with high dose IL-2 was reported to improve response rates and progression-free survival for patients with advanced melanoma (Schwartzentruber et al. 2009). Intratumoral injection of a virus vector encoding granulocyte monocyte colony-stimulating factor (GM-CSF) induced 26 % response rate in a phase II trial in patients with metastatic melanoma (Senzer et al. 2009). A different vaccine, Oncophage (Vitespen, Antigenics) is based on autologous peptides isolated from patient tumor in combination with the heat shock protein 96 (gp96) (Wood and Mulders 2009). An open-labeled trial of Vitespen versus chemotherapy was tested in patients with stage III or stage IV metastatic melanoma. The administration of the vaccine was well tolerated but no statistical differences in OS were observed (Testori et al. 2008). Melacine vaccine (Corixa) is based on tumor lysates combined with monophosphoryl lipid A and mycobacterial cell wall skeleton. A randomized Phase III trial of Melacine combined with high-dose IFN-α2b in malignant melanoma had similar OS when compared with IFN-α2b alone (Mitchell et al. 2007).

The immune response initiated by a vaccine may have potential side effects and multiple vaccinations may induce immunotolerance (Faries et al. 2009; Eggermont 2010). Future trials are warranted to assess the efficacy of cancer vaccine therapy.

A different strategy involves antibodies against cytotoxic T lymphocytes (anti-CTLA-4). Two human IgG monoclonal antibodies that block the interaction between B7 and CTLA-4, ipilimumab (MDX-010, Bristol-Myers Squibb) and tremelimumab (CP-675,206), have been tested in phase II/III trials (Eggermont 2010).

Data from Phase II clinical trials suggest that Ipilimumab at a dose of 10 mg/kg was well tolerated and suggest long term survival effects (Wolchok et al. 2010). Another phase III trial of ipilimumab alone or in combination with a gp100 peptide vaccine was evaluated in 676 patients with unresectable stage III or IV melanoma. An increase in OS (10.0 months in the ipilimumab arm as compared with 6.4 months among patients receiving gp100 was reported. Treatment with ipilimumab was reported to have grade 3 or 4 immune-related adverse events including death (Hodi et al. 2010). Ongoing clinical trials will assess the effect of this therapy in comparison with dacarbazine.

Tremelimumab (CP-675, 206, Pfizer) showed promising clinical activity and was generally well tolerated as single-agent in patients with metastatic melanoma (Camacho et al. 2009). In a phase II clinical study the OS was of 21 % (16 partial responses and 35 stable disease), and median overall survival was 10.0 months (Kirkwood et al. 2010). Trials comparing tremelimumab with dacarbazine and other immunotherapeutic strategies are in progress (Ribas et al. 2009).

CTLA4-blocking therapy resulted in objective clinical responses and represents a promising approach to the immunotherapy of cancer. These results demand further validation to identify of treatment clinical responders.

Key Points

- Single agent chemotherapy remains the back bone treatment in metastatic melanoma.
- Single agent Dacarbazine, the only FDA approved drug, has produced response rates of 10–20 % with complete responses occurring in about 5 % of patients.
- Temozolomide has the advantage of oral administration, acceptable toxicity and good CNS penetration. It is the preferred choice for elderly patients with brain metastases.
- Taxanes are rarely used as first line therapy and have been incorporated as a control arm in some of the recent clinical trials.
- Fotemustine seems to be an active agent, but did not gain in popularity in part due to increased toxicity.
- Cisplatin has a modest clinical activity as a single agent and has been used as part of combination regimens.
- Biochemotherapy for metastatic melanoma is associated with significant toxicity.
- Combination chemotherapy and biochemotherapy has not shown any advantage in response rate or overall survival when compared to DTIC.
- Immunotherapy with high dose IL-2 is associated with durable responses in a small percentage of patients.
- New immunotherapy strategies such as vaccines and CTLA4-blocking therapy resulted in objective clinical responses and represent a promising therapeutic approach.

23.2.4 Summary

The survival of patients with metastatic melanoma is influenced by the extent and the pace of the disease rather than the type of therapeutic interventions. Therefore, an adequate patient selection is important in making treatment decisions. Patients to be considered for treatment with chemotherapy should have a good performance status (ECOG PS 0-1), normal LDH, no evidence of liver, bone or brain metastases and no underline medical conditions that will increase toxicity of chemotherapy. Chemotherapy in metastatic melanoma is associated with low response rate and only a subgroup of patients will achieve a complete response with chemotherapy. Due to the lack of phase III clinical trials showing a survival benefit from any type of chemotherapy over best supportive care, there is no standard chemotherapy regimen accepted for the treatment of metastatic melanoma.

23.3 Treatment of metastatic breast cancer

Despite significant improvement in treatment, metastatic breast cancer remains an incurable disease and is typically associated with a median survival of 18–24 month (Miller and Sledge 1999). The goal of systemic therapy include: prolongation of survival, palliation of symptoms and improvement in quality of life. A single institution (MD Anderson) retrospective study reported the results of 1581 patients treated with doxorubicin. The data showed a complete response (CR) of 17 % and a partial response (PR) of 48 %, with an OS of 41.8 month for the CR group and 24.6 months for the PR group (Sparano 2002).

Tumor heterogeneity is a constant challenge in selecting more appropriate therapeutic interventions that will further improve the clinical outcome in patients with breast cancer. The use of molecular pathology based on gene signature allowed a more precise classification and a better predictive and prognostic outcome to different therapeutic interventions in breast cancer (Eichhorn and Baselga 2010). The choice of first line therapy is becoming increasingly complex and depends to a great extent on tumor molecular signature, patient characteristics and physician preference. Principles of using chemotherapy for patients with metastatic breast cancer are influenced by:

1. Clinical information
   - Type of presentation: Progression following adjuvant treatment versus metastatic disease at the initial presentation
   - Age and menopausal status
   - Medical comorbidities and general performance status
2. Pathological information
   - Type of tumor: invasive ductal (IDC) versus invasive lobular carcinoma (ILC)
   - Proliferative index suggested by tumor grade and K67 index
   - Receptor status for: ER, PR, Her2neu
3. Molecular signature
   - Triple negative (ER-, PR-, Her2-)
   - Basal-like, BRCA1 and Claudin-low (stem cell)
   - Her2 positive
   - Luminal A (ER + and low grade) and luminal B (ER + and high grade)

Patients progressing post adjuvant antracycline-taxane regimens, usually receive single agent chemotherapy for metastatic disease. Those who presented with metastatic disease at the initial diagnosis of breast cancer are more likely to receive 2nd and/or 3rd generation combination chemotherapy (anthracycline and taxane based). Patients younger than 35 years old tend to be triple negative, high grade and benefit more from chemotherapy. Advanced age, 70 years old and more, tend to be strongly ER positive, low or intermediate proliferative index and benefit more from antiestrogen therapy. General performance status and medical comorbidities will influence the choice or the decision to give chemotherapy.

In adjuvant setting, for stage I and II ER positive breast cancer, the clinical benefit of chemotherapy can be predicted by gene signatures (Perou et al. 2000), diagnostic tests such as like *Oncotype* Dx or MammaPrint (O'Toole et al. 2011). In metastatic setting, the presence of Her2 gene amplification will predict clinical benefit from concomitant use of chemotherapy and targeted therapy. For Her2 positive tumors, the choice of chemotherapy combination will be influenced by the cardiac status. Patients with low or borderline ejection fraction (EF%) are more likely to receive antracycline free combination like taxotere, carboplatin, herceptin (TCH) or taxol and herceptin (TH) combination. Young patients are more likely to be treated with adriamycin, cyclophosphamide followed by taxol and herceptin, (AC → TH) regimen. Elderly patients are less suitable to benefit from this regimen and can be offered herceptin and an aromatase inhibitor (Guarneri et al. 2010).

The type of tumor can also influence the therapeutic choice. Invasive ductal type and ER negative breast cancer in younger patients is more likely to respond to chemotherapy. Invasive low grade lobular carcinoma is usually ER positive and develops in atypical metastatic sites (serosa, gall bladder, ovaries, and uterus) (Yeh and Mies 2008; Armes et al. 1998). This type of cancer has a shorter disease free (DFS) but a longer survival rate and responds better to antiestrogen manipulation.

23.3.1 First Line Chemotherapy

A. Previously Untreated Patients First generation combination chemotherapy initially used for the treatment of breast cancer, was cyclophosphamide, methotrexate and 5-florouracil (CMF). The classical CMF regimen (oral cyclophosphamide) showed a superior response rate (48 vs 29 %) and survival (17 vs 12 months) when compared with intravenous CMF in advanced breast cancer, (Engelsman et al. 1991).

Second generation combination chemotherapy are doxorubicin-based. They include cyclophosphamide, adriamycin or epirubicine and 5-florouracil (CAF or CEF) and 5-florouracil, adriomycin or epirubicin and cyclophosphamide (FAC or FEC) combinations. Phase III clinical trials showed an improvement in survival from 14.0 months with CMF to 24.7 months with CAF (Aisner et al. 1987). This therapeutic regimen is associated with cardiac induced toxicity, limiting the cumulative total dose to 340 mg/m^2 for doxorubicine and between 900–1,000 mg/m^2 for epirubicine.

Third generation chemotherapeutic options involve taxanes and anthracyclines for the treatment of advanced breast cancer. Single agent anthracycline as a first line therapy in metastatic breast cancer, showed a response rate between 30–50 % (Beslija et al. 2007). The taxanes have been found equally efficacious in first line (Figgitt and Wiseman 2000; Pacilio et al. 2006; Razis and Fountzilas 2001). Moreover, paclitaxel has shown 35–53 % response rate lasting from 6.8–7.5 months in second and third line settings (Verma et al. 2011; Seidman et al. 1995). Taxanes showed significant activity in phase III trials in patients previously exposed or having failed anthracycline chemotherapy (Nabholtz et al. 1999). In a randomized phase III trial patients receiving doxorubicin and docetaxel experienced a higher response rate as well as a significantly longer time to progression compared to doxorubicin and cyclophosphamide. This results highlight the potential therapeutic effect of this combination in metastatic breast cancer (Nabholtz et al. 2000). Adjuvant trials comparing paclitaxel-anthracycline combinations revealed clinically relevant pharmacokinetic interactions which are sequence and schedule dependent (Conte et al. 2004; Jones et al. 2005).

B. Previously Treated Patients in Adjuvant Setting The optimal treatment of this group is not well established. This group of patients can be divided into three subgroups: patients who priorly received antracycline, priorly received taxane or a combination of anthracycline and taxane therapy.

Theoretical options for the patients previously treated with adjuvant anthracycline include:

- Re-challenge with anthracycline alone or in combination with vinorelbine,
- cyclophosphsmide, gemcitabine
- Taxane therapy alone or in combination with capecitabine, gemcitabine, vinorelbine
- First line anthracyclines (doxorubicin, epirubicin, pegylated liposomal doxorubicine or non-pegylated liposomal doxorubicin) (Ardavanis et al. 2006).

The evidence supporting this approach is limited. The only prospective phase III randomized study designed to evaluate the role of first line anthracycline in previously anthracycline treated breast cancer patients, was prematurely closed due to poor enrolment. Of a total 26 patients, there was a 72 % RR and a median overall survival (MOS) of 15 months (Trudeau et al. 2009).

Another option of first line anthracycline chemotherapy is pegylated liposomal doxorubicine (PLD) which offers the advantage of much lower cardiac toxicity and appear to be active in this setting. In a phase II clinical trial single agent PLD showed a RR of 24 % with a MOS of 12.3 months in a population of patients who received anthracyline chemotherapy in adjuvant or as first line setting. Combination of PLD with vinorelbine, cyclophosphamide or gemcitabine showed a RR ranging from 23–58 % with MOS reported only for vinorelbine of 14.5 months (Jones et al. 2005; Rivera et al. 2003; Batist et al. 2006). Presently, PLD is approved in second line metastatic breast cancer in previously anthracycline treated patients. Non-pegylated liposomal doxorubicine (nPLD) achieved non-conclusive results showing significantly better RR (31 vs 11 % doxorubicin), but no survival benefit (O'Shaughnessy et al. 2002).

Patients who are considered refractory to anthracyclines or achieved the maximum cumulative dose of anthracyclin, are candidates for taxane chemotherapy (docetaxel, paclitaxel, nanoparticle albumin-bound paclitaxel) alone or in combination with other agents (capecitabine, gemcitabine). Head to head comparison of docetaxel vs. paclitaxel showed a significantly longer RR (32 vs. 25 %) and OS (15.4 vs. 12.7 months) in favour of docetaxel (Miles 2008; Soto 2006).

Combination of docetaxel (75 mg/m^2) with capecitabine 1250 mg/m^2 twice per day 14 out of 21 days, showed significant increase in RR (42 vs. 30 %) TTP (6.1 vs. 4.2 months) and OS (14.5 vs. 11.5) when compared with docetaxel alone (Khoo 2004). This combination proved to have significant toxicity, therefore a phase II clinical study analyzed a sequential mode of administration suggesting a better toxicity profile for the sequential docetaxel capecitabine arm (Bayo et al. 2008).

Addition of gemcitabine to different doses of taxanes in a three arms phase III study showed no significant difference among the three dose combinations (Khoo 2004; Levy and Fumoleau 2005). Another phase III trial comparing paclitaxel to the combination gemcitabine and paclitaxel in patients with advanced breast cancer demonstrated superior time to progression and tumor response for the gemcitabine and paclitaxel arm (Albain et al. 2008).

Comparison between the combination capecitabine/docetaxel vs. gemcitabine/docetaxel in a phase III study of metastatic breast cancer patients, showed no survival difference between the two arms, however, gemcitabine-docetaxel appeared to have a more favourable risk-benefit profile than capecitabine-docetaxel, and is an important new treatment option for women with anthracycline-pretreated MBC (Chan et al. 2009).

An improved way of delivering higher doses of paclitaxel could be the binding of the drug to 130-nM nanoparticle albumin (Abraxane). The results of a clinical trial using this compound in patients with previous anthracycline-based adjuvant therapy were reported. This study demonstrated significantly higher response rates and a longer time to tumor progression (23 weeks vs. 16.6 weeks) for patients treated with Abraxane when compared with standard paclitaxel (Gradishar et al. 2005).

The optimal treatment for patients previously treated with anthracycline and taxane in adjuvant setting is not well established. Different treatment options for these patients include re-challenge treatment with taxanes in first line metastatic setting capecitabine or vinorelbine (Zielinski et al. 2010; Verma and Clemons 2007). In a retrospective chart review, single agent capecitabine showed a survival benefit when compared to vinorelbine (median overall survival of 102 days for the vinorelbine group and 188 days for the capecitabine group) (Verma et al. 2007).

Data analysis from phase III clinical trials using combination capecitabine/bevacizumab (Miller et al. 2005) or vinorelbine/gemcitabine vs. capecitabine alone, demonstrated that although combination regimens showed better response rates, they rendered no significant survival benefit (Zielinski et al. 2010).

Other first line treatment options in patients treated with anthracyclines and/or taxanes include paclitaxel (Sawaki et al. 2004; Valero et al. 1998), (nab-paclitaxel, Abraxane^{TM}) (Gradishar et al. 2005) or Docetaxel (Jones et al. 2005). Results reported from a phase III clinical study showed that docetaxel produced a significantly longer TTP and OS time when compared with paclitaxel (Jones et al. 2005). Another study in anthracycline/taxane pretreated patients compared Abraxane at standard dose 260 mg/m^2 every 3 weeks or weekly 150 mg/m^2 and 100 mg/m^2, to Docetaxel 100 mg/m^2 every 3 weeks. This study showed encouraging resulting in a prolongation of more than 6 months for the patients treated in the nab-paclitaxel arm when compared with docetaxel arm (Gradishar et al. 2009).

A group that set itself apart is Her2 positive breast cancer. Although the incidence of this molecular signature is relatively low (12–25 %) the targeted therapy with herceptin or lapatinib reversed the poor outcome of this group into a better one (RR 50 vs. 32 %, MOS 25.1 vs. 20.3 months) (Slamon et al. 2001; Higa and Abraham 2007). Recent data in patients progressing post adjuvant herceptin have shown continued response by maintaining herceptin and changing the chemotherapy (Metro et al. 2008; Jackisch 2006). Equally effective is the switch to lapatinib and capecitabine for women with HER2-positive, advanced breast cancer progressing after treatment with anthracycline, taxane and trastuzumab based therapy (Cameron et al. 2008).

Novel therapeutic approaches include the development of small-molecule kinase inhibitors of HER2. For example, Trastuzumab-DM1 (T-DM1) is a combination of trastuzumab covalently bound to DM1, a derivative of the antimicrotubule chemotherapy maytansanine. This immunoconjugate is directed to HER2-positive tumor cells (Isakoff and Baselga 2011). Results from a phase I clinical study showed that T-DM1 in combination with pertuzumab can establish a complete HER2 receptor blockade. This trial achieved partial responses for women with advanced HER2-positive breast cancers previously treated with trastuzumab (Miller 2010). A subsequent phase II clinical trial with T-DM1 was pursued in patients with HER2-positive metastatic breast cancer who received prior trastuzumab. This study confirmed the safety profile of with T-DM1 and achieved an overall response rate of 25.9 % after more than 12 months of follow-up (Burris et al. 2011). A meta analysis evaluating the benefit of adding concomitant trastuzumab to neoadjuvant (anthracycline and taxane-based) chemotherapy concluded that Trastuzumab significantly reduces the risk of relapse and does not increase the risk of cardiotoxicity (Petrelli et al. 2011).

23.3.2 Summary

The treatment of metastatic breast cancer becomes more and more individualized based on the type of prior adjuvant therapy, time of presentation, location of the metastases, tumor burden, patient's age, co-morbidities, and performance status. Combination chemotherapy, single agent or sequential chemotherapy has become a reality in metastatic melanoma. In the future the decision making process will shift more on molecular tumor signature. HER2 status is being already used in clinical practice to decide the use of herceptin or lapatinib. At present, intense research is being done for triple negative breast cancer tumors subgroups which will serve as an example how tumor molecular signatures can be used to design specific therapeutic interventions.

References

Aamdal S et al (1994) Docetaxel (Taxotere) in advanced malignant melanoma: a phase II study of the EORTC early clinical trials group. Eur J Cancer 30:1061–1064

Ahmann DL, Hahn RG, Bisel HF (1974) Evaluation of 1-(2-chloroethyl-3–4-methylcyclohexyl)-1-nitrosourea (methyl-CCNU, NSC 95441) versus combined imidazole carboxamide (NSC 45338) and vincristine (NSC 67574) in palliation of disseminated malignant melanoma. Cancer 33: 615–618

Aisner J et al (1987) Chemotherapy versus chemoimmunotherapy (CAF v CAFVP v CMF each + /- MER) for metastatic carcinoma of the breast: a CALGB study. Cancer and leukemia Group B. J Clin Oncol 5:1523–1533

Albain KS et al (2008) gemcitabine plus paclitaxel versus paclitaxel monotherapy in patients with metastatic breast cancer and prior anthracycline treatment. J Clin Oncol 26:3950–3957

Al-Sarraf M et al (1982) Cisplatin hydration with and without mannitol diuresis in refractory disseminated malignant melanoma: a southwest oncology group study. Cancer Treat Rep 66:31–35

Anderson CM, Buzaid AC, Legha SS (1995) Systemic treatments for advanced cutaneous melanoma. Oncology (Williston Park) 9:1149–1158, discussion 1163–1144, 1167–1148

Ardavanis A et al (2006) Pegylated liposomal doxorubicin in combination with vinorelbine as salvage treatment in pretreated patients with advanced breast cancer: a multicentre phase II study. Cancer Chemother Pharmacol 58:742–748

Armes JE et al (1998) The histologic phenotypes of breast carcinoma occurring before age 40 years in women with and without BRCA1 or BRCA2 germline mutations. Cancer 83:2335–2345

Atallah E, Flaherty L (2005) Treatment of metastatic malignant melanoma. Curr Treat Options Oncol 6:185–193

Atkins M (ed) (1997) The role of cytotoxic chemotherapeutic agents either alone or in combination with biological response modifiers. (Marcel Dekker, New York)

Atkins MB et al (2002) A phase II pilot trial of concurrent biochemotherapy with cisplatin, vinblastine, temozolomide, interleukin 2, and IFN-α2B in patients with metastatic melanoma. Clin Cancer Res 8:3075–3081

Atkins MB et al (2008) Phase III trial comparing concurrent biochemotherapy with cisplatin, vinblastine, dacarbazine, interleukin-2, and interferon alfa-2b with cisplatin, vinblastine, and dacarbazine alone in patients with metastatic malignant melanoma (e3695): a trial coordinated by the eastern cooperative oncology group. J Clin Oncol 26:5748–5754

Avril MF et al (2004) Fotemustine compared with dacarbazine in patients with disseminated malignant melanoma: a phase III study. J Clin Oncol 22:1118–1125

Balch CM, Houghton AN, Peters LJ (1993) Cutaneous melanoma. In: DeVita VT Jr, Hellman S, Rosenberg SA (eds) Cancer: principles and practice of oncology, 4th edn. Lippincott, Philadelphia, pp 1612–1661

Batist G, Harris L, Azarnia N, Lee LW, Daza-Ramirez P (2006) Improved anti-tumor response rate with decreased cardiotoxicity of non-pegylated liposomal doxorubicin compared with conventional doxorubicin in first-line treatment of metastatic breast cancer in patients who had received prior adjuvant doxorubicin: results of a retrospective analysis. Anticancer Drugs 17:587–595

Bayo J et al (2008) A multicentre phase II study to evaluate sequential docetaxel followed by capecitabine treatment in anthracycline-pretreated HER-2-negative patients with metastatic breast cancer. Clin Transl Oncol 10:817–825

Bedikian AY et al (1995) Phase II trial of docetaxel in patients with advanced cutaneous malignant melanoma previously untreated with chemotherapy. J Clin Oncol 13:2895–2899

Bedikian AY et al (2010) Does complete response to systemic therapy in patients with stage IV melanoma translate into long-term survival? Melanoma Res 21(1):84–90

Beguerie JR, Xingzhong J, Valdez RP (2010) Tamoxifen vs. non-tamoxifen treatment for advanced melanoma: a meta-analysis. Int J Dermatol 49:1194–1202

Beslija S et al (2007) Second consensus on medical treatment of metastatic breast cancer. Ann Oncol 18:215–225

Blach CMHA, Peters LJ (ed) (1993) Cutaneous melanoma 1612–1661 (JB Lippincott, Philadelphia)
Bleehen N et al (1995) Cancer research campaign phase II trial of temozolomide in metastatic melanoma. J Clin Oncol 13:910–913
Brock CS et al (1998) Phase I trial of temozolomide using an extended continuous oral schedule. Cancer Res 58:4363–4367
Burris HA et al (2011) Phase II study of the antibody drug conjugate trastuzumab-DM1 for the treatment of human epidermal growth factor receptor 2 (HER2)–positive breast cancer after prior HER2-directed therapy. J Clin Oncol 29:398–405
Camacho LH et al (2009) Phase I/II trial of tremelimumab in patients with metastatic melanoma. J Clin Oncol 27:1075–1081
Cameron D et al (2008) A phase III randomized comparison of lapatinib plus capecitabine versus capecitabine alone in women with advanced breast cancer that has progressed on trastuzumab: updated efficacy and biomarker analyses. Breast Cancer Res Treat 112:533–543
Carlson RO (2008) New tubulin targeting agents currently in clinical development. Expert Opin Investig Drugs 17:707–722
Chan S et al (2009) Phase III study of gemcitabine plus docetaxel compared with capecitabine plus docetaxel for anthracycline-pretreated patients with metastatic breast cancer. J Clin Oncol 27:1753–1760
Chapman PB et al (1999) Phase III multicenter randomized trial of the dartmouth regimen versus dacarbazine in patients with metastatic melanoma. J Clin Oncol 17:2745
Conte PF et al (2004) Concomitant versus sequential administration of epirubicin and paclitaxel as first-line therapy in metastatic breast carcinoma. Cancer 101:704–712
Crosby T, Fish R, Coles B, Mason MD (2000) Systemic treatments for metastatic cutaneous melanoma. Cochrane Database Syst Rev CD001215
Danson SJ, Middleton MR (2001) Temozolomide: a novel oral alkylating agent. Expert Rev Anticancer Ther 1:13–19
Denny WA (2004) Emerging DNA topoisomerase inhibitors as anticancer drugs. Expert Opin Emerg Drugs 9:105–133
Dorval T et al (1999) Randomized trial of treatment with cisplatin and interleukin-2 either alone or in combination with interferon-α-2a in patients with metastatic melanoma. Cancer 85:1060–1066
Eggermont AMM (2010) Advances in systemic treatment of melanoma. Ann Oncol 21:vii339–vii344
Eichhorn PJ, Baselga J (2010) HER2 signatures in breast cancer: ready to go to print? J Clin Oncol 28:1809–1810
Einzig AI et al (1991) A phase II study of taxol in patients with malignant melanoma. Invest New Drugs 9:59–64
Einzig AI et al (1996) Phase II trial of docetaxel (Taxotere) in patients with metastatic melanoma previously untreated with cytotoxic chemotherapy. Med Oncol 13:111–117
Engelsman E et al (1991) "Classical" CMF versus a 3-weekly intravenous CMF schedule in post-menopausal patients with advanced breast cancer. An EORTC Breast Cancer Co-operative Group Phase III Trial (10808). Eur J Cancer 27:966–970
Eton O et al (2002) Sequential biochemotherapy versus chemotherapy for metastatic melanoma: results from a phase III randomized trial. J Clin Oncol 20:2045–2052
Evans LM, Casper ES, Rosenbluth R (1987) Phase II trial of carboplatin in advanced malignant melanoma. Cancer Treat Rep 71:171–172
Ewesuedo RB, Ratain MJ (1997) Topoisomerase I Inhibitors. Oncologist 2:359–364
Falkson CI et al (1998) Phase III trial of dacarbazine versus dacarbazine with interferon alpha-2b versus dacarbazine with tamoxifen versus dacarbazine with interferon alpha-2b and tamoxifen in patients with metastatic malignant melanoma: an eastern cooperative oncology group study. J Clin Oncol 16:1743–1751
Faries MB, Hsueh EC, Ye X, Hoban M, Morton DL (2009) Effect of granulocyte/macrophage colony-stimulating factor on vaccination with an allogeneic whole-cell melanoma vaccine. Clin Cancer Res 15:7029–7035

Feun LG et al (1995) Phase II trial of recombinant interferon-alpha with BCNU, cisplatin, DTIC and tamoxifen in advanced malignant melanoma. Melanoma Res 5:273–276
Figgitt DP, Wiseman LR (2000) Docetaxel: an update of its use in advanced breast cancer. Drugs 59:621–651
Gajewski TF (2004) Temozolomide for melanoma: new toxicities and new opportunities. J Clin Oncol 22:580–581
Garbe C, Eigentler TK, Keilholz U, Hauschild A, Kirkwood JM (2011) Systematic review of medical treatment in melanoma: current status and future prospects. Oncologist 16:5–24
González Astorga B et al (2009) Biochemotherapy in the treatment of metastatic melanoma in selected patients. Clin Transl Oncol 11:382–386
Goodman LS, Wintrobe MM, Dameshek W, Goodman MJ, Gilman A (1946) Nitrogen mustard therapy—use of methyl-bis(beta-chloroethyl)amine hydrochloride and tris(beta-chloroethyl)amine hydrochloride for hodgkins disease, lymphosarcoma, leukemia and certain allied and miscellaneous disorders. JAMA 132:126–132
Gradishar WJ et al (2005) Phase III trial of nanoparticle albumin-bound paclitaxel compared with polyethylated castor oil–based paclitaxel in women with breast cancer. J Clin Oncol 23:7794–7803
Gradishar WJ et al (2009) Significantly longer progression-free survival with nab-paclitaxel compared with docetaxel as first-line therapy for metastatic breast cancer. J Clin Oncol 27:3611–3619
Guarneri V, Barbieri E, Dieci MV, Piacentini F, Conte P (2010) Anti-HER2 neoadjuvant and adjuvant therapies in HER2 positive breast cancer. Cancer Treat Rev 36:S62–S66
Hamm C, Verma S, Petrella T, Bak K, Charette M (2008) Biochemotherapy for the treatment of metastatic malignant melanoma: a systematic review. Cancer Treat Rev 34:145–156
Harrison MR, Holen KD, Liu G (2009) Beyond taxanes: a review of novel agents that target mitotic tubulin and microtubules, kinases, and kinesins. Clin Adv Hematol Oncol 7:54–64
Higa GM, Abraham J (2007) Lapatinib in the treatment of breast cancer. Expert Rev Anticancer Ther 7:1183–1192
Hill GJ 2nd, Krementz ET, Hill HZ (1984) Dimethyl triazeno imidazole carboxamide and combination therapy for melanoma. IV. Late results after complete response to chemotherapy (Central Oncology Group protocols 7130, 7131, and 7131A). Cancer 53:1299–1305
Hodi FS et al (2010) Improved Survival with Ipilimumab in Patients with Metastatic Melanoma. N Engl J Med 363, 711–723
Hofmann MA, Sterry W, Trefzer U (2007) Complex combination biochemotherapy regimen in advanced metastatic melanoma in a non-intensive care unit: toxicity or benefit? Jpn J Clin Oncol 37:224–229
Huitema AD et al (2000) The clinical pharmacology of alkylating agents in high-dose chemotherapy. Anticancer Drug 11:515–533
Hurley LH (2002) DNA and its associated processes as targets for cancer therapy. Nat Rev Cancer 2:188–200
Hwu W-J et al (2002) Temozolomide plus thalidomide in patients with advanced melanoma: results of a dose-finding trial. J Clin Oncol 20:2610–2615
Isakoff SJ, Baselga J (2011) Trastuzumab-DM1: building a chemotherapy-free road in the treatment of human epidermal growth factor receptor 2–positive breast cancer. J Clin Oncol 29:351–354
Jackisch C (2006) HER-2-positive metastatic breast cancer: optimizing trastuzumab-based therapy. Oncologist 11:34–41
Jacquillat C et al (1990a) Chemotherapy by fotemustine in cerebral metastases of disseminated malignant melanoma. Cancer Chemother Pharmacol 25:263–266
Jacquillat C et al (1990b) Final report of the French multicenter phase II study of the nitrosourea fotemustine in 153 evaluable patients with disseminated malignant melanoma including patients with cerebral metastases. Cancer 66:1873–1878
Jain KK (2010) Personalized cancer vaccines. Expert Opin Biol Ther 10:1637–1647

Jakupec M Galanski M Keppler B (2003) Tumour-inhibiting platinum complexes—state of the art and future perspectives. in Rev Physiol Biochem Pharmacol 146:1–53 (Springer, Berlin Heidelberg)

Jones SE et al (2005) Randomized phase III study of docetaxel compared with paclitaxel in metastatic breast cancer. J Clin Oncol 23:5542–5551

Jordan MA, Kamath K (2007) How do microtubule-targeted drugs work? An overview. Curr Cancer Drug Targets 7:730–742

Kaye SB (1998) New antimetabolites in cancer chemotherapy and their clinical impact. Br J Cancer 78:(Suppl 3):1–7

Keilholz U et al (1997) Interferon alfa-2a and interleukin-2 with or without cisplatin in metastatic melanoma: a randomized trial of the european organization for research and treatment of cancer melanoma cooperative group. J Clin Oncol 15:2579–2588

Keilholz U et al (2005) Dacarbazine, cisplatin, and interferon-Alfa-2b with or without Interleukin-2 in metastatic melanoma: a randomized phase III trial (18951) of the european organisation for research and treatment of cancer melanoma group. J Clin Oncol 23:6747–6755

Khoo K (2004) Randomized phase II trial of three gemcitabine (GEM)-taxane combination in metastatic breast cancer (MBC). J Clin Oncol 22:710

Kirkwood JM et al (1990) Interferon alpha-2a and dacarbazine in melanoma. J Natl Cancer Inst 82:1062–1063

Kirkwood JM et al (2010) Phase II Trial of tremelimumab (CP-675,206) in patients with advanced refractory or relapsed melanoma. Clin Cancer Res 16(3):1042–1048

Kruit WH, Suciu S, Dreno B, Chiarion-Sileni V, Mortier L, Robert C, Maio M, Brichard VG, Lehmann F, Keilholz U (2008) Immunization with recombinant MAGE-A3 protein combined with adjuvant systems AS15 or AS02B in patients with unresectable and progressive metastatic cutaneous melanoma: a randomized open-label phase II study of the EORTC melanoma group. J Clin Oncol 26:16032–18031

Larsen AK, Escargueil AE, Skladanowski A (2003) Catalytic topoisomerase II inhibitors in cancer therapy. Pharmacol Ther 99:167–181

Legha SS, Ring S, Papadopoulos N, Raber M, Benjamin RS (1990) A phase II trial of taxol in metastatic melanoma. Cancer 65:2478–2481

Lens MB, Eisen TG (2003) Systemic chemotherapy in the treatment of malignant melanoma. Expert Opin Pharmacother 4:2205–2211

Levy C, Fumoleau P (2005) Gemcitabine plus docetaxel: a new treatment option for anthracycline pretreated metastatic breast cancer patients? Cancer Treat Rev 31:S17–S22

Maanen MJv, Smeets CJM, Beijnen JH (2000) Chemistry, pharmacology and pharmacokinetics of N, N', N" -triethylenethiophosphoramide (ThioTEPA). Cancer Treat Rev 26:257–268

Marchesi F et al (2007) Triazene compounds: mechanism of action and related DNA repair systems. Pharmacol Res 56:275–287

Maring JG, Groen HJM, Wachters FM, Uges DRA, de Vries EGE (2005) Genetic factors influencing pyrimidine-antagonist chemotherapy. Pharmacogenomics J 5:226–243

Matherly L, Hou Z, Deng Y (2007) Human reduced folate carrier: translation of basic biology to cancer etiology and therapy. Cancer Metastasis Rev 26:111–128

McClay EF, Mastrangelo MJ, Berd D, Bellet RE (1992) Effective combination chemo/hormonal therapy for malignant melanoma: experience with three consecutive trials. Int J Cancer 50:553–556

McDermott DF et al (2000) A phase II pilot trial of concurrent biochemotherapy with cisplatin, vinblastine, dacarbazine, interleukin 2, and interferon α-2B in patients with metastatic melanoma. Clin Cancer Res 6:2201–2208

Metro G, Mottolese M, Fabi A (2008) HER-2-positive metastatic breast cancer: trastuzumab and beyond. Expert Opin Pharmacother 9:2583–2601

Middleton MR et al (2000) Randomized phase III study of temozolomide versus dacarbazine in the treatment of patients with advanced metastatic malignant melanoma. J Clin Oncol18:158

Miles D (2008) Capecitabine and docetaxel in the treatment of metastatic breast cancer: combination, sequence or single agent? Eur J Cancer Suppl 6:5–8
Miller K (2010) A phase Ib/II trial of trastuzumab-DM1 (T-DM1) with pertuzumab (P) for women with HER2-positive, locally advanced or metastatic breast cancer (BC) who were previously treated with trastuzumab (T). J Clin Oncol 28:15s
Miller KD, Sledge GW (1999) The role of chemotherapy for metastatic breast cancer. Hematol Oncol Clin North Am 13:415–434
Miller, KD et al (2005) Randomized phase III trial of capecitabine compared with bevacizumab plus capecitabine in patients with previously treated metastatic breast cancer. J Clin Oncol 23:792–799
Mitchell, MS et al (2007) Randomized Trial of an allogeneic melanoma lysate vaccine with low-dose interferon alfa-2b compared with high-dose interferon alfa-2b for resected stage III cutaneous melanoma. J Clin Oncol 25:2078–2085
Nabholtz J-M et al (1999) Prospective randomized trial of docetaxel versus mitomycin plus vinblastine in patients with metastatic breast cancer progressing despite previous anthracycline-containing chemotherapy. J Clin Oncol 17:1413
Nabholtz JM et al (2000) Docetaxel (Taxotere) in combination with anthracyclines in the treatment of breast cancer. Semin Oncol 27:11–18
O'Shaughnessy J et al (2002) Superior survival with capecitabine plus docetaxel combination therapy in anthracycline-pretreated patients with advanced breast cancer: phase III trial results. J Clin Oncol 20:2812–2823
O'Toole SA., Selinger CI, Millar EK, Lum T, Beith JM (2011) Molecular assays in breast cancer pathology. Pathology 43:116–127
Olszewski U, Hamilton G (2010) A better platinum-based anticancer drug yet to come? Anticancer Agents Med Chem 10:293–301
Ott PA et al (2010) A phase II trial of the epothilone B analog ixabepilone (BMS-247550) in patients with metastatic melanoma. PLoS One 5:e8714
Pacilio C et al (2006) Is epirubicin effective in first-line chemotherapy of metastatic breast cancer (MBC) after an epirubicin-containing adjuvant treatment? A single centre phase III trial. Br J Cancer 94:1233–1236
Perou CM et al (2000) Molecular portraits of human breast tumours. Nature 406:747–752
Petrelli F, Borgonovo K, Cabiddu M, Ghilardi M, Barni S (2011) Neoadjuvant chemotherapy and concomitant trastuzumab in breast cancer: a pooled analysis of two randomized trials. Anticancer Drugs 22:128–135
Pyrhonen S, Hahka-Kemppinen M, Muhonen TA (1992) promising interferon plus four-drug chemotherapy regimen for metastatic melanoma. J Clin Oncol 10:1919–1926
Razis ED, Fountzilas G (2001) Paclitaxel: Epirubicin in metastatic breast cancer—a review. Ann Oncol 12:593–598
Ribas A et al (2009) Dendritic cell vaccination combined with CTLA4 blockade in patients with metastatic melanoma. Clin Cancer Res 15:6267–6276
Rivera E et al (2003) Phase II study of pegylated liposomal doxorubicin in combination with gemcitabine in patients with metastatic breast cancer. J Clin Oncol 21:3249–3254
Rixe O et al (1995) Fotemustine, dacarbazine, vindesine combination chemotherapy in advanced malignant melanoma: a phase II study of 43 patients. Melanoma Res 5:419–424
Rosenberg SA et al (1993) Prospective randomized trial of high-dose interleukin-2 alone or in conjunction with lymphokine-activated killer cells for the treatment of patients with advanced cancer. J Natl Cancer Inst 85:622–632
Rosenberg SA et al (1999) Prospective randomized trial of the treatment of patients with metastatic melanoma using chemotherapy with cisplatin, dacarbazine, and tamoxifen alone or in combination with interleukin-2 and interferon alfa-2b. J Clin Oncol 17:968
Rusthoven JJ (1998) The evidence for tamoxifen and chemotherapy as treatment for metastatic melanoma. Eur J Cancer 34(Suppl 3):S31–36

Sawaki M et al (2004) Paclitaxel administered weekly in patients with docetaxel-resistant metastatic breast cancer: a single-center study. Tumori 90:36–39

Schilcher RB, Wessels M, Niederle N, Seeber S, Schmidt CG (1984) Phase II evaluation of fractionated low and single high dose cisplatin in various tumors. J Cancer Res Clin Oncol 107:57–60

Schultz MZ, Buzaid AC, Poo WJ (1997) A phase II study of interferon-alpha 2b with dacarbazine, carmustine, cisplatin and tamoxifen in metastatic melanoma. Melanoma Res 7:147–151

Schwartzentruber DJ, D Lawson, J Richards, RM Conry, D Miller, J Triesman, F Gailani, LB Riley, D Vena, P Hwu (2009) A phase III multi-institutional randomized study of immunization with the gp100:209–217(210M) peptide followed by high-dose IL-2 compared with high-dose IL-2 alone in patients with metastatic melanoma. J Clin Oncol 27:18s

Seetharamu N, Ott PA, Pavlick AC (2009) Novel therapeutics for melanoma. Expert Rev Anticancer Ther 9:839–849

Seidman AD et al (1995) Paclitaxel as second and subsequent therapy for metastatic breast cancer: activity independent of prior anthracycline response. J Clin Oncol 13:1152–1159

Senzer NN et al. (2009) Phase II clinical trial of a granulocyte-macrophage colony-stimulating factor–encoding, second-generation oncolytic herpesvirus in patients with unresectable metastatic melanoma. J Clin Oncol 27:5763–5771

Serrone L, Zeuli M, Sega FM Cognetti F (2000) Dacarbazine-based chemotherapy for metastatic melanoma: thirty-year experience overview. J Exp Clin Cancer Res 19:21–34

Sessa C, Valota O, Geroni C (2007) Ongoing phase I and II studies of novel anthracyclines. Cardiovasc Toxicol 7:75–79

Slamon DJ et al (2001) Use of chemotherapy plus a monoclonal antibody against HER2 for metastatic breast cancer that overexpresses HER2. N Engl J Med 344:783–792

Soto C (2006) Capecitabine (X) and taxanes in patients (pts) with anthracycline-pretreated metastatic breast cancer (MBC): sequential vs. combined therapy results from a MOSG randomized phase III trial. J Clin Oncol 24(18S):570 (June 20 Supplement)

Sparano JA (ed) (2002) Cytotoxic therapy and other nonhormonal approaches for the treatment of metastatic breast cancer. (Marcel Dekker, New York), pp 417–457

Sparano JA et al (1993) Randomized phase III trial of treatment with high-dose interleukin-2 either alone or in combination with interferon alfa-2a in patients with advanced melanoma. J Clin Oncol 11:1969–1977

Su YB et al (2004) Selective CD4 + Lymphopenia in melanoma patients treated with temozolomide: a toxicity with therapeutic implications. J Clin Oncol 22:610–616

Szyf M, Seley K, Mosley S (2005) Purine analogues and their role in methylation and cancer chemotherapy. In DNA methylation and cancer therapy. Springer, US, pp 178–186

Testori A et al (2008) Phase III comparison of vitespen, an autologous tumor-derived heat shock protein gp96 peptide complex vaccine, with physician's choice of treatment for stage IV melanoma: the C-100–21 Study Group. J Clin Oncol 26:955–962

Trudeau ME, Provencher L, Panasci L, Yelle L, Latreille J, Vandenberg T, Rayson D, Rodgers A, Pouliot J (2009) Phase II multicenter trial of anthracycline rechallenge with pegylated liposomal doxorubicin plus cyclophosphamide for first-line therapy of metastatic breast cancer previously treated with adjuvant anthracyclines. J Clin Oncol 27(35):5906–5910

Valero V et al (1998) A phase II study of docetaxel in patients with paclitaxel-resistant metastatic breast cancer. J Clin Oncol 16:3362–3368

Verma S, Clemons M (2007) First-line treatment options for patients with HER-2 negative metastatic breast cancer: the impact of modern adjuvant chemotherapy. Oncologist 12:785–797

Verma S et al (2007) Survival differences observed in metastatic breast cancer patients treated with capecitabine when compared with vinorelbine after pretreatment with anthracycline and taxane. Am J Clin Oncol 30:297–302

Verma S et al (2011) In the end what matters most? A review of clinical endpoints in advanced breast cancer. Oncologist 16:25–35

Wolchok JD et al (2003) Phase I trial of high dose paracetamol and carmustine in patients with metastatic melanoma. Melanoma Res 13:189–196

Wolchok JD et al (2010) Ipilimumab monotherapy in patients with pretreated advanced melanoma: a randomised, double-blind, multicentre, phase 2, dose-ranging study. Lancet Oncol 11:155–164

Wood AJJ, Rowinsky EK, Donehower RC (1995) Paclitaxel (Taxol). N Engl J Med 332:1004–1014

Wood CG, Mulders P (2009) Vitespen: a preclinical and clinical review. Future Oncol 5:763–774

Yeh I-T, Mies C (2008) Application of Immunohistochemistry to Breast Lesions. Arch Pathol Lab Med 132:349–358

Young AM, Marsden J, Goodman A, Burton A, Dunn JA (2001) Prospective randomized comparison of dacarbazine (DTIC) versus dtic plus interferon-alpha (IFN-[alpha]) in metastatic melanoma. Clin Oncol 13:458–465

Zielinski C, Gralow J, Martin M (2010) Optimising the dose of capecitabine in metastatic breast cancer: confused, clarified or confirmed? Ann Oncol 21(11):2145–2152

Chapter 24
Integrating Chemotherapy to Surgery: Novel Approaches in Regionally Aggressive Cancer Metastasis

Ari Nareg Meguerditchian, Sarkis H. Meterissian and Marissa Grace Ponzo

The focus of this chapter is on exciting new treatment approaches that integrate surgery and directed chemotherapy in the management of patients with metastatic disease outside of classical visceral organs such as the lungs, liver, brain and bones. Two specific clinical situations will be addressed: peritoneal surface carcinomatosis, in-transit extremity recurrence.

24.1 Peritoneal Surface Disease

24.1.1 Introduction

Rather than being an inert virtual space in the abdominal cavity, the peritoneum is an entity with its own anatomy and physiology (Healy and Reznek 1998). These two factors explain the multi-focal and diffuse pattern of metastasis unique to this organ (Sugarbaker 1999).

Peritoneal carcinomatosis represents the secondary extension of a cancer to the peritoneal lining. It is most often seen in the context of gastro-intestinal malignancies, such as colorectal and gastric cancers (Shen et al. 2009b). It can also occur with ovarian carcinoma (Chua et al. 2009a). This type of spread occurs when the tumor invades through the full thickness of the visceral wall or secondary to neoplastic emboli and iatrogenic contamination of the surgical field (Koppe et al. 2006). It is

A. N. Meguerditchian (✉)
Department of Oncology & Surgery, Faculty of Medicine,
McGill University Health Center, McGill University, Montreal, QC, Canada
e-mail: ari.meguerditchian@muhc.mcgill.ca

S. H. Meterissian
Department of Oncology & Surgery, McGill University Health Center,
McGill University, Montreal, QC, Canada

M. G. Ponzo
McGill University, Montreal, QC, Canada

J. V. Burnier, M. N. Burnier, Jr. (eds.), *Experimental and Clinical Metastasis*,
DOI 10.1007/978-1-4614-3685-0_24,

Table 24.1 Common causes of carcinomatosis, incidence and survival

Primary cancer	Incidence (cases/year)	Median survival (in months)
Colorectal	130,000	5.2
Gastric	22,000	3.1
Ovarian	27,000	36
Mesothelioma	1,500	12–17
Appendiceal	500	Not available

estimated that up to 10 % of patients with colorectal cancer present with peritoneal dissemination at the time of initial diagnosis (Glockzin et al. 2009). In addition, about 20 % of patients present with metachronous peritoneal disease during their follow up (Jayne et al. 2002). A proportion of these patients will have disease confined to the peritoneal cavity. Peritoneal carcinomatosis has traditionally been associated with a dismal prognosis (Table 24.1) (Sterward et al. 2005).

In the Evocape 1 prospective study, the mean and median survivals for patients with carcinomatosis were 6.0 and 3.1 months respectively (Sadeghi et al. 2000). More recently, Jayne et al. (2002) have reported similar numbers from a retrospective series of 3,019 patients. In addition, most patients suffer from distressing symptoms such as pain and obstruction.

The management of metastasis to the peritoneal surface has been a challenge. Systemic chemotherapy is largely ineffective, due to limited penetration (Stewart et al. 2009) and conventional surgery is mainly directed at symptom relief through stomas and venting/feeding tubes. However, the localized nature of peritoneal metastasis makes the development of regionally aggressive treatments appealing. Cytoreductive surgery (CS) combined with hyperthermic intraperitoneal chemotherapy (HIPEC) has recently emerged as a novel approach to successfully combine aggressive surgical therapy to directly applied cytotoxic therapy.

24.1.2 Regional Therapy

Spatt et al. first described a system to deliver chemotherapy directly into the peritoneum (where the disease is located) in 1980 (Spratt et al. 1980a, b). Since then, the concept of multimodal regional therapy for the management of peritoneal surface malignancies has evolved significantly. In its current form, it consists of the following three essential components:

- Maximal surgical cytoreduction
- Administration of intraperitoneal chemotherapy: intra-operative or early post-operative (EPIC)
- Addition of hyperthermia.

24.1.2.1 Maximal Surgical Cytoreduction

A.1) Intra-operative disease scoring Classically, the surgeon will begin with a thorough examination of the abdomen. The extent of disease spread to the peritoneum

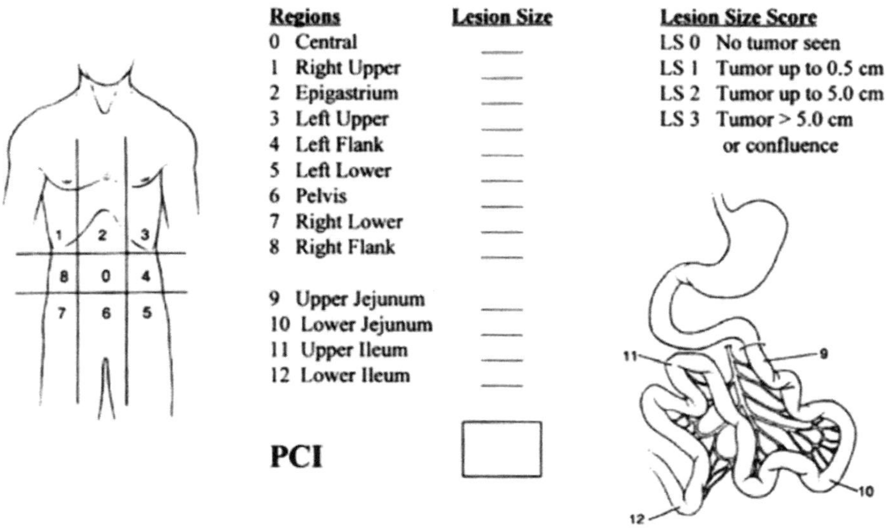

Fig. 24.1 Peritoneal carcinomatosis index (PCI). The abdomen is divided into 13 regions. Lesions are scored in size (0–3). Summation is a numerical score between 1 and 39. (Adapted from Harmon and Sugarbaker 2005)

is assessed and scored. Particular attention is paid to sites and structures that are at high risk of harboring metastatic disease. These include: the incision site, the left and right hemidiaphragm, the falciform ligament, the lesser omentum, the greater omentum, the lesser cavity, the mesentery of the small bowel, the anastomotic site, the paracolic gutters and the pelvic inlet (at the level of the anterior and posterior reflection of the peritoneum near the pelvic brim).

Intraoperative staging of the extent of tumor burden is a critical component of the procedure. There are a few systems to quantitate peritoneal carcinomatosis at surgery. Gilly's classification consists of four groups (Gilly et al. 1999; Porcheron et al. 2000; Glehen et al. 2004):

- Stage I: nodules < 5 mm and localized to one part of the abdomen;
- Stage II: nodules < 5 mm diffuse to the whole abdomen;
- Stage III: nodules 5–2 cm;
- Stage IV: tumor deposits > 2 cm.

The Japanese Society for Gastric Cancer has generated its own classification for peritoneal disease originating from a gastric primary which has been correlated with survival in many studies (Fujimoto et al. 1997; Ouchi et al. 1998; Hagiwarw et al. 1999). Sugarbaker's scoring system, the Peritoneal Cancer Index (PCI) seems to have a more widespread acceptance in North America (Jacquet and Sugarbaker 1996). Described in (Fig. 24.1) (Jacquet and Sugarbaker 1996; Gilly et al. 1994; Harmon and Sugarbaker 2005), the PCI is based on dividing the abdomen and pelvis into 13 regions. In each one, the size of the largest lesion is graded from 0 to 3. These are then summated to generate a numerical score between 1 and 39. The PCI has been shown to be both predictive of resectability and survival (Chereau et al. 2010).

Table 24.2 Organs resected during cyotreductive surgery

Organ	Frequency (%)
Small bowel	58
Omentum	55
Colon	31
Ovary	18
Spleen	9
Gallbladder	9
Uterus	7
Rectum	7
Appendix	5
Kidney	5
Liver	5
Diaphragm	4
Pancreas	4
Bladder	2
Lung	2
Stomach	2

A.2) Resection The goal of cytoreduction is to remove all gross disease within the abdominal cavity, as well as involved organs and peritoneum. Improved surgical techniques and anesthetic monitoring allow for an aggressive approach with the goal of complete cytoreduction. This often results in multivisceral resections (Table 24.2) (Chereau et al. 2010).

In a series of 121 patients with peritoneal carcinomatosis treated with cytoreductive surgery and intraperitoneal chemotherapy, the most frequently sacrificed organs included the small bowel and colon (Shen et al. 2008). Routine omentectomy is also performed. Any tumor adherent or invasive to vital structures that cannot be safely resected should be removed using an ultrasonic surgical aspirator (CUSA, Valleylab, Boulder CO). The completeness of resection is graded using the following classification (Stewart et al. 2009; Shen et al. 2009a):

- R0: complete removal of all visible tumor and negative cytology or microscopic margins;
- R1: complete removal of all visible tumor and positive cytology or microscopic margins;
- R2a: minimal residual tumor, nodule(s) ≤ 0.5 cm;
- R2b: gross residual tumor, nodule > 0.5 cm but ≤ 2 cm;
- R2c: extensive disease remaining, nodules > 2 cm.

Some surgeons prefer using the completion of cytoreduction (CC) score:

- CC-0: no residual disease;
- CC-1: $\leq$0.25 cm residual disease;
- CC-2: 0.25–2.5 cm residual disease;
- CC-3: ≥ 2.5 cm residual disease.

Aggressive surgical cytoreduction is critical in the management of peritoneal surface malignancies, as even the most optimal chemotherapy perfusion will penetrate only a few millimeters. The importance of achieving maximal cytoreduction cannot be

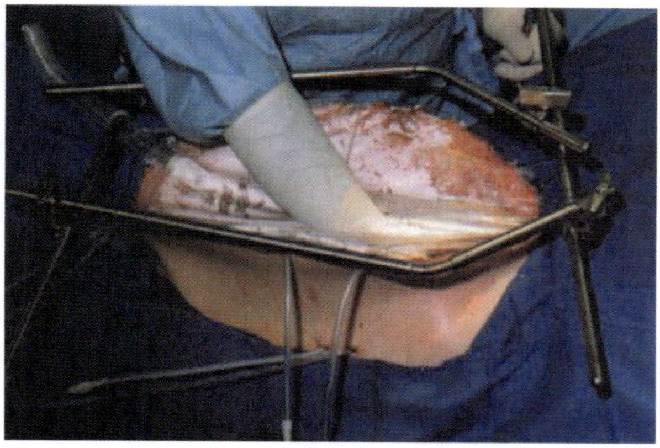

Fig. 24.2 Coliseum technique. (Adapted with permission from Glehen et al. 2008)

underestimated (Yan et al. 2006). Shen et al. (2008), report a 36 % difference in 5-year survival rates between an R0 resection and an R2c resection. Their findings are echoed by Glenhen's 506 patients multicenter study (Glehen et al. 2004).

24.1.2.2 Intraperitoneal Chemotherapy Perfusion

The goal of intraperitoneal chemoperfusion is to expose the entire peritoneal surface to antineoplastic agents. Direct tumor absorption of drugs reaches a maximum of only 5 mm beneath tissue surface (Los et al. 1991), highlighting the importance of maximal cytoreduction. Peritoneal chemotherapy is administered intraoperatively (HIPEC), although some also advocate the use of early post-operative intraperitoneal chemotherapy (EPIC) as well.

B.1) Hyperthermic intraperitoneal chemotherapy (HIPEC) HIPEC can be performed via an open or closed technique. The open technique, also known as the "Coliseum technique", consists of leaving the abdominal cavity open. A Silastic sheet can be sutured to the skin over a Thompson retractor, suspending the abdominal wall and creating a coliseum-like container for the chemoperfusate (Fig. 24.2) (Glehen et al. 2008).

There are several advantages and disadvantages of this approach (Table 24.3) (Shen et al. 2009b).

In the closed technique, once maximal cytoreduction is completed, inflow and outflow catheters are placed into the abdominal cavity. The former are positioned near the diaphragmatic recess whereas the later are secured at the pelvic inlet (Fig. 24.3) (Shen et al. 2008). Temperature probes are placed in the catheters, and the abdominal wall is closed temporarily. A perfusion circuit is established with Ringer's Lactate and once a flow of 600–900 mL/min is achieved using a roller pump, the chemotherapeutic agent is added. The temperature probes allow constant temperature monitoring. Chemotherapy is not instilled until a minimum of 40°C has been reached and a heat exchanger is used to maintain such a target temperature. The abdomen is gently massaged during the 90–120 min of perfusion.

Table 24.3 Coliseum technique: advantages and disadvantages

Advantages	Disadvantages
Optimal thermal homogeneity	Heat dissipation
Maximal spatial diffusion, as the perfusate is manually spread in the abdominal cavity	Potential exposure of the operating room personnel to toxic chemotherapy

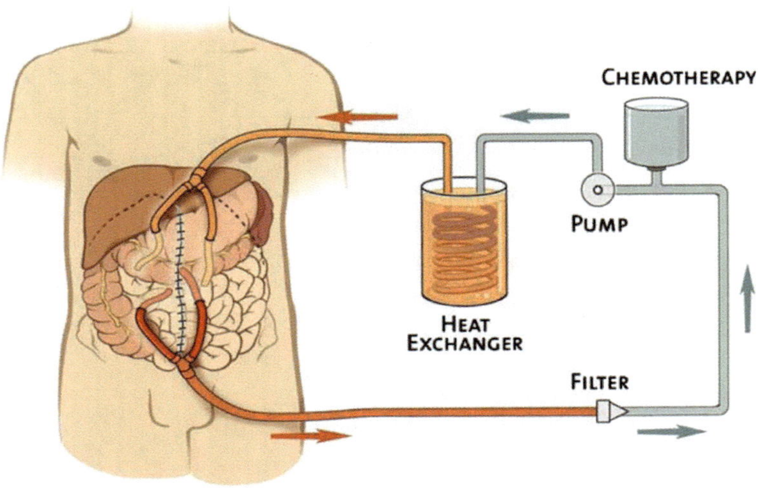

Fig. 24.3 Closed technique: schematic of intraperitoneal hyperthermic chemotherapy setup (closed technique). (Adapted with permission from Shen et al. 2008)

Advocates of the closed technique note the following advantages (Shen et al. 2009b; Esquis et al. 2006):

- Minimized chemotherapy exposure to operating room personnel
- Deeper penetration of agents into tissue due to increased intra-abdominal pressure;
- More stable temperature during the length of the treatment
- The main disadvantage is the need for additional equipment and personnel to manage to heat exchanger roller pump. No prospective trial has validated the superiority of one technique over the other.

The most frequently used chemotherapeutic agent for HIPEC is Mitomycin C, with a variety of dosages from 10–120 mg/m^2 reported (Chua et al. 2009e). Usually, the total dose of Mitomycin C does not exceed 40 mg. Other agents and combinations that are gaining increased popularity include cisplatin + mitomycin C, cisplatin + doxorubicin or cisplatin alone. (Chua et al. 2009e; Yan et al. 2009; Kerscher et al. 2010; Elias et al. 2010; Cohen et al. 2010).

B.2) Early post-operative intraperitoneal chemotherapy (EPIC) In this variation, the surgical procedure ends with the placement of Tenckhoff catheters after maximal cytoreduction. Chemotherapy is then administered into the peritoneal cavity during days 1–5 of the post-operative period, classically consisting of Fluorouracil at 15 mg/kg/day in 1 L of dialysis solution (Glehen et al. 2004). The main argument against EPIC is the unevenness of drug distribution, due to early postoperative adhesions. As demonstrated by Jacquet et al. (1995), fibrin deposits decrease tumor cell exposure to chemotherapy. In addition, there are non-negligible complications related to intra-abdominal catheters (Topuz et al. 1998). This issue of complications related to postoperative peritoneal access devices has also been noted in the management of carcinomatosis of ovarian origin (Robindon and Beyer 2010). Nevertheless, there has never been a study comparing HIPEC to EPIC. Some surgeons proceed to EPIC after completing HIPEC and not encountering serious complications. Ultimately, the lack of clear consensus as to the value of EPIC leaves the decision to use this technique to the surgeon's preference (Esquivel et al. 2007).

B.3) Pharmacology of intraperitoneal (IP) chemotherapy The anatomic and physiologic particularities of the peritoneum have been used for treatment delivery for a long time. In fact, the first report of IP drug administration was in 1744. However, the use of IP chemotherapy for the management of cancer dates back to 1955, following the discovery of the antineoplastic potential of nitrogen mustard (Weisberger et al. 1955). The successful use of IP chemotherapy in the management of cancer metastasis must satisfy three basic conditions:

- Providing high local drug concentration for a significant duration
- Ensuring adequate penetration into the tumor
- Targeting specifically tumor cells.

As described initially by Dedrick and collegues (1978), the existence of a peritoneal-plasma barrier consisting of the mesothelium and underlying submesothelial tissue defines the pharmacokinetic rationale for IP chemotherapy administration (Jones et al. 1978). The presence of this barrier results in a peritoneal drug clearance that is much slower than the plasma clearance, allowing IP drug concentrations higher than systemic concentrations (Markman 2008). Within this barrier, the main element delaying transperitoneal passage is the glycocalyx of the endothelial lining of the peritoneal microvascular network (Flessner 2008). Since the peritoneum extensively covers visceral surfaces, the transfer of drugs from peritoneal to vascular compartments occurs principally through the portal circulation (Ceelen and Flessner 2010).

High concentrations of IP chemotherapy help overcome the specific biological features of IP cancer cells that make them a challenging therapeutic target. First, peritoneal carcinomatosis follows the principles of Gompertzian cellular kinetics: tumor growth is initially exponential, however, as the cancer enlarges, its blood supply and growth slowdown, and a larger proportion of cells enter a non-proliferative phase which makes them less responsive to antineoplastic agents (Shen et al. 2009b; Simpson-Herren 1976). Second, peritoneal cancer deposits are characterized by pronounced hypoxia and a poorly developed vasculature that lacks functional lymphatics (Li et al. 2007; Jain 2001a; Jain 2001b), making drug penetration into tumor tissue a major problem. Finally, the high interstitial pressure within tumor deposits further decreases tumor penetration (Bajaj and Yeo 2010; Heldin et al. 2004). Achieving high

IP drug concentrations is even more critical when using molecules such as alkylating agents and platinum derivatives, which are cell-cycle independent.

Significant duration to drug exposure is another critical aspect of IP therapy success. Dedrick demonstrated that the regional pharmacokinetic advantage of IP chemotherapy is inversely proportional to its peritoneal clearance. This can be summarized by the ratio of the area under the concentration versus time curve (AUC) in peritoneal perfusate versus plasma (Dedrick 1985). This notion is particularly important in prolonged IP chemotherapy administration models such as EPIC. Experiments at preventing rapid IP chemotherapy clearance are currently being conducted using particulate formations of varying sizes, hydrogel-base systems and lipid encapsulation (Lu et al. 2008; Tsai et al. 2007; Yeo et al. 2007; Gelderblom et al. 2002).

Key Points

- The main element delaying drug transperitoneal passage is the glycocalyx of the endothelial lining of the peritoneal microvascular network.
- The transfer of drugs from peritoneal to vascular compartments occurs principally through the portal circulation.
- Non-proliferative phase of IP cancer cells makes them less responsive to antineoplastic agents.
- Peritoneal cancer deposits are characterized by pronounced hypoxia and an underdeveloped vasculature that lacks functional lymphatics, resulting in poor drug penetration.
- High interstitial pressure within tumor deposits decreases tumor drug penetration.
- Regional pharmacokinetic advantage of IP chemotherapy is inversely proportional to its peritoneal clearance.

24.1.3 Morbidity and Mortality

Deaths and complications HIPEC is a technically involved procedure, requiring multiple resections and exposure to high doses of cytotoxic therapy in patients otherwise weakened by recurrent disease and multiple other forms of treatment. These issues are clearly reflected in the non-negligible morbidity and mortality rates associated to the procedure (Ahmad et al. 2004). In a review of case series reported from 24 institutions performing HIPEC, Chua et al noted perioperative mortality rates between 0 and 17 % (Chua et al. 2009e). Most contemporary series report similar treatment-related death rates (Shen et al. 2009a; Elias et al. 2010). Common causes of multi-organ system failure leading to death within 30 days of the procedure include:

- Sepsis (frequently from bowel perforation or anastomotic leakage)
- Marrow failure
- Respiratory failure due to pulmonary embolus or pneumonia

Table 24.4 Complication grading scale

Grade	Definition
I	Any minor derivation from normal post-op course
II	Requires pharmacologic intervention
III	Requires surgical, endoscopic, radiologic intervention
IIIa	Without general anesthesia
IIIb	Under general anesthesia
IV	Life-threatening complication with ICU stay
IVa	Single-organ dysfunction
IVb	Multi-organ dysfunction
V	Death

- Cardiac failure
- Renal failure
- Factors predicting mortality include (Shen et al. 2003)
- Presence of ascites
- Poor performance status
- Bowel obstruction.

Morbidity related to HIPEC can be classified according to the scale proposed in Table 24.4 (Shen et al. 2008; Dindo et al. 2004). The overall perioperative complication rate is close to 40 % (Shen et al. 2009a; Smeenk et al. 2006; Verwaal et al. 2004), although grade III/ IV toxicity rates as high as 52 % have been reported (Elias et al. 2007; Smeenk et al. 2007). Up to 23 % of patients require reoperation (Chua et al. 2009e; Elias et al. 2007; Schmidt et al. 2005; Helm et al. 2007).

The most frequently occurring complications that are related to surgery and chemotherapy are presented in (Table 24.5) (Piso et al. 2009; Glockzin et al. 2009). Several groups have noted that the incidence of post-operative complications is related to (Stephens et al. 1999):

- Carcinomatosis stage
- Duration of operation (>7 h)
- Number of anastomoses
- Location of anastomoses (colon)
- Number of peritonectomy procedures.

It is important to note that morbidity and mortality are also related to the learning curve (Yan et al. 2007a). Not only does the toxicity of the treatment itself decrease over time, but also the outcome of the complications improve as well (Moran et al. 2006). A recent study reported the feasibility of HIPEC in a community hospital setting with equivalent morbidity and mortality rates (Kerscher et al. 2010).

Table 24.5 Frequently observed complications of IP therapy

Surgical complications	Chemotherapy complications
Gastrointestinal obstruction (dynamic or mechanical)	Leucopenia
Anastomotic leakage or intestinal perforation	Anemia
Wound infection	Thrombopenia
Bleeding or thromboemboli	Heart, liver and renal toxicity

Quality of life McQuellon et al have reported extensively on the quality of life of patients undergoing HIPEC. Using the FACT-C scale as a measuring instrument, they have shown a significant initial decrease in overall wellness, with a sustained subsequent increase at 3, 6 and 12 months follow up. In fact, most patients in their series returned to baseline or better levels of functioning within 3 months of treatment. At 12 months, 74 % of patients resumed over 50 % of their normal activities. Interestingly, 38 % of patients had depressive symptoms at baseline and 29 % persisted at 1 year. At 3 years, no limitations on moderate activity were reported by 94 % of surviving patients. It can be argued that while a significant decrease in the quality of life occurs early on, an acceptable quality of life can be reached by 6–12 months (McQuellon et al. 2001, 2003, 2007, 2008). The main challenges impacting quality of life in patients undergoing this form of invasive treatment include the presence of ostomies, fatigue, insomnia, and pain (Helm et al. 2007).

Patient Selection The most common entities for HIPEC treatment are colorectal cancer, gastric cancer; ovarian cancer; peritoneal mesothelioma ; and appendiceal cancer (Stewart et al. 2005). Proper patient selection is an important component of treatment success.

The following criteria have been proposed (Shen et al. 2009b; Yan et al. 2007b):

- No significant cardiopulmonary disease. In terms of comorbidities, an ECOG performance score of 0 or 1 has been associated to better survival than a score of 2 or 3. Additionally, patients with bowel obstruction or malignant ascites represent poor candidates for HIPEC (Sugarbaker 1995);
- No evidence of extra-abdominal disease and peritoneal disease should be
- Peritoneal disease potentially completely resectable;
- Absence of bulk retroperitoneal disease.

Liver metastases were initially viewed as contraindications to HIPEC. However, there are more and more reports of a similar overall survival for patients with an isolated liver metastasis undergoing HIPEC (Varban et al. 2009; Elias et al. 2010). In a recent consensus statement on HIPEC up to three small, resectable hepatic metastases are not considered a contraindication.

Modern imaging techniques are practical in preventing unwarranted laparotomies. Nevertheless, CT scanning has limited sensitivity in assessing non-visceral small volume peritoneal disease (de Bree et al. 2004). The same has been shown for PET scan imaging for peritoneal surface disease (Sobhani et al. 2008). Interestingly, a small prospective study showed a more accurate pre-operative detection rate for small volume peritoneal disease with the use of MRI with dilute oral barium and IV gadolinium (Low et al. 1997).

The peritoneal surface disease severity score (PSDS) is a recently developed tool that may help in minimizing overtreatment with aggressive multimodality therapy (Pelz et al. 2009). It takes into account clinical symptoms, extent of carcinomatosis and primary tumor histology. Patients are then staged from I to IV, based on the summation of their scores. Chua et al have shown that even in the context of maximal cytoreduction and completed intraperitoneal chemotherapy, patients who were PSDS stage IV had a median survival of 7 months (Chua et al. 2009c).

Outcomes The Evocape study defined the average survival of patients with carcinomatosis against which all new therapeutic approaches are compared (Sadeghi et al. 2000). In 2003 Vic Verwaal and colleagues published a trial on the use of maximal cytoreduction and intraperitoneal chemotherapy. Patients were treated either with systemic therapy alone or with systemic therapy plus HIPEC. While often criticized, this paper has the unique advantage of being the only randomized trial assessing this novel yet morbid form of treatment. When compared with the standard IV chemotherapy alone, patients having received HIPEC lived twice as long, with a median survival of 22.3 months instead of 12.6 months ($p = 0.032$). The authors have now published their 8 year follow up data, demonstrating that cytoreduction followed by HIPEC does significantly add survival time up to (45 %) 5 year survival rate in a selected group of patients (Verwaal et al. 2008). While not as strong as a randomized trial, two other publications reporting outcomes are worth mentioning. In a retrospective multicentric study from France, Elias et al. reported an overall median survival of 30.1 months in a group of 523 patients, with a five-year overall and disease free survivals of 27 and 10 % respectively. In a different multicenter retrospective trial with 506 patients Glehen et al. (2004) reported at a median follow up of 53 months a median survival of 32.4 months for patients in whom complete cytoreductive surgery was performed. Factors associated with a favorable outcome included, complete cytoreduction, limited carcinomatosis, absence of invaded lymph nodes and use of adjuvant chemotherapy (Elias et al. 2010). Factors independently associated with a worse outcome were incomplete of cytoreduction, presence of bowel obstruction, malignant ascites and poor histological differentiation (Glehen et al. 2004; Shen et al. 2008).

24.1.3.1 Hyperthermia

The addition of hyperthermia to IP chemotherapy to maximize its efficacy was first proposed by Spratt (1980a). The rationale for this is based on the thermal enhancement of the cytotoxicity of drugs such as alkylating agents and platinum compounds (Cho et al. 2008; Issels 2008). The following benefits have been attributed to moderate hyperthermia:

- Increased tumor blood supply and oxygenation (Sun et al. 2008);
- Enhanced drug penetration into tumors and consequent increase in intratumoral drug concentration (Los et al. 1991; Jacquet et al. 1998; Pestieau et al. 2001)
- Enhanced drug avidity and chemosensitivity through increased cellular accumulation and alteration of DNA damage repair capacity (Teicher et al. 1981; Watanabe et al. 1992).

Drugs for which thermal enhancement has been documented are detailed in (Table 24.6) (Ceelen and Flessner 2010). Current consensus is that a constant intraperitoneal temperature of 39–40°C should be achieved (Esquivel et al. 2007). This explains the use of a recirculating perfusion circuit during intraoperative IP chemoperfusion.

Table 24.6 Drug penetration into peritoneum. (Ceelen and Flessner 2010)

Drug	Drug penetration distance (mm)	Thermal enhancement
Alkylating agents		
Mitomycin	2	+
Platinum compounds		
Cisplatin	1–3	+
Carboplatin	0.5	+
Oxaliplatin	1–2	+
Taxanes		
Paclitaxel	> 80 cell layers	Not studied
Docetaxel	Unknown	+
Antimetabolites		
5-fluorouracil	0.2	–

24.1.4 Summary

Cancer recurrence in the form of peritoneal carcinomatosis is an aggressive and challenging disease. In addition to significantly shortening survival, carcinomatosis is associated with debilitating symptoms such as obstruction and pain. Maximal cytoreduction and intraperitoneal chemotherapy is associated with improved survival, however, this comes at the cost of a high rate of complications and prolonged recovery. As this novel approach in addressing peritoneal metastases evolves, a greater degree of standardization of eligibility criteria, technical steps and chemotherapy administration modes will emerge. In addition, we can expect to see an expansion of its indication to other types of diseases such as advanced small bowel malignancies (Chua et al. 2009d) and thorax (Chua et al. 2009b).

24.2 In-transit Disease of the Extremities

24.2.1 Introduction

More than half of the newly diagnosed cases of melanoma occur in the extremities. Close to 40 % of these patients will present with loco-regional recurrence. From this group, about 10 % will recur between the primary tumor site and the regional lymph nodes (Koops et al. 1998; Pawlik et al. 2005; Kretschmer et al. 2006). These so-called "in-transit metastases" are defined by the American Joint Committee on Cancer (AJCC) as any dermal or sub-dermal metastases that are more than 2 cm from the primary lesion, but not beyond the regional lymph node basin (Balch et al. 2001). In a review of 1,000 patients, 5 % were localized to the head and neck, 8 % to the upper extremities, 9 % to the trunk, and 19 % to the lower extremities (Calabro et al. 1989). Other studies confirm that in-transit melanoma is particularly common to the lower extremities (Pawlik et al. 2005; Calabro et al. 1989; Wong et al. 1990).

According to the seventh edition of the AJCC cancer staging system, in-transit metastases are classified as N2c or N3 (depending on the presence of lymph node disease) both of which correspond to Stage III and consequently potentially salvageable disease. Five-year survival rates for these patients range between 30 and 50 % (Edge et al. 2010). Additionally, at least half of them are expected to survive 2 years without evidence of distant metastases, making curative treatment of these lesions a reasonable objective (Balch et al. 1998). More importantly, these lesions can result in significant morbidity, such as bleeding, ulceration, infection, pain and psychological distress.

Unfortunately, most non-surgical approaches for treating in-transit disease have failed, including radiation, chemotherapy, immunotherapy and injections. From a surgical perspective, the number and distribution of these lesions often preclude excision and closure, and while amputation provides a definitive solution its impact on patient functionality makes it a prohibitive choice.

24.2.2 Isolated Limb Perfusion

A) A historical perspective ILP was first described by Creech and Krementz at the Charity Hospital in New Orleans in 1958 (Creech et al. 1958). Chemotherapy had already been in use for over 15 years at that time to treat a variety of malignancies, and its side effects were well known. The principle was to establish circulatory isolation of a tumor-bearing region, with subsequent exposure to high dose chemotherapy. By isolating a given tumor-bearing extremity, Creech and Krementz believed they could expose the tumor tissue to maximal concentrations of chemotherapy, while minimizing the systemic side effects. This idea of isolating the circulation was inspired by the success of the heart-lung apparatus in the treatment of intracardiac defects (Gibbon 1954). Creech and Krementz performed experimental studies to determine the extent of which circulatory isolation could be achieved, the maximal dose of chemotherapeutic agents (nitrogen mustard and phenylalanine mustard or *melphalan*) that can be used safely in perfusion, the effects of chemotherapeutic agents on blood oxygenation, and their duration of action (Creech et al. 1958; Ryan et al. 1958).

Anti-tumor activity of melphalan was demonstrated in animal-based models (Luck 1956, 1957). In the original report, clinical studies were performed on 24 patients with a variety of neoplasms including malignant melanoma, sarcoma and carcinoma, involving the transverse colon, thumb, lung, breast, rectum and scapula using either nitrogen mustard or melphalan (Creech et al. 1958).

The first ILP procedure was performed on a 76 year old male with a small black mole on the dorsum of his left foot, which had been initially asymptomatic, but subsequently began to become irritated and bleeding. Following a wide local excision with skin grafting, histological analysis confirmed the suspicion of melanoma. A left groin dissection was performed 1 week later and revealed no nodal involvement although tumor cells were noted in the lymphatic vessels. The patient experienced extensive satellitosis (approximately 175 metastatic lesions) with many pigmented lesions appearing on the medial aspect of his left leg and thigh within 1 year. Due to his age, and the extensiveness of the metastases, he was not a candidate for amputation and was offered ILP with melphalan for palliation. The patient experienced a complete response as determined by regression of the cutaneous metastases both grossly and histologically, and the patient died 16 years later, of unrelated causes (Creech et al. 1958; Krementz et al. 1994).

B) Current technical principles The technique for ILP has largely remained unchanged since its formal introduction by Creech and Krementz (1958) (Ross 2008). The artery and vein supplying the tumor-bearing area are surgically dissected and cannulas of appropriate size are inserted (typically 18–20 French in the vein and 12–18 French in the artery) while collaterals are ligated (Ross 2008; Brady et al. 2006). An Esmarch tourniquet is placed as proximal to the cannulated vessels as possible to isolate the limb from the systemic circulation. Circulatory isolation not only minimizes systemic toxicity, but also aids in maintaining the desired chemotherapeutic concentration within the limb. Chemotherapeutic doses of up to ten times those tolerated by the systemic circulation can be achieved with this method. Circulation time is approximately 1 h, and flow rates are generally 400–600 mL/min for the leg, and 200–400 mL/min for the arm (Ross 2008). Cannulas are connected to an extra-corporeal circuit, which generates a high-flow, hyperoxic perfusate, provides adequate tissue perfusion pressures and allows for relatively long treatment duration. The bubble oxygenator, which is part of the extra-corporeal circuit, gives rise to a partial pressure of oxygen of approximately 400 mmHg and is thought to have its own tumoricidal effect and potentiate the effect of the alkylating agent (Krementz and Knudson 1961).

A potential side effect of this method is leakage of the chemotherapeutic agent into the systemic circulation. This is monitored by radiolabeling the patient's erythrocytes with Technetium 99m, and giving back the radiolabelled erythrocytes in two aliquots to the patient: one in the systemic circulation, and one in the isolated circulation. A gamma probe is used to detect leakage of the erythrocytes from the isolated circuit into the systemic circulation by holding the probe over the precordium and detecting a rise in radioactive count over time. This method can also detect a leak of the systemic circulation into the isolated limb, as this would dilute the concentration of the chemotherapy in the limb.

C) Hyperthermia The initial ILP procedures were performed under normothermic conditions. However Cavaliere (Cavaliere et al. 1967) and Stehlin (Stehlin 1969) showed that mild hyperthermia (38.5–40°C) can increase the uptake of chemotherapy agent within cells, while true hyperthermia (>41°C) is associated with increased regional toxicity. Although ILP with mild hyperthermia has become the standard, no direct comparisons in prospective randomized controlled trials have been conducted to evaluate the benefit of increasing perfusate temperatures. Mild hyperthermia is achieved by wrapping the limb with a thermal blanket and using heated perfusate, while temperature is monitored using thermistor probes placed in the subcutaneous and intramuscular portions of the limbs.

Table 24.7 Wieberdink toxicity scale. (Wieberdink et al. 1982)

Grade	Description
I	No reaction
II	Slight erythema and/or edema
III	Considerable erythema and/or edema with some blistering, slight disturbance of motility
IV	Extensive epidermolysis and/or obvious damage to deep tissues, causing definite functional disturbances threatening or manifest compartmental syndrome
V	Reaction which may necessitate amputation

D) Chemotherapy agents used Melphalan is the standard medication used because of its efficacy and low toxicity profile. Dosing is determined by the volume of the limb to be perfused, and doses typically range from 10 mg/L for the leg to 13 mg/L for the arm (Wieberdink et al. 1982). In a modification to the original procedure by Creech and Krementz, actinomycin-D is administered in combination with melphalan, showing favorable response rates when administered by ILP (Thompson et al. 1997; Sanki et al. 2007). A recently completed trial, the ACOSOG Z0020, evaluated the efficacy of adding tumor necrosis factor (TNF) to melphalan in ILP (Cornett et al. 2006). One hundred and three patients were randomized to hyperthermic ILP with melphalan and TNF-alpha versus hyperthermic ILP with melphalan alone. The results showed that there was no significant advantage with the addition of TNF-alpha as complete response (CR) rates were similar in both arms; 25 % in patients receiving melphalan alone, and 26 % in patients receiving melphalan and TNF-alpha. A recent systematic review of 22 studies including 2,018 ILP procedures evaluated the clinical response, survival and toxicity data of normo or hyperthermic ILP with melphalan either with or without TNF, and other drugs (Moreno-Ramirez et al. 2010). Interestingly, this data is inconsistent with the results of ACOSOG Z0020, suggesting a benefit when combining melphalan and TNF-alpha (CR of 68.50 %) in comparison to melphalan alone (CR of 46.50 %). Other drugs have been studied in the setting of hyperthermic ILP such as dimethyltriazenoimidazole carboxamide, cisplatin, carboplatin and thiotepa. However none of these have undergone Phase I or II clinical trials and thus, melphalan remains the standard chemotherapeutic.

E) Toxicity Toxicity was routinely assessed in ILP studies using the Wieberdink toxicity scale (Table 24.7) (Wieberdink et al. 1982). Patients can expect transient toxicity lasting a few weeks, which may include erythema, desquamation, alopecia, onycholysis, skin color changes, peripheral neuropathy and pain (Thompson et al. 1998). Patients undergoing either normo- or hyperthermic ILP may develop lymphedema (30–40 %), compartment syndrome (10–15 %), and long-term peripheral neuropathy (5–8 %) (Coleman et al. 2009). Post-operatively, the risk of developing compartment syndrome is assessed by serum creatine phosphokinase analysis and clinical assessment. Values exceeding 1,000 IU/L have been shown to correlate with severe limb toxicity (Kroon et al. 2009). There is also a small risk (1–2 %) of severe toxicity requiring amputation (Beasley et al. 2009a).

F) Clinical Outcomes Complete response, (CR) is defined as the resolution of all visible disease, and partial response (PR) is defined as a decrease in ≥ 50 % of the diameter of all lesions, without the appearance of new lesions (Ariyan and Brady 2008). CR rates range from 39–82 %, with an overall survival of 42–55 % at 5 years (Sanki et al. 2007; Cornett et al. 2006; Minor et al. 1985, Storm and Morton 1985; Kroon et al. 1987, 1993; Di Filippo et al. 1989; Klaase et al. 1994; Aloia et al. 2005). There is a trend for single-center studies to have higher CR rates compared with multicenter randomized trials.

This wide variation in CR rates can be attributed to (Ariyan and Brady 2008):

- The lack of standard staging;
- The absence of objective and reproducible criteria for assessment of clinical response;
- Variations in procedural details.

Although achieving a CR following ILP treatment has been shown to be associated with a long-term survival, no randomized controlled trials have demonstrated that ILP actually prolongs survival (Sanki et al. 2007; Bryant et al. 1995; Noorda et al. 2004). Nevertheless, more than 50 years of evidence have made hyperthermic ILP with melphalan the standard of treatment.

Key Points

- ILP principle is to establish circulatory isolation of a tumor-bearing region, with subsequent exposure to high dose chemotherapy.
- Circulation time is approximately 1 h, and flow rates are usually 400–600 mL/min for the leg, and 200–400 mL/min for the arm.
- High chemotherapeutic doses of up to ten times the dosage tolerated by the systemic circulation can be administered.
- A potential side effect is leakage of the chemotherapeutic agent into the systemic circulation, which can be monitored by erythrocyte radiolabeling with Technetium 99m.
- ILP with mild hyperthermia (38.5–40°C) can increase the uptake of chemotherapy agent.
- Melphalan is the standard medication used because of its efficacy and low toxicity profile.
- ILP transient toxicity may include erythema, desquamation, alopecia, onycholysis, peripheral neuropathy and pain.
- Complete response rates to ILP range from 39–82 %, with an overall survival of 42–55 % at 5 years.

24.2.3 Isolated Limb Infusion

Studies from the Sydney Melanoma Unit in the early 1990s, led by John Thompson, gave rise to the development of isolated limb infusion (ILI) as a minimally invasive, low-morbidity and less complex alternative to ILP (Thompson et al. 2008). ILI

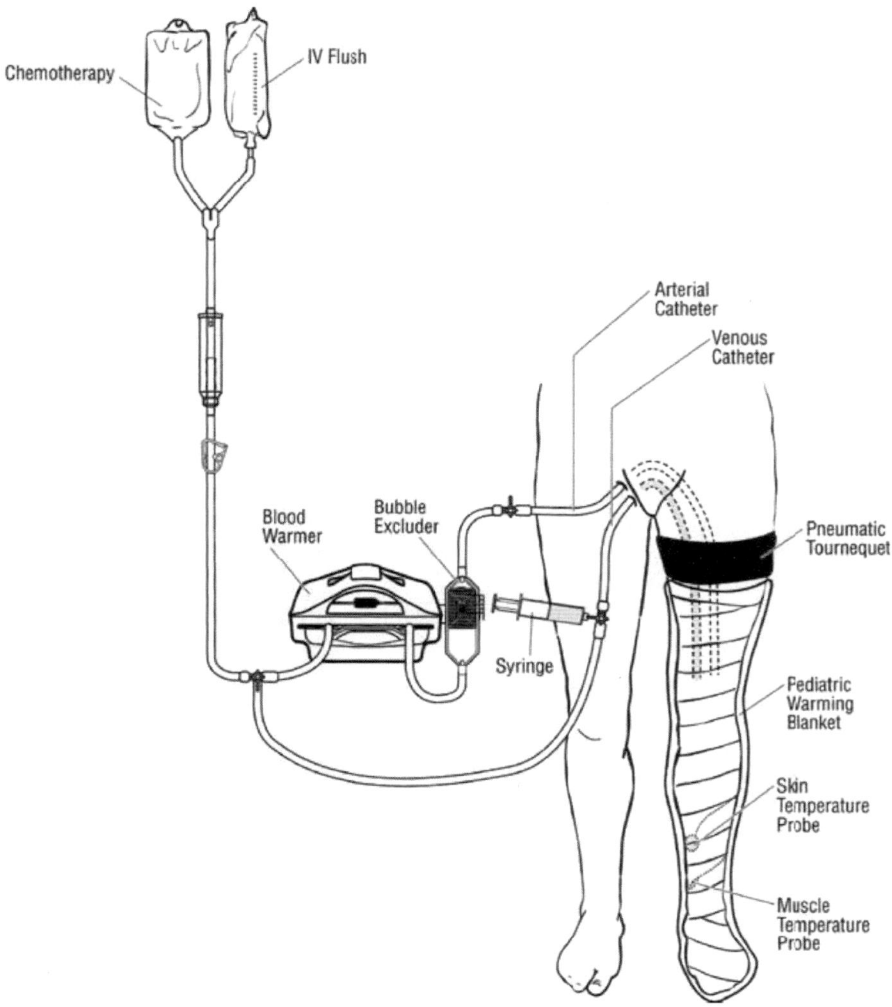

Fig. 24.4 Isolated limb infusion. (Adapted with permission from Brady et al. 2006 and Ross 2008)

differs from ILP in that it is a low-flow method, performed without oxygenation of the perfusate, and involves percutaneous insertion of vascular catheters rather than surgical placement (Thompson et al. 1994; Brady et al. 2006, 2009).

A) Technical aspects: simplified circuitry, benefits of hyperthermia and hypoxia (Fig. 24.4) Interventional radiology is utilized for the insertion of multiholed arterial and venous catheters via the contralateral groin using the Seldinger technique, and in the case of the lower extremities, they are threaded around the aortic and vena cava bifurcations into the femoral artery and vein of the tumor-bearing extremity (Seldinger 1953). The location of the catheters is subsequently verified by X-ray.

A low flow heparin infusion is used to ensure catheter patency. Once the patient is moved to the operating suite and anesthetized, an Esmarch tourniquet is placed at the most proximal aspect of the affected limb, similar to ILP, allowing for a high dose of chemotherapeutic agent to be administered (Thompson et al. 1994). The cardiopulmonary bypass machine is not used in ILI, making the procedure not only technically simpler, but also more cost-effective in that the equipment, disposables and personnel to operate the extracorporeal circulator are not needed. Furthermore, a blood transfusion is not required to prime the circuit, thus minimizing the risks incurred by transfusion of blood products. The circuit simply consists of a blood warmer/bubble excluder that circulates blood from the arterial to the venous catheter. The temperature of the patient's extremity is increased to about 40°C using warming blankets.

The chemotherapeutic agent is delivered by a pressure bag and intravenous fluid pump via the arterial catheter at a concentration of 5–10 μg/L for melphalan and 50–100 μg/L for actinomycin-D. The infusate is not oxygenated as in ILP. In fact, is maintained acidotic and hypoxic, which potentiates the anti-tumor activity of melphalan (Siemann et al. 1991; van de Merwe et al. 1993). Circulation is manually maintained using a syringe and a high-flow, three-way stopcock, and has an average flow rate of 50–100 mL/min. The infusion circulates for about 20–30 min and requires an operative block time of about 2–3 h, which is significantly less than conventional ILP which requires up to 6 h (Thompson et al. 1998). Notably, increased length of infusion is not associated to better clinical outcomes in the literature (Parsons et al. 1981). Most of melphalan's cellular uptake takes place in the first 20 min of treatment. At the end of the procedure, the hypoxic blood is evacuated from the extremity prior to taking down the Esmarch tourniquet.

B) Advantages of ILI over ILP ILI presents multiple advantages over ILP, although no head-to head prospective comparison has ever been performed in the context of a clinical trial. These advantages include:

- No vascular dissection involved, minimally invasive percutaneous access only.
- Technical simplicity, resulting in shorter operative times.
- No need for extracorporeal circulation and associated staff/equipment;
- Easily repeatable technique.
- Wider patient eligibility (elderly, patients with peripheral vascular disease).

C) Clinical Outcomes The Sydney Melanoma Unit (SMU) was the first to publish data on the clinical outcomes of ILI. In a study involving 128 ILI procedures, Lindner et al. reported a CR of 41, PR of 44, and overall response rate (OR) of 85 % (Lindner et al. 2002). More recently, the same group expanded their study by addition 57 ILI procedures, and reported a CR of 38 and PR of 46 % (Kroon et al. 2008). However, these clinical outcomes seem to be lower when performed in other institutions. Two sites in the United States, Duke University Hospital and Memorial Sloan Kettering Cancer Center (MSKCC) have published their experience with ILI, with lower clinical outcomes, namely a CR of 23–30 % and a PR of 33 % (Brady et al. 2006; Beasley et al. 2008). Similarly, a review of 128 ILI procedures done at eight different institutions reported a CR of 31, a PR in 36, and no response in

36 % (Beasley et al. 2009a). There are several reasons explaining the discrepancy between the Australian and American data. Differences in technique (i.e. differences in tourniquet and infusion time), healthcare team experience, and methods of reporting clinical outcomes may have played a significant role in determining clinical outcome data. Furthermore, the SMU patients overall had a higher disease stage, and when they were stratified by disease stage and tumor burden, response rates were comparable to those from the American data (Beasley et al. 2009a).

In patients who experience a CR or PR, the risk of recurrence is significant, and no study has shown that ILI or ILP improve overall survival in patients with in-transit extremity melanoma (Kroon et al. 2008). MKSCC and Duke reported a 12 month median duration of CR (Brady et al. 2006; Beasley et al. 2008), while the SMU reported a median overall duration of response of 13 months, and a 22 month median duration of CR (Kroon et al. 2008). Unfortunately, no randomized controlled trials exist that directly compare the efficacy and side effects of ILI and ILP. However, using the data available, response rates from ILI (23–41 %) seem to be on the lower end of the range compared to those for ILP (25–82 %) (Lindner et al. 2002; Kroon et al. 2008).

Patients may be offered a second ILI procedure if they are nonresponsive to the initial treatment, experience a progression of disease within the ILI perioperative period, or after experiencing a CR or PR. Unfortunately, the SMU reported OR rates (83 %) that were not significantly different after a second ILI procedure with melphalan and actinomycin-D compared the first ILI (Kroon et al. 2009a). Furthermore, a repeat ILI was associated with greater rates of limb toxicity (increased number of patients with grade IV toxicities) and a low CR (23 vs 38 %) (Kroon et al. 2009a).

D) Toxicity Limb toxicity rates are similar between ILI and ILP, however wound complications, post-operative vascular problems, and long-term morbidity are less likely with ILI. ILI-associated toxicities include transient lymphedema, erythema, desquamation, alopecia, skin color changes, onycholysis and discomfort (Thompson et al. 1998). The likelihood of amputation is reduced with ILI (0.3 %, compared with 2 % in ILP) (Beasley et al. 2009a). Overall, ILI is considered to be a low morbidity procedure and it may also be used as a palliative method to achieve control of in-transit extremity disease in patients with distant metastases (Kroon et al. 2009b). Patients with painful, ulcerating, bleeding, foul-smelling melanoma lesions and who were expected to suffer significantly in their near future, underwent ILI with the purpose of palliation and local disease control. Investigators observed a limb salvage rate of 86 % (which included all patients with CR, PR or stable disease response) and OR of 76 % (Kroon et al. 2009b).

E) Other applications ILI or ILP may be offered to patients with soft tissue sarcoma (STS) that are confined to an extremity and are not resectable. The results from ILI in the treatment of STS have been comparable to melanoma (Hegazy et al. 2007; Moncrieff et al. 2008; Hoekstra and van Ginkel 2003).A study conducted at the SMU evaluated the effect of ILI on STS in 21 patients. Seven patients underwent ILI to treat inoperable recurrences or for palliation and fourteen patients underwent ILI as neoadjuvant therapy prior to surgery. Limb salvage was achieved in 76, and 57 %

experienced a CR. Patients that achieved CR had a significantly longer duration of response than patients with a PR, but survival time was not significantly different. The procedure was well tolerated with fourteen patients experiencing Wieberdink grade II toxicity. Importantly, response rates were not significantly different among patients with different stages of disease; however a lower stage was significantly associated with longer survival (Moncrieff et al. 2008).

Key Points

- ILI is a low-flow method, performed without oxygenation of the perfusate, and involves percutaneous insertion of vascular catheters.
- The circuit consists of a blood warmer/bubble excluder that circulates blood from the arterial to the venous catheter.
- The temperature of the patient's extremity is increased to up to 40°C.
- The infusate is maintained acidotic and hypoxic, which potentiates the anti-tumor activity of the chemotherapeutic agent.
- The infusion circulates for about 20–30 min which is significantly less than conventional ILP.
- The reported CR median duration is between 13–22 months.
- Post-operative vascular problems, and long-term morbidity are less frequent with ILI compared to ILP.
- ILI is considered to be a low morbidity procedure and is also used as a palliative method.

24.2.4 Chemotherapeutics in ILP and ILI

Established chemotherapeutic agents: Melphalan Melphalan has been the chemotherapeutic agent of choice since its use for the first ILP by Krementz and Creech, and subsequently by Thompson for ILI. Other agents have been tested in the setting of ILP and ILI such as cisplatin (Benckhuijsen et al. 1988; Fletcher et al. 2004; Hoekstra et al. 1993; Thompson and Gianoutsos 1992; Krementz and Ryan 1972), dacarbazine (Bonenkamp et al. 2004; Lejeune and Ghanem 1987), and nitrogen mustard (Briele et al. 1985). However, melphalan remains the mainstay of treatment. Optimization studies have been done to determine an appropriate therapeutic index without incurring excessive toxicity. Studies have been done to determine what variables are associated with excessive toxicities and tumor response. In the initial days of ILP, melphalan drug dosing was based on body weight, and the drug dose typically fell in the range of 1.0–2.8 mg/kg (Fraker 1998). However, using this method does not take into account differences in weight distribution among individuals.

Melphalan dosing was subsequently based on limb volume calculations. Generally, the optimal therapeutic index of melphalan is achieved when the lower limbs are perfused with 10 mg per liter of limb volume, and the upper limbs are perfused with 13 mg per limb volume (Krementz et al. 1994; Wieberdink et al. 1982; Fraker

1998). Interestingly, a study of 14 hyperthermic ILPs showed that there was a four-fold difference in plasma concentration of melphalan among patients using a similar calculation for dosing based on limb volume (Cheng et al. 2003).

Elevated levels of melphalan plasma concentration was correlated with increasing toxicity, where five patients experienced major toxicities of grade III and IV, although there was no benefit to tumor response (Cheng et al. 2003). This suggested that overestimation of melphalan dosing based on limb volume calculations may be associated with increased toxicity. These data are reproducible among other studies (Vrouenraets et al. 1998, 1999), and also in the setting of ILI (Beasley et al. 2008). When the dosing was corrected for ideal body weight (IBW), there was less variation in the mean melphalan concentrations and less toxicity was observed (10 % with grade III toxicities or greater with doses adjusted for IBW, versus 33 % with more than grade III toxicities with doses not adjusted for IBW). Furthermore, another study by McMahon and colleagues supports that correcting for IBW in ILI results in lower toxicity rates without affecting tumor response (McMahon et al. 2009). In a multi-institutional review, Beasley et al. demonstrated that adjusting for IBW in 162 ILI cases decreased toxicity and did not alter CR (Beasley et al. 2009a). However, it remains a matter of debate on whether to recommend correcting for IBW when using melphalan in either ILP or ILI at the present time.

B) Agents that reduce chemoresistance of melphalan Overcoming chemoresistance is a challenge for multiple chemotherapeutic agents, and melphalan is no different in this respect. Melphalan acts by alkylating DNA bases, resulting in DNA cross-linkages that render the DNA unable to be replicated or transcribed in a regular manner required for cell survival. The cell is inefficient at repairing DNA cross-linkages using cellular mechanisms, and thus the cell undergoes faulty DNA replication at best, eventually resulting in cell death or apoptosis. Neoplastic cells have developed resistance mechanisms to overcome chemotherapeutic treatment, including enhanced repair of DNA cross-links, decreased drug uptake into the cell, increased drug efflux from the cell, and inactivation of the drug once inside the cell. The latter mechanism is believed to be most significant and involves the molecule glutathione (GSH). GSH has been shown to give rise to GSH S-alkylating agent conjugates which cause melphalan to be rendered inactive and unable to alkylate DNA (Grubbs et al. 2004a). This process is enhanced by a major group of detoxification enzymes, the glutathione-S-transferases (GST) (Hayes and Pulford 1995), which catalyze the conjugation of GSH to various toxic agents, including melphalan. Using various human and murine cell-based models, elevated GSH levels (Suzukake et al. 1982; Green et al. 1984) and increased GST activity (Robson et al. 1987) have been correlated with resistance to chemotherapy.

Butathione sulfixime (BSO) Various chemosensitizing agents have been tested with the goal of rendering neoplastic cells sensitive to melphalan. Butathione sulfixime (BSO) is one such agent. BSO is a small molecule inhibitor of a key enzyme, γ-glutamylcysteine-synthetase, required in the synthesis of GSH, which is involved in melphalan resistance (Green et al. 1984; Suzukake et al. 1982). Using a xenograft model of extremity melanoma, the Tyler group showed that treating animals with peritoneal BSO along with melphalan via ILI resulted in delayed tumor growth and decreased levels of GSH, without increased toxicity (Grubbs et al. 2004b). Phase I clinical trials are underway where patients will be treated with BSO with a 3-day infusion during the time of melphalan ILI (Coleman et al. 2009).

Bevacizumab (Avastin) Dysfunctional tumor vasculature poses a challenge in efficient delivery of chemotherapeutic agent to the tumor. A key endothelial cell specific growth factor involved in the formation of new tumor vasculature, also known as angiogenesis, is Vascular Endothelial Growth Factor (VEGF) (Kim et al. 1993; Presta et al. 1997). Bevacizumab is a monoclonal antibody targeted to human VEGF, which has been shown to transiently "normalize" tumor vasculature, and suppress tumor growth (Kim et al. 1993; Jain 2001b). Inducing a transient normalization of tumor vasculature may facilitate the delivery of melphalan within extremity melanoma. Pretreatment of orthotopic neuroblastoma xenografts with bevacizumab allowed for efficacious delivery of chemotherapeutic agent topotecan to tumors as evidence by greater tumor growth inhibition compared to either drug alone or both administered concurrently (Dickson et al. 2007).

ADH-1 (Exherin) ADH-1 is another agent that has been shown to improve clinical response to melphalan in preclinical models of extremity melanoma. E-cadherin is a transmembrane protein involved in maintaining cell-cell interactions within a monolayer of epithelial cells. During the malignant transformation of a melanoma, E-cadherin expression is thought to be switched to N-cadherin. This results in a diversification of not only the cell-cell contacts, but also in downstream intracellular signaling pathways that regulate cellular proliferation, survival and angiogenesis. ADH-1 is a cyclic pentapeptide that disrupts cell-cell adhesions mediated by N-cadherin and thus, is specific to malignant cells that aberrantly express N-cadherin (Augustine et al. 2008). Recently, a Phase I study was conducted to assess the safety, toxicity, pharmacokinetics, and efficacy of systemic ADH-1 in combination with melphalan administered by ILI in patients with in-transit extremity melanoma (Beasley et al. 2009b). The study reported a CR of 50 %, and a PR of 12.5 % in 16 patients with minimal toxicities. The group reported that as opposed to bevacizumab treatment, ADH-1 treatment resulted in increased vascular permeability which may result in better delivery of melphalan to the tissues, however further studies are needed to investigate this (Coleman et al. 2009; Beasley et al. 2009a). Phase II clinical trials are currently in progress (Coleman et al. 2009).

Other chemotherapy agents Although melphalan has been the mainstay of treatment for the last 50 years, some do not respond to treatment, and others experience a recurrence following ILP and ILI. Thus, there remains room for improvement in selecting novel chemotherapeutic agents with acceptable efficacies and toxicities. Below we discuss other chemotherapeutic agents and their clinical efficacies and toxicities.

Temozolomide Temozolomide (TMZ) is a cytotoxic second generation DNA-alkylating agent and a prodrug of the active metabolite 3-methyl-(triazen-1-yl)imidazole-4-carboxamide. It is commonly used in the treatment of anaplastic astrocytoma, and glioblastoma multiforme and is approved for the treatment of advanced melanoma in >20 countries worldwide (Trinh et al. 2009). When used systemically as a single agent in the management of metastatic melanoma, TMZ produces a response rate 12–14 % for both the monthly dosing regimen (200 mg/m^2/day for 5 days once every 4 weeks) (Middleton et al. 2000), and extended-dosing regimen (75 mg/m^2/day for 6 weeks once every 8 weeks) (Rietschel et al. 2008). However, TMZ has not yet been tested for its efficacy as a regional chemotherapeutic agent in patients with in-transit disease. The Tyler group performed ILI using a human melanoma xenograft model where 5×10^6 cultured human melanoma cells (DM6) were injected in the hindlimbs of irradiated athymic nude rats and allowed to grow to a size of 10 mm^3 before commencement of treatment. These preclinical studies showed prolonged tumor growth delay when TMZ was infused regionally within the lower limb using an ILI approach, compared to systemic administration (Ueno et al. 2004). Using the same animal model, the Tyler group later showed that the cytotoxicity of TMZ was increased when used in hyperthermic conditions (Ko et al. 2006). These preclinical studies are optimistic, and clinical trials are currently under review to test the efficacy of TMZ administered regionally for locally advanced in-transit melanoma (Coleman et al. 2009).

Agents that reduce chemoresistance of TMZ: O6-benzylguanine Similar to the pathway of resistance to melphalan outlined previously, a mechanism of resistance downstream of TMZ has also been identified and characterized. TMZ is an alkylating agent, and melanoma cells counteract the action of TMZ by efficiently repairing damaged DNA. O6-alkylguanine-DNA alkyltransferase (AGT) is a major DNA repair enzyme involved in nucleotide repair following DNA damage downstream of TMZ treatment (Ueno et al. 2006). O6-benzylguanine (O6BG) is an inhibitor of AGT. Using five different rat xenograft human melanoma models, it was shown that pretreatment of animals with peritoneal O6BG resulted in a significant reduction of AGT activity (by 93.5 %) and that subsequent treatment with TMZ by ILI resulted in a marked reduction of tumor growth (Ueno et al. 2006; Yoshimoto et al. 2007). This data suggest that chemomodulation of TMZ with O6BG leads to increased efficacy of the anti-tumor treatment.

Sorafenib (Nexavar) The RAS/RAF/MEK/ERK/MAP kinase pathway is known to mediate cellular proliferation downstream from growth factor signalling. A landmark study showed that B-Raf mutations are found in 66 % of malignant melanomas, whereas they occur at lower frequency in other tumor types (Davies et al. 2002).A single missense mutation (V600E) in the kinase domain accounts for approximately 80 % of all B-raf mutations in melanoma. B-raf is a serine/threonine kinase that is among one of the targets of the multi-kinase inhibitor, sorafenib. Sorafenib is FDA-approved for the treatment of advanced renal cell carcinoma, and advanced heptocellular carcinoma. Various Phase I and II clinical trials have been conducted either with systemic sorafenib alone or in combination with chemotherapeutic agents carboplatin, dacarbazine, paclitaxel and TMZ with mixed results (Hauschild et al. 2009; McDermott et al. 2008; Amaravadi et al. 2009; Eisen et al. 2006). Novel BRAF kinase inhibitors that are selective for the oncogenic V600E mutation are under development and are showing promising results (Poulikakos et al. 2010). Given the predominance of B-raf mutations in melanoma, targeted therapy would potentially be an ideal agent either alone or in combination with melphalan in the treatment of in-transit extremity melanoma. Further studies are necessary to test this hypothesis.

24.2.5 Summary

In transit melanoma is a challenging metastatic recurrence of cancer both for the oncologist and the patient. ILP and ILI are effective in controlling disease progression, without proceeding to amputation. Although no randomized clinical trial exists to compare the two, studies suggest that ILP is marginally more effective than ILI but that ILI has much lower toxicity. The indications for ILP and ILI are expanding, including STS and other tumors. Melphalan remains the chemotherapeutic of choice, although clinical trials are in progress to test the efficacy of novel agents, including targeted therapeutics.

References

Ahmad SA et al (2004) Reduced morbidity following cytoreductive surgery and intraperitoneal hyperthermic chemoperfusion. Ann Surg Oncol 11:387–392

Aloia TA et al (2005) Predictors of outcome after hyperthermic isolated limb perfusion: role of tumor response. Arch Surg 140:1115–1120

Amaravadi RK et al (2009) Phase II trial of Temozolomide and Sorafenib in advanced melanoma patients with or without brain metastases. Clin Cancer Res 15:7711–7718

Ariyan CE, Brady MS (2008) History of regional chemotherapy for cancer of the extremities. Int J Hyperthermia 24:185–192

Augustine CK et al (2008) Targeting N-cadherin enhances antitumor activity of cytotoxic therapies in melanoma treatment. Cancer Res 68:3777–3784

Bajaj G, Yeo Y (2010) Drug delivery systems for intraperitoneal therapy. Pharm Res 27:735

Balch CM et al (2001) Final version of the American Joint Committee on Cancer staging system for cutaneous melanoma. J Clin Oncol 19:3635–3648

Balch CM, Houghton AN, Sober A, Soong S (1998) Recurrent regional metastases and their management. Quality medical, Missouri.

Beasley GM et al (2008) Isolated limb infusion for in-transit malignant melanoma of the extremity: a well-tolerated but less effective alternative to hyperthermic isolated limb perfusion. Ann Surg Oncol 15:2195–2205

Beasley GM et al (2009a) A multi-institutional experience of isolated limb infusion: defining response and toxicity in the US. J Am Coll Surg 208:706–715 (discussion 715–707)

Beasley GM et al (2009b) A phase 1 study of systemic ADH-1 in combination with melphalan via isolated limb infusion in patients with locally advanced in-transit malignant melanoma. Cancer 115:4766–4774

Benckhuijsen C, Kroon BB, van Geel AN, Wieberdink J (1988) Regional perfusion treatment with melphalan for melanoma in a limb: an evaluation of drug kinetics. Eur J Surg Oncol 14:157–163

Bonenkamp JJ et al (2004) Isolated limb infusion with fotemustine after dacarbazine chemosensitisation for inoperable loco-regional melanoma recurrence. Eur J Surg Oncol 30:1107–1112

Brady MS, Brown K, Patel A, Fisher C, Marx W (2006) A phase II trial of isolated limb infusion with melphalan and dactinomycin for regional melanoma and soft tissue sarcoma of the extremity. Ann Surg Oncol 13:1123–1129

Brady MS, Brown K, Patel A, Fisher C, Marx W (2009) Isolated limb infusion with melphalan and dactinomycin for regional melanoma and soft-tissue sarcoma of the extremity: final report of a phase II clinical trial. Melanoma Res 19:106–111

Briele HA et al (1985) Pharmacokinetics of melphalan in clinical isolation perfusion of the extremities. Cancer Res 45:1885–1889

Bryant PJ, Balderson GA, Mead P, Egerton WS (1995) Hyperthermic isolated limb perfusion for malignant melanoma: response and survival. World J Surg 19:363–368

Calabro A, Singletary SE, Balch CM (1989) Patterns of relapse in 1001 consecutive patients with melanoma nodal metastases. Arch Surg 124:1051–1055

Cavaliere R et al (1967) Selective heat sensitivity of cancer cells. Biochemical and clinical studies. Cancer 20:1351–1381

Ceelen WP, Flessner MF (2010) Intraperitoneal therapy for peritoneal tumors: biophysics and clinical evidence. Nat Rev Clin Oncol 7:108–115

Cheng TY et al (2003) Marked variability of melphalan plasma drug levels during regional hyperthermic isolated limb perfusion. Am J Surg 186:460–467

Chereau E et al (2010) Comparison of peritoneal carcinomatosis scoring methods in predicting resectability and prognosis in advanced ovarian cancer. Am J Obstet Gynecol 202:178 e171–178 e110

Chua TC et al (2009a) Intraoperative hyperthermic intraperitoneal chemotherapy after cytoreductive surgery in ovarian cancer peritoneal carcinomatosis: systematic review of current results. J Cancer Res Clin Oncol 135:1637–1645

Chua TC et al (2009b) Thoracic cytoreductive surgery and intraoperative hyperthermic intrathoracic chemotherapy for pseudomyxoma peritonei. J Surg Oncol 99:292–295

Chua TC, Morris DL, Esquivel J (2009c) Impact of the peritoneal surface disease severity score on survival in patients with colorectal cancer peritoneal carcinomatosis undergoing complete cytoreduction and hyperthermic intraperitoneal chemotherapy. Ann Surg Oncol 17:1330

Chua TC, Koh JL, Yan TD, Liauw W, Morris DL (2009d) Cytoreductive surgery and perioperative intraperitoneal chemotherapy for peritoneal carcinomatosis from small bowel adenocarcinoma. J Surg Oncol 100:139–143

Chua TC, Yan TD, Saxena A, Morris DL (2009e) Should the treatment of peritoneal carcinomatosis by cytoreductive surgery and hyperthermic intraperitoneal chemotherapy still be regarded as a highly morbid procedure?: a systematic review of morbidity and mortality. Ann Surg 249:900–907

Cho CH et al (2008) Regional hyperthermia of the abdomen in conjunction with chemotherapy for peritoneal carcinomatosis: evaluation of two annular-phased-array applicators. Int J Hyperthermia 24:399–408

Coleman A, Augustine CK, Beasley G, Sanders G, Tyler D (2009) Optimizing regional infusion treatment strategies for melanoma of the extremities. Expert Rev Anticancer Ther 9:1599–1609

Cohen MS et al (2010) Combination intraperitoneal chemotherapy is superior to mitomycin C or oxaliplatin for colorectal carcinomatosis in vivo. Ann Surg Oncol 17:296–303

Cornett WR et al (2006) Randomized multicenter trial of hyperthermic isolated limb perfusion with melphalan alone compared with melphalan plus tumor necrosis factor: American College of Surgeons Oncology Group trial Z0020. J Clin Oncol 24:4196–4201

Creech O Jr, Krementz ET, Ryan RF, Winblad JN (1958) Chemotherapy of cancer: regional perfusion utilizing an extracorporeal circuit. Ann Surg 148:616–632

Davies H et al (2002) Mutations of the BRAF gene in human cancer. Nature 417:949–954

de Bree E et al (2004) Peritoneal carcinomatosis from colorectal or appendiceal origin: correlation of preoperative CT with intraoperative findings and evaluation of interobserver agreement. J Surg Oncol 86:64–73

Dedrick RL (1985) Theoretical and experimental bases of intraperitoneal chemotherapy. Semin Oncol 12:1–6

Dedrick RL, Myers CE, Bungay PM, DeVita VT Jr (1978) Pharmacokinetic rationale for peritoneal drug administration in the treatment of ovarian cancer. Cancer Treat Rep 62:1–11

Dickson PV et al (2007) Bevacizumab-induced transient remodeling of the vasculature in neuroblastoma xenografts results in improved delivery and efficacy of systemically administered chemotherapy. Clin Cancer Res 13:3942–3950

Di Filippo F et al (1989) Prognostic variables in recurrent limb melanoma treated with hyperthermic antiblastic perfusion. Cancer 63:2551–2561

Dindo D, Demartines N, Clavien PA (2004) Classification of surgical complications: a new proposal with evaluation in a cohort of 6336 patients and results of a survey. Ann Surg 240:205–213

Edge SB et al (2010) AJCC cancer staging manual. Springer, New York.

Eisen T et al (2006) Sorafenib in advanced melanoma: a Phase II randomised discontinuation trial analysis. Br J Cancer 95:581–586

Elias D et al (2007) Optimization of hyperthermic intraperitoneal chemotherapy with oxaliplatin plus irinotecan at 43 degrees C after compete cytoreductive surgery: mortality and morbidity in 106 consecutive patients. Ann Surg Oncol 14:1818–1824

Elias D et al (2010) Peritoneal colorectal carcinomatosis treated with surgery and perioperative intraperitoneal chemotherapy: retrospective analysis of 523 patients from a multicentric French study. J Clin Oncol 28:63–68

Elias D et al (2010) Pseudomyxoma peritonei: a French multicentric study of 301 patients treated with cytoreductive surgery and intraperitoneal chemotherapy. Eur J Surg Oncol 36:456

Esquis P et al (2006) High intra-abdominal pressure enhances the penetration and antitumor effect of intraperitoneal cisplatin on experimental peritoneal carcinomatosis. Ann Surg 244:106–112

Esquivel J et al (2007) Cytoreductive surgery and hyperthermic intraperitoneal chemotherapy in the management of peritoneal surface malignancies of colonic origin: a consensus statement. Society of Surgical Oncology. Ann Surg Oncol 14:128–133

Flessner MF (2008) Endothelial glycocalyx and the peritoneal barrier. Perit Dial Int 28:6–12

Fletcher WS, Pommier R, Small K (2004) Results of cisplatin hyperthermic isolation perfusion for stage IIIA and IIIAB extremity melanoma. Melanoma Res 4:17–19

Fraker DL (1998) Hyperthermic regional perfusion for melanoma of the limbs. In: Balch CM, Houghton AN, Sober AJ, Soong S (eds) Cutaneous melanoma. Quality Medical, St. Louis. pp 281–300

Fujimoto S et al (1997) Improved mortality rate of gastric carcinoma patients with peritoneal carcinomatosis treated with intraperitoneal hyperthermic chemoperfusion combined with surgery. Cancer 79:884–891

Gelderblom H et al (2002) Influence of Cremophor El on the bioavailability of intraperitoneal paclitaxel. Clin Cancer Res 8:1237–1241

Gibbon JH Jr (1954) Application of a mechanical heart and lung apparatus to cardiac surgery. Minn Med 37:171–185 (passim)

Gilly FN et al (1994) Regional chemotherapy (with mitomycin C) and intra-operative hyperthermia for digestive cancers with peritoneal carcinomatosis. Hepatogastroenterology 41:124–129

Gilly FN et al (1999) Peritonectomy combined with intraperitoneal chemohyperthermia in abdominal cancer with peritoneal carcinomatosis: phase I-II study. Anticancer Res 19:2317–2321

Glehen O et al (2004) Cytoreductive surgery combined with perioperative intraperitoneal chemotherapy for the management of peritoneal carcinomatosis from colorectal cancer: a multi-institutional study. J Clin Oncol 22:3284–3292

Glehen O et al (2008) Hyperthermic intraperitoneal chemotherapy: nomenclature and modalities of perfusion. J Surg Oncol 98:242–246

Glockzin G, Schlitt HJ, Piso P (2009) Peritoneal carcinomatosis: patients selection, perioperative complications and quality of life related to cytoreductive surgery and hyperthermic intraperitoneal chemotherapy. World J Surg Oncol 7:5

Glockzin G, Ghali N, Lang SA, Schlitt HJ, Piso P (2009) Results of cytoreductive surgery and hyperthermic intraperitoneal chemotherapy for peritoneal carcinomatosis from colorectal cancer. J Surg Oncol 100:306–310

Green JA et al (1984) Potentiation of melphalan cytotoxicity in human ovarian cancer cell lines by glutathione depletion. Cancer Res 44:5427–5431

Grubbs EG et al (2004a) In-transit melanoma: the role of alkylating-agent resistance in regional therapy. J Am Coll Surg 199:419–427

Grubbs EG et al (2004b) Modulation of resistance to regional chemotherapy in the extremity melanoma model. Surgery 136:210–218

Hagiwara A et al (1999) Extensive gastrectomy and carbon-adsorbed mitomycin C for gastric cancer with peritoneal metastases. Case reports of survivors and their implications. Hepatogastroenterology 46:1673–1677

Harmon RL, Sugarbaker PH (2005) Prognostic indicators in peritoneal carcinomatosis from gastrointestinal cancer. Int Semin Surg Oncol 2:3

Hayes JD, Pulford DJ (1995) The glutathione S-transferase supergene family: regulation of GST and the contribution of the isoenzymes to cancer chemoprotection and drug resistance. Crit Rev Biochem Mol Biol 30:445–600

Hauschild A et al (2009) Results of a phase III, randomized, placebo-controlled study of sorafenib in combination with carboplatin and paclitaxel as second-line treatment in patients with unresectable stage III or stage IV melanoma. J Clin Oncol 27:2823–2830

Healy JC, Reznek RH (1998) The peritoneum, mesenteries and omenta: normal anatomy and pathological processes. Eur Radiol 8:886–900

Hegazy MA et al (2007) Preoperative isolated limb infusion of Doxorubicin and external irradiation for limb-threatening soft tissue sarcomas. Ann Surg Oncol 14:568–576

Heldin CH, Rubin K, Pietras K, Ostman A (2004) High interstitial fluid pressure—an obstacle in cancer therapy. Nat Rev Cancer 4:806–813

Helm CW et al (2007) Hyperthermic intraperitoneal chemotherapy in conjunction with surgery for the treatment of recurrent ovarian carcinoma. Gynecol Oncol 105:90–96

Hoekstra HJ, van Ginkel RJ (2003) Hyperthermic isolated limb perfusion in the management of extremity sarcoma. Curr Opin Oncol 15:300–303

Hoekstra HJ, Schraffordt Koops H, de Vries LG, van Weerden TW, Oldhoff J (1993) Toxicity of hyperthermic isolated limb perfusion with cisplatin for recurrent melanoma of the lower extremity after previous perfusion treatment. Cancer 72:1224–1229

Issels RD (2008) Hyperthermia adds to chemotherapy. Eur J Cancer 44:2546–2554

Jacquet PSP (1995) Abdominal adhesions causing intestnal obstruction following cytoreduction surgery and early postoperative intraperitoneal chemotherapy. Acta Chirurgica Australica 27:92–95

Jacquet P, Sugarbaker PH (1996) Clinical research methodologies in diagnosis and staging of patients with peritoneal carcinomatosis. Cancer Treat Res 82:359–374

Jacquet P, Averbach A, Stuart OA, Chang D, Sugarbaker PH (1998) Hyperthermic intraperitoneal doxorubicin: pharmacokinetics, metabolism, and tissue distribution in a rat model. Cancer Chemother Pharmacol 41:147–154

Jain RK (2001a) Delivery of molecular medicine to solid tumors: lessons from in vivo imaging of gene expression and function. J Control Release 74:7–25

Jain RK (2001b) Normalizing tumor vasculature with anti-angiogenic therapy: a new paradigm for combination therapy. Nat Med 7:987–989

Jayne DG, Fook S, Loi C, Seow-Choen F (2002) Peritoneal carcinomatosis from colorectal cancer. Br J Surg 89:1545–1550

Jones RB et al (1978) High volume intraperitoneal chemotherapy ("belly bath") for ovarian cancer. Pharmacologic basis and early results. Cancer Chemother Pharmacol 1:161–166

Kerscher AG, Mallalieu J, Pitroff A, Kerscher F, Esquivel J (2010) Morbidity and mortality of 109 consecutive cytoreductive procedures with hyperthermic intraperitoneal chemotherapy (HIPEC) performed at a community hospital. World J Surg 34:62–69

Klaase JM et al (1994) Limb recurrence-free interval and survival in patients with recurrent melanoma of the extremities treated with normothermic isolated perfusion. J Am Coll Surg 178:564–572

Kim KJ et al (1993) Inhibition of vascular endothelial growth factor-induced angiogenesis suppresses tumour growth in vivo. Nature 362:841–844

Ko SH et al (2006) Optimizing a novel regional chemotherapeutic agent against melanoma: hyperthermia-induced enhancement of temozolomide cytotoxicity. Clin Cancer Res 12:289–297

Koops HS et al (1998) Prophylactic isolated limb perfusion for localized, high-risk limb melanoma: results of a multicenter randomized phase III trial. European Organization for Research and Treatment of Cancer Malignant Melanoma Cooperative Group Protocol 18832, the World Health Organization Melanoma Program trial 15, and the North American Perfusion Group Southwest Oncology Group-8593. J Clin Oncol 16:2906–2912

Koppe MJ, Boerman OC, Oyen WJ, Bleichrodt RP (2006) Peritoneal carcinomatosis of colorectal origin: incidence and current treatment strategies. Ann Surg 243:212–222

Krementz ET, Ryan RF (1972) Chemotherapy of melanoma of the extremities by perfusion: fourteen years clinical experience. Ann Surg 175:900–917

Krementz ET, Knudson L (1961) The effect of increased oxygen tension on the tumoricidal effect of nitrogen mustard. Surgery 50:266–273

Krementz ET et al (1994) Regional chemotherapy for melanoma. A 35-year experience. Ann Surg 220:520–534 (discussion 534–525)

Kretschmer L et al (2006) Factors predicting the risk of in-transit recurrence after sentinel lymphonodectomy in patients with cutaneous malignant melanoma. Ann Surg Oncol 13:1105–1112

Kroon BB et al (1993) Results of a double perfusion schedule with melphalan in patients with melanoma of the lower limb. Eur J Cancer 29A:325–328

Kroon BB, Van Geel AN, Benckhuijsen C, Wieberdink J (1987) Normothermic isolation perfusion with melphalan for advanced melanoma of the limbs. Anticancer Res 7:441–442

Kroon HM, Moncrieff M, Kam PC, Thompson JF (2009) Factors predictive of acute regional toxicity after isolated limb infusion with melphalan and actinomycin D in melanoma patients. Ann Surg Oncol 16:1184–1192

Kroon HM, Moncrieff M, Kam PC, Thompson JF (2008) Outcomes following isolated limb infusion for melanoma. A 14-year experience. Ann Surg Oncol 15:3003–3013

Kroon HM, Lin DY, Kam PC, Thompson JF (2009a) Efficacy of repeat isolated limb infusion with melphalan and actinomycin D for recurrent melanoma. Cancer 115:1932–1940

Kroon HM, Lin DY, Kam PC, Thompson JF (2009b) Isolated limb infusion as palliative treatment for advanced limb disease in patients with AJCC stage IV melanoma. Ann Surg Oncol 16:1193–1201

Lejeune FJ, Ghanem GE (1987) A simple and accurate new method for cytostatics dosimetry in isolation perfusion of the limbs based on exchangeable blood volume determination. Cancer Res 47:639–643

Li XF et al (2007) Visualization of hypoxia in microscopic tumors by immunofluorescent microscopy. Cancer Res 67:7646–7653

Lindner P, Doubrovsky A, Kam PC, Thompson JF (2002) Prognostic factors after isolated limb infusion with cytotoxic agents for melanoma. Ann Surg Oncol 9:127–136

Los G, Verdegaal EM, Mutsaers PH, McVie JG (1991) Penetration of carboplatin and cisplatin into rat peritoneal tumor nodules after intraperitoneal chemotherapy. Cancer Chemother Pharmacol 28:159–165

Low RN et al (1997) Peritoneal tumor: MR imaging with dilute oral barium and intravenous gadolinium-containing contrast agents compared with unenhanced MR imaging and CT. Radiology 204:513–520

Lu Z et al (2008) Tumor-penetrating microparticles for intraperitoneal therapy of ovarian cancer. J Pharmacol Exp Ther 327:673–682

Luck JM (1956) Action of p-[di(2-chloroethyl)]-amino-l-phenylalanine on Harding-Passey mouse melanoma. Science 123:984–985

Luck JM (1957) The action of the phenylalanine mustards and of several homologs on mouse melanoma. Cancer Res 17:1071–1076

Markman M (2008) Strategies to examine new compounds for intraperitoneal use in ovarian cancer. Int J Gynecol Cancer 18(Suppl 1):33–35

McDermott DF et al (2008) Double-blind randomized phase II study of the combination of sorafenib and dacarbazine in patients with advanced melanoma: a report from the 11715 study group. J Clin Oncol 26:2178–2185

McMahon N et al (2009) Optimizing melphalan pharmacokinetics in regional melanoma therapy: does correcting for ideal body weight alter regional response or toxicity? Ann Surg Oncol 16:953–961

McQuellon RP et al (2001) Quality of life after intraperitoneal hyperthermic chemotherapy (IPHC) for peritoneal carcinomatosis. Eur J Surg Oncol 27:65–73

McQuellon RP et al (2003) Long-term survivorship and quality of life after cytoreductive surgery plus intraperitoneal hyperthermic chemotherapy for peritoneal carcinomatosis. Ann Surg Oncol 10:155–162

McQuellon RP et al (2007) Monitoring health outcomes following cytoreductive surgery plus intraperitoneal hyperthermic chemotherapy for peritoneal carcinomatosis. Ann Surg Oncol 14:1105–1113

McQuellon RP et al (2008) Survival and health outcomes after cytoreductive surgery with intraperitoneal hyperthermic chemotherapy for disseminated peritoneal cancer of appendiceal origin. Ann Surg Oncol 15:125–133

Middleton MR et al (2000) Randomized phase III study of temozolomide versus dacarbazine in the treatment of patients with advanced metastatic malignant melanoma. J Clin Oncol 18:158–166

Minor DR et al (1985) A clinical and pharmacokinetic study of isolated limb perfusion with heat and melphalan for melanoma. Cancer 55:2638–2644

Moncrieff MD et al (2008) Isolated limb infusion for advanced soft tissue sarcoma of the extremity. Ann Surg Oncol 15:2749–2756

Moran BJ, Mukherjee A, Sexton R (2006) Operability and early outcome in 100 consecutive laparotomies for peritoneal malignancy. Br J Surg 93:100–104

Moreno-Ramirez D, de la Cruz-Merino L, Ferrandiz L, Villegas-Portero R, Nieto-Garcia A (2010) Isolated limb perfusion for malignant melanoma: systematic review on effectiveness and safety. Oncologist 15:416

Noorda EM et al (2004) Isolated limb perfusion for unresectable melanoma of the extremities. Arch Surg 139:1237–1242

Ouchi K et al (1998) Therapeutic significance of palliative operations for gastric cancer for survival and quality of life. J Surg Oncol 69:41–44

Parsons PG, Carter FB, Morrison L, Regius Mary S (1981) Mechanism of melphalan resistance developed in vitro in human melanoma cells. Cancer Res 41:1525–1534

Pawlik TM et al (2005) Predictors and natural history of in-transit melanoma after sentinel lymphadenectomy. Ann Surg Oncol 12:587–596

Pelz JO, Stojadinovic A, Nissan A, Hohenberger W, Esquivel J (2009) Evaluation of a peritoneal surface disease severity score in patients with colon cancer with peritoneal carcinomatosis. J Surg Oncol 99:9–15

Pestieau SR, Belliveau JF, Griffin H, Stuart OA, Sugarbaker PH (2001) Pharmacokinetics of intraperitoneal oxaliplatin: experimental studies. J Surg Oncol 76:106–114

Piso P et al (2009) Quality of life after cytoreductive surgery and hyperthermic intraperitoneal chemotherapy for peritoneal surface malignancies. J Surg Oncol 100:317–320

Porcheron J et al (2000) Intraperitoneal chemohyperthermia for peritoneal carcinomatosis: original modeling, clinical tolerance and results study about 30 patients. Hepatogastroenterology 47:1411–1418

Poulikakos PI, Zhang C, Bollag G, Shokat KM, Rosen N (2010) RAF inhibitors transactivate RAF dimers and ERK signalling in cells with wild-type BRAF. Nature 464:427–430

Presta LG et al (1997) Humanization of an anti-vascular endothelial growth factor monoclonal antibody for the therapy of solid tumors and other disorders. Cancer Res 57:4593–4599

Rietschel P et al (2008) Phase II study of extended-dose temozolomide in patients with melanoma. J Clin Oncol 26:2299–2304

Robinson WR, Beyer J (2010) Factors affecting the completion of intraperitoneal chemotherapy in women with ovarian cancer. Int J Gynecol Cancer 20:70–74

Robson CN et al (1987) Reduced levels of drug-induced DNA cross-linking in nitrogen mustard-resistant Chinese hamster ovary cells expressing elevated glutathione S-transferase activity. Cancer Res 47:6022–6027

Ross MI (2008) Current status of hyperthermic limb perfusion for in-transit melanoma. Int J Hyperthermia 24:205–217

Ryan RF, Winblad JN, Krementz ET, Creech O Jr (1958) Treatment of malignant neoplasms with chemotherapeutic agents utilizing a pump-oxygenator: technics and early results. Bull Tulane Univ Med Fac 17:133–143

Sadeghi B et al (2000) Peritoneal carcinomatosis from non-gynecologic malignancies: results of the EVOCAPE 1 multicentric prospective study. Cancer 88:358–363

Sanki A, Kam PC, Thompson JF (2007) Long-term results of hyperthermic, isolated limb perfusion for melanoma: a reflection of tumor biology. Ann Surg 245:591–596

Schmidt U, Dahlke MH, Klempnauer J, Schlitt HJ, Piso P (2005) Perioperative morbidity and quality of life in long-term survivors following cytoreductive surgery and hyperthermic intraperitoneal chemotherapy. Eur J Surg Oncol 31:53–58

Seldinger SI (1953) Catheter replacement of the needle in percutaneous arteriography; a new technique. Acta radiol 39:368–376

Shen P et al (2003) Factors predicting survival after intraperitoneal hyperthermic chemotherapy with mitomycin C after cytoreductive surgery for patients with peritoneal carcinomatosis. Arch Surg 138:26–33

Shen P et al (2008) Peritoneal surface disease from colorectal cancer: comparison with the hepatic metastases surgical paradigm in optimally resected patients. Ann Surg Oncol 15:3422–3432

Shen P, Stewart JH, Levine EA (2009a) The role of cytoreductive surgery and hyperthermic intraperitoneal chemotherapy for metastatic colorectal cancer with peritoneal surface disease. Curr Probl Cancer 33:154–167

Shen P, Stewart JH, Levine EA (2009b) Cytoreductive surgery and hyperthermic intraperitoneal chemotherapy for peritoneal surface malignancy: overview and rationale. Curr Probl Cancer 33:125–141

Siemann DW, Chapman M, Beikirch A (1991) Effects of oxygenation and pH on tumor cell response to alkylating chemotherapy. Int J Radiat Oncol Biol Phys 20:287–289

Simpson-Herren L, Sanford AH, Holmquist JP (1976) Effects of surgery on the cell kinetics of residual tumor. Cancer Treat Rep 60:1749–1760

Smeenk RM, Verwaal VJ, Zoetmulder FA (2006) Toxicity and mortality of cytoreduction and intraoperative hyperthermic intraperitoneal chemotherapy in pseudomyxoma peritonei—a report of 103 procedures. Eur J Surg Oncol 32:186–190

Smeenk RM, Verwaal VJ, Zoetmulder FA (2007) Learning curve of combined modality treatment in peritoneal surface disease. Br J Surg 94:1408–1414

Spratt JS, Adcock RA, Muskovin M, Sherrill W, McKeown J (1980a) Clinical delivery system for intraperitoneal hyperthermic chemotherapy. Cancer Res 40:256–260

Spratt JS, Adcock RA, Sherrill W, Travathen S (1980b) Hyperthermic peritoneal perfusion system in canines. Cancer Res 40:253–255

Sobhani I et al (2008) Early detection of recurrence by 18FDG-PET in the follow-up of patients with colorectal cancer. Br J Cancer 98:875–880

Stehlin JS Jr (1969) Hyperthermic perfusion with chemotherapy for cancers of the extremities. Surg Gynecol Obstet 129:305–308

Stephens AD et al (1999) Morbidity and mortality analysis of 200 treatments with cytoreductive surgery and hyperthermic intraoperative intraperitoneal chemotherapy using the coliseum technique. Ann Surg Oncol 6:790–796

Stewart JH, Shen P, Levine EA (2005) Intraperitoneal hyperthermic chemotherapy for peritoneal surface malignancy: current status and future directions. Ann Surg Oncol 12:765–777

Stewart JH, Levine EA, Shen P (2009) The current role of hyperthermic intraperitoneal chemotherapy for peritoneal dissemination of appendiceal tumors. Curr Probl Cancer 33:142–153

Storm FK, Morton DL (1985) Value of therapeutic hyperthermic limb perfusion in advanced recurrent melanoma of the lower extremity. Am J Surg 150:32–35

Sugarbaker PH (1995) Peritonectomy procedures. Ann Surg 221:29–42

Sugarbaker PH (1999) Management of peritoneal-surface malignancy: the surgeon's role. Langenbecks Arch Surg 384:576–587

Sun X et al (2008) Changes in tumor hypoxia induced by mild temperature hyperthermia as assessed by dual-tracer immunohistochemistry. Radiother Oncol 88:269–276

Suzukake K, Petro BJ, Vistica DT (1982) Reduction in glutathione content of L-PAM resistant L1210 Cells confers drug sensitivity. Biochem Pharmacol 31:121–124

Teicher BA, Kowal CD, Kennedy KA, Sartorelli AC (1981) Enhancement by hyperthermia of the in vitro cytotoxicity of mitomycin C toward hypoxic tumor cells. Cancer Res 41:1096–1099

Thompson JF, Gianoutsos MP (1992) Isolated limb perfusion for melanoma: effectiveness and toxicity of cisplatin compared with that of melphalan and other drugs. World J Surg 16:227–233

Thompson JF, Hunt JA, Shannon KF, Kam PC (1997) Frequency and duration of remission after isolated limb perfusion for melanoma. Arch Surg 132:903–907

Thompson JF, Kam PC (2008) Current status of isolated limb infusion with mild hyperthermia for melanoma. Int J Hyperthermia 24:219–225

Thompson JF, Kam PC, Waugh RC, Harman CR (1998) Isolated limb infusion with cytotoxic agents: a simple alternative to isolated limb perfusion. Semin Surg Oncol 14:238–247

Thompson JF, Waugh RC, Saw RPM, Kam PCA (1994) Isolated limb infusion with melphalan for recurrent limb melanoma: a simple alternative to isolated limb perfusion. Reg Cancer Treat 7:188–192

Topuz E et al (1998) Catheter complications associated with intraperitoneal chemotherapy. Eur J Gynaecol Oncol 19:275–279

Trinh VA, Patel SP, Hwu WJ (2009) The safety of temozolomide in the treatment of malignancies. Expert Opin Drug Saf 8:493–499

Tsai M et al (2007) Effects of carrier on disposition and antitumor activity of intraperitoneal Paclitaxel. Pharm Res 24:1691–1701

Ueno T et al (2004) Temozolomide is a novel regional infusion agent for the treatment of advanced extremity melanoma. Am J Surg 188:532–537

Ueno T et al (2006) Modulation of chemotherapy resistance in regional therapy: a novel therapeutic approach to advanced extremity melanoma using intra-arterial temozolomide in combination with systemic O6-benzylguanine. Mol Cancer Ther 5:732–738

Varban O, Levine EA, Stewart JH, McCoy TP, Shen P (2009) Outcomes associated with cytoreductive surgery and intraperitoneal hyperthermic chemotherapy in colorectal cancer patients with peritoneal surface disease and hepatic metastases. Cancer 115:3427–3436

van de Merwe SA et al (1993) Modification of human tumour and normal tissue pH during hyperthermic and normothermic antiblastic regional isolation perfusion for malignant melanoma: a pilot study. Int J Hyperthermia 9:205–217

Verwaal VJ et al (2003) Randomized trial of cytoreduction and hyperthermic intraperitoneal chemotherapy versus systemic chemotherapy and palliative surgery in patients with peritoneal carcinomatosis of colorectal cancer. J Clin Oncol 21:3737–3743

Verwaal VJ, van Tinteren H, Ruth SV, Zoetmulder FA (2004) Toxicity of cytoreductive surgery and hyperthermic intra-peritoneal chemotherapy. J Surg Oncol 85:61–67

Verwaal VJ, Bruin S, Boot H, van Slooten G, van Tinteren H (2008) 8-year follow-up of randomized trial: cytoreduction and hyperthermic intraperitoneal chemotherapy versus systemic chemotherapy in patients with peritoneal carcinomatosis of colorectal cancer. Ann Surg Oncol 15:2426–2432

Vrouenraets BC, Klaase JM, Nieweg OE, Kroon BB (1998) Toxicity and morbidity of isolated limb perfusion. Semin Surg Oncol 14:224–231

Vrouenraets BC et al (1999) Relation between limb toxicity and treatment outcomes after isolated limb perfusion for recurrent melanoma. J Am Coll Surg 188:522–530

Watanabe M, Tanaka R, Hondo H, Kuroki M (1992) Effects of antineoplastic agents and hyperthermia on cytotoxicity toward chronically hypoxic glioma cells. Int J Hyperthermia 8:131–138

Wieberdink J, Benckhuysen C, Braat RP, van Slooten EA, Olthuis GA (1982) Dosimetry in isolation perfusion of the limbs by assessment of perfused tissue volume and grading of toxic tissue reactions. Eur J Cancer Clin Oncol 18:905–910

Weisberger AS, Levine B, Storaasli JP (1955) Use of nitrogen mustard in treatment of serous effusions of neoplastic origin. J Am Med Assoc 159:1704–1707

Wong JH, Cagle LA, Kopald KH, Swisher SG, Morton DL (1990) Natural history and selective management of in transit melanoma. J Surg Oncol 44:146–150

Yan TD, Black D, Savady R, Sugarbaker PH (2006) Systematic review on the efficacy of cytoreductive surgery combined with perioperative intraperitoneal chemotherapy for peritoneal carcinomatosis from colorectal carcinoma. J Clin Oncol 24:4011–4019

Yan TD et al (2007a) Learning curve for cytoreductive surgery and perioperative intraperitoneal chemotherapy for peritoneal surface malignancy—a journey to becoming a Nationally Funded Peritonectomy Center. Ann Surg Oncol 14:2270–2280

Yan TD, Sim J, Morris DL (2007b) Selection of patients with colorectal peritoneal carcinomatosis for cytoreductive surgery and perioperative intraperitoneal chemotherapy. Ann Surg Oncol 14:1807–1817

Yan TD et al (2009) Cytoreductive surgery and hyperthermic intraperitoneal chemotherapy for malignant peritoneal mesothelioma: multi-institutional experience. J Clin Oncol 27:6237–6242

Yeo Y et al (2007) In situ cross-linkable hyaluronan hydrogels containing polymeric nanoparticles for preventing postsurgical adhesions. Ann Surg 245:819–824

Yoshimoto Y et al (2007) Defining regional infusion treatment strategies for extremity melanoma: comparative analysis of melphalan and temozolomide as regional chemotherapeutic agents. Mol Cancer Ther 6:1492–1500

Chapter 25
Palliative Radiation Therapy

Fabio Luis Cury and George Shenouda

25.1 Introduction

Radiation therapy is the field of oncology that uses ionizing radiation to kill malignant cells, by disturbing cellular processes, preventing a perfect cell division and, consequently, inducing cellular death (Barnes et al. 2010). The deleterious effects of radiation started to be used in cancer treatment soon after Wilhelm Roentgen discovered X-rays in 1896. But only in the 1950's, treatment machines similar to those used today started to be produced, wide spreading the use of radiation therapy in cancer treatment. Further popularization occurred in the 1990's after the development of modern CT-scanners and the use of up to date computer software, allowing better understanding and visualization of radiation distribution within the human body.

Treatment is usually delivered with photons, although superficial lesions, such as skin cancer and rib metastases, can also be effectively treated with electrons. The dose of radiation delivered to a tumor is measured in gray (Gy), and varies depending on the type of cancer being treated, tumor location and treatment intent, i.e., curative or palliative. The total dose of radiation is usually delivered in a number of fractions. Fractionation gives time to cells to recover, and since normal cells have a better DNA repair system than cancer cells, the deleterious effects of radiation will be more effective on damaging malignant cells. Fractionation also gives time to cells to move from a radioresistant cell cycle phase (S-phase) to a more radiosensitive one (G2-M phase). Also, hypoxic tumors can experience reoxygenation and become more radiosensitive, as a consequence of reduction of acute and/or chronic hypoxia between fractions Currently, it is estimated that approximately 60–70 % of patients diagnosed with cancer will undergo radiation therapy during the course of their treatment, with either curative or palliative intent. Curative radiation therapy, as the name suggests, has the objective of cure by eradicating both macroscopic and microscopic disease. Palliative radiation therapy has the main objective to relieve

F. L. Cury (✉) · G. Shenouda
Department of Oncology, Division of Radiation Oncology, Montreal General Hospital, McGill University Health Center, McGill University, Montreal, QC, Canada
e-mail:fabio.cury@muhc.mcgill.ca

J. V. Burnier, M. N. Burnier, Jr. (eds.), *Experimental and Clinical Metastasis*,
DOI 10.1007/978-1-4614-3685-0_25, © Springer Science+Business Media New York 2013

symptoms, recover loss of function caused by tumor compression, and improve quality of life in patients who have metastatic disease. The objective of this chapter is to examine the use of radiation therapy in the treatment of the most common sites of metastases, and to present novel techniques that may improve therapy in a patient population with limited options.

25.2 Brain Metastases

Brain metastases are a common clinical entity that the oncologist encounters in more than 20–40 % of patients with cancer (Barnes et al. 2010). Brain metastases are the most common CNS malignant involvement as they outnumber the primary CNS primary neoplasms by a factor of 10–1. Metastatic spread to the brain has an annual incidence of 170,000–200,000 cases per year. Approximately 15 % of adults who die of cancer will have parenchymal brain metastases (Patchell and Posner 1985). The most common cancers to metastasize to the brain are lungs (40 %), breast (25 %), melanoma (10 %), unknown primary site (10 %), and other sites (15 %). Autopsy series demonstrate a 10–30 % incidence rate for all patients with a diagnosis of cancer (Li and Poon 1988; Wen et al. 2001). Even though it is common for patients with brain metastases to have active primary and other systemic metastatic disease, progression of brain metastases is the cause of death in approximately 50 % of this group of patients (Borgelt et al. 1981; Kurtz et al. 1981; Chatani et al. 1986). The incidence of brain metastases has increased over time, probably as a result of advances in neuro-imaging procedures and improvements in the treatment of primary tumor and systemic disease, which has led to an increase of survival. Treatment for brain metastases patients includes corticosteroids, anticonvulsants to control seizures, surgery, radiotherapy, radiosurgery and chemotherapy. The appropriate aim of treatment is improvement or maintenance of quality of life.

25.2.1 Clinical Presentation

The majority of the patients will present with one or more of the following symptoms: headaches, nausea and vomiting, blurred vision, mental status and speech disturbances. They can also complain of motor or sensory changes as well convulsions. On examination the following signs can be elicited: hemiparesis, neurocognitive deficits, papilledema, ataxia, and apraxia. The presence of these symptoms and signs in any patient with known malignancy should be considered highly suspicious for brain metastases and urgent investigations initiated at once to determine the possible etiology of the patient's complaints. The differential diagnosis includes infectious process, cerebro-vascular accidents, metabolic and paraneoplastic manifestations of malignancy. Moreover, any of these differential diagnoses can coexist with brain metastases at the same time and may lead to difficulties in making the diagnosis. The patient with suspected brain metastases should be evaluated by a multidisciplinary team of expert medical professionals to evaluate the patients and to recommend the best approach to making the diagnosis and to initiating the appropriate and timely interventions.

The standard of care for imaging the central nervous system (CNS) in cancer patients is the MRI with Gadolinium contrast infusion. MRI has a higher resolution and accuracy as compared to CT scans of the brain. MRI will frequently disclose smaller lesions not detected on CT scans. The detection of multiple lesions by MRI will have a major impact on the prognosis and on the subsequent management of patients who otherwise were considered to have a single lesion on CT scan. Care must be taken to identify leptomeningeal spread if present as well as any other metastatic process to the spinal cord that may complicate the clinical presentation.

Positron emission tomography (PET) and CT scans are important investigative tools for the systemic evaluation of the disease status. Furthermore, the use of PET-CT scans will help to identify the primary site of the malignancy if the patient presents with brain metastases with no previous history of cancer.

25.2.2 Prognosis

The prognosis is determined by many factors including patient's age, status of the primary disease control, and the Karnofsky performance status (KPS). Gaspar et al. (1997) who analysed the Radiation Therapy Oncology Group (RTOG) experience have reported these prognostic factors in the treatment of more than a thousand patients with brain metastases. A recursive partition analysis (RPA) revealed three different prognostic classes. RPA class 1 included patients who were younger than 65 years, with a KPS of 70 or higher, and a controlled primary disease. RPA class 3 included patients with a KPS less than 70. RPA class 2 included patients who did not belong to either class 1 or 3. The median survival of patients in the three RPA classes was as follows: patients with an RPA class 1 had a median survival of 7.1 months; patients with an RPA class 2 had a median survival of 4.2 months, while patients with an RPA class 3 had a median survival of 2.3 months.

25.2.3 Medical Treatment

Corticosteroids The initial treatment for patients with brain metastases consists of corticosteroids in order to reduce the vasogenic edema and to improve the neurological deficits. The introduction of corticosteroids in the form of Dexamethasone results in overall improvement in the neurological function and KPS in two-thirds of the patients. Patient receiving corticosteroids should also receive concurrent proton pump inhibitor to reduce the chances of corticosteroids induced peptic ulcer. The usual dosage of corticosteroids in patients with brain metastases is a 10 mg intravenous or oral bolus, followed by a 4–6 mg, q.6.h–q.8.h of Dexamethasone equivalent dose. The dose of Dexamethasone should be tapered off over a period of 4 weeks.

Anticonvulsants Based on four negative randomized trials for prophylactic use of anticonvulsants in patients with brain tumors, the American Academy of Neurology recommends that prophylactic anticonvulsants not be initiated in newly diagnosed patients who have not experienced seizure (Glantz et al. 2000). It is important to recognize the fact that anticonvulsants are known to impact negatively on neurocognitive functions. Klein et al. (2002) correlated seizure burden with quality of life and neurocognitive functions. The study demonstrates the significant correlation between the increase in the number of anticonvulsants with a decrease in quality of life and neurocognitive functions. It is safe to taper a patient off of anticonvulsants if they have been started prophylactically, provided that they had not experienced any seizure activity.

25.2.4 Whole Brain Radiotherapy

Whole brain radiotherapy (WBRT) is considered to be the standard of care in patients with newly diagnosed brain metastases. In general, whole brain radiotherapy should be started shortly after the diagnosis of brain metastases is made. A total dose of 30 Gy in ten fractions is considered the most appropriate dose fractionation for most patients with brain metastases (Gaspar et al. 2010). A similarly acceptable radiotherapy schedule of 37.5 Gy in 17 fractions is another alternative. There is still no agreement on the dose fractionation despite numerous studies designed to determine the optimal dose fractionation schedule. In patients with RPA Class III, a shorter course of 20 Gy in five fractions should be considered as an acceptable scheme. The natural history of patients with brain metastases as the presenting event in the cancer diagnosis is frequently unpredictable. These patients may live sufficiently long, enough to experience late radiation toxicity; therefore a less hypofractionated radiotherapy schedule is preferable. Whole brain irradiation to a dose of 45–50 Gy in 2 Gy fractions over 5 weeks should be considered in patients with brain metastases from germ cell tumors metastatic to the brain, as these patients are potentially curable with long survival.

The post-operative delivery of WBRT for such patients aims to sterilize residual disease in the tumor bed as well as other sites of occult disease in the brain. For patients who have undergone removal of solitary brain metastases, the addition of WBRT results in a lower incidence of brain recurrence. The University of Kentucky randomized patients with single brain metastases to surgery (S) alone (46 patients), or surgery followed by WBRT (49 patients) (Patchell et al. 1998). The overall survival times were not statistically significant different between the two arms of the trial with a median survival time of 48 weeks in the S+WBRT group versus 43 weeks in patients who had surgery alone. The addition of WBRT to S reduced the rate of death due to neurological causes (14 %) as compared to surgery alone (44 %). The addition of post-operative WBRT also delayed death due to neurological disease progression.

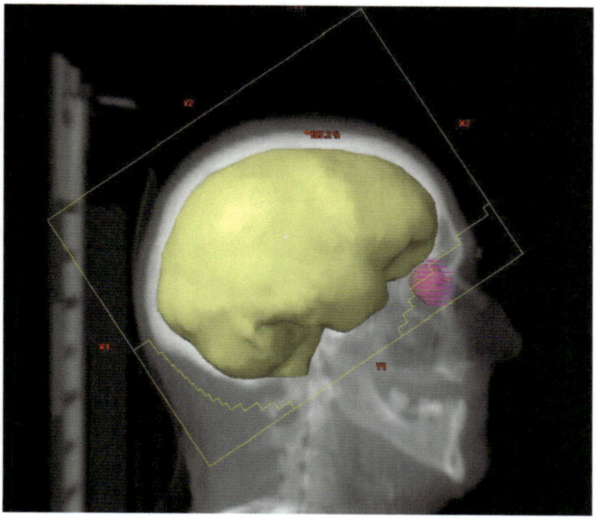

Fig. 25.1 Example of whole brain radiotherapy for multiple brain metastases with appropriate shielding of the eyes (*red*)

Figure 25.1 depicts a typical example of whole brain radiotherapy for a patient with multiple brain metastases from a primary lung cancer.

25.2.5 Surgical Resection

There is extensive literature on the surgical management of brain metastases. Surgical resection of solitary brain metastases is increasingly performed on patients with favorable prognostic factors, accessible lesions, and/or metastatic lesions from relatively radio-resistant tumors such as renal cell carcinoma and melanoma. Due to the fact that metastases are usually well demarcated from surrounding brain, gross total resection with a minimum of morbidity and mortality is often possible. Relief of symptoms of intracranial hypertension and focal brain dysfunction has been demonstrated. Patient survival is also dependent on the extent of extra-cranial disease. Three prospective randomized trials in which surgical excision followed by WBRT compared to WBRT alone in patients with single metastases have been done. Patchell and colleagues (1990) randomized patients with single metastases to either surgical excision followed by WBRT (25 patients) or biopsy followed by WBRT (23 patients). The median survival times of patients who underwent surgical resection compared to those who had biopsy were 40 and 15 weeks, respectively. Vecht et al. (1993) randomized 63 patients to the same regimens with similar results. Although a third randomized trial failed to show the same survival advantage (Mintz et al. 1996), the preponderance of available evidence suggests that surgical removal of solitary metastases followed by WBRT is superior to WBRT alone for selected patients. The results of the three randomized clinical trials are summarized in Table 25.1.

Controversy exists regarding the role of surgery in the management of multiple metastases. Bindal et al. (1993) analyzed patients with multiple metastases who had

Table 25.1 Whole brain radiotherapy versus surgery plus whole brain

Radiotherapy for single brain metastasis

Reference	Treatment arms	N	Median survival	Length of functional independence (week)	CNS death (%)
Patchell et al. (1990)	S + WBRT	25	40	38	29
	WBRT	23	15	8	50
Vecht et al. (1993)	S + WBRT	32	43	33	35
	WBRT	31	26	15	33
Mintz et al. (1996)	S + WBRT	41	24	8	46
	WBRT	43	27	9	63

S surgery, *WBRT* whole brain radiotherapy, *CNS* central nervous system

all the tumors resected and compared these with patients with multiple metastases who had some but not all of their brain metastases resected. A further comparison was made in patients with single metastases that were treated with complete resection plus WBRT. The authors found that the group with completely resected multiple metastases did relatively well (median survival, 14 months) and was similar to the group with single resected metastases (median survival, 14 months). The patients who did not have all of their brain tumors removed did less well (median survival, 6 months). The 1-month mortality rate for the multiple metastases group was only 4 %.

Hazuka et al. (1993) reported a retrospective surgical series with 18 patients with multiple metastases and 28 patients with single metastases. The group with multiple metastases had a median survival of 5 months; those with single metastases had a median survival of 12 months. Overall, only 50 % of patients had complete resections, and the complete resection rate in the multiple metastases group was not reported.

Occasionally, surgery is necessary in patients with multiple metastases who have a single life-threatening brain lesion. The intent of surgery in these cases is to remove the single life-threatening lesion without resecting the other lesions. The standard of care for most patients with brain metastases is WBRT alone. The best results from surgery are found in patients with a single surgically accessible lesion and either no remaining systemic disease (true solitary metastasis) or controlled systemic cancer limited to the primary site only. A study from Memorial Sloan-Kettering Cancer Center (Burt 1992) has suggested that in patients undergoing resection of brain metastases from non-small cell lung carcinoma, survival is increased significantly in patients with complete resection of the primary lung disease. There was no correlation of survival with initial cancer stage per se. Also, surgical treatment may be indicated in patients without known systemic cancer (to obtain a tissue diagnosis) and in patients with impending herniation resulting from pressure effects.

25.2.6 Radiosurgery

Stereotactic radiosurgery (SRS) is a radiotherapeutic technique that delivers high dose irradiation to a small target in a single session with a steep dose fall off. There are two major delivery techniques, gamma knife SRS or linac-based SRS. The linac-based SRS systems are of two types: those with a tracking system such as cyberknife and those without tracking system such as the trilogy system. The attractive property of SRS in the treatment of brain metastases is that SRS will focus the dose on the tumor target, and at the same time spares the surrounding normal tissues from toxicity. A stereotactic radiosurgery was designed to treat intracranial targets such as primary and metastatic brain tumors, acoustic neuromas, meningiomas, brain adenomas and craniopharyngiomas, as well as vascular diseases, such as arteriovenous malformation and cavernous angiomas. Stereotactic radiosurgery was also used to treat functional disorders of the CNS such as, trigeminal neuralgia, involuntary movements and epilepsy. Stereotactic radiosurgery is minimally invasive and can be performed as an outpatient procedure with important implication for quality of life and health care economics when compared with surgery (Mehta et al. 1992; 1997).

Most of the evidence supporting the use of SRS for metastatic brain tumor comes from prospective non-randomized trials and retrospective studies (Sawaya et al. 1994; Lippitz et al. 2004; Bhatnagar et al. 2002; Simonova et al. 2000). These reports suggest that SRS is more effective than WBRT and it is comparable to or superior to surgery. Stereotactic radiosurgery as the sole initial management or as a boost technique before or after WBRT has emerged as a widely practiced modality for brain metastases. The goal of SRS with WBRT is to achieve brain control without the possible long-term neurotoxicity or neurocognitive side effects associated with WBRT. The rationale for SRS, when used as a boost in combination with WBRT, is to improve local control. Stereotactic radiosurgery boost seems to improve survival of selected patients in whom the problem is prominent brain metastases rather than extracranial disease. Stereotactic radiosurgery has its role as a salvage treatment for local recurrence and/or new brain lesions after surgery or WBRT or even after previous SRS. Radiosurgery provides an additional boost to WBRT in patients with brain metastases that are not surgical candidates or because of deep-seated unresectable brain lesions.

Three randomized clinical trials have been reported examining the role of SRS. One study, reported by Kondziolka et al. (1999) randomized patients with two to four lesions to WBRT (30 Gy in 12 fractions) or to WBRT + SRS boost. The study was stopped at an interim evaluation at 60 % accrual. Twenty-seven patients were randomized (14 to WBRT alone and 13 to WBRT plus SRS). The groups were well matched to age, sex, tumor type, number of tumors, and extent of extracranial disease. The rate of local failure at 1 year was 100 % after WBRT alone but only 8 % in patients who had boost SRS. The median time to local failure was 6 months after WBRT alone (95 % confidence interval [CI], 3.5–8.5) in comparison to 36 months (95 % CI, 15.6–57) after WBRT plus SRS ($p = 0.0005$). The median time to any brain failure was improved in the SRS + WBRT group ($p = 0.002$). Tumor control did not depend on histology ($p = 0.85$), number of initial brain metastases ($p = 0.25$), or extent of extracranial disease ($p = 0.26$). Patients who received WBRT alone lived a median of 7.5 months, while those who received WBRT plus radiosurgery lived 11 months ($p = 0.22$). Survival did not depend on histology or number of tumors, but was related to extent of extracranial disease ($p = 0.02$). There was no neurologic or systemic morbidity related to SRS. The authors concluded that combined WBRT and SRS for patients with two to four brain metastases significantly improve control of brain disease. WBRT alone does not provide lasting and effective care for most patients.

A second study was reported by Andrews et al. (2004) (RTOG 9508), where randomized patients with brain metastases, with one to three lesions, treated with WBRT alone were compared with patients treated with WBRT + SRS boost. The median survival rate of patients who received WBRT alone ranged from 5.5 to 7.5 months and was not statistically different from the WBRT + SRS group who showed a median survival rate of 5–11 months. However, on multivariate analysis, WBRT + SRS improved survival in patients with RPA class I and in patients with non-small cell lung cancer. In patients with unresectable or inoperable lesions, SRS resulted in a median survival of 6.5 months compared to 4.9 months in the WBRT group ($p = 0.039$). There was less steroid dependence in the group of patients who received SRS + WBRT as compared to those who received WBRT alone. There was a statistically non-significant increase of late grade 3 and 4 CNS toxicities (6 %) in patients who received the SRS boost. Another trial randomized patients with one to three brain metastases to WBRT, WBRT + SRS, or SRS alone. The local control was higher in the group of patients who received WBRT + SRS or SRS alone, and was better than the group of patients who were treated with WBRT alone (Chougule et al. 2000). Similar results were reported from the Japanese Radiotherapy Oncology Study Group (Aoyama et al. 2006). The study randomized patients to WBRT + SRS versus SRS alone showing that the addition of SRS to WBRT significantly improved local control rate for patients up to four brain metastases. The trial also showed that the tapering of steroid doses and the improvement in KPS were significantly better in the SRS boost arm at 6 months. This was accomplished without a significant increase in acute or late radiation-induced side effects. The study also demonstrated that the omission of WBRT resulted in decreased local control both at the sites of SRS and also in the remaining untreated brain.

In conclusion, SRS alone or in combination with WBRT has emerged as a widely practice treatment modality for brain metastases. The ideal treatment approach may be surgical, resection of the larger or more symptomatic lesions combined with SRS for the surgically inaccessible lesions. Clinical trials have shown the mandatory need for WBRT (Patchell et al. 1990, 1998).

25.2.7 Concurrent Radiosensitizers

In order to improve the efficacy of WBRT in patients with brain metastases, many chemotherapeutic agents and radiosensitizers were used in clinical trials. Radiotherapy was delivered to the whole brain in doses that varied from 30 Gy in ten fractions, 37.5 Gy in 17 fractions, or 40 Gy in 20 fractions in addition to one of the following agents used as a radiosensitizer including: Misonidazole, Nitrosourea, Bromodeoxyuridine, Carboplatin, Motexafin Gadolinium, and Temozolomide (TMZ)

(Patchell et al. 1990; Guerrieri et al. 2004; Komarnicky et al. 1991; Mehta et al. 2003; Suh et al. 2006; Ushio et al. 1991; Verger et al. 2005). No clinical trial has demonstrated any survival benefit when a radiosensitizer was administered during WBRT.

The concurrent administration of TMZ with conventional WBRT was investigated in a phase II study from the Metaxas Cancer Hospital (Antonadou et al. 2002a). In this trial, 52 patients with brain metastases from a variety of primary tumors (among whom 31 had non-small cell lung cancer, nine small cell lung cancer and five had breast cancer) were randomized to WBRT and a total dose of 40 Gy with a daily fraction of 2 Gy, with or without concurrent administration of TMZ. Temozolomide was administered orally at a dose of 75 mg/m^2 during radiation treatment and 200 mg/m^2/day for 5 days every 28 days for a maximum of six additional cycles. Treatment response was assessed on the basis of CT scanning or MRI 2 months after completion of radiation treatment according to the World Health Organization (WHO) criteria for response. Forty-five patients were assessable for response. The objective response rate in the group receiving TMZ (96 %) was significantly superior ($p = 0.017$) to that achieved with WBRT alone (67 %). Another measure of treatment efficacy is the requirement for medication to palliate neurological symptoms. The proportion of patients who required corticosteroids in the TMZ plus WBRT group decreased from 100 to 67 % 2 months after the completion of WBRT, compared with a decrease from 100 to 91 % in the WBRT group. Patients treated with TMZ plus WBRT had a slight improvement in overall survival (8.6 months) compared with WBRT alone (7.0 months). The addition of TMZ to WBRT was generally well tolerated.

In a phase III study concurrent administration of TMZ with WBRT was investigated further. In this trial, 123 patients with brain metastases were randomized to TMZ and WBRT or WBRT alone. The total radiation dose was 30 Gy, with a daily fraction of 3 Gy. TMZ was administered with the same schedule as in the previous trial. Treatment response was assessed with CT scanning or MRI 3 months after completion of the radiation treatment. A total of 123 patients were assessable for response, among them 103 lung cancer patients. The objective response rate in the group receiving TMZ (50 %) was significantly higher ($p = 0.028$) than that achieved with WBRT alone (31 %). The evaluation of lung cancer patients gave similar results; the response rate in the TMZ group (48 %) was significantly superior ($p = 0.031$) to that of the WBRT alone group (27 %). The hazard ratio for death from any cause in the TMZ group compared with the control group was 0.69 (95 % confidence interval (CI): 0.46–1.02, $p = 0.06$). The median survival in the TMZ plus WBRT group was 7.87 months, while in the WBRT group it was 4.93 months. In the subgroup analysis for the lung cancer patients, median time to progression in the brain was 4.8 months (95 % CI: 1.71–9.18) for the WBRT group, while more than 50 % of the patients in the TMZ plus WBRT group were disease-free. There was a significant difference between the two groups ($p < 0.001$) (Antonadou et al. 2002b).

25.2.8 Neurocognitive Decline in Patients with Brain Metastases

Unfortunately, WBRT leads to cognitive impairment in long-term survivors, especially in the elderly. In a recent study using more conventional fractionation, 33 % of the patients developed late neurocognitive toxicity with a median follow-up of 10 months. Memory impairment was the most common symptom in 50 % of the patients. The actuarial rate of neurocognitive toxicity at 2 years was 49 % with 20 % of the patients showing a decline in the KPS of greater than 10 % (Nieder et al. 1999). The first large prospective study to evaluate neurocognitive functions in patients with brain metastases was performed using a battery of cognitive tests at baseline, monthly for 6 months and then every 3 months until death before and after WBRT. Ninety percent of the patients showed an impaired performance in one or more of the neurocognitive tests at baseline. The majority of the patients showed a decline of neurocognitive function after WBRT with 59 % of the patients experiencing greater than 2 standard deviation decline in their performance at 6 months (Meyers et al. 2004).

Current understanding of the effect of radiotherapy on neurocognitive function is very limited. It is becoming increasingly clear that the pathophysiology of late radiotherapy injury is a dynamic, complex and a result of inter and intra cellular interactions between the vasculature and the parenchymal cells (Monje and Palmer 2003). Histological studies reveal that the death of endothelial cells begins during radiotherapy and continues over the next few months. Over weeks to months, small vessels become partially or completely occluded by thrombi from platelet clusters. This mechanism results in a histopathological picture similar to the small vessel disease seen with vascular dementia (Belka et al. 2001).

Hippocampal dependant functions of learning memory and special information processing seem to be preferentially affected by radiotherapy (Armstrong et al. 2000, 2002; Monje et al. 2002). Radiation exposure induces microglial inflammatory response in the neurogenic region of the hippocampus that appears to inhibit the neurogenesis of stem cells.

Current clinical research is underway to determine whether the use of Memantine would reduce the neurocognitive deficit encountered in patients who receive WBRT for brain metastases. Memantine, an N-methyl-D-asparate (NMDA) receptor antagonist, may be neuroprotective agent against neural injury associated with radiation-induced ischemia. Memantine has been shown to improve cognitive functions in patients with mild to moderate vascular dementia and in patients with moderate to severe Alzheimer's type dementia. Currently there is a Phase II study by the RTOG where patients are randomized to Memantine versus placebo started on the first day of WBRT. The results of the study are awaited and may lead to an improvement in neurocognitive preservation and quality of life in this group of patients.

In addition to the impact of WBRT on neurocognitive function in patients with brain metastases, other factors may co-exist and contribute to the cognitive dysfunction in this group of patients. Such factors include anticonvulsants, opioids, chemotherapy, surgery, and the presence of the brain metastases itself.

25.2.9 Recurrent Brain Metastases

Brain metastases often recur. In general, the same therapeutic options used for patients with newly diagnosed brain metastases are available for those with recurrent disease. The type of the initial treatment will limit the therapeutic options available at recurrence. Other factors contributing to the decision on what modality should be used are functional status, extension of disease, recurrence/progression, and treatment must be individualized accordingly (Ammirati et al. 2010). Most frequently, patients have already received WBRT at the time of the initial diagnosis of brain metastases. The amount of WBRT that can be safely delivered in these patients at the time of recurrence is in the range of 15–20 Gy, and is usually ineffective for adequate tumor control. Retrospective studies of re-irradiation showed poor impact on overall survival of this group of patients with recurrent brain metastases (Kurtz et al. 1981; Hazuka and Kinzie 1988; William et al. 1996).

Conventional surgery for recurrent tumors is an option in patients who have a single recurrence and a good performance status. A retrospective study (Sundaresan et al. 1988) examined 48 patients treated with reoperation for recurrent brain metastases and revealed a median survival of 6.7 months after reoperation. In another report of 109 patients with non-small cell lung cancer and recurrent brain metastases, 32 had surgery for their recurrences and survived longer compared to patients with recurrence that did not undergo surgery (Arbit et al. 1995). In all of these studies, the patients were a select group with relatively little systemic disease and a single recurrent metastasis.

In conclusion, stereotactic radiosurgery has been used to treat recurrent brain metastases. Radiosurgery has the theoretical advantage of being able to deliver large doses of additional radiation to small areas of the brain. It is usually delivered to a highly select group of patients who had small recurrent tumors and limited systemic disease. Further studies are needed to determine the true value of stereotactic radiosurgery in the management of recurrent brain metastases.

Key Points

- The most common primary tumors that metastasize to the brain are lungs, breast, and melanoma.
- Progression towards brain metastases indicates a poor overall survival rate.
- The median survival rate of patients with brain metastases, depending on the prognostic class according to a recursive partitioning analysis, is between 2.3–7.1 months.
- Surgical resection is performed in selective cases of solitary brain metastases.
- The addition of whole brain radiotherapy to surgery may increase the survival rate and reduce the incidence of recurrence of brain metastases.
- Stereotactic radiosurgery alone or in combination with whole brain radiotherapy is widely accepted treatment options for patients with brain metastases.
- Concurrent administration of chemotherapeutic agents with whole brain radiotherapy seems to improve the overall survival rate of patients with brain metastases when compared to whole brain radiotherapy alone.

25.3 Bone Metastases

25.3.1 Introduction

After lung and liver, bone is the third most common site of metastases from many types of solid tumors (Clezardin and Teti 2007) with a particularly high incidence in breast, prostate and lung malignancies. Although breast and lung tumors are usually responsible for osteolytic bone lesions, prostate cancer originates osteoblastic lesions. The only tumor that causes only one type of lesion is myeloma that is always associated with osteolytic lesions. All other types of tumors have a combination of osteolytic and osteoblastic components (Roodman 2004).

Bone metastases are common and frequently incapacitating cancer patients. Prognosis for patients diagnosed with bone metastases is generally poor, but survival depends on the primary cancer site, ranging from months for lung cancer (Coleman 2006) to years for prostate and breast cancer (Coleman 2006; Coleman and Ruben 1987; Ibrahim et al. 2010). Although not an imminent life-threatening situation by itself, skeletal involvement causes a detrimental impact on quality of life. A wide range of symptoms and complications are associated with bone metastases, including pain, pathologic fractures, spinal cord compression and, in extreme situations, hypercalcemia (Coleman 2001). As a consequence of the diversity of problems caused by bone metastases, its treatment becomes a challenge and convenes for a multidisciplinary team for adequate management.

25.3.2 Evaluation

Pain is not a patognomonic sign of bone metastasis and by itself should not be interpreted as disease progression. Differential diagnosis has to be made from new and progressive nonmalignant conditions, such as arthritis, osteoporosis, musculoskeletal conditions, as well as treatment-related complications. Therefore, a comprehensive medical history is required, and a thorough physical examination must be performed, including a neurological examination to rule out the possibility of spinal cord, cauda equina or nerve root compression. Biopsies are not performed in all patients, but when necessary, image-guided percutaneous bone biopsies were shown to be safe and cost-effective (Coleman 2001; Jelinek et al. 2002).

Correlation between findings on physical exam with imaging studies is essential to determine the possible cause and extent of disease. When patients present with localized tenderness on physical exam the first imaging study is plain radiography, given its high specificity in comparison to other modalities, such as bone scan. Plain radiographs, are also useful to diagnose impending or established pathologic fractures, or as a confirmatory study after questionable bone scan results. The main weakness of plain radiographs in the assessment of bone metastases is that small lesions are not always seen.

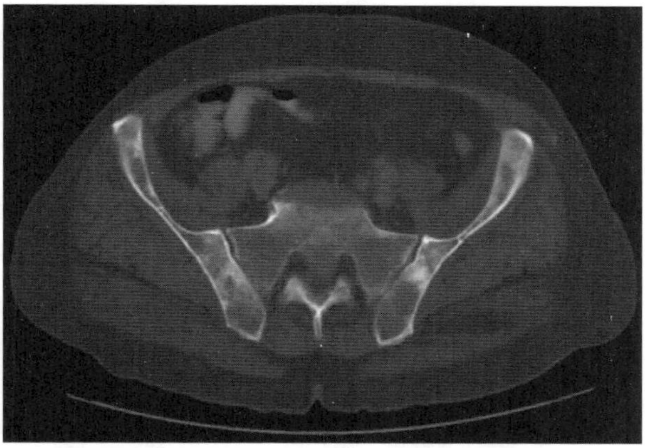

Fig. 25.2 Pelvic CT-scan of a 76 year-old men with metastatic prostate cancer, showing osteoblastic and osteolytic lesions

Computed tomography (CT) scans (Fig. 25.2) are more sensitive than plain radiographs in depicting small lesions, defining extension of cortical destruction and evaluating the risk of pathologic fracture. Moreover, the visualization of soft tissue extension of disease is possible with the use of CT-scan, helping to better understand symptoms, otherwise not explained by plain radiographs alone. Its use in the screening of bone metastases is not cost-effective, given the time needed to perform a whole-body CT-scan.

Similarly to CT-scan, magnetic resonance imaging (MRI) (Fig. 25.3) is very useful as a confirmatory study in the evaluation of suspicious lesions, which are unclear on plain radiographs and unspecific on bone scan. It also provides excellent soft tissue

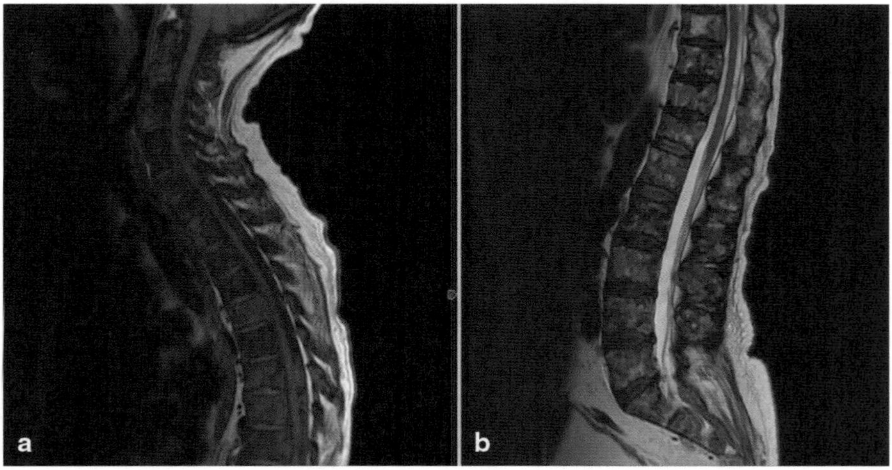

Fig. 25.3 MRI of (**a**) cervical, thoracic, and (**b**) lumbar spine on a patient with prostate cancer, presenting with diffuse metastastic disease to vertebral bodies and multilevel pathologic fractures. No spinal cord or cauda equina compression is present

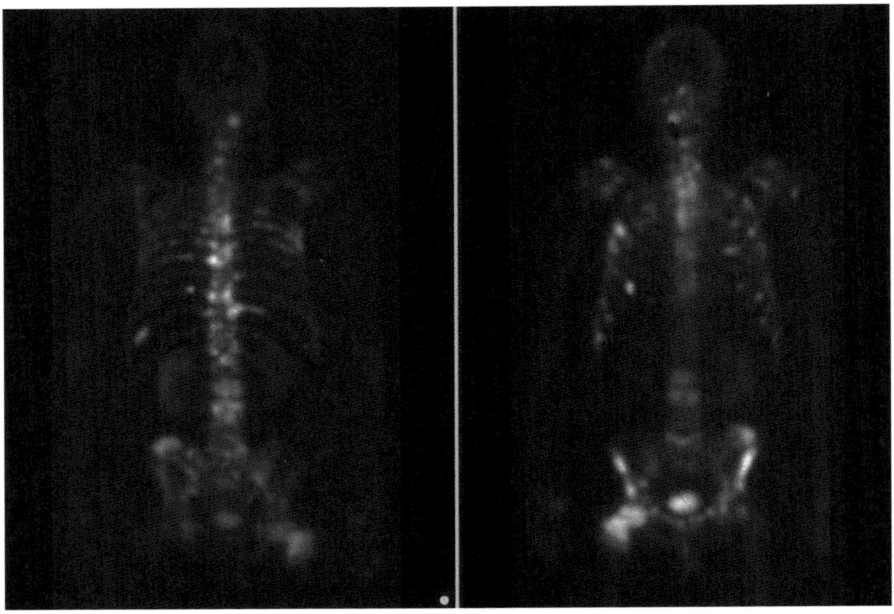

Fig. 25.4 Bone scan of a 76 year-old men with diffuse bone metastases

contrast, allowing for better visualization of soft tissue extension and compression of nervous structures. Along with myelography, it is the study of choice to investigate spinal cord compression.

Bone scintigraphy (radionuclide bone scan using Technetium-99) is very sensitive in the detection of bone metastases (Fig. 25.4), but its sensitivity is limited to the detection of osteoblastic lesions–cancerous or not. Although not specific for bone metastases, with false-positive results frequently associated with degenerative processes, trauma, or Paget's disease, bone scan is the most useful modality to investigate the existence and distribution of bone metastases, and, therefore, part of the screening process of metastatic bone disease.

Positron emission tomography (PET) scan usually uses 18-Fluorodeoxyglucose (FDG) isotope to identify areas of increased metabolic activity in the body (Fig. 25.5). Increased metabolism is usually detected on osteolytic bone lesions (Cook et al. 1998) in which cases PET scan can be more sensitive than bone scan in detecting bone metastases (Even-Sapir et al. 2006). Its use is not widespread given its lack of ability to detect osteoblastic lesions and cost.

25.3.3 External Beam Radiation Therapy

The pain mechanism that is not associated with fracture in patients with bone metastases is poorly understood, as well as the mechanism by which the use of radiation

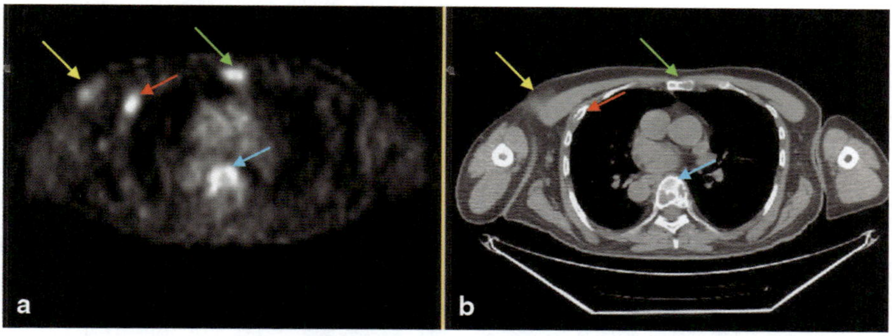

Fig. 25.5 Axial image from a PET/CT scan with *arrows* showing the correlation between findings on (**a**) PET-scan and (**b**) CT-scan of metastatic lesions to the sternum (*green*), rib, with soft tissue extension (*red*), thoracic vertebrae (*blue*) and enlarged axillary's lymph node metastasis (*yellow*)

therapy will provide a pain relief (Saarto et al. 2002). Radiation therapy effectively alleviates pain induced by metastatic bone disease, improving quality of life, and reducing the need of analgesics. Moreover, radiation therapy has potential to prevent pathologic fractures, and treat/prevent spinal cord compression. Localized external beam radiation therapy (EBRT) is the most commonly used form of radiation therapy for bone metastases. An example of EBRT planning for painful thoracic spine metastases is given in Fig. 25.6.

Painful Bone Metastases Radiation therapy improves pain control in 80–90 % of patients with painful bone metastases, with complete pain response in 50–60 % of cases (Berk 1995; Sze et al. 2003, 2004; Ratanatharathorn et al. 1999; Steenland et al. 1999).

Several EBRT fractionation schedules were investigated in clinical trials. The most important subject investigated is how many fractions of radiation therapy are needed to provide adequate pain control, without disrupting patient's quality of life with new side effects associated with treatment and dislocation to the hospital to receive prolonged daily treatments. The largest trials are summarized on Table 25.2. Generally, comparisons were made between single fraction and multiple fraction treatment schedules, and the results are quite similar among all trials indicating that single fraction is equivalent to multi fraction EBRT in terms of pain control, narcotic relief, time to pain improvement and pain recurrence, incidence of pathologic fractures, and quality of life. A common difference between both schedules is the rate of retreatment, which is usually double for patients undergoing single fraction treatment. However, it has been shown that after one 8 Gy fraction, retreatment with a repeat 8 Gy fraction to the same area is safe and efficient (Yarnold 1999). Another difference between both schedules is a significant difference in acute toxicity favoring single fraction radiation therapy, shown by Hartsell et al. (2005). A meta-analysis (Jackson Sai-Yiu 2003) as well as systematic (Sze 2003; Chow et al. 2007) and critical (Pradier et al. 2003) reviews, reveal a fairly consistency of results among randomized controlled trials that investigated the subject fractionation (Table 25.2).

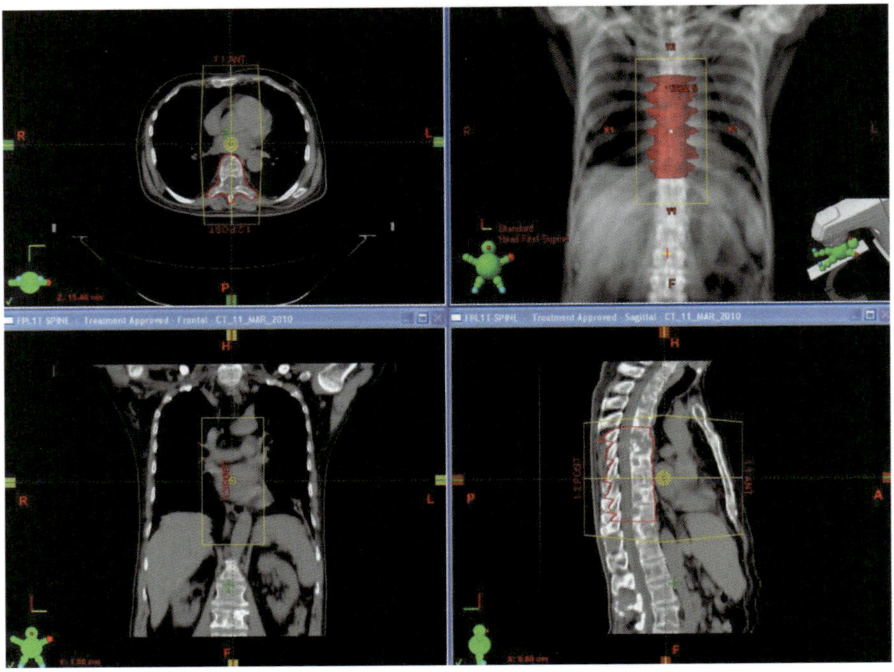

Fig. 25.6 External beam radiation therapy planning for a patient with cutaneous melanoma and diffuse metastatic disease with painful bone metastases in the thoracic spine. Treatment plan was performed to deliver 8 Gy in one fraction to the painful area using 2 EBRT fields (*anterior and posterior*)

Although the rate of bone recalcification was shown to be lower after single dose RT (120 %), compared to fractionated RT (173 %) (Koswig and Budach 1999), what is observed clinically is that the rate of pathologic fractures is somewhat similar after single or multiple-fraction treatment, ranging from 2 to 5 % (Hartsell et al. 2005; Nielson et al. 1998; Roos et al. 2005). The exception was the study by Steenland et al. (1999), showing a higher incidence of pathologic fracture (4 vs. 2 %) in patients who underwent single fraction treatment.

Immediately after radiation therapy for pain relief, up to 40 % of patients can present a pain flare in the treatment field (Hird et al. 2009) defined as an augmentation of pain intensity by two points on the visual analog scale. Pain flare can last up to 7 days, but there are some suggestions that it can be prevented with the prophylactic use of 8 mg dexamethasone before radiotherapy (Chow et al. 2007). The antialgic effects of EBRT on painful bone metastasis are usually seen at a median time of 1–4 weeks after treatment (Yarnold 1999; Koswig et al. 1999; Tong et al. 1982) and the duration of response ranges from 12 to 24 weeks (Pradier et al. 2008).

Pathologic fractures Radiation therapy has a role in preventing pathologic fractures in patients with bone metastases. However, when a patient presents with impending

Table 25.2 Randomized trials for painful bone metastases

Trial	Patients	Fractionation schedules	Primary endpoint (results in percentage)	Other endpoints (results in percentage)
Nielsen et al. (1998)	241	8 Gy/1 fr vs. 20 Gy/5 fr	Pain control (49 vs. 55 at 4 weeks) (60 vs. 60 at 12 weeks)	Quality of life (similar) Analgesic consumption (similar) Side effects (similar) Pathologic facture (5 vs. 5) Retreatment (21 vs. 12)
Steenland et al. (1999) (Dutch trial)	1,171	8 Gy/1 fr vs. 24 Gy/6 fr	Pain control (72 vs. 69)	Complete pain control (37 vs. 33) Use of analgesics (similar) QoL (similar) Side effects (similar) Pathologic fractures (4 vs. 2) Retreatment rate (25 vs. 7)
Yarnold et al. (1999) BPTWP (British trial)	765	8 Gy/1 fr vs. 20 Gy/5 fr or 30 Gy/10 fr	Pain relief (78 vs. 78)	Complete pain control (57 vs. 58) Time to first pain improvement (similar) Time to complete pain relief (similar) Time to pain recurrence (similar) Toxicity (similar) Pathologic fractures (2 vs. <1) Retreatment rate (23 vs. 10)
Hartsell et al. (2005) (RTOG 9714)	898	8 Gy/1 fr vs. 30 Gy/10 fr	Pain relief (50 vs. 48)	Complete pain relief (15 vs. 18) Narcotic relief (similar) Acute toxicity (10 vs. 17, $p=0.002$) Chronic toxicity (4 vs. 4) Pathologic fractures (5 vs. 4) Retreatment (18 vs. 9)

fr number of RT fractions, *BPTWP* bone pain trial working party

or existing pathologic fracture of a weight-bearing bone, little can be done with radiation therapy alone. Whenever possible, surgical fixation should be performed to decrease pain and facilitate rehabilitation, restoring limb function in more than 80 % of patients (Harrington 1997) and improving quality of life. Unfortunately, surgery frequently does not result in complete tumor removal, and EBRT is often indicated postoperatively, as it reduces the need of further orthopedic procedures to the same site (Townsend et al. 1995) and improves bone recalcification (Koswig and Budach 1999) EBRT is usually performed 2–4 weeks following surgery, after complete healing of surgical incision. As there are no randomized trials on total dose and fractionation schedule for this situation, most centers use the same schedules used for painful bone metastasis.

Spinal cord compression Spinal cord compression is a medical emergency that occurs in 5–10 % of patients with bone metastases (Elte et al. 1986; Käkönen and Mundy 2003; Mercadante 1997; Halfdanarson et al. 2006) with debilitating and catastrophic complications, if not dealt with within reasonable time. Spinal cord or cauda equina compressions result from direct tumor extension or direct pressure by an unstable fractured vertebral body against these neurological structures. As a consequence, patients may present in addition to back pain, weakness, sensory deficits and/or autonomic dysfunction, characterized by urinary retention and fecal incontinence.

Treatment consists of corticosteroid therapy, followed by surgery and/or radiation therapy, and its main objectives are pain control and preservation or improvement of neurologic function. Patients, who are surgical candidates, i.e., with good life expectancy and medically fit, should undergo aggressive treatment with surgical decompression followed by EBRT. As shown by Patchell et al. (2005) on a randomized clinical trial, combined therapy consisting of surgery plus EBRT significantly improves pain control and neurological function in patients with spinal cord compression, compared to radiation therapy alone.

Patients, who are not good surgical candidates, are treated with corticoids and radiation therapy. In this situation, single fraction and multi-fraction EBRT provide similar response rates in terms of pain control and neurologic function. Once again, the main difference between fractionation schedules was the rate of local recurrence, higher with single fraction (8 Gy) and with low-total dose (20 Gy) schedules, in comparison to schedules delivering higher total doses (30–40 Gy) (Rades et al. 2005, 2006). Decision of fractionation schedule is usually based upon patient's life expectancy.

25.3.4 Stereotactic Body Radiosurgery

When the total dose delivered by previous course(s) of EBRT reached the tolerance dose of adjacent normal structures (Emami et al. 1991), more radiotherapy cannot be safely delivered without serious side effects. In such cases, high-precision techniques can be used to spare normal healthy tissues and minimize side effects.

Stereotactic body radiosurgery (SBRT) is a technique that emerged as a non-invasive option for retreatment of bone metastasis, especially lesions close to important nervous structures, such as the vertebral spine and skull base. One of the largest series using this technique was published by Gerszten et al. (2007), with 500 cases of spinal metastases in 393 patients using SBRT, most of them previously treated with EBRT. In his cohort, doses ranged from 12.5 to 25 Gy in a single fraction, providing of long term pain and tumor control at a median follow-up of 21 months, with no late neurologic complications.

In conclusion, the potential benefits of SBRT in the treatment of bone metastasis are short treatment time in an outpatient setting with good quality symptomatic response, using higher doses of radiation than those delivered by EBRT. Similarly to all new technologies, one must be careful when using SBRT, since long term follow-ups and randomized clinical trails are not available. But despite of this, SBRT can be considered a novel treatment option for the treatment of bone metastasis in previously irradiated sites.

Key Points

- Bones are the third most common sites of metastases.
- Survival rate depends on the primary malignant site and other sites of metastases and ranges from months to years.
- Bone metastases have a detrimental impact on the quality of life.
- Bone metastases are investigated by a combination of different imaging techniques including plain X-Rays, CT-scans, and MRIs.
- Localized external beam radiation therapy (EBRT) is the most commonly used form of radiation therapy for bone metastases.
- Single-fraction radiotherapy with 1 × 8 Gy is an effective therapeutic strategy for pain relief equivalent to multi-fraction radiotherapy for metastases without pathological fractures or spinal cord compression.
- In patients with pathological fractures EBRT is often indicated postoperatively to reduce the need of further orthopedic procedures.
- In patients with spinal cord compression therapy consisting of surgery plus EBRT improves pain control and neurological function.

25.3.5 Stereotactic Body Radiation Therapy for Liver Metastases

Metastatic disease represents a significant burden in the care of patients with malignancy, especially those patients with breast, colorectal and lung cancers. For example, the combined incidence of breast, and Colorectal Cancer (CRC) is approximately 360,000 cases per year, with 19 % of breast, and 39 % of CRC patients dying from their disease (Jema et al. 2005). Although chemotherapy is the standard of care for metastatic disease, the value of chemotherapy is limited and recent studies showed that those patients who appear to have few sites of involvement may benefit from the addition of local therapy, such as surgical resection of metastases or stereotactic body radiotherapy (SBRT) (Greenberg et al. 1996; Falkson et al. 1990).

Hepatic resection, or metastatectomy, is an accepted standard therapy for medically and technically operable hepatic oligometastases from colorectal cancer (CRC). Several retrospective trials have demonstrated long-term survival in selected group of patients with metastatectomy (Fong et al. 1999; Shah et al. 2007; Aloi et al. 2006). One study (Fong et al. 1999) reported a 10-year survival of 22 % in 1,000 patients with CRC who underwent hepatic resection for hepatic metastases. In a study reported by Aloia et al. (2006) hepatic resection was compared with radiofrequency ablation of the hepatic lesions. It showed a several fold increase of local failure in the radiofrequency ablation versus hepatic resection.

Only a subset of liver metastases is resectable because of factors such as disease location, proximity to blood vessels and or other critical structures. A significant group of patients are deemed surgical risks because of poor general medical status. Stereotactic radiation therapy is an alternative approach in unresectable lesions, medically unfit patients, or patients who do not desire surgery.

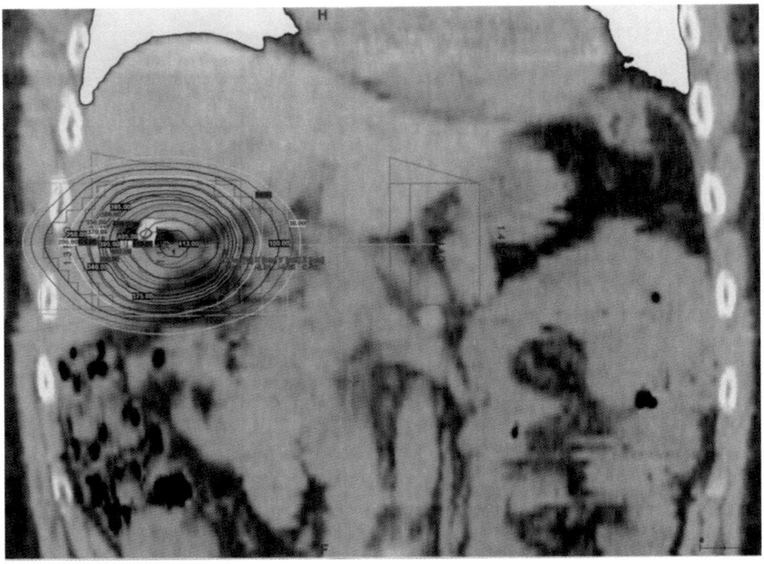

Fig. 25.7 SBRT for the treatment of a single metastatic hepatic lesion, showing the sharply treated lesion with sparing of the rest of the normal liver parenchyma. (Courtesy of Dr. D. Roberge)

Stereotactic body radiation therapy involves a brief, intensified regimen of radiotherapy tightly focused on targets in extracranial neoplastic lesions. The term stereotactic relates to the correlation of tumor target position to reliable fiducials with readily known position. The fiducials define a coordinate system that can be used to target the tumor, orient the treatment planning process, and ultimately guide the therapy toward the intended target location in the body.

Patients selected for SBRT should have a limited number of demarcated tumors whose extent can be identified directly on treatment-planning image or reliably fused by image registration techniques. Patient positioning should be reproducible and comfortable because of the longer treatment sessions as compared with conventional external beam radiotherapy. The avoidance of large safety margins around the target is very important in order to avoid toxicity to normal tissues. This is accomplished by the use of different target motion control techniques to minimize organ motion during the delivery of SBRT. The different target motion control techniques include gating, tracking, and dampening. Gating involves the monitoring of the respiratory cycle and the delivering of the treatment during one specific phase of the respiratory cycle, typically at the end of expiration, while the beam is turned off in the other phase of breathing. Tracking involves physically moving a beam of irradiation to coincide with tumor motion in the beam's eye view. Generally, a fiducial marker is used in tracking techniques to activate the beam delivery. Dampening is another method to reduce tumor motion, and it is done by abdominal compression or by breath holding techniques. These dampening techniques will reduce the cephalo-caudal diaphragmatic excursion and thereby help to reduce the motion of the target, especially in the lower lungs and the liver. An example of SBRT for a single liver metastasis from a primary nasopharyngeal cancer is illustrated in Fig. 25.7.

Rusthoven and colleagues (2009a) reported the results of a multi-institutional Phase I/II trial of SBRT for patients with one to three liver metastases. The trial objectives were to evaluate the efficacy and tolerability of high dose SBRT in this group of patients, with a maximum individual lesion diameter of 6 cm. The SBRT was delivered in three fractions, and the dose was escalated from 36 to 60 Gy during the phase I of the study, and established at 60 Gy for the Phase II. A secondary end point of the study was survival. Forty-seven patients were included in the trial and were treated for a total of 63 hepatic lesions. Only one patient (2 %) suffered from grade 3 soft tissue toxicity in the form of tissue breakdown of the anterior abdominal wall in close proximity to the high dose region of the SBRT plan. The authors of the study reported no grade 4 or 5 toxicity. The local control was defined by imaging in patients who lived 6 months or longer following SBRT. Patients who died prior to the 6-month time point were not considered accessible for local control, but were analyzed for overall survival. Forty-nine out of the 63 lesions were accessible for local control analysis. Actuarial local controls at 1 and 2 years were 95 and 92 %, respectively. The observed local control of lesions treated to 60 Gy was 94 %. The local control for lesions with a diameter less than 3 cm was 100 % compared to 77 % for those lesions with a diameter larger than 3 cm. The median and 2-year overall survivals were 20.5 months and 30 %, respectively. The site of the primary disease was found to be significantly predictive of survival, both on univariate and multivariate analysis. Primary tumors of the lung, ovary, and non-colorectal gastrointestinal sites were associated with a worse outcome with a median of 12 months, as compared to favorable sites, such as colorectal, breast, renal, and carcinoids who showed a median survival of 32 months. The authors concluded that SBRT is an effective and safe non-invasive method of treatment in selected patients with oligometastatic disease to the liver.

The Heidelberg group reported the results of a dose escalation study of single-dose SBRT for hepatic metastases (Herfarth et al. 2001). The study included 37 patients with a total of 60 hepatic lesions, four primary hepatic tumors, and 56 metastatic lesions, with a median tumor volume of 10 cc. The most common primary sites were breast, and colorectal primaries. The dose was escalated from 14 to 26 Gy in a single fraction. The reported actuarial freedom from local progression was 67 % for the whole group at 18 months. The same investigators described transient radiographic changes typically observed after SBRT (Herfarth et al. 2003). These changes consisted of a sharply demarcated hypodense area surrounding the treated lesion on non-enhanced CT scans. These changes can potentially obscure the evaluation of response if it is done within the first few months after SBRT.

Investigators from the University of Colorado and from Indiana University (Tracey et al. 2005) reported their results for a dose escalation study for patients with one to three hepatic metastases from any solid tumor, with a cumulative maximum diameter of 6 cm, and a KPS equal or better than 60. The first cohort of patients was treated to a dose of 36 Gy to the planning target volume (PTV) in three fractions. No patient developed any grade 3 dose limiting toxicity (DLT) and the dose was escalated to 60 Gy in three fractions. The PTV included the lesion plus a 5 mm radial margin and a 10 mm cephalo-caudad margin, allowing a minimum of 700 cc of normal liver tissue to receive a cumulative dose not exceeding 15 Gy from the entire course of treatment. Sixteen out of the 18 accrued patients had received at least one type of systemic therapy before liver SBRT; 8 patients had received three or more types of chemotherapeutic agent. Twelve patients remained alive at the time of analysis, a median of 7.1 months after enrollment in the protocol (range, 3.8–12.3 months). Six patients died within 3.1–18.9 months after enrollment.

In conclusion, stereotactic body radiotherapy is used more and more as an effective treatment modality today. The results of prospective well-designed studies will help to refine SBRT. Further work in radiobiology will help to better our understanding of the biological effects of large dose per fraction used in SBRT. Strict dose volume constraints for SBRT will continue to be established and will improve the safety of such an effective and a noninvasive treatment.

25.3.6 Stereotactic Body Radiotherapy for Lung Metastases

Stereotactic body radiotherapy (SBRT) is an attractive technique to treat lung metastases as it involves a brief, intensified delivery of tightly focused external radiotherapy targeting one or more discreet lung lesions. This allows a high dose of radiation to be focally administered without excessive risk of radiation pneumonitis. This property opened the door for the initial application of SBRT in the treatment of patients with early stage non-small cell lung cancer (NSCLC). This principle was tested in a dose escalation study in patients with medically inoperable Stage I NSCLC. The maximum tolerated dose was 66 Gy in three fractions (McGarry et al. 2005; Fakiris et al. 2009) with a dose response relationship and better local control with the higher dose. Timmerman and colleagues (2006) reported a 2-year actuarial local control of 95 % with SBRT of 60–66 Gy in three fractions. Other investigators (Nagata et al. 2005; Xia et al. 2006) reported similar results in other series using high-dose SBRT in patients with Stage I NSCLC. An example of SBRT for a single lung metastasis is shown in Fig. 25.8.

Rusthoven et al. (2009b) reported the results of a multi-institutional Phase I/II trial of stereotactic body radiotherapy for patients with 1–3 lung metastases. For this study, patients with a cumulative maximum diameter, smaller than 7 cm were enrolled and treated in a multi-institutional phase I/II clinical trial. The SBRT was delivered in three fractions. The phase I study established a total dose of 60 Gy as safe. The primary endpoint of the phase II study was local control with lesions with at least 6 months of radiographic follow-up were accessible for local control. The secondary endpoints included toxicity and overall survival. Sixty-three lesions in 38 patients were treated according to this study. There was no grade IV toxicity. The incidence of any grade III toxicity was 8 % with symptomatic pneumonitis in 2.6 %. Local control was accessible in 50 lesions with a median follow-up of 15.4 months. The actuarial local control at 1 and 2 years after SBRT was 100 and 96 % respectively. Local disease progression occurred in one patient, 13 months after SBRT. The median survival of patients on study was 19 months.

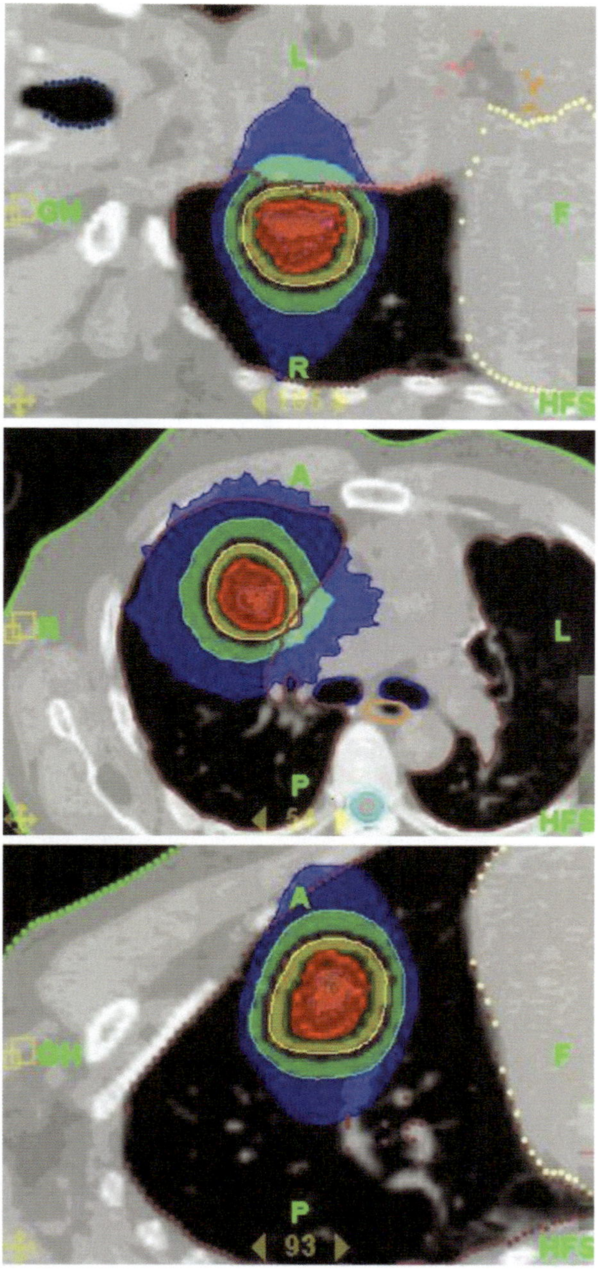

Fig. 25.8 Dose distributions in coronal, axial, and sagital views of a SBRT plan of a patient with a solitary lung metastasis. The target volume received a dose of 60 Gy in three fractions (*red*), while the normal lung at the periphery of the lesion received < 20 Gy (*blue*). (Courtesy of Dr. J. Wan)

Milano and colleagues (2008) reported the result of a phase II clinical trial using SBRT to a dose of 50 Gy in ten fractions in the treatment of patient with oligo-metastatic disease. The 2-year local control for all treated lesions was 67 %. Similarly, investigators from Heidelberg treated 61 patients with 71 lung metastases using single fractions SBRT to a dose of 12–30 Gy and reported actuarial local control of 74 % in 2 years (Hof et al. 2007).

The most frequent grade III toxicity consisted of chest wall pain, rib fracture, skin toxicities and pneumonitis. A recent combined analysis of patients treated with thoracic SBRT revealed that the volume of chest wall receiving at least 30 Gy in three fractions (V30) was the best predictor of chest wall toxicity (Dunlap et al. 2008). The incidence and severity of chest wall pain increased with increasing V30, and no chest wall toxicity was observed with V30 less than 10 cc. The skin constraints limiting the dose to the skin surface to less than 21 Gy in three fractions is an acceptable constraint. The low rate of radiation pneumonitis observed in SBRT for NSCLC and lung metastases suggests that the dose constraints of V15 less than 35 % are unacceptable constraint. A recent report by Dunlap et al. (2010) recommends that a chest wall (CW) volume receiving 30 Gy in three to five fractions should be limited to 30 cc in order to reduce the risk of toxicity without compromising tumor coverage. Other authors also cautioned about the delivery of large doses to the heart, esophagus, and bronchi (Wulf et al. 2004; Fukumoto et al. 2002; Lee et al. 2003).

25.3.7 Summary

Any therapeutic intervention is associated with side effects, both acute and long term. The long-term side effects of therapy were of major concern in patients with curative disease, as these patients are expected to live long enough to express the side effects of the treatment. This concern is also an important issue for patients with metastatic disease; however it is not of the same relative importance because of the expected short survival of these patients. The main objective of the palliative treatment is to control symptoms, such as bleeding, pain, or increased intracranial pressure as fast as possible. Most of the time large doses of radiotherapy are utilized and result in good immediate response. Nowadays, because of the improved survival in patients with metastatic disease, the long-term treatment-related side effects have become a real and significant concern. Due to new medical, technical advances of cancer diagnosis and treatment, patients with metastatic cancer disease live longer than many decades ago. Patients must receive the palliative therapy that will benefit them using state-of–the-art technical advances in treatment delivery and based on properly executed clinical trials. A multidisciplinary team of experts must perform management of patients with metastatic disease, to ensure that patients are receiving the best possible treatment.

References

Aloia TA et al (2006) Solitary colorectal liver metastasis: resection determines outcome. Arch Surg 141:460–466 (discussion 466–467)

Ammirati M et al (2010) The role of retreatment in the management of recurrent/progressive brain metastases: a systematic review and evidence-based clinical practice guideline. J Neurooncol 96:85–96

Andrews DW et al (2004) Whole brain radiation therapy with or without stereotactic radiosurgery boost for patients with one to three brain metastases: phase III results of the RTOG 9508 randomised trial. Lancet 363:1665–1672

Antonadou D et al (2002a) Phase II randomized trial of temozolomide and concurrent radiotherapy in patients with brain metastases. J Clin Oncol 20:3644–3650

Antonadou D et al (2002b) Whole brain radiotherapy alone or in combination with temozolomide for brain metastases. a phase III study. Int J Radiat Oncol Biol Phys 54:93–94

Aoyama H et al (2006) Stereotactic radiosurgery plus whole-brain radiation therapy vs stereotactic radiosurgery alone for treatment of brain metastases: a randomized controlled trial. JAMA 295:2483–2491

Arbit E et al (1995) The treatment of patients with recurrent brain metastases. A retrospective analysis of 109 patients with nonsmall cell lung cancer. Cancer 76:765–773

Armstrong CL et al (2000) Radiotherapeutic effects on brain function: double dissociation of memory systems. Neuropsychiatry Neuropsychol Behav Neurol 13:101–111

Armstrong CL et al (2002) Late cognitive and radiographic changes related to radiotherapy: initial prospective findings. Neurology 59:40–48

Barnes EA et al (2010) Physician expectations of treatment outcomes for patients with brain metastases referred for whole brain radiotherapy. Int J Radiat Oncol Biol Phys 76:187–192

Belka C, Budach W, Kortmann RD, Bamberg M (2001) Radiation induced CNS toxicity—molecular and cellular mechanisms. Br J Cancer 85:1233–1239

Berk L (1995) Prospective trials for the radiotherapeutic treatment of bone metastases. Am J Hosp Palliat Care 12:24–28

Bhatnagar A, Heron DE, Kondziolka D, Lunsford LD, Flickinger JC (2002) Analysis of repeat stereotactic radiosurgery for progressive primary and metastatic CNS tumors. Int J Radiat Oncol Biol Phys 53:527–532

Bindal RK, Sawaya R, Leavens ME, Lee JJ (1993) Surgical treatment of multiple brain metastases. J Neurosurg 79:210–216

Borgelt B et al (1981) Ultra-rapid high dose irradiation schedules for the palliation of brain metastases: final results of the first two studies by the Radiation Therapy Oncology Group. Int J Radiat Oncol Biol Phys 7:1633–1638

Burt M, Wronski M, Arbit E, Galicich JH (1992) Resection of brain metastases from non-small-cell lung carcinoma. Results of therapy. Memorial Sloan-Kettering Cancer Center Thoracic Surgical Staff. J Thorac Cardiovasc Surg 103:399–410 (discussion 410–411)

Chatani M, Teshima T, Hata K, Inoue T (1986) Prognostic factors in patients with brain metastases from lung carcinoma. Strahlenther Onkol 162:157–161

Chougule PB et al (2000) Randomized treatment of brain metastasis with gamma knife radiosurgery, whole brain radiotherapy or both. Int J Radiat Oncol Biol Phys 48:114

Chow E, Harris K, Fan G, Tsao M, Sze WM (2007) Palliative radiotherapy trials for bone metastases: a systematic review. J Clin Oncol 25:1423–1436

Clezardin P, Teti A (2007) Bone metastasis: pathogenesis and therapeutic implications. Clin Exp Metastasis 24:599–608

Coleman RE (2001) Metastatic bone disease: clinical features, pathophysiology and treatment strategies. Cancer Treat Rev 27:165–176

Coleman RE (2006) Clinical features of metastatic bone disease and risk of skeletal morbidity. Clin Cancer Res 12:6243s–6249s

Coleman RE, Rubens RD (1987) The clinical course of bone metastases from breast cancer. Br J Cancer 55:61–66

Cook GJ, Houston S, Rubens R, Maisey MN, Fogelman I (1998) Detection of bone metastases in breast cancer by 18FDG PET: differing metabolic activity in osteoblastic and osteolytic lesions. J Clin Oncol 16:3375–3379

Dunlap NE et al (2008) Chest wall volume receiving more than 30 Gy predicts risk of severe pain and/or rib fracture following lung SBRT. Int J Radiat Oncol Biol Phys 72:S36

Dunlap NE et al (2010) Chest wall volume receiving > 30 Gy predicts risk of severe pain and/or rib fracture after lung stereotactic body radiotherapy. Int J Radiat Oncol Biol Phys 76:796–801

Elte JW, Bijvoet OL, Cleton FJ, van Oosterom AT, Sleeboom HP (1986) Osteolytic bone metastases in breast carcinoma pathogenesis, morbidity and bisphosphonate treatment. Eur J Cancer Clin Oncol 22:493–500

Emami B et al (1991) Tolerance of normal tissue to therapeutic irradiation. Int J Radiat Oncol Biol Phys 21:109–122

Even-Sapir E et al (2006) The detection of bone metastases in patients with high-risk prostate cancer: 99mTc-MDP planar bone scintigraphy, single- and multi-field-of-view SPECT, 18F-Fluoride PET, and 18F-Fluoride PET/CT. J Nucl Med 47:287–297

Fakiris AJ et al (2009) Stereotactic body radiation therapy for early-stage non-small-cell lung carcinoma: four-year results of a prospective phase II study. Int J Radiat Oncol Biol Phys 75:677–682

Falkson G, Gelman RS, Leone L, Falkson CI (1990) Survival of premenopausal women with metastatic breast cancer. Long-term follow-up of Eastern Cooperative Group and Cancer and Leukemia Group B studies. Cancer 66:1621–1629

Fong Y, Fortner J, Sun RL, Brennan MF, Blumgart LH (1999) Clinical score for predicting recurrence after hepatic resection for metastatic colorectal cancer: analysis of 1001 consecutive cases. Ann Surg 230:309–318 (discussion 318–321)

Fukumoto S-i et al (2002) Small-volume image-guided radiotherapy using hypofractionated, coplanar, and noncoplanar multiple fields for patients with inoperable Stage I nonsmall cell lung carcinomas. Cancer 95:1546–1553

Gaspar L et al (1997) Recursive partitioning analysis (RPA) of prognostic factors in three radiation therapy oncology group (RTOG) brain metastases trials. Int J Radiat Oncol Biol Phys 37:745–751

Gaspar LE et al (2010) The role of whole brain radiation therapy in the management of newly diagnosed brain metastases: a systematic review and evidence-based clinical practice guideline. J Neurooncol 96:17–32

Gerszten PC, Burton SA, Ozhasoglu C, Welch WC (2007) Radiosurgery for spinal metastases: clinical experience in 500 cases from a single institution. Spine (Phila Pa 1976) 32:193–199

Glantz MJ et al (2000) Practice parameter: anticonvulsant prophylaxis in patients with newly diagnosed brain tumors. Report of the Quality Standards Subcommittee of the American Academy of Neurology. Neurology 54:1886–1893

Greenberg PA et al (1996) Long-term follow-up of patients with complete remission following combination chemotherapy for metastatic breast cancer. J Clin Oncol 14:2197–2205

Guerrieri M et al (2004) A randomised phase III study of palliative radiation with concomitant carboplatin for brain metastases from non-small cell carcinoma of the lung. Lung Cancer 46:107–111

Halfdanarson TR, Hogan WJ, Moynihan TJ (2006) Oncologic emergencies: diagnosis and treatment. Mayo Clin Proc 81:835–848

Harrington KD (1997) Orthopedic surgical management of skeletal complications of malignancy. Cancer 80:1614–1627

Hartsell WF et al (2005) Randomized trial of short- versus long-course radiotherapy for palliation of painful bone metastases. J Natl Cancer Inst 97:798–804

Hazuka MB, Kinzie JJ (1988) Brain metastases: results and effects of re-irradiation. Int J Radiat Oncol Biol Phys 15:433–437

Hazuka MB et al (1993) Multiple brain metastases are associated with poor survival in patients treated with surgery and radiotherapy. J Clin Oncol 11:369–373

Herfarth KK et al (2001) Stereotactic single-dose radiation therapy of liver tumors: results of a phase I/II trial. J Clin Oncol 19:164–170

Herfarth KK et al (2003) Assessment of focal liver reaction by multiphasic CT after stereotactic single-dose radiotherapy of liver tumors. Int J Radiat Oncol Biol Phys 57:444–451

Hird A et al (2009) Determining the incidence of pain flare following palliative radiotherapy for symptomatic bone metastases: results from three canadian cancer centers. Int J Radiat Oncol Biol Phys 75:193–197

Hof H, Hoess A, Oetzel D, Debus J, Herfarth K (2007) Stereotactic single-dose radiotherapy of lung metastases. Strahlenther Onkol 183:673–678

Ibrahim T et al (2010) Pathogenesis of osteoblastic bone metastases from prostate cancer. Cancer 116:1406–1418

Jackson Sai-Yiu W, Rebecca W, Mary J, Andrea B, Timothy W (2003) Meta-analysis of dose-fractionation radiotherapy trials for the palliation of painful bone metastases. Int J Radiat Oncol Biol Phys 55:594–605

Jelinek JS et al (2002) Diagnosis of primary bone tumors with image-guided percutaneous biopsy: experience with 110 tumors. Radiology 223:731–737

Jemal A et al (2005) Cancer statistics, 2005. CA Cancer J Clin 55:10–30

Käkönen S-M, Mundy GR (2003) Mechanisms of osteolytic bone metastases in breast carcinoma. Cancer 97:834–839

Klein M et al (2002) Effect of radiotherapy and other treatment-related factors on mid-term to long-term cognitive sequelae in low-grade gliomas: a comparative study. Lancet 360:1361–1368

Komarnicky LT et al (1991) A randomized phase III protocol for the evaluation of misonidazole combined with radiation in the treatment of patients with brain metastases (RTOG-7916). Int J Radiat Oncol Biol Phys 20:53–58

Kondziolka D, Patel A, Lunsford LD, Kassam A, Flickinger JC (1999) Stereotactic radiosurgery plus whole brain radiotherapy versus radiotherapy alone for patients with multiple brain metastases. Int J Radiat Oncol Biol Phys 45:427–434

Koswig S, Budach V (1999) Remineralization and pain relief in bone metastases after after different radiotherapy fractions (10 times 3 Gy vs. 1 time 8 Gy). A prospective study. Strahlenther Onkol 175:500–508

Koswig S, Buchali A, Bohmer D, Schlenger L, Budach V (1999) Palliative radiotherapy of bone metastases. A retrospective analysis of 176 patients. Strahlenther Onkol 175:509–514

Kurtz JM, Gelber R, Brady LW, Carella RJ, Cooper JS (1981) The palliation of brain metastases in a favorable patient population: a randomized clinical trial by the Radiation Therapy Oncology Group. Int J Radiat Oncol Biol Phys 7:891–895

Lee SW et al (2003) Stereotactic body frame based fractionated radiosurgery on consecutive days for primary or metastatic tumors in the lung. Lung Cancer 40:309–315

Li KC, Poon PY (1988) Sensitivity and specificity of MRI in detecting malignant spinal cord compression and in distinguishing malignant from benign compression fractures of vertebrae. Magn Reson Imaging 6:547–556

Lippitz BE et al (2004) Gamma knife radiosurgery for patients with multiple cerebral metastases. Acta Neurochir Suppl 91:79–87

McGarry RC, Papiez L, Williams M, Whitford T, Timmerman RD (2005) Stereotactic body radiation therapy of early-stage non-small-cell lung carcinoma: phase I study. Int J Radiat Oncol Biol Phys 63:1010–1015

Mehta M et al (1997) A cost-effectiveness and cost-utility analysis of radiosurgery vs. resection for single-brain metastases. Int J Radiat Oncol Biol Phys 39:445–454

Mehta MP et al (1992) Defining the role of radiosurgery in the management of brain metastases. Int J Radiat Oncol Biol Phys 24:619–625

Mehta MP et al (2003) Survival and neurologic outcomes in a randomized trial of motexafin gadolinium and whole-brain radiation therapy in brain metastases. J Clin Oncol 21:2529–2536

Mercadante S (1997) Malignant bone pain: pathophysiology and treatment. Pain 69:1–18

Meyers CA et al (2004) Neurocognitive function and progression in patients with brain metastases treated with whole-brain radiation and motexafin gadolinium: results of a randomized phase III trial. J Clin Oncol 22:157–165

Milano MT et al (2008) A prospective pilot study of curative-intent stereotactic body radiation therapy in patients with 5 or fewer oligometastatic lesions. Cancer 112:650–658

Mintz AH et al (1996) A randomized trial to assess the efficacy of surgery in addition to radiotherapy in patients with a single cerebral metastasis. Cancer 78:1470–1476

Monje ML, Palmer T (2003) Radiation injury and neurogenesis. Curr Opin Neurol 16:129–134

Monje ML, Mizumatsu S, Fike JR, Palmer TD (2002) Irradiation induces neural precursor-cell dysfunction. Nat Med 8:955–962

Nagata Y et al (2005) Clinical outcomes of a phase I/II study of 48 Gy of stereotactic body radiotherapy in 4 fractions for primary lung cancer using a stereotactic body frame. Int J Radiat Oncol Biol Phys 63:1427–1431

Nieder C et al (1999) Late radiation toxicity after whole brain radiotherapy: the influence of antiepileptic drugs. Am J Clin Oncol 22:573–579

Nielsen OS, Bentzen SM, Sandberg E, Gadeberg CC, Timothy AR (1998) Randomized trial of single dose versus fractionated palliative radiotherapy of bone metastases. Radiother Oncol 47:233–240

Patchell RA, Posner JB (1985) Neurologic complications of systemic cancer. Neurol Clin 3:729–750

Patchell RA et al (1990) A randomized trial of surgery in the treatment of single metastases to the brain. N Engl J Med 322:494–500

Patchell RA et al (1998) Postoperative radiotherapy in the treatment of single metastases to the brain: a randomized trial. JAMA 280:1485–1489

Patchell RA et al (2005) Direct decompressive surgical resection in the treatment of spinal cord compression caused by metastatic cancer: a randomised trial. Lancet 366:643–648

Pradier O, Bouchekoua M, Albargach N, Muller M, Malhaire JP (2008) Radiothérapie des métastases osseuses: quel est le meilleur schéma de radiothérapie? Cancer/Radiothérapie 12:837–841

Rades D et al (2006) Defining the appropriate radiotherapy regimen for metastatic spinal cord compression in non-small cell lung cancer patients. Eur J Cancer 42:1052–1056

Rades D et al (2005) Evaluation of five radiation schedules and prognostic factors for metastatic spinal cord compression. J Clin Oncol 23:3366–3375

Ratanatharathorn V, Powers WE, Moss WT, Perez CA (1999) Bone metastasis: review and critical analysis of random allocation trials of local field treatment. Int J Radiat Oncol Biol Phys 44:1–18

Roodman GD (2004) Mechanisms of bone metastasis. N Engl J Med 350:1655–1664

Roos DE et al (2005) Randomized trial of 8 Gy in 1 versus 20 Gy in 5 fractions of radiotherapy for neuropathic pain due to bone metastases (Trans-Tasman Radiation Oncology Group, TROG 96.05). Radiother Oncol 75:54–63

Rusthoven KE et al (2009a) Multi-institutional phase I/II trial of stereotactic body radiation therapy for liver metastases. J Clin Oncol 27:1572–1578

Rusthoven KE et al (2009b) Multi-institutional phase I/II trial of stereotactic body radiation therapy for lung metastases. J Clin Oncol 27:1579–1584

Saarto T, Janes R, Tenhunen M, Kouri M (2002) Palliative radiotherapy in the treatment of skeletal metastases. Eur J Pain 6:323–330

Sawaya R, Ligon BL, Bindal RK (1994) Management of metastatic brain tumors. Ann Surg Oncol 1:169–178

Shah SA et al (2007) Survival after liver resection for metastatic colorectal carcinoma in a large population. J Am Coll Surg 205:676–683

Simonova G, Liscak R, Novotny J Jr, Novotny J (2000) Solitary brain metastases treated with the Leksell gamma knife: prognostic factors for patients. Radiother Oncol 57:207–213

Steenland E et al (1999) The effect of a single fraction compared to multiple fractions on painful bone metastases: a global analysis of the Dutch bone metastasis study. Radiother Oncol 52:101–109

Suh JH et al (2006) Phase III study of Efaproxiral as an adjunct to whole-brain radiation therapy for brain metastases. J Clin Oncol 24:106–114

Sundaresan N, Sachdev V, DiGiacinto G, Hughes J (1988) Reoperation for brain metastases. J Clin Oncol 6:1625–1629

Sze WM, Shelley MD, Held I, Wilt TJ, Mason MD (2003) Palliation of metastatic bone pain: single fraction versus multifraction radiotherapy—a systematic review of randomised trials. Clin Oncol 15:345–352

Sze WM, Shelley M, Held I, Mason M (2004) Palliation of metastatic bone pain: single fraction versus multifraction radiotherapy—a systematic review of the randomised trials. Cochrane Database System Review CD004721

Timmerman R et al (2006) Excessive toxicity when treating central tumors in a phase II study of stereotactic body radiation therapy for medically inoperable early-stage lung cancer. J Clin Oncol 24:4833–4839

Tong D, Gillick L, Hendrickson FR (1982) The palliation of symptomatic osseous metastases: final results of the study by the radiation therapy oncology group. Cancer 50:893–899

Townsend PW, Smalley SR, Cozad SC, Rosenthal HG, Hassanein RE (1995) Role of postoperative radiation therapy after stabilization of fractures caused by metastatic disease. Int J Radiat Oncol Biol Phys 31:43–49

Tracey ES et al (2005) A phase I trial of stereotactic body radiation therapy (SBRT) for liver metastases. Int J Radiat Oncol Biol Phys 62:1371–1378

Ushio Y et al (1991) Chemotherapy of brain metastases from lung carcinoma: a controlled randomized study. Neurosurgery 28:201–205

Vecht CJ et al (1993) Treatment of single brain metastasis: radiotherapy alone or combined with neurosurgery? Ann Neurol 33:583–590

Verger E et al (2005) Temozolomide and concomitant whole brain radiotherapy in patients with brain metastases: a phase II randomized trial. Int J Radiat Oncol Biol Phys 61:185–191

Wen PY, Black PM, Loeffler JS (ed) (2001) Treatment of metastatic cancer. Lippincott Williams & Wilkins, Philadelphia

William WW, Steven ES, Timothy ES, Edward GS (1996) Analysis of outcome in patients reirradiated for brain metastases. Int J Radiat Oncol Biol Phys 34:585–590

Wulf J et al (2004) Stereotactic radiotherapy for primary lung cancer and pulmonary metastases: a noninvasive treatment approach in medically inoperable patients. Int J Radiat Oncol Biol Phys 60:186–196

Xia T et al (2006) Promising clinical outcome of stereotactic body radiation therapy for patients with inoperable Stage I/II non-small-cell lung cancer. Int J Radiat Oncol Biol Phys 66:117–125

Yarnold JR (1999) 8 Gy single fraction radiotherapy for the treatment of metastatic skeletal pain: randomised comparison with a multifraction schedule over 12 months of patient follow-up on behalf of the bone pain trial working party. Radiother Oncol 52:111–121

Chapter 26
Role of Surgery in the Diagnosis and Management of Metastatic Cancer

Peter Metrakos, Eli Kakiashvili, Murad Aljiffry, Mazen Hassanain and Prosanto Chaudhury

26.1 Introduction

Surgery gained an important role in the context of multidisciplinary management of metastatic disease. In the last decade there have been tremendous advances in the field of surgical oncology. These therapeutic modalities are employed not only in the palliative care of the patients with advanced metastatic cancer but also aim to improve the survival rates. Modern invasive techniques such as thoracoscopy and laparoscopy are effective treatments with lower morbidity rates allowing faster recovery. These techniques can be employed nowadays in conjunction with chemotherapeutic options.

P. Metrakos (✉)
Multi-Organ Transplant Program, McGill University Health Center,
McGill University, Montreal, QC, Canada

Hepatic, Pancreatic and Biliary Surgery, McGill University Health Center,
McGill University, Montreal, QC, Canada
e-mail: peter.metrakos@muhc.mcgill.ca

E. Kakiashvili
Department of Surgery, McGill University Health Center, McGill University,
Montreal, QC, Canada

M. Aljiffry
Department of Surgery, Transplant Surgery and Hepatobiliary/Pancreatic Surgery, McGill University Health Center, McGill University, Montreal, QC, Canada

Department of Surgery, King Abdul Aziz University, Jeddah, Saudi Arbia

M. Hassanain
Department of Surgery, McGill University Health Center, McGill University,
Montreal, QC, Canada

Department of Surgery, King Saud University, Riyadh, Saudi Arabia

P. Chaudhury
Department of Surgery, McGill University Health Center, McGill University,
Montreal, QC, Canada

J. V. Burnier, M. N. Burnier, Jr. (eds.), *Experimental and Clinical Metastasis*,
DOI 10.1007/978-1-4614-3685-0_26, © Springer Science+Business Media New York 2013

Advances in imaging techniques such as computed tomography (CT), magnetic resonance imaging (MRI) and positron emission tomography (PET) scanning, allow a better diagnosis and eligibility for surgical resection of metastases for selected patients.

Various minimally invasive techniques are employed to treat metastatic disease in different sites. For example metastatic brain lesions are operated with highly effective gamma knife and stereotactic radiotherapy (Kienast and Winkler 2010). Thoracic metastatic lesions are treated with video assisted thoracoscopic surgery (VATS), a procedure proven to be less morbid when compared to open lobectomy (Rueth and Andrade 2010). Another example are surgical options for metastatic lesions to the bone which include bone fixations and arthroplasties, radiosurgery, radiofrequency ablation (RFA), and percutaneous cementoplasty (Aboulafia et al. 2007).

Furthermore, new strategies are developed for the treatment of liver metastasis. This organ is the most common site for hematogenous metastatic dissemination from primary tumors including colorectal cancer, gastrointestinal tumors, breast, lung, pancreas, and melanoma. A variety of techniques have been described including resection, cryosurgery, radiofrequency thermal ablation and hepatic artery embolization (Dimitroulis et al. 2010).

In the following section we will address more in depth the role of surgery in the context of a multidisciplinary approach including chemotherapy and radiotherapy for the management of liver metastasis from colorectal cancer.

26.2 Current Management for Liver Metastases From Colorectal Cancer

Liver metastasis is encountered in nearly half of patients with stage III colorectal cancer (CRC) and in majority of cases is the only site of metastases (Taylor et al. 1990; Gilbert and Kagan 1976; Manfredi et al. 2006). Surgical intervention for colorectal liver metastases (CRLM) is an effective therapy for a significant number of patients. Due to a better understanding of liver anatomy and advances in perioperative management, the operative mortality is now well below 5 % (Fong et al. 1999; Nordlinger et al. 1996; Rees et al. 2008). The 5-year survival after resection of CRLM is 30 % but recurrence is common in approximately two-third of patients (Fong et al. 1995; Ito et al. 2010).

Only 10–20 % of patients are candidates for surgery and patient selection should include careful evaluation and delineation of metastases, exclusion of non-resectable extrahepatic disease and general physiological fitness tests (Welsh et al. 2008).

Synchronous metastatic lesions may be detected during preoperative evaluation or identified intraoperatively. Suspicious liver lesions should be biopsied and sent to pathological evaluation to confirm metastatic disease. Metachronous liver metastases may be diagnosed after colorectal surgery and confirmed on follow-up radiological imaging.

Preoperative hepatic assessment involves advanced imaging techniques employed to delineate hepatic anatomy and to detect accurately all intrahepatic lesions before resection. These modalities include transabdominal sonography, helical and multidetector-row CT (MDCT), FDG- PET and gadolinium-enhanced MR imaging and superparamagnetic iron oxide (SPIO)-enhanced MR imaging (Martinez et al. 2007; Nesbitt et al. 2007; Bipat et al. 2005). Laparoscopic ultrasound emerged as a valuable technique for detection of liver metastases and significantly improves the selection of candidates for resection (Rahusen et al. 1999). The use of enhanced MR imaging increased detection of small metastases and translates in a lower incidence of unresectable metastases during laparotomy (Senéterre et al. 1996; Yoon and Tanabe 1999).

The evaluation of visible lesions should include an assessment of both the number, extent of the lesions and post-surgical volume of the remnant liver parenchyma. The remaining functional liver volume is an important factor that should be considered before surgery. Current recommendations suggest that if remnant liver parenchyma is normal, 75 % of the volume of the liver can be resected (Pawlik and Choti 2007; Abdalla et al. 2006; Nordlinger et al. 2009). In addition, vascular invasion should also be assessed as the resection is contraindicated when both branches of liver pedicle, vena cava or all hepatic veins are affected.

Indications and contraindications for liver resection of colorectal cancer liver metastases have changed during the past few years. Some of the traditional criteria are now outdated and resections are performed in patients with more than four or bilobar locations. Although the presence of extrahepatic disease is considered a contraindication, recent studies suggest that resection may be performed in selected cases (Pawlik and Choti 2007; Hubbard and Alberts 2010). Recently, the European Colorectal Metastasis Treatment Group (ECMTG) proposed a new CRC staging system in order to take into account patients with potentially resectable liver metastases (Nordlinger et al. 2007, 2009). A clinical risk score may assess the long term outcome for patients undergoing resection for CRLM. The number and size of metastases, disease-free interval, preoperative carcinoembryonic (CEA), stage of the primary tumor, number of liver nodules, and resection margin of more than 1 cm or less than1 cm are the main prognostic factors that predict long term survival after resection (Fong et al. 1999; Blumgart 2007). This scoring system has been independently validated and is useful as a staging system for determining which patients may benefit from liver resection. The only contraindication for hepatic resection is the inability to achieve margin-negative resection with an adequate hepatic volume reserve (Fong et al. 1999; Blumgart 2007; Timmerman et al. 2009).

In recent years, comprehensive knowledge of liver anatomy led to the development of better surgical techniques and improved outcomes for resection of CRLM. Liver resections are still performed based on the functional anatomy of the liver as described by Couinaud (1957), who divided the liver into eight sectors or segments (Huang et al. 2008; Fig. 26.1).

Some authors recommend that the surgical decision should be individualized based on number, size, location and distribution of metastases (Pawlik and Choti 2007; Pawlik et al. 2005). They suggested that smaller metastases can be removed

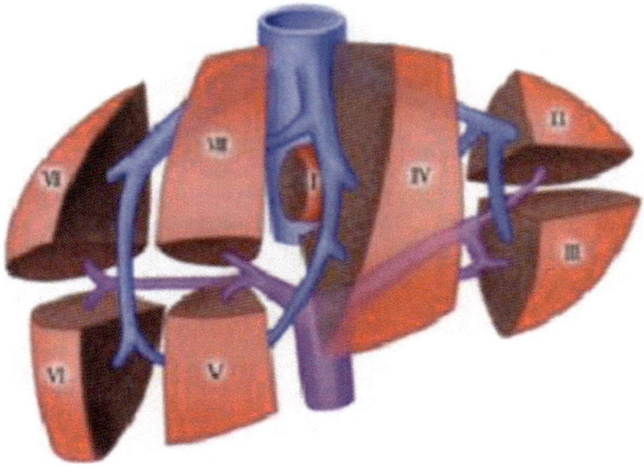

Fig. 26.1 Segmental anatomy of the liver according to Couinaud. (Adapted from Huang et al. 2008)

without respecting anatomical lines (wedge resection). Large, deep metastases should be resected along anatomical lines in which one or more segments are removed providing that 20–25 % of hepatic parenchyma is maintained (Chun and Vauthey 2007).

The standardized future liver remnant (FLR) ratio is defined as the ratio of measured FLR to the calculated total liver volume (TLV) (Johnson et al. 2005). This parameter allows a better comparison between patients and estimates prognosis after resection. The surgical decision regarding FLR should be done on individual bases taking in consideration patient's comorbidities, such as diabetes, obesity and metabolic syndrome which may impair hepatic regeneration (Abdalla et al. 2006). An expert consensus statement regarding the percentages of future liver remnant (FLR) after resection, established a cut-off point of 20 % FLR for patients with healthy liver, of 30 % for patients who received extensive chemotherapy and of 40 % for patients with hepatic fibrosis or cirrhosis (Abdalla et al. 2006).

In approximately 20 % of cases liver metastases are present at the time of CRC diagnosis and they are considered synchronous. In these cases a combined resection of primary tumor and liver metastases is associated with increased mortality and morbidity (Memon and Beckingham 2001). At present, strategies for the management of synchronous liver metastases are changing. Resection techniques will vary according to metastatic location and hepatic functional reserve (Li Destri et al. 2008). The surgical decision should be individualized according to the clinical situation and experience of the centre and should be made in consultation with the multidisciplinary team.

The alternatives to be taken in consideration are simultaneous or staged resection with a recovery period or a course of chemotherapy between resections (Nordlinger et al. 2007). Recent evidence suggests that simultaneous resections are safe, with shorter hospitalization time and better patient outcomes (Mansour and Fong 2007). The surgical decision is influenced by the primary tumor and the potential resectability of CRLM (Mansour and Fong 2007; Adam 2007). A symptomatic primary tumor may preclude the possibility of simultaneous resection of liver metastases. In contrast, in the case of a asymptomatic primary tumor the approach depends more on the resectability of the liver metastases (Adam 2007). Contraindications for simultaneous resection are based on medical comorbidities, an advanced primary tumor and the need of extensive liver resection (Mansour and Fong 2007; Adam 2007). However, experienced surgical centres for metastatic colorectal cancer resections are now reporting similar survival rates between simultaneous and staged resections (Mansour and Fong 2007).

The surgical resection of colorectal cancer liver metastases involves intraoperative assessment for metastases and signs of extrahepatic disease. Intraoperative ultrasound (IOUS) is a minimally invasive approach which allows the real-time visualization during surgery. It is standard part of the procedure and it is used for the location of previously unknown lesions, for guiding the line of transection and mark important vascular patterns (Roh 1998). Different studies emphasise the role of intraoperative ultrasound (IOUS) with regard to the management of patients with liver metastases. In fact, IOUS has a significant impact on surgical decisions-making and is comparable to open procedures with respect to the detection of CRLM (Foley et al. 1998; Cervone et al. 2000; Zacherl et al. 2002). In some cases, this procedure in combination with laparoscopy was reported to provide useful information regarding resectability and to avoid inadequate laparotomies in 24 out of 47 (51 %) of patients (Rahusen et al. 1999).

The goal of surgical resection is the complete removal of all macroscopically detectable metastatic lesions if possible with cancer free margin (R0 resection; Ito et al. 2010; Hubbard and Alberts 2010; Cady et al. 1998; Garden et al. 2006). The ability to achieve a margin-negative resection is very important leading to improved outcomes (Van Cutsem et al. 2006; Pawlik and Vauthey 2008). Currently, there is no agreed consensus concerning the extent of the tissue resection. In general liver metastases should be resected with at least a 1-cm tumor-free margin but smaller margins are not contraindications to resection (Poultsides et al. 2010; Figueras et al. 2007).

Blood loss following liver resection has a major impact on morbidity and mortality (Hamady et al. 2004). Surgical strategies should include modern transection techniques, various clamping methods and hemodynamic monitoring in order to minimize the risk for blood loss. For example, water-jet cutters and ultrasonic scalpel technologies are effective methods for transection (Holt et al. 2000; Nguyen et al. 2009; Rau et al. 2001). Different clamping techniques such as interrupted portal triad clamping seem to preserve vascular and biliary structures and postoperative liver function (Chiappa et al. 2001; Crenesse et al. 2001; Kimura et al. 2002).

Other options include total vascular exclusion technique (TVE) which is a method that completely isolates the liver from the circulatory system. Data from a series of 45 consecutive major liver resections has shown that this technique was well tolerated and had limited intraoperative blood loss (MacKenzie et al. 2005). Due to the strong correlation between central venous pressure (CVP) and the extent of blood loss (Johnson et al. 1998), another method to manipulate the bleeding is to lower the CVP to 5 mmHg or less (Johnson et al. 1998; Smyrniotis et al. 2004).

In rare cases, the resection entails total vascular exclusion and subsequent vascular reconstruction. This complex major reconstruction of hepatic vessels requires *in situ*, *ante situ* or *ex situ* surgical approaches and in rare cases results in autotransplantation of the remnant liver (Lodge 2004; Lodge et al. 2000; Oldhafer et al. 2001). Although these techniques are associated with a considerable surgical risk, they remain a viable therapeutic alternative in patients with vascular tumor involvement.

Several strategies to improve resectability potential in patients who fail to meet the usual criteria for resection include portal vein embolization (PVE) and two-stage resection technique. These decisions are carefully assessed and depend on the individual clinical situation.

Portal vein embolization (PVE) is employed in patients with insufficient FLR criteria for resectability. This surgical technique redirects the blood flow of the segments to be resected to the non-embolized healthy segments of the liver (de Baere et al. 2007). Additionally, portal vein embolization is used to induce an increase in the volume of non-embolized liver due liver hypertrophy (Abdalla et al. 2006; Chun and Vauthey 2007).

A two-stage resection consists of two sequential hepatectomies performed in patients with advanced bilobar or multinodular disease that cannot be resected in a single procedure (Wicherts et al. 2007). The second stage of this technique is potentially curative and may involve PVE and additional chemotherapeutic courses (Chun and Vauthey 2007; Wicherts et al. 2007).

Although, the 5-year survival rate after resection of CRLM has improved to rates ranging between 40 % and 58 % the reported morbidity rates are up to 39 % (Abdalla et al. 2004).

In several studies the perioperative mortality ranged from 0 to 7 % and was influenced by the extent of liver resection. The most common causes of morbidity included hepatic failure, haemorrhage, sub- phrenic abscesses, biliary fistula, wound infection, pneumonia and myocardial infarction (Fong et al. 1997; Schlag et al. 1990; Doci et al. 1991; Scheele and Altendorf-Hofmann 1999; Cummings et al. 2007)

Recurrence of liver metastasis was reported in up to 65 % within 2 year after surgery following liver resection for CRLM. The most common sites of recurrence following resection of colorectal cancer liver metastases are the liver and lung (Fong et al. 1997; de Jong et al. 2009). Repeat liver resections are feasible and several groups showed that morbidity, mortality and overall survival (OS) were comparable with the outcomes of the initial hepatectomy (Adam et al. 2003; Petrowsky et al. 2002). Liver reoperation in these cases is technically more challenging due to formation of dense adhesions around the subhepatic space and due to an increased risk of vascular injuries and haemorrhages (Aramaki et al. 2000).

26.3 Locoregional Methods

1. Cryotherapy Regional therapies for liver metastases, such as hepatic cryosurgery and radiofrequency ablation are promising surgical techniques that attempt to destroy the tumors in situ. Hepatic cryotherapy involves freeze/thaw cycles administered to the liver tumors by means of a cryoprobe inserted into the lesion (Whittaker 1984). The cryogenic approach is suitable for patients with unresectable but isolated liver metastases and results in avascular lesions and necrosis of cancer cells. This procedure spares the surrounding liver tissues and can be repeated. In some centers, cryosurgery is performed instead of hepatic resection or as an adjunct to surgery (Gruenberger et al. 2001; Ruers et al. 2001). Different techniques such as hepatic inflow or outflow occlusion may be employed to prevent inadequate freezing of the lesions situated adjacent to blood vessels (Seifert et al. 1998). However, cryosurgical ablation is frequently associated with complications such as subsequent haemorrhage of cracking frozen liver, biloma, biliary fistula and liver abscess. In one study the recurrence rate was as high as 53 % (Adam et al. 2002) and overall morbidity ranged from 6 to 29 % with an overall mortality rate of 1.6 %. Intraoperative ultrasound technology and an improved liquid nitrogen delivery system allows better control of freezing (Subar et al. 2003).

2. Radiofrequency ablation Radiofrequency ablation (RFA) of liver metastases is yet another evolving technology employed to treat patients with unresectable lesions and with no evidence of extrahepatic disease (Curley 2001). During this technique a RFA needle electrode is introduced into the centre of the lesion. This method induces coagulative necrosis through tissue heating to temperatures that exceed 60°C (Goldberg et al. 1995). One of the limitations of radiofrequency ablation is the size of the lesion. Tumors less than 2.5 cm can be ablated with the placement of a needle electrode in the center of the tumor. For larger tumors repositioning of the needle and multiple deployments are needed (Abdalla et al. 2004; Goldberg et al. 1995; Livraghi et al. 2001). A percutaneous approach may be used in patients with a limited number of small metastases while a laparoscopic approach under ultrasonography guidance offers an accurate positioning of the RF needle and is recommended in lesions less than 4.0 cm in diameter. However, percutaneous ablation has been reported to achieve worse local control rates than the open surgical approach (Kuvshinoff and Ota 2002; Mulier et al. 2005). Larger lesions are less likely to be successfully ablated completely and RF can be used as a part of an open surgical procedure (Hamady et al. 2004). In patients with multilobar disease this procedure can be combined with resection (Oshowo et al. 2003; Pawlik et al. 2003; Evrard et al. 2004). A significantly higher local recurrence rate was reported with large tumors more than 4 cm in diameter (Kuvshinoff and Ota 2002; Solbiati et al. 2001; Wood et al. 2000).

The effects of RFA in the proximity of the major hepatic vessels could be diminished due to heat dissipation resulting in a cooling effect dependent on blood circulation. In these cases vascular occlusion techniques such as hepatic inflow occlusion may prevent heat dissipation (Delis et al. 2007; Goletti et al. 2000). Additional complications can be encountered if the procedure is performed in tumors close to the hepatic hilum because of the increased risk of bile duct stricture and fistula. In these cases vascular occlusion techniques such as hepatic inflow occlusion may prevent heat dissipation (Curley 2001; Karmali and Dixon 2004). The overall complication rates after cryoablation range from 15 to 60 %, and include damage to the diaphragm or colon, pleural effusion, hemorrhage, biloma, liver abscess and arterioportal venous (Giorgio et al. 2005). Radiofrequency ablation for CRLM provides survival rates in between 35 and 57 % (Oshowo et al. 2003; Solbiati et al. 2001; Iannitti et al. 2002; Gillams and Lees 2005). However, has a significantly lower survival rate when compared to surgical resection alone (Hamady et al. 2004; Abdalla et al. 2004). Currently this procedure has roles in treating unresectable disease and in combination with surgery to extend the limits of resection and for recurrent CRLM.

26.4 Chemotherapy for Patients with Colorectal Cancer Liver Metastases

The chemotherapeutic treatment of CRC has the potential of inducing tumor downstaging and may permit resection of about 15 % of metastases which have been initially considered unresectable. Several groups reported the results of resection in patients who did not initially meet the criteria for resectability (Bismuth et al. 1996; Giacchetti et al. 1999). In a series of 1,104 initially unresectable patients, (12.5 %) underwent secondary hepatic resection after an average of 10 courses of chemotherapy. In this group the survival rate at five-year follow-up was of 33 % and 52 patients had repeat hepatectomies because of recurrences (Adam et al. 2004).

Chemotherapeutic regimens based on fluorouracil (5-FU) in combination with leucovorin (LV) are standard theraphies for CRLM, yielding a response rate (RR) of 20–30 % and median survival time of 11–12 months (Kemeny 2006). Newer systemic chemotherapy regimens including oxaloplatin and irinotecan increased the response rates in CRLM patients leading to and an OS of 33–62 % (Saltz et al. 2000; Venook et al. 2006). Modulated infusional 5-FU regimens combined with oxaloplatin (FOLFOX regimen) or irinotecan (FOLFIRI regimen) produce high response rates of more than 50 % (Tournigand et al. 2004; Pozzo et al. 2004). In these cases successful secondary resections have been reported (Tanaka et al. 2003). With the use of the FOLFOX or a capecitabine and oxaliplatin-regimen, Gruenberger et al. (2004) reported a peri-operative mortality of 0 % in 50 patients. In a large ($n = 364$) phase III clinical trial, European Organization for the Research and Treatment of Cancer (EORTC) 40983 study, the preoperative FOLFOX4 (six cycles before and six cycles after surgery) regimen was associated with a longer PFS in patients who underwent metastases resection (Nordlinger et al. 2008). A phase III, randomised, open-label multicentre study compared standard treatment with FUFIRI (irinotecan, 5-fluorouracil) to mIROX which uses an identical schedule of irinotecan plus oxaliplatin. Both regimens induced a similar response. However, the combination of high-dose 5-FU/folinic acid and irinotecan remains standard of care in first-line treatment of metastatic colorectal cancer due to a better tolerability (Fischer von Weikersthal et al. 2011).

Further development of targeted therapy agents such as the monoclonal antibodies against the epidermal growth factor receptor (EGFR) such as cetuximab and panitumumab, and bevacizumab, which targets the vascular endothelial growth factor (VEGF), has clearly improved the outcomes of CRLM (Reidy and Saltz 2007). The recent recognition of the role of KRAS in predicting response to cetuximab may have a role in further selection of patients (Lievre et al. 2008). More recently, clinical trials have shown that the addition of cetuximab translated into high response rates when added to oxaloplatin and irinotecan-based combination regimens (Tabernero et al. 2007; Arnold et al. 2008; Saltz et al. 2004). When cetuximab was combined with an infusional 5-FU/LV plus irinotecan regimen, five out of 19 patients became candidates for secondary resection that was successfully performed in four patients (Folprecht et al. 2006).

The anti-VEGF antibody bevacizumab is also able to enhance the activity of cytotoxic chemotherapy and several studies have demonstrated a role for bevacizumab in either first or second line therapy of CRLM. In addition to inhibitory effect on angiogenesis, this agent possibly acts through an enhanced delivery of chemotherapeutic agents by lowering intratumoral tissue pressure (Saltz et al. 2008; Hurwitz et al. 2004). These effects were evaluated in a larger phase III trial where bevacizumab combined with IFL (irinotecan/5FU/leucovorin) was compared with IFL and placebo in patients with CRLM. Median OS was significantly increased to 20.3 months in the IFL and bevacizumab arm. Complications including wound healing delays, hepatocellular insufficiency, infections, and bleeding were observed in patients who undergo surgery while receiving bevacizumab (Tamandl et al. 2010) raising concern that the use of bevacizumab may increase the risk for wound-related complications (Ellis et al. 2005). However, a subsequent study showed that the postoperative morbidity and mortality after resection of CRLM did not increase in patients treated with Bevacizumab and standard chemotherapy as compared with resection after chemotherapy alone (Tamandl et al. 2010). There is no general consensus regarding the timing of surgery after therapy with bevacizumab. In one study, a median time of 58 days from bevacizumab discontinuation to surgery was not associated with increased surgical complications (Kesmodel et al. 2008).

The issue of the optimal timing and duration of neoadjuvant chemotherapy still remains controversial. When the liver metastases are considered unresectable, the ECMTG recommends the resection of primary tumor if possible. However, if the primary tumor is essentially asymptomatic, then a course of chemotherapy should be administered first. In general, short curses of chemotherapy (up to six cycles) are recommended, with surgery being performed as soon as a response to chemotherapy is observed (Kemeny et al. 2006).

This approach permits insight into the responsiveness to therapy and also allows a thorough monitoring of the effects of therapy on tumor progression (Nordlinger et al. 2007).

When the liver metastases are resectable, the potential benefits of neoadjuvant chemotherapy include the opportunity to test for chemoresponsiveness (Leonard et al. 2005) and may allow immediate treatment of microscopic disease (Mandala et al. 2007). Moreover, the response to neoadjuvant chemotherapy for synchronous CRLM may have prognostic implications and has a role in patient selection for further therapy (Allen et al. 2003). However, peri-operative chemotherapy may damage the liver and impair the functioning of the remaining hepatic tissue after surgery.

Chemotherapy -associated liver injury results in vascular changes and steatohepatitis (Aloia and Fahy 2010). Vascular changes include sinusoidal dilatation with erythrocytic congestion, accompanied by presinusoidal fibrosis and fibrotic venular occlusion (Rubbia-Brandt et al. 2004). Evidence suggests that oxaloplatin-based regimens are associated with higher risk for hepatic vascular lesions (Rubbia-Brandt et al. 2004; Karoui et al. 2006), whereas irinotecan-based regimens are associated with higher risk for steatosis and steatohepatitis (Vauthey et al. 2006).

Safety data from the EORTC 40983 study, which compared surgery alone with perioperative chemotherapy showed very low mortality rates (about 1 %) and acceptable rate of reversible complications (Taïeb et al. 2005).

Although chemotherapy contributes to downsizing tumors, this approach can negatively impact the quality of life of patients due to a greater toxicity. The clinical significance of liver injury associated with perioperative chemotherapy remains uncertain. Patients should be carefully assessed for their ability to undergo chemotherapy as well as surgery.

26.5 Adjuvant Therapy

Clinical trials have demonstrated the benefit of adjuvant chemotherapy following resection in order to treat microscopic metastatic disease.

Hepatic Arterial Infusion Hepatic arterial infusion (HAI) delivers high concentrations of cytotoxic drugs by localized infusion. Data from different trials suggest higher response rates for HAI when compared with systemic chemotherapy alone (Kemeny et al. 1999; Hebbar et al. 2009). This data was confirmed in a meta-analysis of seven randomized controlled trials in 1,098 patients which showed median OS durations of 16.04 months and 12.64 months for HAI and systemic chemotherapy respectively (Mocellin et al. 2007, 2009). HAI with oxaliplatin or irinotecan-based chemotherapy also achieved encouraging results in approximately 15–20 % of the patients (Boige et al. 2008). A recent phase II trial assessed the potential benefit of systemic oxaliplatin and capecitabine alternating with HAI of floxuridine. In this trial alternating HAI and systemic capecitabine and oxaliplatin rendered survival rates of 85 % at 2 years and was clinically tolerable (Alberts et al. 2010). New randomized trials with anti-angiogenic and anti-epidermal growth factor receptor agents are needed to determine the clinical benefit of HAI (Biasco et al. 2006; Alberts and Wagman 2008).

Systemic Adjuvant Chemotherapy Systemic adjuvant chemotherapy after resection of liver metastases aims to reduce the risk of relapse and death (Figueras et al. 2001). Data analysis from clinical trials comparing postsurgical chemotherapy to chemotherapy alone showed that in a pool of 278 patients the adjuvant chemotherapy group had a significantly reduced risk of relapse and a modest increase in OS (Mitry et al. 2008). Significant improvement was reported with oxaliplatin and the 5-Fluorouracil/Leucovorin schedule in terms of both disease free survival (DFS) and OS at 3 years in the MOSAIC (Multicenter International Study of Oxaliplatin/5-Fluorouracil/Leucovorin in the Adjuvant Treatment of Colon Cancer) trial (André et al. 2009). The update at 6-year follow-up confirmed these results and chemotherapy with FOLFOX for 6 months has been adopted worldwide as the standard of care in stage III colon cancer patients. Adjuvant chemotherapy with irinotecan was also assessed after complete resection of liver metastases. However, phase III clinical trials evaluating the addition of irinotecan to LV5FU2 failed to show an improvement in OS or disease DFS (Ychou et al. 2009; Van Cutsem et al. 2009; Saltz et al. 2007). Preliminary data from a phase III study which assessed adjuvant capecitabine plus oxaliplatin (XELOX) versus bolus FU/LV (Mayo Clinic or Roswell Park regimen), (Schmoll et al. 2007) showed that the 3 year DFS for patients receiving XELOX was superior to DFS in 5-FU/LV arm (Lindsay and Cassidy 2011). An ongoing phase III trial is evaluating patients randomized after resection to receive adjuvant oxaliplatin plus capecitabine (CAPOX) combined with bevacizumab versus CAPOX alone (Snoeren et al. 2010).

The roles of targeted agents associated with adjuvant systemic chemotherapy following resection of liver metastases as well as the optimal duration of adjuvant therapy are currently evaluated in ongoing clinical trials.

Immunotherapy Emerging data supports the role of immunotherapy as neoadjuvant therapy in association with resection of CRLM. Treatment with interleukin 2 before hepatectomy was shown to prevent the postoperative immunodepression (Okuno et al. 1999, 2000). Vaccination with autologous tumor-derived heat-shock protein 96, induced a CD8-mediated tumor-specific response and prolonged survival in metastatic colorectal patients after liver resection (Mazzaferro et al. 2003; Pilla et al. 2005). Also, adjuvant therapy with OncoVAX (Vaccinogen, Inc.) an autologous tumor vaccine, significantly improved OS and recurrence-free survival in stage II colon cancer (Hanna et al. 2006).

Recently, a meta- analysis investigating the role of active specific immunotherapy (ASI) in advanced colorectal cancer and suspected minimal residual colorectal cancer indicated that ASI may provide a promising therapeutic approach in suspected minimal residual CRC (Rao et al. 2011).

Future work is needed to evaluate the implication of cancer vaccines and neoadjuvant immunotherapy in the treatment of hepatic colorectal metastases.

Radiotherapy Selective internal radiation therapy (SIRT) is a new promising treatment for metastases to the liver (Stubbs and Wickremesekera 2004). SIRT is a technique that delivers a single dose of 90Yttrium microspheres into the hepatic artery, resulting in selective tumor uptake and irradiation. Encouraging results have been reported in different studies utilizing this technique for the treatment of CRC liver metastases (Dancey et al. 2000; Campbell et al. 2000). A recent analysis showed a significant improvement in progression free survival (PFS) and median survival associated with SIRT, when compared with chemotherapy. However this method is associated with potential side effects. Further clinical trials are warranted to assess the effect of SIRT in conjunction with chemotherapeutic modalities and surgery (Townsend et al. 2009).

26.6 Key Points

- Liver resection is an effective therapy with potentially curative intent for colorectal liver metastases
- Patient selection should include careful evaluation and delineation of metastases, exclusion of non-resectable extrahepatic disease and general physiological fitness tests
- Resection techniques will vary according to the number and location of metastases and hepatic functional reserve
- The only contraindication for resection is the inability to achieve margin-negative resection while maintaining an adequate hepatic volume reserve
- Resectability may be achieved using portal vein embolization, two stage hepatectomy, or a combination of surgery and ablation
- Patients with unresectable tumors may benefit from tumor ablation techniques such as cryotherapy or radiofrequency ablation
- Systemic chemotherapies regimens based on 5-fluorouracil, oxaliplatin and irinotecan are well tolerated and may downstage unresectable tumors into potentially resectable ones
- Adjuvant chemotherapy improves survival after resection of hepatic colorectal metastases
- The surgical decision should be individualized according to clinical situation, experience of the surgical centre and should be made in consultation with a multidisciplinary team.

26.7 Summary

Patients with liver metastases from CRC that are potentially resectable should be evaluated by an experienced team. Today it is clear that surgical resection remains the best treatment for long-term survival. Although a minority of patients are amenable to this therapeutic modality, resectability with curative intent is rapidly becoming the standard of care. With the new surgical techniques and advances in chemotherapy, an increased number of patients can benefit from this procedure. A therapeutic decision to proceed with resection should be individualized based on a thorough clinical assessment of the patient.

Only two absolute contraindications to liver resection preclude this therapeutically decision. The first is inadequate FLR following resection. However, as FLR can be augmented using PVE, no clinical situation should be ruled out without a careful assessment of available alternatives. The second is tumor invasion of all three hepatic veins or invasion of both portal pedicles. Patients who are not suitable to surgical resection and who have no extrahepatic disease are amenable to several newer therapies such as cryosurgery and radiofrequency ablation (RFA). Hepatic artery catheter chemotherapy and portal vein embolization can be alternatively performed in cases of extensive hepatic metastases. Systemic chemotherapy has therapeutic roles in patients with extrahepatic disease as contributes to improved outcomes when compared with surgery alone. In unresectable disease, consideration should be given to immunotherapy in combination with antitumor cytotoxic agents in order to amplify the therapeutic efficacy of anticancer agents. SIRT is beneficial in patients without extrahepatic metastases who failed chemotherapeutic regimens.

The timing between chemotherapy and surgery is very important for optimal outcome of patients. All patients should be managed by a multidisciplinary team and final therapeutically strategies should be guided by a thorough clinical assessment.

References

Abdalla EK et al (2004) Recurrence and outcomes following hepatic resection, radiofrequency ablation, and combined resection/ablation for colorectal liver metastases. Ann Surg 239:818–825 (discussion 825–817)

Abdalla EK et al (2006) Improving resectability of hepatic colorectal metastases: expert consensus statement. Ann Surg Oncol 13:1271–1280

Aboulafia AJ, Levine AM, Schmidt D, Aboulafia D (2007) Surgical therapy of bone metastases. Semin Oncol 34:206–214

Adam R (2007) Colorectal cancer with synchronous liver metastases. Br J Surg 94:129–131

Adam R et al (2002) A comparison of percutaneous cryosurgery and percutaneous radiofrequency for unresectable hepatic malignancies. Arch Surg 137:1332–1339 (discussion 1340)

Adam R et al (2003) Liver resection for colorectal metastases: the third hepatectomy. Ann Surg 238:871–883 (discussion 883–874)

Adam R et al (2004) Rescue surgery for unresectable colorectal liver metastases downstaged by chemotherapy: a model to predict long-term survival. Ann Surg 240:644–657 (discussion 657–648)

Alberts SR et al (2010) Alternating systemic and hepatic artery infusion therapy for resected liver metastases from colorectal cancer: a North Central Cancer Treatment Group (NCCTG)/National Surgical Adjuvant Breast and Bowel Project (NSABP) phase II intergroup trial, N9945/CI-66. J Clin Onc 28:853–858

Alberts SR, Wagman LD (2008) Chemotherapy for colorectal cancer liver metastases. Oncologist 13:1063–1073

Allen PJ et al (2003) Importance of response to neoadjuvant chemotherapy in patients undergoing resection of synchronous colorectal liver metastases. J Gastrointest Surg 7:109–115 (discussion 116–107)

Aloia TA, Fahy BN (2010) Chemotherapy-associated hepatotoxicity: how concerned should we be? Exp Rev Anticancer Ther 10:521–527

André T et al (2009) Improved overall survival with oxaliplatin, fluorouracil, and leucovorin as adjuvant treatment in stage II or III colon cancer in the MOSAIC trial. J Clin Onc 27:3109–3116

Aramaki M et al (2000) Postoperative complications of repeat hepatectomy for liver metastasis from colorectal carcinoma. Hepatogastroenterology 47:478–480

Arnold D et al (2008) Cetuximab in combination with weekly 5-fluorouracil/folinic acid and oxaliplatin (FUFOX) in untreated patients with advanced colorectal cancer: a phase Ib/II study of the AIO GI Group. Ann Onc 19:1442–1449

Biasco G et al (2006) Treatment of hepatic metastases from colorectal cancer: many doubts, some certainties. Cancer Treat Rev 32:214–228

Bipat S et al (2005) Colorectal liver metastases: CT, MR imaging, and PET for diagnosis—meta-analysis1. Radiology 237:123–131

Bismuth H et al (1996) Resection of nonresectable liver metastases from colorectal cancer after neoadjuvant chemotherapy. Ann Surg 224:509–520 (discussion 520–502)

Blumgart LH (ed) (2007) Surgery of the liver, biliary tract and pancreas, 4th edn. Saunders, Philadelphia

Boige V et al (2008) Hepatic arterial infusion of oxaliplatin and intravenous LV5FU2 in unresectable liver metastases from colorectal cancer after systemic chemotherapy failure. Ann Surg Onc 15:219–226

Cady B et al (1998) Surgical margin in hepatic resection for colorectal metastasis: a critical and improvable determinant of outcome. Ann Surg 227:566–571

Campbell AM, Bailey IH, Burton MA (2000) Analysis of the distribution of intra-arterial microspheres in human liver following hepatic yttrium-90 microsphere therapy. Phys Med Biol 45:1023–1033

Cervone A, Sardi A, Conaway GL (2000) Intraoperative ultrasound (IOUS) is essential in the management of metastatic colorectal liver lesions. Am Surg 66:611–615

Chiappa A et al (2001) Comparison of continuous versus intermittent hepatic pedicle clamping in an experimental model. Hepatogastroenterology 48:1416–1420

Chun YS, Vauthey JN (2007) Extending the frontiers of resectability in advanced colorectal cancer. Eur J Surg Oncol 33(Suppl 2):52–S58

Couinaud C (ed) (1957) Le foie; études anatomiques et chirurgicales. Masson, Paris

Crenesse D et al (2001) Intermittent ischemia reduces warm hypoxia-reoxygenation-induced JNK(1)/SAPK(1) activation and apoptosis in rat hepatocytes. Hepatology 34:972–978

Cummings LC, Payes JD, Cooper GS (2007) Survival after hepatic resection in metastatic colorectal cancer. Cancer 109:718–726

Curley SA (2001) Radiofrequency ablation of malignant liver tumors. Oncologist 6:14–23

Dancey JE et al (2000) Treatment of nonresectable hepatocellular carcinoma with intrahepatic 90Y-microspheres. J Nucl Med 41:1673–1681

de Baere T, Denys A, Madoff DC (2007) Preoperative portal vein embolization: indications and technical considerations. Tech Vasc Interv Radiol 10:67–78

de Jong MC et al (2009) Rates and patterns of recurrence following curative intent surgery for colorectal liver metastasis: an international multi-institutional analysis of 1,669 patients. Ann Surg 250:440–448

Delis SG, Madariaga J, Bakoyiannis A, Dervenis C (2007) Current role of bloodless liver resection. World J Gastroenterol 13:826–829

Dimitroulis D et al (2010) Role of surgery in colorectal liver metastases: too early or too late? World J Gastroenterol 16:3484–3490

Doci R et al (1991) One hundred patients with hepatic metastases from colorectal cancer treated by resection: analysis of prognostic determinants. Br J Surg 78:797–801

Ellis LM, Curley SA, Grothey A (2005) Surgical resection after downsizing of colorectal liver metastasis in the era of bevacizumab. J Clin Oncol 23:4853–4855

Evrard S et al (2004) Surgical treatment of liver metastases by radiofrequency ablation, resection, or in combination. Eur J Surg Oncol 30:399–406

Figueras J et al (2001) Resection rate and effect of postoperative chemotherapy on survival after surgery for colorectal liver metastases. Br J Surg 88:980–985

Figueras J et al (2007) Effect of subcentimeter nonpositive resection margin on hepatic recurrence in patients undergoing hepatectomy for colorectal liver metastases. Evidences from 663 liver resections. Ann Oncol 18:1190–1195

Fischer von Weikersthal L et al (2011) Phase III trial of irinotecan plus infusional 5-fluorouracil/folinic acid versus irinotecan plus oxaliplatin as first-line treatment of advanced colorectal cancer. Eur J Cancer 47:206–214

Foley EF, Kolecki RV, Schirmer BD (1998) The accuracy of laparoscopic ultrasound in the detection of colorectal cancer liver metastases. Am J Surg 176:262–264

Folprecht G et al (2006) Cetuximab and irinotecan/5-fluorouracil/folinic acid is a safe combination for the first-line treatment of patients with epidermal growth factor receptor expressing metastatic colorectal carcinoma. Ann Onc 17:450–456

Fong Y, Blumgart LH, Cohen AM (1995) Surgical treatment of colorectal metastases to the liver. CA Cancer J Clin 45:50–62

Fong Y et al (1997) Liver resection for colorectal metastases. J Clin Oncol 15:938–946

Fong Y, Fortner J, Sun RL, Brennan MF, Blumgart LH (1999) Clinical score for predicting recurrence after hepatic resection for metastatic colorectal cancer: analysis of 1,001 consecutive cases. Ann Surg 230:309–318 (discussion 318–321)

Garden OJ et al (2006) Guidelines for resection of colorectal cancer liver metastases. Gut 55(Suppl 3):1–8

Giacchetti S, Itzhaki M, Gruia G (1999) Long-term survival of patients with unresectable colorectal cancer liver metastases following infusional chemotherapy with 5-fluorouracil, leucovorin, oxaliplatin and surgery. Ann Onc 10:663–669

Gilbert H, Kagan AR (ed) (1976) Metastases: incidence, detection, and evaluation without histologic confirmation. Amsterdam, North Holland, pp 385–405

Gillams AR, Lees WR (2005) Radiofrequency ablation of colorectal liver metastases. Abdom Imaging 30:419–426

Giorgio A, Tarantino L, de Stefano G, Coppola C, Ferraioli G (2005) Complications after percutaneous saline-enhanced radiofrequency ablation of liver tumors: 3-year experience with 336 patients at a single center. Am J Roentgenol 184:207–211

Goldberg SN et al (1995) Tissue ablation with radiofrequency using multiprobe arrays. Acad Radiol 2:670–674

Goletti O et al (2000) Laparoscopic radiofrequency thermal ablation of hepatocarcinoma: preliminary experience. Surg Laparosc Endosc Percutan Tech 10:284–290

Gruenberger T, Jourdan JL, Zhao J, King J, Morris DL (2001) Reduction in recurrence risk for involved or inadequate margins with edge cryotherapy after liver resection for colorectal metastases. Arch Surg 136:1154–1157

Gruenberger T, Schuell B, Kornek G, Scheithauer W (2004) Neoadjuvant chemotherapy for resectable colorectal cancer liver metastases: impact on magnitude of liver resection and survival. J Clin Onc 22(Suppl):3598 (Meeting Abstracts no. 14)

Hamady ZZR, Kotru A, Nishio H, Lodge JPA (2004) Current techniques and results of liver resection for colorectal liver metastases. Br Med Bull 70:87–104

Hanna MG Jr, Hoover HC Jr, Pinedo HM, Finer M (2006) Active specific immunotherapy with autologous tumor cell vaccines for stage II colon cancer: logistics, efficacy, safety and immunological Pharmacodynamics. Hum Vaccin 2:185–191

Hebbar M, Pruvot F-R, Romano O, Triboulet J-P, de Gramont A (2009) Integration of neoadjuvant and adjuvant chemotherapy in patients with resectable liver metastases from colorectal cancer. Cancer Treat Rev 35:668–675

Holt DR, Thiel DV, Edelstein S, Brems JJ (2000) Hepatic resections. Arch Surg 135:1353–1358

Huang S-H et al (2008) A fast method to segment the liver according to Couinaud's classification. In Gao X, Müller H, Loomes M, Comley R, Luo S (eds) Medical imaging and informatics, vol 4987. Springer, Berlin, pp 270–276

Hubbard JM, Alberts SR (2010) Treatment of liver-limited metastatic colorectal cancer. Cancer J 16:235–240

Hurwitz H et al (2004) Bevacizumab plus irinotecan, fluorouracil, and leucovorin for metastatic colorectal cancer. N Eng J Med 350:2335–2342

Iannitti DA, Dupuy DE, Mayo-Smith WW, Murphy B (2002) Hepatic radiofrequency ablation. Arch Surg 137:422–426 (discussion 427)

Ito K, Govindarajan A, Ito H, Fong Y (2010) Surgical treatment of hepatic colorectal metastasis: evolving role in the setting of improving systemic therapies and ablative treatments in the 21st century. Cancer J 16:103–110 (110.1097/PPO.1090b1013e3181d1097e1098e1095).

Johnson M, Mannar R, Wu AVO (1998) Correlation between blood loss and inferior vena caval pressure during liver resection. Br J Surg 85:188–190

Johnson TN, Tucker GT, Tanner MS, Rostami-Hodjegan A (2005) Changes in liver volume from birth to adulthood: a meta-analysis. Liver Transplant 11:1481–1493

Karmali S, Dixon E (2004) Biliary stricture resulting from radiofrequency ablation. Am J Surg 188:76–77

Karoui M et al (2006) Influence of preoperative chemotherapy on the risk of major hepatectomy for colorectal liver metastases. Ann Surg 243:1–7

Kemeny N (2006) Management of liver metastases from colorectal cancer. Oncology (Williston Park) 20:1161–1176, 1179 (discussion 1179–1180, 1185–1166)

Kemeny N et al (1999) Hepatic arterial infusion of chemotherapy after resection of hepatic metastases from colorectal cancer. N Engl J Med 341:2039–2048

Kemeny NE et al (2006) Hepatic arterial infusion versus systemic therapy for hepatic metastases from colorectal cancer: a randomized trial of efficacy, quality of life, and molecular markers (CALGB 9481). J Clin Oncol 24:1395–1403

Kesmodel SB et al (2008) Preoperative bevacizumab does not significantly increase postoperative complication rates in patients undergoing hepatic surgery for colorectal cancer liver metastases. J Clin Onc 26:5254–5260

Kienast Y, Winkler F (2010) Therapy and prophylaxis of brain metastases. Expert Rev Anticancer Ther 10:1763–1777

Kimura F et al (2002) Evaluation of total hepatic vascular exclusion and pringle maneuver in liver resection. Hepatogastroenterology 49:225–230

Kuvshinoff BW, Ota DM (2002) Radiofrequency ablation of liver tumors: influence of technique and tumor size. Surgery 132:605–611 (discussion 611–602)

Leonard GD, Brenner B, Kemeny NE (2005) Neoadjuvant chemotherapy before liver resection for patients with unresectable liver metastases from colorectal carcinoma. J Clin Oncol 23:2038–2048

Li Destri G et al (2008) Metachronous liver metastases and resectability: Fong's score and laparoscopic evaluation. HPB (Oxford) 10:13–17

Lievre A et al (2008) KRAS mutations as an independent prognostic factor in patients with advanced colorectal cancer treated with cetuximab. J Clin Oncol 26:374–379

Lindsay CR, Cassidy J (2011) XELOX in colorectal cancer: a convenient option for the future? Exp Rev Gastr Hepatol 5:9–19

Livraghi T et al (2001) Percutaneous radio-frequency ablation of liver metastases from breast cancer: initial experience in 24 patients. Radiology 220:145–149

Lodge JPA (2004) Hemostasis in liver resection surgery. Semin Hematol 41:70–75

Lodge JP, Ammori BJ, Prasad KR, Bellamy MC (2000) Ex vivo and in situ resection of inferior vena cava with hepatectomy for colorectal metastases. Ann Surg 231:471–479

MacKenzie S, Dixon E, Bathe O, Sutherland F (2005) Intermittent hepatic vein—total vascular exclusion during liver resection: anatomic and clinical studies. J Gastrointest Surg 9:658–666

Mandala M, Mosconi S, Quadri A, Milesi L, Labianca R (2007) Neoadjuvant chemotherapy for patients with liver metastases from colorectal cancer. Expert Rev Anticancer Ther 7:887–897

Manfredi S et al (2006) Incidence and patterns of recurrence after resection for cure of colonic cancer in a well defined population. Br J Surg 93:1115–1122

Mansour J, Fong Y (2007) Timing of the liver resection for patients with synchronous metastases: practical and outcome considerations. Ann Surg Oncol 14:2435–2436

Martinez L, Puig I, Valls C (2007) Colorectal liver metastases: radiological diagnosis and staging. Eur J Surg Oncol 33(Suppl 2):S5–16

Mazzaferro V et al (2003) Vaccination with autologous tumor-derived heat-shock protein gp96 after liver resection for metastatic colorectal cancer. Clin Cancer Res 9:3235–3245

Memon MA, Beckingham IJ (2001) Surgical resection of colorectal liver metastases. Colorectal Dis 3:361–373

Mitry E et al (2008) Adjuvant chemotherapy after potentially curative resection of metastases from colorectal cancer: a pooled analysis of two randomized trials. J Clin Onc 26:4906–4911

Mocellin S, Pasquali S, Nitti D (2009) Fluoropyrimidine-HAI (hepatic arterial infusion) versus systemic chemotherapy (SCT) for unresectable liver metastases from colorectal cancer. Cochrane Database Syst Rev 8:CD007823

Mocellin S, Pilati P, Lise M, Nitti D (2007) Meta-analysis of hepatic arterial infusion for unresectable liver metastases from colorectal cancer: the end of an era? J Clin Onc 25:5649–5654
Mulier S et al (2005) Local recurrence after hepatic radiofrequency coagulation: multivariate meta-analysis and review of contributing factors. Ann Surg 242:158–171
Nesbitt C, Glendinning RJ, Byrne C, Poston GJ (2007) Factors that influence treatment strategies in advanced colorectal cancer. Eur J Surg Oncol 33(Suppl 2):88–94
Nguyen KT, Gamblin TC, Geller DA (2009) World review of laparoscopic liver resection-2,804 patients. Ann Surg 250:831–841
Nordlinger B et al (1996) Surgical resection of colorectal carcinoma metastases to the liver. A prognostic scoring system to improve case selection, based on 1,568 patients. Association Francaise de Chirurgie. Cancer 77:1254–1262
Nordlinger B et al (2007) Does chemotherapy prior to liver resection increase the potential for cure in patients with metastatic colorectal cancer? A report from the European colorectal metastases treatment group. Eur J Cancer 43:2037–2045
Nordlinger B et al (2008) Perioperative chemotherapy with FOLFOX4 and surgery versus surgery alone for resectable liver metastases from colorectal cancer (EORTC Intergroup trial 40983): a randomised controlled trial. The Lancet 371:1007–1016
Nordlinger B et al (2009) Combination of surgery and chemotherapy and the role of targeted agents in the treatment of patients with colorectal liver metastases: recommendations from an expert panel. Ann Oncol 20:985–992
Okuno K, Kaneda K, Yasutomi M (1999) Regional IL-2-based immunochemotherapy of colorectal liver metastases. Hepatogastroenterology 46(Suppl 1):1263–1267
Okuno K, Hirai N, Takemoto Y, Kawai I, Yasutomi M (2000) Interleukin-2 as a modulator of 5-fluorouracil in hepatic arterial immunochemotherapy for liver metastases. Hepatogastroenterology 47:487–491
Oldhafer KJ, Lang H, Malago M, Testa G, Broelsch CE (2001) Ex situ resection and resection of the in situ perfused liver: are there still indications? Chirurg 72:131–137
Oshowo A, Gillams A, Harrison E, Lees WR, Taylor I (2003) Comparison of resection and radiofrequency ablation for treatment of solitary colorectal liver metastases. Br J Surg 90:1240–1243
Pawlik TM, Choti MA (2007) Surgical therapy for colorectal metastases to the liver. J Gastrointest Surg 11:1057–1077
Pawlik TM, Vauthey JN (2008) Surgical margins during hepatic surgery for colorectal liver metastases: complete resection not millimeters defines outcome. Ann Surg Oncol 15:677–679
Pawlik TM, Izzo F, Cohen DS, Morris JS, Curley SA (2003) Combined resection and radiofrequency ablation for advanced hepatic malignancies: results in 172 patients. Ann Surg Oncol 10:1059–1069
Pawlik TM et al (2005) Effect of surgical margin status on survival and site of recurrence after hepatic resection for colorectal metastases. Ann Surg 241:715–722 (discussion 722–714)
Petrowsky H et al (2002) Second liver resections are safe and effective treatment for recurrent hepatic metastases from colorectal cancer: a bi-institutional analysis. Ann Surg 235:863–871
Pilla L et al (2005) Natural killer and NK-Like T-cell activation in colorectal carcinoma patients treated with autologous tumor-derived heat shock protein 96. Cancer Res 65:3942–3949
Poultsides GA, Schulick RD, Pawlik TM (2010) Hepatic resection for colorectal metastases: the impact of surgical margin status on outcome. HPB (Oxford) 12:43–49
Pozzo C et al (2004) Neoadjuvant treatment of unresectable liver disease with irinotecan and 5-fluorouracil plus folinic acid in colorectal cancer patients. Ann Onc 15:933–939
Rahusen FD et al (1999) Selection of patients for resection of colorectal metastases to the liver using diagnostic laparoscopy and laparoscopic ultrasonography. Ann Surg 230:31–37
Rao B et al (2011) Clinical outcomes of active specific immunotherapy in advanced colorectal cancer and suspected minimal residual colorectal cancer: a meta-analysis and system review. J Translat Med 9:17
Rau HG et al (2001) Dissection techniques in liver surgery. Chirurg 72:105–112

Rees M, Tekkis PP, Welsh FK, O'Rourke T, John TG (2008) Evaluation of long-term survival after hepatic resection for metastatic colorectal cancer: a multifactorial model of 929 patients. Ann Surg 247:125–135

Reidy D, Saltz L (2007) Targeted therapy for metastatic colorectal cancer: current challenges and future directions. Curr Colorec Cancer Rep 3:109–115

Roh MS (ed) (1998) Colorectal cancer metastatic to the liver: resection and other techniques. Mosby Inc, St. Louis, pp 352–355

Rubbia-Brandt L et al (2004) Severe hepatic sinusoidal obstruction associated with oxaliplatin-based chemotherapy in patients with metastatic colorectal cancer. Ann Oncol 15:460–466

Ruers TJ, Joosten J, Jager GJ, Wobbes T (2001) Long-term results of treating hepatic colorectal metastases with cryosurgery. Br J Surg 88:844–849

Rueth NM, Andrade RS (2010) Is VATS lobectomy better: perioperatively, biologically and oncologically? Ann Thorac Surg 89:2107–2111

Saltz LB et al (2000) Irinotecan plus fluorouracil and leucovorin for metastatic colorectal cancer. Irinotecan Study Group. N Engl J Med 343:905–914

Saltz LB et al (2004) Phase II trial of cetuximab in patients with refractory colorectal cancer that expresses the epidermal growth factor receptor. J Clin Onc 22:1201–1208

Saltz LB et al (2007) Irinotecan fluorouracil plus leucovorin is not superior to fluorouracil plus leucovorin alone as adjuvant treatment for stage III colon cancer: results of CALGB 89803. J Clin Onc 25:3456–3461

Saltz LB et al (2008) Bevacizumab in combination with oxaliplatin-based chemotherapy as first-line therapy in metastatic colorectal cancer: a randomized phase III study. J Clin Onc 26:2013–2019

Scheele J, Altendorf-Hofmann A (1999) Resection of colorectal liver metastases. Langenbeck's Arch Surg 384:313–327

Schlag P, Hohenberger P, Herfarth C (1990) Resection of liver metastases in colorectal cancer-competitive analysis of treatment results in synchronous versus metachronous metastases. Eur J Surg Oncol 16:360–365

Schmoll H-J et al (2007) Phase III trial of capecitabine plus oxaliplatin as adjuvant therapy for stage III colon cancer: a planned safety analysis in 1,864 patients. J Clin Onc 25:102–109

Seifert JK, Junginger T, Morris DL (1998) A collective review of the world literature on hepatic cryotherapy. J R Coll Surg Edinb 43:141–154

Senéterre E et al (1996) Detection of hepatic metastases: ferumoxides-enhanced MR imaging versus unenhanced MR imaging and CT during arterial portography. Radiology 200:785–792

Smyrniotis V, Kostopanagiotou G, Theodoraki K, Tsantoulas D, Contis JC (2004) The role of central venous pressure and type of vascular control in blood loss during major liver resections. Am J Surg 187:398–402

Snoeren N et al (2010) A randomized two arm phase III study in patients post radical resection of liver metastases of colorectal cancer to investigate bevacizumab in combination with capecitabine plus oxaliplatin (CAPOX) vs CAPOX alone as adjuvant treatment. BMC Cancer 10:545

Solbiati L et al (2001) Percutaneous radio-frequency ablation of hepatic metastases from colorectal cancer: long-term results in 117 patients. Radiology 221:159–166

Stubbs RS, Wickremesekera SK (2004) Selective internal radiation therapy (SIRT): a new modality for treating patients with colorectal liver metastases. HPB (Oxford) 6:133–139

Subar DA, Sheen AJ, Sherlock DJ (2003) Cryoablation for liver tumors—is there clinical utility? MedGenMed 5:19

Tabernero J et al (2007) Phase II trial of cetuximab in combination with fluorouracil, leucovorin, and oxaliplatin in the first-line treatment of metastatic colorectal cancer. J Clin Onc 25:5225–5232

Taïeb J et al (2005) Intensive systemic chemotherapy combined with surgery for metastatic colorectal cancer: results of a phase II study. J Clin Onc 23:502–509

Tamandl D et al (2010) Liver resection remains a safe procedure after neoadjuvant chemotherapy including bevacizumab: a case-controlled study. Ann Surg 252:124–130

Tanaka K et al (2003) Role of neoadjuvant chemotherapy in the treatment of multiple colorectal metastases to the liver. Br J Surg 90:963–969

Taylor I, Mullee MA, Campbell MJ (1990) Prognostic index for the development of liver metastases in patients with colorectal cancer. Br J Surg 77:499–501

Timmerman RD et al (2009) Local surgical, ablative, and radiation treatment of metastases. CA Cancer J Clin 59:145–170

Tournigand C et al (2004) FOLFIRI followed by FOLFOX6 or the reverse sequence in advanced colorectal cancer: a randomized GERCOR study. J Clin Oncol 22:229–237

Townsend A, Price T, Karapetis C (2009) Selective internal radiation therapy for liver metastases from colorectal cancer. Cochrane Database Syst Rev 4:CD007045

Van Cutsem E et al (2006) Towards a pan-European consensus on the treatment of patients with colorectal liver metastases. Eur J Cancer 42:2212–2221

Van Cutsem E et al (2009) Randomized phase III trial comparing biweekly infusional fluorouracil/leucovorin alone or with irinotecan in the adjuvant treatment of stage III colon cancer: PETACC-3. J Clin Onc 27:3117–3125

Vauthey JN et al (2006) Chemotherapy regimen predicts steatohepatitis and an increase in 90-day mortality after surgery for hepatic colorectal metastases. J Clin Oncol 24:2065–2072

Venook A, Niedzwiecki D, Hollis D, Sutherland S, Goldberg R, Alberts S, Benson A, Wade J, Schilsky R, Mayer R (2006) Phase III study of irinotecan/5FU/LV (FOLFIRI) or oxaliplatin/5FU/LV (FOLFOX)±cetuximab for patients (pts) with untreated metastatic adenocarcinoma of the colon or rectum (MCRC): CALGB 80203 preliminary results. J Clin Onc 24(Suppl):3509 (Meeting Abstracts no. 18)

Welsh FK, Tekkis PP, John TG, Rees M (2008) Predictive models in colorectal liver metastases—can we personalize treatment and outcome? Dig Surg 25:406–412

Whittaker DK (1984) Mechanisms of tissue destruction following cryosurgery. Ann R Coll Surg Engl 66:313–318

Wicherts DA, de Haas RJ, Adam R (2007) Bringing unresectable liver disease to resection with curative intent. Eur J Surg Oncol 33(Suppl 2):42–51

Wood TF et al (2000) Radiofrequency ablation of 231 unresectable hepatic tumors: indications, limitations, and complications. Ann Surg Oncol 7:593–600

Ychou M et al (2009) A phase III randomised trial of LV5FU2 + irinotecan versus LV5FU2 alone in adjuvant high-risk colon cancer (FNCLCC Accord02/FFCD9802). Ann Onc 20:674–680

Yoon SS, Tanabe KK (1999) Surgical treatment and other regional treatments for colorectal cancer liver metastases. Oncologist 4:197–208

Zacherl J et al (2002) Current value of intraoperative sonography during surgery for hepatic neoplasms. World J Surg 26:550–554

Part VII
Targeted Therapy for Metastatic Disease

Editor:
Dana Faingold

Chapter 27
Prerequisite Genetic Traits for Metastasis

Dana Faingold, Dawn Russell-Hermanns and Silvin Bakalian

The genetic and epigenetic abnormalities in tumors influence the metastatic traits of disseminated cells by activation of oncogenes and inactivation of tumor-suppressor genes. Tumor-suppressor genes affect genome stability, cancer-cell survival and growth while also being involved in the response and repair of DNA. They are a part of the prerequisites for metastasis and determine initiation and continuous development of the oncogenic process resulting in unrestricted proliferation and resistance to cell death signals. Inactivation of tumor suppressor genes can occur through various mechanisms such as loss of heterozygosity and chromosomal damage as well as by genetic mutations and epigenetic mechanisms such as promoter hypermethylation (Nguyen and Massague 2007; Eccles 2005). The amplification and mutation of oncogenes in primary tumors, together with the selective pressures of the tumor microenvironment play a key role in the formation of metastasis (Bernards and Weinberg 2002).

27.1 Tumor Suppressor Genes

27.1.1 Retinoblastoma Pathway

The p16Ink4a–CyclinD1-CDK4-RB pathway regulates the cell cycle at the G1/S transition. Absent or mutated components of the RB pathway lead to the subsequent loss of the G1/S checkpoint in multiple cancers, thus promoting aberrant

D. Faingold (✉) · S. Bakalian
Department of Pathology, Henry C. Witelson Ocular Pathology Laboratory,
McGill University, Montreal, QC, Canada
e-mail: faingolddana@yahoo.com

D. Russell-Hermanns
Henry C. Witelson Ocular Pathology Laboratory, McGill University, Montreal, QC, Canada

S. Bakalian
e-mail: sbakalian@hotmail.com

J. V. Burnier, M. N. Burnier, Jr. (eds.), *Experimental and Clinical Metastasis*,
DOI 10.1007/978-1-4614-3685-0_27,

proliferation (Sherr and McCormick 2002). The unphosphorylated state of RB is maintained by p16INK4a which competes with the activity of cyclin D- dependent kinases (CDK), thus blocking the entry into S phase and the E2F (E2 transcription factor) transcriptional program (Knudsen and Wang 2010). Mutations in this pathway occur frequently in many cancers and the RB protein is functionally inhibited in 25 % of primary tumors. Once RB is hyperphosphorylated by the CyclinD1/CDK4 complex, it results in E2F-regulated gene expression, stimulating G1 to S transition. Persistent mitogenic stimulation could lead to overexpression of either CDK4 or Cyclin D1 resulting in inhibition of the RB pathway function by blocking the growth-suppressing activity of p16INK4a (Ortega et al. 2002). Transcription of the *cyclin D1* gene, its synthesis and assembly with CDK4, is regulated by ras (reticular activating system) and phosphatidylinositol 3-kinase (PI3-K) signaling (Kim and Diehl 2009).

Therapeutic Options Several therapeutic strategies are employed against defects in the RB-pathway and encouraging results are emerging in preclinical studies inducing the expression of p16Ink4a by means of adenoviral vectors containing human p16 cDNA (Craig et al. 1998). Additionally, positive results for reactivation of the RB-pathway are reported in studies using inhibitors of DNA methylation or histone deacetylases, which lead to the activation of epigenetically silenced p16Ink4a. The authors reported that DNA methyltransferase inhibitor 5-aza-2′-deoxycytidine (5–7aza-CdR) and the histone deacetylase inhibitor 4-phenylbutyric acid (PBA) caused cell cycle arrest, apoptosis and induced p16 (CDKN2A/INK4) and p21 (CIP1/SDI1/WAF1) in bladder carcinoma cells (Egger et al. 2007). Together, these studies suggest that RB-pathway activation could be used therapeutically.

Inhibition of Cdk4/6 kinase activity is another therapeutic option which was evaluated with second-generation CDK4/6 inhibitors in pre-clinical studies. Oral administration of these compounds induced tumour regression in xenograft animal models of human colon carcinoma causing elimination of phospho-RB. This therapeutic strategy of activating RB is currently under investigation in phase I-II trials (Knudsen and Wang 2010; Fry et al. 2004).

Flavopiridol is a semisynthetic flavone CDK inhibitor that interferes with CDK9-cyclin complex binding resulting in apoptosis. Phase I studies have revealed favorable responses in metastatic breast cancer carcinoma in combination with doxetacel (Freyer et al. 2003). Flavopiridol was also shown to have a synergistic effect with Herceptin, a drug active against Her2/neu (human epidermal growth factor receptor 2) in breast cancer cell lines (Nahta et al. 2002).

The cross talk between p53 status and levels of E2F activity influences the overall response to therapy. Therapeutic approaches that target p53 include stimulation of E2F-activity and restoration of the pro-apoptotic activity of p53 (Polager and Ginsberg 2009). It has been previously shown that RB-deficient tumor lines or those exhibiting deregulated E2F activity can be good targets for compounds that have the capacity to activate p53 (Kitagawa et al. 2008). Gene therapy using virus-activated E2F-regulated gene expression (pESM6), was shown to induce tumor reduction in preclinical studies. These studies affirm the potential of pESM6 as a viable agent for gene therapy of DNA tumor virus-associated cancers (Lim et al. 2006). Also, gene transfer of a truncated variant of the retinoblastoma gene, (RB94), has been proven to inhibit proliferation of several human tumor cell types including pancreatic cancer (Roig et al. 2004).

Key Points Therapeutic strategies for reactivation of the retinoblastoma pathway

- Retinoblastoma gene transfer therapy
- Induction of the expression and activation of epigenetically silenced p16Ink4a
- Inhibition of Cdk4/6 kinase activity
- Stimulation of E2F-dependent apoptosis

27.1.2 The p53 Tumor Suppressor Gene

The p53 tumor suppressor gene maintains genomic integrity. Its transcription factor is induced in response to DNA damage, hypoxia, and oncogene activation. P53 regulates a number of downstream genes including p21, MDM2 (Mouse Double Minute 2), GADD45 (Growth Arrest and DNA Damage), BAX (Bcl2- associated X protein), as well as cell cycle (G1/S) and G2/M DNA check-points. This allows for cellular repair mechanisms or initiation of apoptosis through both extrinsic and intrinsic pathways (Sherr and McCormick 2002). The p53 tumor suppressor gene is the most frequently mutated gene in human tumors resulting in loss of its biological responses and inhibition of apoptotic mechanisms.

Therapeutic options Several strategies for restoration of wild-type p53 function and induction of apoptosis in tumors have been explored. These have included p53 gene–replacement therapy in which the E1 adenoviral region is replaced with the cDNA of the p53 gene, driven by a cytomegalovirus promoter (Ad-p53, ADVEXIN [Introgen Therapeutics, Inc.]) (Invitrogen 2007). Preclinical studies have shown encouraging results for this treatment modality with regard to antitumor activity and feasibility of gene therapy (Bianco et al. 2007). Evidence of clinical activity was also observed in clinical trials, where re-expression of wild type p53 by viral-mediated gene transfer induced tumor regression and stabilization in patients with NSCLC (non-small-cell lung cancer) and squamous cell carcinoma of the head and neck (HNCC) (Vecil and Lang 2003; Wiman 2007; Roth 1996; Nemunaitis et al. 2000; Clayman et al. 1999). However, no significant benefit was observed in patients with primary stage III ovarian cancer when treated with intraperitoneal delivery of a replication-deficient adenoviral vector expressing wild-type p53 (Zeimet and Marth 2003).

A different strategy employs a genetically modified adenovirus, (Onyx-015) which eliminates p53 by producing the early region protein E1B 55K. This protein binds p53 and targets it for destruction by inducing apoptosis in the cells expressing mutant p53. Evidence of clinical activity was reported after intra-tumor injection in clinical trials in combination with chemotherapeutic agents in head and neck cancer as well as in pancreatic adenocarcinoma (Khuri et al. 2000; Hecht et al. 2003). Adenoviral vascular delivery for systemic metastases is also currently under investigation. Positive results have also emerged from additional therapeutic modalities involving small molecule therapy that functions through reactivation of mutant p53. In preclinical studies, p53 C-terminus derived semisynthetic peptides were shown to induce p53-dependent apoptosis in tumor cells (Haupt and Haupt 2004). Other methods exploit the p53- MDM2-mediated inhibition with drugs that interrupt the p53–MDM 2 interaction. For example, a synthetic class of cis-imidazoline analogs (Nutlins) interferes with the p53-MDM2 complex inhibiting tumor cell cycle and triggering apoptosis (Vassilev et al. 2004). Anti-sense mRNA therapy directed towards *MDM2* was shown to induce down regulation of the MDM2 and p53-mediated anti proliferative effects in human cancers cells, *in vitro* and *in vivo* (Wang et al. 2003). Other strategies include Hsp90 (heat shock protein-90) inhibitors where drug exposure was shown to induce destabilization of the mutant p53 protein in breast and prostate tumor cell lines (Blagosklonny et al. 1995).

Key Points Therapeutic strategies involving tumor suppressor p53

- Adenovirus-mediated p53 gene therapy
- Introduction of wild-type *p53* gene into tumor cells using viral vectors
- Interference with p53–MDM2 and down-regulation of MDM2 expression
- Targeting mutant p53 (Hsp90 inhibitors)
- Adenovirus-mediated inactivation of mutant p53
- Restoration of inactive or suppressed wild type p53
- Reactivation of mutant p53 with small molecule therapy

27.1.3 BRCA1 and BRCA2 Tumor Suppressor Genes

The tumor suppressor genes *BRCA1* (Breast Cancer 1) and *BRCA2* (Breast Cancer 2) are involved in DNA repair and have been identified in breast cancer and ovarian cancer. In 80 % of the cases mutations in the *BRCA1 and BRCA2* genes involve abnormal truncation of the BRCA protein (Sobol et al. 1996; Welcsh and King 2001). Individuals with mutations in these genes have a 15–20 fold increase in risk of breast cancer compared with the general population (Wooster et al. 1995). *BRCA2* mutation carriers are at an increased risk of developing breast cancer (in both males and females), as well as melanoma, ovarian, prostatic, pancreatic, and carcinoma of the gall bladder. *BRCA1* gene replacement therapies have shown anti-tumor responses in preclinical studies. Additionally, responses were seen in Phase I trials of patients with extensive metastatic breast cancer when treated with retroviral *LXSN-BRCA1sv* gene therapy. However, a phase II trial in ovarian patients showed no response, and no vector stability in response to *BRCA1*gene therapy (Tait et al. 1999)

27.1.4 PTEN Tumor Suppressor Gene

PTEN (phosphatase and tensin homolog) functions as a tumor suppressor through its lipid phosphatase activity negatively influencing Akt through the dephosphorylation of phosphatidylinositol-3,4,5-trisphosphate (PIP3). Loss of PTEN is a common event in cancer and occurs through mutation, deletion, or epigenetic silencing inducing PI3K/Akt pathway hyperactivation. PTEN is mutated or deleted in about 30–40 % of tumors including brain, bladder, breast, prostate, and endometrial cancers. It correlates with poor prognosis and metastatic disease. Gene therapy with wild-type PTEN has been attempted in preclinical studies, however, clinical-translational therapeutic strategies focus in targeting PI3K-Akt-mTOR pathway in tumors with PTEN functional loss (Zhang and Yu 2010).

27.1.5 Other Tumor Suppressor Genes

The *FHIT* (fragile histidine triad) gene located on 3p14.2 is homozygously deleted and targeted by genomic alterations leading to a decrease or loss of gene and protein expression in many cancers (Joannes et al. 2009). Lack of FHIT expression correlates with tumor progression to metastasis as *FHIT* controls the invasive phenotype of lung tumor cells by regulating the expression of genes associated with epithelial–mesenchymal transition (Joannes et al. 2009). FHIT gene, re-expression by a recombinant adenoviral vector, resulted in apoptosis and reduced tumorigenicity in lung cancer (Ji et al. 1999). Additionally, gene therapy involving administration of the *FUS1* (cell fusion 1) tumor suppressor gene might have applicability in lung cancer (Ji and Roth 2008). Intravenous administration of nanoparticle encapsulated FUS1 expression plasmid had antitumor effects in human lung cancer xenograft models (Deng et al. 2008).This treatment was well tolerated in a Phase I clinical trial of FUS1-nanoparticles in patients with chemotherapy refractory stage IV lung cancer (Ji and Roth 2008; Lu et al. 2009).

27.1.6 Metastatic Suppressor Genes

Metastatic suppressor genes are differentially expressed between metastatic and non-metastatic cells and interfere with several signaling pathways involved in metastatic colonization. Examples include nm23 (non-metastatic gene 23) modulation of the ERK (extracellular signal-regulated kinase) pathway, BRMS1 (Breast cancer metastasis suppressor 1) alteration of phosphoinositide signaling, and MKK4 (mitogen-activated protein kinase kinase 4) activation of JNK (c-Jun NH(2)-terminal protein kinase) and p38 stress pathways (Rinker-Schaeffer et al. 2006). Silence inactivation or loss of heterozygozity of metastatic suppressor genes and low expression in tumors were associated with a higher risk of metastatic disease (Martins et al. 2008;

Bakalian et al. 2007). Therefore, re-expression of metastatic suppressor genes may have therapeutic effects on micrometastatic tumor cells (Steeg 2004). Several compounds that can elevate nm23 have been identified including indomethacin, gamma Linolenic Acid, trichostatin A, 5-aza-deoxycytidine, and medroxyprogesterone acetate. Results from in vivo models of lung metastasis demonstrated a reduction of the metastatic potential with administration of high doses of medroxyprogesterone acetate (Marshall et al. 2009). This therapeutic strategy is currently evaluated in a phase II clinical study investigating the effect of nm23 re-expression in breast cancer cells and subsequent metastatic colonization (Steeg et al. 2008).

27.2 Prerequisites for Metastasis: Oncogenes

Genetic instability in primary tumors increases the chance of further oncogenic mutational events and results in the induction of unrestricted proliferative capabilities and resistance to apoptotic signals. The amplification and mutation of oncogenes in primary tumors, together with the selective pressures of the tumor microenvironment play a key role in the formation of metastasis. This suggests that metastatic potential might be pre-programmed in tumors, whereas a selective population of cells might require additional alterations in tumor suppressor genes and oncogenes to initiate the metastatic cascade (Bernards and Weinberg 2002).

27.2.1 Myc

Oncogene amplifications affect distinct genetic programs leading to cell cycle progression, invasiveness and metastasis, for example downstream EGFR (epithelial growth factor receptor), C-ERbB2, Myc (myelocytomatosis viral oncogene) and ras signaling (Nguyen and Massague 2007). The *Myc* proto-oncogene family encodes nuclear products which are deregulated as a result of point mutations, gene amplification and translocation. *Myc* family genes are activated in a wide variety of human hematological malignancies and solid tumors as a consequence of activation of one or more signalling pathways. These include RAS-RAF-MAPK, PI3K, WNT- β catenin pathways and STAT (signal transducer and activator of transcription) pathways (Pelengaris et al. 2002). *Myc* is a key regulator for many biological activities including cell-cycle progression, apoptosis, tumor growth, angiogenesis, cell adhesion and motility. It is associated with poor prognosis and metastasis (Nesbit et al. 1999).

Strategies currently employed for targeting *Myc* include antisense oligonucleotides resulting in tumor cell growth arrest and induction of apoptosis in a variety of tumor cell lines. Experiments in xenograft models of breast carcinoma, melanoma and neuroblastoma resulted in prevention of tumor formation (Vita and Henriksson 2006).

Phosphorodiamidate morpholino oligomers (PMOs) are DNA antisense oligonucleotides that inhibit *Myc* gene expression by preventing its mRNA translation. This agents inhibited tumor growth and induced apoptosis in prostate cancer xenografts. Further clinical studies evaluated them in adenocarcinoma of prostate and breast tumor tissues (Devi et al. 2005) and assessed its safety in human trials (Iversen et al. 2003).

Other agents which interfere with *Myc* promoter and transcription are DNA analogs. These compounds specifically hybridize to DNA and/or RNA in a complementary manner thus inhibiting transcription and translation of the *Myc* target gene (Pession et al. 2004).

Cationic porphyrin (TMPyP4), which inhibits *Myc* transcription by blocking G quadruplexes, inhibited the *in vitro* transcription of *Myc* and decreased tumor growth rates in xenograft models (Grand et al. 2002)

The regulatory effect on gene transcription of *Myc* is dependent on dimerization and complex formation with a b-HLH-LZ protein Max. Targeting Myc–Max complex with small molecules is another therapeutic option (Berg et al. 2002). Small interfering RNA (siRNA) against *Myc* resulted in apoptotic effects and tumor growth reduction in xenograft models (Shen et al. 2005). Therefore targeting expression or function of Myc shows interesting promise and development of agents with improved delivery and efficacy is further anticipated in clinical settings (Ponzielli et al. 2005).

27.2.2 HER-2

The human epidermal growth factor receptor (HER, ERB) family consists of EGFR (HER1 or ERBB1), HER2 (EGFR2 or ERBB2/NEU), HER3 (EGFR3 or ERBB3), and HER4 (EGFR4 or ERBB4) (Rowinsky 2004). The *HER-2* (human epithelial receptor 2, also known as *HER-2/neu* or *ER*B-2) gene is located on chromosome 17q and encodes a 185-kDa trans-membrane receptor tyrosine kinase with a key role in normal cell growth and differentiation. The amplification and over-expression of the *HER-2* gene results in malignant transformation of cells and affects up to 30 % of patients with metastatic breast cancer correlating with increased metastatic potential in ovarian, breast cancer and in NSCLC (Yarden and Sliwkowski 2001; Slamon et al. 1989).

Trastuzumab (Herceptin®; Genentech, Inc.; South San Francisco, CA), is the first approved humanized monoclonal antibody designed to block the receptor extracellular domain of human epidermal growth factor receptor-2 (HER2) that is over expressed in metastatic breast cancer and affects intracellular signaling and tumor cell growth. Trastuzumab therapy alone or in combination with taxanes chemotherapy provided the proof of principle that targeting HER-2 receptors results in cytotoxic and cytostatic effects. This combination demonstrated clinical benefit in terms of response rate and survival for patients with HER-2-positive disease and represents the first-line therapy for these patients (Cobleigh et al. 1999; Slamon et al. 2001; Vogel et al. 2002). Other combinations of trastuzumab with chemotherapy are also

Table 27.1 Monoclonal antibody therapies targeting EGFR (ERB-1 and ERB-2)

Trastuzumab (Herceptin, Genentech Inc)	Breast cancer
Cetuximab (Erbitux, ImClone Systems)	Colorectal, NSCLC, pancreatic, breast cancer and HNSCC
Panitumumab (Vectibix, Amgen)	Colorectal cancer
ABX-EGF (Amgen)	NSCLC, colorectal, prostate, renal, HNSCC
Matuzumab (EMD 72000, Pharma)	NSCLC, colorectal, ovarian cancer, HNSCC, pancreas
Pertuzumab (Omnitarg;)	Prostate, ovarian, breast and NSCLC
Nimotuzumab (hR3)	Squamous cell carcinoma of head and neck

currently under investigation. Clinical data indicate that the therapy with trastuzumab may induce a decrease in ejection fraction, cardiac dysfunction in about 1–4 % of patients treated with trastuzumab and this side effect may be augmented in combination with chemotherapy (Perez and Rodeheffer 2004).

Clinical trials evaluating the response to trastuzumab and other cytotoxic agents such as vinorelbine (Burstein et al. 2003), gemcitabine (Loesch et al. 2008), and capecitabine (Tevaarwerk and Kolesar 2009) have shown positive response rates and increased overall survival times in patients with metastatic breast cancer. Tanespimycin a new 17-AAG analog has demonstrated promising antitumor activity and tolerability in a Phase II clinical trial in patients with HER 2-neu positive metastatic breast cancer. These results were reported for a combination of 17-AAG with trastuzumab in patients previously nonresponsive to Herceptin alone (Modi et al. 2007).

Other humanized anti-EGFR (ERB-1 and ERB-2) monoclonal antibodies cetuximab and panitumumab bind to the extracellular domain of EGFR, thus leading to inhibition of its downstream signaling. These agents are currently being investigated in phase II and III clinical trials in NSCLC (Jatoi et al. 2010). Cetuximab and panitumumab have shown evidence of activity in combination with cytotoxic chemotherapy and radiotherapy in the treatment of metastatic colorectal cancer or as monotherapy for the treatment of metastatic head and neck squamous cell carcinoma (HNSCC). It is indicated for the treatment of KRAS wild-type metastatic colorectal cancer in combination with chemotherapy or as a single agent in patients refractory to chemotherapy (Cutsem et al. 2009; Bokemeyer et al. 2009). The presence of activating K-ras mutations has been identified as a potent predictor of resistance to cetuximab or panitumumab therapy (Tol and Punt 2010; Keating 2010). Cetuximab monotherapy is currently the only approved molecular target therapy in patients with recurrent or metastatic HNSCC, and has been shown as a radiation-sensitizing agent in primary radiation therapy of this disease (Jackisch 2006; Cripps et al. 2010). Other monoclonal antibodies targeting HER-2 include humanized antibodies matuzumab (EMD72000), nimotuzumab (hR3), and pertuzumab (Genentech),which are currently in preclinical or phase I and II clinical studies in low HER-2-expressing breast cancers, NSCLC, colorectal, ovarian cancer, pancreas, prostate and ovarian cancer (Bianco et al. 2007). Examples of monoclonal antibody agents are shown in Table 27.1.

The HER, ERB family of trans-membrane receptors forms dimers upon ligand binding, resulting in activation of the intracellular tyrosine kinase domain, and

Table 27.2 EGFR tyrosine kinase inhibitors that are currently under investigation for various malignancies

Inhibitor	Specificity	Selected tumor types
Gefitinib (Iressa®; AstraZeneca)	ErbB-1 tyrosine kinase inhibitor	Metastatic NSCLC, head and neck squamous cell carcinoma, breast, ovarian, prostate, glioma, pancreatic, colorectal cancer
Erlotinib (Tarceva™; Genentech)	ErbB-1 tyrosine kinase inhibitor	NSCLC, metastatic pancreatic cancer, HNSCC, breast, ovarian, prostate, colorectal, glioma
Lapatinib (GlaxoSmithKline)	Dual effect ErbB-1 and ErbB-2	Colorectal cancer and HNSCC

triggering of the downstream effector pathways involved in cellular proliferation, angiogenesis, and metastasis. Mutations in the EGFR tyrosine kinase receptor family of receptors have been associated with poor prognosis in breast cancer, ovarian and NSCLC (Paez et al. 2004; Lassus et al. 2006; Generali et al. 2007). Tyrosine kinase inhibitors bind to the intracellular ATP-binding site on the receptor and inhibit cell proliferation by blocking intracellular signals that stimulate gene expression. The mechanisms of action include inhibition of cancer cell proliferation via G_0/G_1 cell cycle arrest, anti-angiogenic effects and inhibition of invasion and metastasis (Olayioye et al. 2000). These agents are reported to be able to cross into the CNS and have excellent oral bioavailability (Roy and Perez 2009; Gril et al. 2008).

Novel treatment regimens under investigation for patients with advanced breast cancer and NSCLC include HER tyrosine kinase inhibitors, gefitinib (Iressa®; AstraZeneca Pharmaceuticals) and erlotinib, (Tarceva™; Genentech) which are specific for EGFR and lapatinib (Tykerb, GlaxoSmithKline) a dual EGFR and HER-2 inhibitor (Table 27.2). In a phase III clinical trial that led to FDA approval for erlotinib, 731 patients with NSCLC previously treated with one or two chemotherapy regimens were randomized to receive erlotinib or placebo. Erlotinib treatment was shown to be superior to placebo in survival, quality of life, and related symptoms in advanced and metastatic NSCLC patients (Shepherd et al. 2005). However, the combination of erlotinb with first-line chemotherapy such as carboplatin and paclitaxel has failed to show additional benefit when compared with chemotherapy alone (Herbst et al. 2005; Gridelli et al. 2007). Also, the results of a phase III clinical study with combination therapy between erlotinib and gemcitabine in pancreatic cancer patients showed a modest improvement in the median overall survival (Moore et al. 2007).

Small molecule therapy with lapatinib, a dual oral inhibitor for EGFR and HER2 showed antitumor activity in preclinical studies (Rusnak et al. 2007). Lapatinib combined with capecitabine (Xeloda; Roche) demonstrated significant improvements in the time to progression and response rate when compared with capecitabine alone in breast cancer patients and this combination is currently approved for treatment of HER-2-overexpressing chemorefractory breast cancer patients (Tevaarwerk and Kolesar 2009; Jackisch 2006; Higa and Abraham 2007). Lapatinib was proven to have manageable side effects including diarrhea and skin rash.

A phase III, randomized, open-label study comparing the efficacy of gefitinib for first line therapy with carboplatin–paclitaxel demonstrated an increase in objective response rates, significantly longer progression-free survival times and improved quality of life among EGFR mutation–positive patients who received gefitinib alone (Jiang 2009). Positive results are also emerging from other phase III clinical trials that investigated the clinical efficacy of gefitinib as monotherapy and in combination with chemotherapy for the treatment of NSCLC. These trials have revealed the comparable efficacy of gefitinib compared with docetaxel, (Douillard et al. 2010; Kim et al. 2008).

HER-2 inhibitors have been proven in clinical trials as beneficial therapeutic strategies for metastatic disease. Insights into future development of drugs that target this biochemical pathway will determine optimal sequence of administration as well as markers for the group of patients most likely to respond.

27.3 Growth Factor Receptors and Their Effector Pathways

Identification of oncogenic kinases has paved the way for further development of anticancer agents. Specifically, inhibitors of receptor tyrosine kinases (RTKs), such as BCR-ABL, c-KIT, PDGFR, EGFR, IGF1R, Met and Src, may have a role in the treatment of cancer.

27.3.1 KIT

KIT (c-KIT receptor) gene encodes a trans-membrane receptor tyrosine kinase which activates downstream signaling pathways involved in cellular proliferation and survival. Mutation and activation of *KIT* oncogene have been described in a variety of malignancies, such as gastrointestinal stromal tumors (GIST), acute myelogenous leukemia (AML) and result in aberrant signaling, increased proliferation and antiapoptotic effects. Imatinib (imatinib mesylate, Gleevec) targets the c-KIT tyrosine kinase, the Bcr–Abl tyrosine kinase and PDGFR (platelet-derived growth factor receptor) (Druker 2008). Clinical studies in patients with advanced GIST, where mutations in *KIT* have been reported in 75–80 % of tumors, demonstrated the efficacy and safety of imatinib mesylate treatment, leading to its approval for targeted therapy (Demetri et al. 2002). However, phase II clinical studies of imatinib mesylate in patients with metastatic melanoma and an activating *KIT* mutation, showed insufficient therapeutic effect. (Wyman et al. 2006). Also, although the drug was generally well tolerated, it had minimal activity in recurrent or persistent uterine carcinoma (Huh et al. 2010), recurrent ovarian cancer (Alberts et al. 2007) or primary peritoneal carcinoma (Schilder et al. 2008).

Other small molecule tyrosine kinase inhibitors that affect c-KIT are in various stages of clinical development. Examples include sorafenib, and sunitinib which have potent KIT inhibitory effect while also inhibiting other tyrosine kinases involved in oncogenic growth and progression, such as vascular endothelial growth factor receptors (VEGFR 1, 2, and 3), and PDGFR. Sunitinib was FDA approved for second-line therapy in GIST and RCC (renal cell carcinoma) (Faivre et al. 2007) whereas Sorafenib demonstrated potent effects in RCC and hepatocellular carcinoma (HCC) (Hahn and Stadler 2006).

Recently, a small-molecule multikinase inhibitor Dasatinib, (BMS 354825), an orally available therapeutic agent was shown to inhibit Bcr-Abl and Src-family kinases, but also c-KITand PDGFR. This drug demonstrated potent effects and was approved for the treatment of patients with Bcr-Abl-positive chronic myeloid leukemia (CML) as well as acute lymphoblastic leukemia (ALL) resistant or intolerant to imatinib. Given its activity against c-KIT, PDGFR and Src kinases, this drug was evaluated and demonstrated favorable effects on several human solid tumor lines (González et al. 2006; Buettner et al. 2008; Coluccia et al. 2006). It is currently being investigated in clinical trials in patients with metastatic breast cancer to the bone (Rose and Siegel 2010) and in patients with metastatic prostate cancer (Yu et al. 2009).

27.3.2 Insulin-Like Growth Factor

The insulin-like growth factor (IGF) signaling axis is a prerequisite for oncogenic transformation and mediates tumor growth in a variety of human malignancies through its effects on proliferation and anti-apoptosis. The biological actions of the insulin-like growth factors, IGFI and IGFII, are mediated by activation of the IGFI receptor (IGFIR), a tyrosine kinase trans-membrane linked to the RAS-RAF-MAPK and PI3K-PKB/AKT signal transduction cascades. The IGF1R is over-expressed by tumors such as melanomas, colon cancer, pancreatic, prostate and renal cancer (Chitnis et al. 2008). This occurs as a result of loss-of-function and mutation of tumor suppressors such as wild-type p53, BRCA1 and VHL (von Hippel Lindau) resulting in transcriptional deregulation of the *IGFIR* gene (Werner and Roberts 2003). Stimulation of IGF1R-pathway results in activation of the RAS/RAF/MAPK pathway and induces differentiation and survival signals leading to tumor proliferation (Riedemann and Macaulay 2006). Anti-apoptotic effects are mediated through interaction of the IGF-1R with one of its major substrates, insulin receptor substrate 1 (IRS-1) which activates the PI3K-AKT pathway (Kulik et al. 1997).

IGF1R activation is linked to cancer progression and metastasis through multiple signaling intermediates. IGF1R-mediated signaling enhances ß-catenin transcriptional activity and interferes with E-cadherin expression, actin polymerization and focal adhesion complex formation, thus inducing loss of cellular adhesion (Morali et al. 2001; Playford et al. 2000). Another possible way in which IGF1 pathway induces the metastatic phenotype is interaction with integrin-mediated signaling pathways. These include $\alpha_v\beta_3$ (Shen et al. 2006) and IGF-induced secretion of matrix metalloproteinases (MMPs) as well as regulation of the urokinase plasminogen activator/plasmin (uPA) system of proteolysis resulting in degradation of the extracellular matrix (ECM) (Bahr and Groner 2005). These mechanisms were confirmed by several models which demonstrated that IGF1R over-expression confers anchorage-independent growth and promotes an invasive, metastatic phenotype (All-Ericsson et al. 2002; Economou et al. 2008; Lopez and Hanahan 2002; Chernicky et al. 2000).

Table 27.3 Examples of IGF1R tyrosine kinase inhibitors that are currently under investigation

Small molecule inhibitor	Specificity	Selected tumor types
OSI-906 (OSI Pharmaceuticals)	IGF1R	Phase I advanced solid tumors
	IR	Phase III Adrenocortical, Phase I ovarian
Insm-18 (NDGA) Insmed	IGF1R	Phase I advanced solid tumors
	HER2-Neu	
NVP-AEW54 1(Novartis)	IGF1R	Preclinical
NVP-ADW742	IGF1R	Preclinical
BMS-536924 (Bristol-Myers-Squibb)	IGF1R	Phase I
	IR	
AG1024 (Calbiochem-EMD Biosciences)	IGF1R	Preclinical
	IR	
Picropodophyllin PPP (Karolinska Institute/Biovitrum)		Uveal melanoma
PQIP (OSI Pharmaceuticals)	IGF1R	
XL 228	IGF1R	Phase I study of patients with solid malignancies
	SRC	

Altering IGF1R function might inhibit tumor cell growth and also has effects on anchorage-independent growth, survival, migration, invasion and colonization of tumor cells. Different strategies in blocking the IGF-1R signaling pathway include small molecule inhibitors, blocking antibodies, antisense oligonucleotides and plasmids, antisense and siRNA. In preclinical models as well as in early phase clinical trials down-regulation of IGF-1R revealed favorable results (Chitnis et al. 2008; Bahr and Groner 2005; Li et al. 2009).

A. IGF1R tyrosine kinase inhibitors The development of tyrosine kinase inhibitors downstream of the IGFI receptor has led to the development of compounds with a high degree of selectivity for IGF1R (Table 27.3). However, as there is a high degree of sequence homology between the insulin receptor (IR) and IGF1R, this type of inhibition could potentially result in metabolic changes (Pollak et al. 2004). Examples of small molecules that compete for the ATP binding pocket of IGF1R are NVP-ADW742 and NVP-AEW54 1(Novartis). Preclinical data for these compounds reported anti-proliferative activity in cancer cells by interfering with cell cycle progression (Martins et al. 2006) and anti-tumor effects in multiple myeloma xenografts (Mitsiades et al. 2004) and fibrosarcoma xenografts (Garcia-Echeverria et al. 2004).

OSI-906 (OSI pharmaceutical) is a new small molecule, dual kinase inhibitor of both IGF-1R and IR. Data from a phase I clinical trial in patients with advanced solid tumors indicated that OSI-906 was well-tolerated and showed that at a low dosing schedule retained strong anti-tumor activity, with reduced incidence of IR-mediated side effects (Macaulay et al. 2010). This drug is currently evaluated in a Phase III clinical trial in adrenocortical carcinoma and in a Phase I/II clinical trial in ovarian cancer [1].

[1] NIH's ClinicalTrials.gov. Available from (http://www.clinicaltrials.gov/) and ClinicalTrialsFeeds.org (http://www.clinicaltrialsfeeds.org/) web sites.

Insm-18 (NDGA) (Nordihydroguaiaretic Acid) (Insmed), is an orally available small molecule IGF-1 tyrosine kinase inhibitor that has demonstrated anti-tumor activity in preclinical studies of breast, lung, pancreatic and prostate tumors (Chitnis et al. 2008; Hewish et al. 2009). This agent is currently evaluated in phase I clinical studies with non-metastatic recurrent prostate cancer (Harzstark et al. 2007).

Another small-molecule inhibitor, BMS-536924, (Bristol-Myers-Squibb) had an effect on insulin receptor kinase activity and reduced tumor cell proliferation of breast cancer cell lines *in vitro* (Litzenburger et al. 2009) and was also effective in reducing tumor xenograft size in vivo (Haluska et al. 2006)

Tyrphostin (AG1024), a substrate competitive, specific inhibitor of IGF-1R was proven to inhibit tumor cell growth in prostate, breast cancer and melanoma cell lines (Hewish et al. 2009).

Cyclolignans are selective inhibitors of tyrosine phosphorylation of the IGF-1R. Xenograft data has shown efficacy for one of these compounds, picropodophyllin (PPP), in Ewing's sarcoma cells, melanoma cells, and prostate carcinoma cells (Girnita et al. 2004).

PQIP (OSI pharmaceutical) is a 1,3-disubstituted-8-amino-imidazopyrazine derivative inhibitor of IGF-1R kinase. It has recently been reported to be particularly effective in breast cancer (Zeng et al. 2009), pancreatic cancer, and ovarian cell lines as well as in HNSCC and NSCLC. In xenograft models, this agent inhibited IGF-1R dependent tumor growth in colorectal cancer which correlated with the degree and duration of inhibition of IGF-IR phosphorylation (Hewish et al. 2009; Ji et al. 2007).

B. Monoclonal Antibodies IGF1R neutralizing monoclonal antibodies block the receptor–ligand interactions subsequently resulting in receptor internalization and degradation blocking intracellular signaling. The antibody-induced IGF1R down-regulation is selective against the IGF1R without interfering with IR and possibly induces less metabolic toxicity than that seen with the IGF1R small molecule inhibitors (Gualberto and Pollak 2009).

IMC-A12 (cixutumumab), Imclone, has the ability to induce IGF1R down-regulation and has shown promising activity in human tumor xenograft models of breast, lung, colon, and pancreatic cancers (Rowinsky et al. 2007). This agent was well tolerated evidence of stable disease were reported in a phase I clinical trial in patients with advanced solid tumors (Higano et al. 2007; Rothenberg et al. 2007). A similar study combining an IMC-A12 and a mTOR inhibitor (temsirolimus) in patients with solid tumors or lymphoma reported that the combination is well tolerated and demonstrated prolonged stable disease in two patients with metastatic prostate cancer and breast cancer (Naing et al. 2009). IMC-A12 is currently evaluated in patients with prostate cancer, metastatic colorectal cancer, Ewing's sarcoma and in a pediatric population with refractory solid tumors (Atzori et al. 2009).

CP-751871 (figitumumab, Pfizer) a fully human IgG2 monoclonal antibody, that blocks IGFI binding, and prevents activation of IGF1 causing down-regulation of IGF1R *in vitro* and in tumor xenografts of breast cancer, colon cancer, and multiple myeloma (Cohen et al. 2005). Phase I studies have suggested a favorable toxicity profile and signs of disease stabilization in patients with advanced solid tumors (Molife et al. 2010). Clinical trials are ongoing and include prostate, breast, colorectal and melanoma patients. Preliminary data from a Phase II clinical trial in NSCLC evaluating CP-751871 in combination with paclitaxel and carboplatin (Karp et al. 2008) suggested promising results showing a 46 % response after addition of CP-751871 in comparison with a response rate of 32 % for patients treated with chemotherapy alone (Karp et al. 2009). However, results from a phase III study conducted to test the efficacy of the combination of paclitaxel, carboplatin, and CP-751871 reported that the addition of CP-751871 did not increase overall survival and resulted in adverse side effects resulting in discontinuation of this trial (Jassem et al. 2010). Further evaluation of CP-751871 in combination with chemotherapy or erlotinib is currently in progress for patients with advanced NSCLC. Other clinical trials in progress include phase I- II studies of CP-751871 as monotherapy or in conjunction with chemotherapy in patients with metastatic colorectal cancer, Ewing's sarcoma and in breast cancer (Atzori et al. 2009; Rodon et al. 2008).

R1507 (robatumumab, Roche), is a fully human IgG1 type monoclonal antibody also selective against IGFIR. Xenograft data has shown efficacy in osteosarcoma cancer models (Kolb et al. 2010). The results of a phase I study evaluating R1507 administered weekly in patients with advanced solid neoplasms in particular Ewing's sarcoma revealed partial responses and evidence of stable disease (Kurzrock et al. 2010).

AMG 479 (Amgen) is a fully IgG1 human monoclonal antibody selective to IGF1R that exhibited broad antitumor activity in xenograft models (Beltran et al. 2009). Furthermore, AMG 479 administration was proven safe in phase I clinical trials in patients with advanced solid tumors and demonstrated preliminary efficacy with one durable complete response and a partial response in two patients with Ewing-primitive neuroectodermal tumors (Tolcher et al. 2009a). Assessments of a combination of AMG 479 with panitumumab or gemcitabine in patients with advanced solid tumors, reported that the combination was well tolerated with very few side effects. There was a partial response and signs of stable disease were observed (Sarantopoulos et al. 2008; Puzanov et al. 2010). Further trials include evaluation of this agent in a Phase II double blind randomised study in hormone receptor positive metastatic breast, colorectal and lung cancer patients[2]. Results from a phase II clinical trial assessing safety, tolerability and maximum tolerated dose of a combination of AMG 479 with gemcitabine in patients with pancreatic cancer were promising with regard to tolerability. The second stage of this trial randomised the treatment between gemcitabine and AMG 479, versus gemcitabine and placebo, resulting in improved overall survival rate at six months (57 % in AMG 479 arm versus 50 % in gemcitabine plus placebo arm) (Kindler et al. 2010).

Sch717454 (Robatumumab), (19D12, Schering-Plough), a human IgG1 anti-IGFIR antibody demonstrated antitumor activity in solid tumor xenografts, including Ewing sarcoma, rhabdomyosarcoma, glioblastoma, neuroblastoma, and osteosarcoma panels (Kolb et al. 2008; Wang et al. 2010). This drug is currently under

[2] NIH's ClinicalTrials.gov. Available from (http://www.clinicaltrials.gov/) and ClinicalTrials-Feeds.org (http://www.clinicaltrialsfeeds.org/) web sites.

Table 27.4 Examples of novel IGF1R monoclonal antibodies

Monoclonal antibodies	Specificity	Selected tumor types
GSK 621659A (GSK)		Preclinical
CP 751–871 (Pfizer)	IgG2	Phase I–II in prostate, breast, colorectal and melanoma Phase III in NSLC with paclitaxel and carboplatin
IMC-A12 (ImClone)	Fully human IgG1	Phase I–II in prostate cancer, Ewing's sarcoma, colorectal cancer
AVE1642 (Sanofi-Aventis)		Phase I in patients with advanced solid tumors
MK 0646 (Merck)		Phase I in advanced solid tumors Phase–II in pancreatic cancer and colorectal cancer
AMG 479 (Amgen)		Phase I advanced solid tumors Sarcoma, breast cancer patients, colorectal cancer and lung cancer Phase II–II pancreatic cancer in combination with gemcitabine
R 1507 (Roche)	IgG1	Phase I in patients with advanced solid tumors and I–II in Ewing's sarcoma
SCH-717454 (19D12, Schering-Plough)		Phase I–II metastatic osteosarcoma

evaluation in phase II clinical trials in patients with metastatic relapsed osteosarcoma.[3]

MK-0646, dalotuzumab (Merck) is an anti-IGFIR antibody that was investigated in a phase I clinical trial which suggested favorable toxicity in patients with advanced solid tumors (Hidalgo et al. 2008). Further results and signs of antitumor activity were reported from a Phase I study of MK-0646, in combination with gemcitabine for advanced previously untreated pancreatic cancer (Javle et al. 2010). This agent is currently being evaluated in combination with cetuximab and irinotecan in an ongoing randomised phase II/III study in patients with refractory metastatic colorectal cancer. Preliminary data showed that the combination was tolerable with no overlapping toxicities (Watkins et al. 2009).

AVE1642, (Axelar), a humanized monoclonal antibody, specific for human IGF1R was reported to be well tolerated as a single agent in a phase I clinical trial in patients with advanced solid tumors (Tolcher et al. 2008).

A summary of novel IGF1R monoclonal antibodies therapies is given in Table 27.4.

27.4 Limitless Replicative Potential: Telomerase

Telomerase is an enzyme that maintains the ability of cancer cells to achieve limitless proliferation thus allowing them to divide an indefinite number of times.

This process is the result of the addition of TTAGGG nucleotide repeats onto the telomers of chromosomal DNAs maintaining their length. Telomerase activation

[3] (http://www.clinicaltrials.gov/)

is not found in somatic cells, however, is an early event during oncogenesis and has been detected in 85–90 % of tumors correlating with poor prognosis (Kim et al. 1994). Telomerase has important roles in angiogenesis, metastasis and cancer stem cells in addition to its classical function in telomere length maintenance (Dikmen et al. 2009). Therefore a growing number of anti-telomerase strategies have emerged against the RNA component hTERC (human telomerase RNA component) and the protein component of hTERT (human telomerase reverse transcriptase) (Blackburn et al. 2006). The main strategies are targeting the RNA component hTERC and hTERT by antisense oligonucleotides.

Other methods target the telomerase associated proteins TP1(telomerase associated protein 1) and TRF1 (human tekomeric-repeat binding factor) (Burger 2007).

Imetelstat (GRN163L, Geron) is a 13-mer oligonucleotide that targets the active site of the enzyme TERC- RNA template. It has exhibited promising anti-tumor effects including antiangiogenic and anti-metastatic effects. Imetelstat was effective in preclinical studies in breast and lung cancer tumor cell lines and xenograft models (Dikmen et al. 2005; Hashizume and Gupta 2010). It entered phase I and II clinical trials in patients with chronic lymphocytic leukemia, multiple myeloma, and advanced solid tumors (NSCL and breast cancer).

Several small molecules, BRACO19 and RHPS4 that target single stranded telomeric repeat sequences (G-quadruplex), have shown very promising anticancer activity in tumour xenograft models (Neidle 2010).

27.5 Resistance to Apoptosis

Evasion of apoptosis is yet another crucial step in the overall process of tumor development. Anti-apoptotic mechanisms are up-regulated in tumors due to overexpression of anti-apoptotic proteins. Additionally, resistance to apoptosis and anoikis are important characteristics of metastatic cells. Apoptosis is the result of several key events that include inactivation of p53, activation of survival pathways (PI3k), and the upregulation of MMPs (which down-regulate death receptors, release growth factors, and prepare the extracellular matrix for invasion). Overexpression of anti-apoptotic proteins such as BCL-2, BCL-XL or focal adhesion kinase (FAK) also play a role (Vaux et al. 1988; Cory and Adams 2002).

The BCL-2 family is an important regulator of the mitochondria-dependent apoptotic pathways. It consists of pro-apoptotic proteins such as the BH3 family, two multi-domain pro-apoptotic proteins BAX and BAK as well as several multi-domain anti-apoptotic proteins (BCL-2, BCL-XL, BCL-W, MCL-1 and A1) (Cotter 2009). The anti-apoptotic BCL-2 promotes cell survival by impeding the activation of pro-apoptotic caspase proteins thereby contributing to the pathogenesis and progression of human cancers. Increased expression of BCL-2 is common in a number of tumors such as melanoma, lung, renal, colo-rectal, head and neck and brain cancer. Increased expression has also been seen in B cell lymphomas, NHL and chronic myelogenous leukemia (CML) (Cotter 2009; Maurer et al. 1998; Ravandi et al. 2001; Sharma et al. 2004; Shabnam et al. 2004; Sharma et al. 2005; Gradilone et al. 2003). Overexpression of BCl-2 in tumors has a negative impact on anticancer therapy as a result of increased resistance to drugs and radiotherapy (Sartorius and Krammer 2002).

Alterations in the expression and function of BCL-2 occur for various reasons. These include chromosomal abnormalities, gene hypomethylation, altered epigenetic regulation of the *BCL-2* gene (Hanada et al. 1993) and down-regulation of inhibitory mechanisms of the microRNAs *miR-15* and *miR-16* (Cimmino et al. 2005). Other factors, such as p53 mutation contribute to anti-apoptotic mechanisms in tumors through regulation of pro-apoptotic targets in the BCL-2 family including BAX and the BH3 proteins PUMA (p53 up-regulated modulator of apoptosis) and NOXA (Cotter 2009; Yu et al. 2001; Nakano and Vousden 2001; Miyashita and Reed 1995). Additionally, deregulations in many signal-transduction pathways in cancers affect the expression of the BCL-2 family members (e.g. RAS pathway, PI3-K and nuclear factor-κB (NF-κB) transcription factors) (Mayo and Baldwin 2000; Cox and Der 2003). Each of the biological steps of the apoptotic process has been therapeutically targeted resulting in the development of specialized apoptosis-modulatory therapy. These agents are currently under investigation in various clinical trials.

Therapeutic opportunities Inactivation of BCL-2 has been shown to induce apoptosis in malignant cells and to increase their sensitivity to chemotherapy (Guo et al. 2003). BCL-2 antisense oligonucleotide therapy showed anti-tumor responses and increased apoptosis in melanoma biopsies (Jansen et al. 1988).

Oblimersen sodium (G3139, Genasense) is an antisense phosphorothioate oligodeoxynucleotide (ODN) that is designed to be complementary to the first six codons of the human BCL-2 mRNA sequence. It is currently being extensively evaluated in clinical trials in CLL, AML, advanced melanoma (Patel et al. 2009). This therapy induces pro-apoptotic effects through an increase in BAX and PARP as well as through the release of cytochrome **c** with subsequent activation of the caspase cascade (Nicholson 2000). Furthermore, several studies have indicated that this compound has modulatory effects on the immune system. Results from phase I and III clinical trials using this agent in combination with classic chemotherapeutic agents demonstrated modest anti-tumor responses (Jansen et al. 1988; Nicholson 2000; Kang and Reynolds 2009).

Addition of BCL-2 anti-sense therapy to dacarbazine was evaluated in a randomized phase III clinical trial in patients with cutaneous melanoma, and revealed an improvement in clinical outcomes (Bedikian et al. 2006). BCl-2 antisense drug therapy has shown chemosensitizing effects in CLL patients when combined with cyclophosphamide (O'Brien et al. 2007, 2009). In metastatic prostate cancer it has been used in combination with mitoxantrone (Tolcher et al. 2005). In breast cancer it has been used as an adjuvant to docetaxel (Moulder et al. 2008) and in colorectal cancer in combination with irinotecan (Mita et al. 2006). However, addition of oblimersen to etoposide did not improve overall clinical outcome in patients with SCLC (Rudin et al. 2008).

Table 27.5 Examples of BCL-2 inhibitors that are currently in clinical development

Drug	Target	Clinical Trial
Oblimersen	Anti-sense BCL-2	CLL, AML, multiple myeloma, SCLC, non-Hodgkin's lymphoma and melanoma
Gossypol (AT-101)	BCL-2 small molecule inhibitor BH3 mimetic	Phase I/II CLL, prostate cancer
ABT-737	BCL-2, BCL-XL, BCL-W	
(ABT-263)	BH3 mimetic	Phase I in chronic myelogenous leukemia and (SCLC)
GX15–070	Pan apoptotic inhibitor BCL-2, BCL-XL, BCL-W, MCL-1	Phase I in SCLC and NSCLC

An alternative strategy inclusive of the BCL-XL antisense oligonucleotide targeting a specific BCL-XL sequence has been shown to induce even further chemosensitization of the tumor cells (Zangemeister-Wittke et al. 2000).

Other therapeutic modalities affecting gene or protein expression are small molecules that act as BH3 mimetics and bind to BCL2 neutralizing its activity and inducing pro-apoptotic effects. Several agents targeting the BCL-2 family and demonstrating inhibition of BCL-2, BCL-XL, and MCL-1 are currently being evaluated in clinical trials. An example is Gossypol which is a drug that entered Phase II clinical trials in CLL and in prostate cancer (Kang and Reynolds 2009; MacVicar et al. 2008) and was also tested in patients with advanced cancers (Saleh et al. 2009). Other pan-apoptotic inhibitors have been developed, for example the ABT-737 (A-779024, Abbott Laboratories), a small-molecule inhibitor of BCL-2, BCL-XL and BCL-W (Oltersdorf et al. 2005). Yet another example is ABT-263 which is an oral compound of ABT-737 that was shown to induce tumor regression in xenograft models of SCLC and acute lymphoblastic leukemia (ALL) (Tse et al. 2008). Lastly, GX15-070 (Obatoclax, Gemin X), also an inhibitor of BCL-2 family is currently in preliminary trials in patients with small cell lung cancer (SCLC) (Chiappori et al. 2009). A summary of BCL-2 inhibitors that are currently in preclinical and clinical development is shown in Table 27.5 (Nicholson 2000; Kang and Reynolds 2009).

27.6 Abnormalities in Growth-Stimulatory Signaling Pathways

27.6.1 RAS/RAF/MEK/ERK

Advancements in the field of molecular and genomic technology have led to the identification of various pathways that are deregulated in human cancers. This has paved the way for further investigation of additional targets for anticancer therapy.

The *RAS* family of oncogenes (*HRAS*, *KRAS*, and *NRAS*) encodes 21-kDa plasma membrane–associated G-proteins that regulate signaling cascades involved in normal cellular differentiation, proliferation, and survival (Downward 2003). Activating

Table 27.6 A summary of novel therapies that s target Ras-Raf-MEK-ERK pathway

Inhibitor	Specificity	Selected tumor types
Tipifarnib (Zarnestra™; Ortho Biotech Products, Lonafarnib (Sarasar™; Schering-Plough), BMS-214662 (Bristol-MyersSquibb, FTI-277 (Calbiochem). L744832 (Biomol International L.P., Biosciences.)	Inhibitors of the farnesyl-transferase enzyme	NSCLC, HNSCC, breast, ovarian, prostate, glioma, pancreatic, colorectal cancer
Sorafenib (BAY 43–9006, Nexavar®)	Raf-1, wild-type B-Raf, and *b-raf* V600E RAF kinase, VEGFR2, PDGFR-α and PDGFR-β, FLT3 and c-Kit	Metastatic RCC, HCC, melanoma, NSCLC, breast, ovarian, prostate, pancreatic, colorectal, glioma
PLX4032, PLX4720	B-Raf	Melanoma
Selumetinib (AZD6244; ARRY-142886)	MEK inhibitor	Melanoma
Tanespimycin (KOS-953, 17-AGG) Hsp90 inhibitor	B-Raf, AKT/PKB, ERBB2, CDK4, HER2, HIF-1α	Melanoma, breast cancer
Vaccination with mutant KRAS peptides		Pancreatic adenocarcinoma
RAS antisense treatment, ISIS2503, ISIS5132	HRAS, c-RAF1	NSCLC

oncogenic mutations in the all three *RAS* genes are common in several human cancers (Lowy and Willumsen 1993; Davies et al. 2002) and approximately 50 % of metastatic tumors contain RAS mutations (Chambers and Tuck 1993). RAS oncogenes contribute to tumor growth, invasion, angiogenesis and metastasis through Ras binding to Raf protein kinases, Raf-MEK-extracellular signal-regulated kinase family, and PI3K pathway. Additionally, RAS oncogenes function through Ral-specific guanine nucleotide exchange factors (RalGEFs), (Chambers and Tuck 1993; Shields et al. 2000; Ward et al. 2001) RAC, RHO and NFkB pathways (Downward 2003). A number of drugs that specifically target KRAS function have been developed and are currently under investigation in clinical trials (Table 27.6) (Downward 2003; Bos 1989).

Maturation of Ras proteins is a process that relies on farnesylation through covalent attachment of the enzyme coupling a 15-carbon isoprenyl group to Ras proteins. (Adjei et al. 2000). Inhibitors of the farnesyl-transferase enzyme are currently being investigated as potential therapeutic agents in the treatment of various cancers (Johnston 2001). Farnesyl-transferase enzyme inhibitors (FTIs) mimic the carboxy-terminal motif of RAS and compete for binding to farnesyltransferase. These compounds for example tipifarnib (Zarnestra™; Ortho Biotech Products),lonafarnib (Sarasar™; Schering-Plough Corporation), BMS-214662 (Bristol-Myers Squibb), FTI-277(Calbiochem),EMD and L744832 (Biomol International L.P., Biosciences) were demonstrated to have apoptotic and anti-angiogenic effects. They were also effective in achieving inhibition of tumor cell growth in various cancers such as that of colon, bladder, lung, prostate, and pancreas (Johnston 2001). FTIs initially showed significant promise in preclinical studies (Appels et al. 2005) and were subsequently tested in combination with cytotoxic drugs in clinical trials for lung cancer (Isobe et al. 2005). However, the results gathered from other phase II clinical trials revealed only moderate effects. Further studies are required for a complete understanding of the biological activities of FTIs (Brunner et al. 2003).

The RAF–MEK–ERK signaling cascade has an important role in tumor pathogenesis, and aberrant signaling through RAF (a downstream effector of the RAS pathway) occurs in approximately 30 % of human cancers (Bos 1989). Activating mutations of *BRAF* occur in approximately 8 % of human tumors, most frequently in melanoma (66 %), colorectal, and thyroid cancers. The three *RAF* somatic missense mutations code for cytoplasmic serine/threonine kinases which were shown to be related to proliferation and resistance to apoptosis. Therefore BRAF protein serine/threonine kinase could be used as an important and specific therapeutic target (Davies et al. 2002).

A. Kinase inhibitors targeting RAS effector pathway Sorafenib (BAY 43–9006, Nexavar®), is a multikinase inhibitor which was designed as an inhibitor for Raf-1, wild-type B-Raf and *b-raf* V600E. Sorafenib also inhibits several receptor tyrosine kinases on the intracellular domain of VEGFR1, VEGFR2, VEGFR3, PDGF receptors FMS-like tyrosine kinase 3 (Flt-3), stem cell factor receptor (KIT), and the glial cell-line derived neurotrophic factor receptor (RET) (Downward 2003). Sorafenib demonstrated good safety, tolerability and clinical activity in several tumor types particularly in patients with RCC and HCC (Strumberg et al. 2007; Lombardi et al. (in press); Escudier et al. 2007; Llovet et al. 2008). Further phase II and III studies evaluating sorafenib demonstrated an increased median overall survival and delayed the median time to progression in patients with advanced HCC and metastatic RCC (Lombardi et al. (in press); Cheng et al. 2009; Keating and Santoro 2009; Reeves and Liu 2009). However, a phase III clinical trial of sorafenib in combination with carboplatin and paclitaxel in patients with metastatic melanoma did not have an impact on improvement in overall survival (Hauschild et al. 2009).

Other small-molecule inhibitors of Raf kinases including Raf265 (Novartis), XL281 (Exelixis/Bristol Myers Squibb), AZ628 (AstraZeneca), SB-590885 (GlaxoSmithkline) and PLX-4032 (Plexxikon/Roche) a highly selective inhibitor for BRAF(V600E) has demonstrated a greater selectivity and antitumor activity in preclinical trials and phase I studies (Wellbrock and Hurlstone 2010; Pratilas and Solit 2010).

PLX-4032 is currently under clinical investigation as a single agent in metastatic cutaneous melanoma. The results from a phase I trial, reported good oral bioavailability, tumor regression and a median increased survival in metastatic melanoma patients (Flaherty et al. 2009). This therapeutic agent is currently being investigated in phase III clinical trials. However, PLX4032 may paradoxically enhance the proliferation of tumors through ERK activation in tumor cells that co-express BRAF(V600E) and mutant RAS (Pratilas and Solit 2010; Poulikakos et al. 2010).

Other drugs targeting the RAS/RAF- ERK–MAPK pathway include inhibitors of Hsp90 and its target proteins. Some of these client proteins such as RAF, AKT,

ERK, PI3K, VEGF, uPA, and MMPs are involved in promoting cancer invasion and angiogenesis. Inhibition of Hsp90 results in destabilization of the client proteins with antitumor effects (Koga et al. 2009). Tanespimycin (KOS-953) an inhibitor of Hsp90, was evaluated in a phase II clinical trial in cutaneous melanoma (Solit et al. 2008) and in combination with trastuzumab in breast cancer (Modi et al. 2007). The combination of sorafenib and tanespimycin resulted in pharmacodynamic activity in kidney cancer and melanoma meeting the criteria for further evaluation (Vaishampayan et al. 2010).

B. MEK inhibitors Mitogen-activated protein kinase (MAPK) pathway activation can result from mutations of *BRAF* and *RAS* oncogenes or upstream deregulation of growth factor receptors.

Inhibitors of the RAF–MEK–ERK signaling could modulate tumor cells growth, differentiation, and proliferation. MEK inhibitor, PD0325901(Pfizer), significantly suppresses pERK levels in certain tumors in preclinical studies (Barrett et al. 2008) and showed preliminary clinical activity in patients with advanced cancers (LoRusso et al. 2010). The specific MEK 1/2 inhibitor AZD6244 (ARRY-142886) (AstraZeneca)) is an ATP noncompetitive, allosteric inhibitor of MEK1/MEK2 and has shown tumor suppressive activity in pre-clinical models including melanoma, pancreatic, colon, lung, and breast cancers (Pratilas and Solit 2010; Bennouna et al. 2010). The results reported from a phase II clinical trial in cutaneous melanoma have shown lasting remissions in patients with BRAF mutations and this agent is currently being evaluated in Phase II clinical trials (Bennouna et al. 2010; Board et al. 2009). However, the activity of this agent was comparable to disease-specific standard chemotherapy. AZD6244 is currently undergoing evaluation in Phase II trials in combination with other chemotherapeutic agents in selected patients with active mutations in BRAF and/or RAS.

Another therapeutic approach is the development of antisense synthetic oligonucleotides that are specific for sequences in the mRNAs for HRAS (ISIS2503) or c-RAF1 (ISIS5132). These agents are now being evaluated for clinical activity in phase II trials NSCLC (Sato et al. 2007). However, their high level of specificity for one target is likely to be less effective in a tumor modulated by pleiotropic mechanisms.

Immunotherapy via vaccination with mutant KRAS peptides induced a transient Ras-specific T-cell response, a long-term immune response and increased survival in patients with pancreatic carcinoma following surgical resection (Wedén et al. 2010)

27.6.2 *Phosphatidylinositide 3-Kinase (PI3K) Pathway*

The PI3K pathway is a major cellular signal transduction pathway involved in cell growth, survival, angiogenesis and metabolism (Vivanco and Sawyers 2002). Activation of the PI3K pathway occurs through stimulation of RTKs which results in the assembly of receptor–PI3K complexes. Based on their structure PI3Ks are classified as class I (class IA p110α, p110β, p110δ and class IB, p110γ), class II (PI3KC2α,

PI3KC2β and PI3KC2γ) and class III (lipid kinases VPS34; homologue of the yeast vacuolar protein sorting-associated protein 34) which mediates signaling through mammalian target of rapamycin (mTOR) (Cantley 2002; Workman et al. 2010). The activation of the catalytic subunit of class I- PI3Ks is followed by the phosphorylation of phosphatidylinositol-4, 5-bisphosphate (PIP2) to phosphatidylinositol-3, 4, 5-trisphosphate (PtdIns(3,4,5)P_3).They recruit PDK1 and AKT to the plasma membrane followed by AKT phosphorylation at Thr308 by PDK1 and at Ser473 by mammalian target of rapamycin (mTOR) complex 2 (TORC2), (Wullschleger et al. 2006; Sarbassov et al. 2005). PTEN is a major limiting factor of this step and antagonizes this process by dephosphorylating PIP_3 to inhibit activation of AKT (Zhang and Yu 2010; Blanco-Aparicio et al. 2007). *PTEN* tumor suppressor gene is frequently inactivated in cancers by mutation, resulting in accumulation of PIP3 thus triggering the activation of its downstream effectors PDK1 and AKT/PKB (Yuan and Cantley 2008). One of the consequences of AKT activation is mTOR activation. The signaling complex downstream mTOR include ribosomal protein S6 kinase 1(p70S6K) and eukaryotic translation initiation factor 4E-binding protein 1 (4EBP1) which are important factors in protein synthesis, cell growth, metabolism and angiogenesis (Wang et al. 2006; Sabatini 2006). Phosphorylated AKT mediates the activation and inhibition of several targets, promoting cell cycle progression, proliferation and inhibition of apoptosis through various mechanisms (Yuan and Cantley 2008). Mutations in both PI3K and mTOR pathway are critical for tumor growth and survival and are involved in a wide range of tumors including breast, prostate, colon carcinomas and malignant brain tumors (Blume-Jensen and Hunter 2001).

The signalling of the PI3K pathway triggers tumor progression through multiple effects on cellular growth, proliferation, survival, motility and modulates tumor drug resistance (Vivanco and Sawyers 2002).The PI3K–AKT pathway also modulates angiogenic effects through upregulation of hypoxia-inducible factor (HIF)-1α and VEGF (Eccles and Welch 2007; Kong and Yamori 2008).

PI3K -AKT activation in cancer can occur at multiple points including activation of receptors or oncogenes upstream of PI3K or accumulation of PtdIns(3,4,5)P_3. Additionally this pathway can be deregulated through mutation or loss of the tumor suppressor PTEN, PI3K or of the downstream elements such as AKT and mTOR (Yuan and Cantley 2008; Abdel-Rahman et al. 2006; Watters and Huang 2009). Several studies indicated that targeting the PI3K-AKT pathway caused a reduction of tumor cell proliferation as well as their migratory and invasive capacity (Vivanco and Sawyers 2002). Therefore, the PI3K/AKT/mTOR pathway is considered an attractive target for novel anti-cancer therapeutic strategies. Several pathway components including AKT, PI3K and mTOR represent potential therapeutic targets. Many of these inhibitors are currently being evaluated preclinically or in early clinical trials (Liu et al. 2009).

A. PI3K inhibitors All PI3K isoforms are mutated in several cancers (Samuels et al. 2004) and are proven to induce oncogenic transformation in xenograft animal models. They are involved in cancer cell proliferation, growth, apoptosis, cytoskeletal rearrangement and tumor angiogenesis while also being a therapeutic target in tumors with PI3K mutations (Kang et al. 2006).

Table 27.7 Examples of several PI3K inhibitors currently being evaluated in preclinical and patient trials

Inhibitor	Specificity	Selected tumor types
PX-866 (Oncothyreon, Bellevue, WA, USA)	PI3 K (p110α, -δ and -γ)	Ovarian and lung carcinoma, colon xenografts Phase I clinical trial in patients with advanced metastatic solid cancer
CAL-101	PI3 K δ	Non-Hodgkin's lymphoma, mantle cell lymphoma, and CLL
PI-103(Novartis, Basel)	Class I PI3 K and mTOR	Preclinical studies in ovarian, breast, glioblastoma
XL765	Dual class I PI3K and mTOR	Patients with advanced tumors
SF1126 (Semafore, Indianapolis, IN, USA)	PI3K class I mTORC1/2	Antitumor and antiangiogenic effects in preclinical studies Phase I clinical trials
GDC-0941	pan PI3 K inhibitor	Breast, ovarian, lung, prostate xenografts Phase I clinical trials
GSK1059615	PI3K inhibitor	Phase I clinical trial
XL114	Pan PI3K inhibitor	Preclinical studies in breast, lung, ovarian, prostate and glioma tumors Phase I clinical trials
ZSTK474 (Zenyaku Kogyo, Tokyo, Japan)	Pan PI3 K inhibitor	Tumor xenografts of prostate adenocarcinoma, colorectal carcinoma and lung adenocarcinoma
XL184	PI3 K (p110α, -δ and –γ) and (TORC1, TORC2) MET, VEGFR2, and RET	Phase I-III clinical trials in patients with patients with progressive glioblastoma and medullary thyroid cancer
NVP-BEZ235 (Novartis)	Pan-PI3K/mTOR	Phase I and II clinical trials in patients with advanced breast, prostate, and brain cancers
NVP-BGT226	Dual class I PI3K and mTOR inhibitor	Phase I

The first PI3K inhibitors to be extensively researched were the fungal metabolite wortmannin (Arcaro and Wymann 1993) and LY294002 (Vlahos et al. 1994) which block the enzymatic activity of PI3Ks through an ATP-binding competitive mechanism (Liu et al. 2009).These compounds showed dose-dependent cell growth inhibition and antitumor and antiangiogenic efficacy in preclinical studies, but high levels of toxicity (dermal and liver toxicity), combined with poor solubility and low bioavailability, prevented their evaluation in clinical trials. However, wortmannin and LY294002 were widely used as tools for further elucidating the biological roles of PI3Ks in tumorigenesis (Workman et al. 2010). Several PI3K inhibitors have been developed and are currently being evaluated in preclinical and patient trials (Table 27.7)

New generation of PI3K inhibitors include PX-866 (Oncothyreon, Bellevue, WA, USA), a compound similar to wortmanin which demonstrated activity as an oral irreversible PI3K inhibitor with selectivity for class I PI3K isoforms α, γ and δc in lung carcinoma, ovarian and colon carcinoma xenografts (Ihle et al. 2004). This drug is currently being investigated in a phase I clinical trial in patients with advanced metastatic cancers and preliminary results indicated signs of disease stabilization (Jimeno et al. 2009).

Pan-specific PI3K inhibitors (for example PI-103, NVP-BEZ235, GDC-0941 and ZSTK474), occupy the ATP-binding site of the enzyme and have improved properties to modulate PI3K kinases.

GDC-0941 is a pan PI3K inhibitor that demonstrated signs of antitumor activity in multiple xenograft models such as breast, ovarian, lung and prostate cancer (Folkes et al. 2008). In a phase I clinical trial in patients with advanced solid tumors this agent was well tolerated, with signs of biological activity (Hoff et al. 2010). Recent studies with GDC-0941 have shown promising results by combining this agent with trastuzumab (Yao et al. 2009) and MEK inhibitors (Hoeflich et al. 2009).

ZSTK474 (Zenyaku Kogyo, Tokyo, Japan) is a triazine derivative with selective pan-PI3K inhibitory activity that showed favorable responses in preclinical studies with tumor xenografts of prostate adenocarcinoma, colorectal carcinoma and lung adenocarcinoma, (Yaguchi et al. 2006).

PI-103 (Novartis) is a synthesized molecule of the pyridofuropyrimidine that shares a similar structure with LY294002 and has the ability to target both PI3K-p110α and mTOR. It demonstrated antiproliferative and antitumor effects in pre-clinical studies in, breast and ovarian cells xenografts and enhanced chemotherapy-induced cell death of glioblastoma GBM cells (Raynaud et al. 2007; Westhoff et al. 2009). Further studies are ongoing to determine the efficacy and the pharmacological properties of PI-103 agent to target both mTOR and PI3Ks in cancer (Raynaud et al. 2007; Fan et al. 2006).

SF1126 (Semafore) is a LY294002 pro-drug that targets all PI3 K class I isoforms including mTORC1/2 and has proven antitumor and antiangiogenic responses in preclinical studies of brain, neuroblastoma, NSCLC, prostate, myeloma, RCC. It is currently being evaluated in phase I and dose escalation clinical studies (Garlich et al. 2008).

Encouraging results have been described for XL765 compound which is a dual PI3K and mTOR inhibitor which is currently in phase I studies in patients with solid tumors. Preliminary results showed that XL765was well tolerated and demonstrated pharmacodynamic modulation of PI3K and ERK pathway with evidence of stable disease in patients with advanced cancer (Papadopoulos et al. 2008; Brana et al. 2010). Other multikinase PI3K inhibitors, XL184, XL147, XL765 and XL147 (Exelixis) are currently in development. Clinical data from patients treated with XL184 a MET, VEGFR2, and RET inhibitor, has demonstrated activity in phase I-III clinical trials in patients with progressive glioblastoma and medullary thyroid cancer (Wen et al. 2010; Sugawara et al. 2009).

XL-765, a pan-class I- PI3K inhibitor has an inhibitory effect also on DNA-PK and MTOR and has the ability to induce delays in tumor growth in xenograft models. This agent has been well tolerated as monotherapy in a phase I clinical trial when administered orally to patients with advanced solid tumors, (Papadopoulos et al. 2008) or in combination with temozolomide (TMZ), (Nghiemphu et al. 2010).

Interim analyses of an ongoing phase I clinical trial in patients with advanced cancer showed that the XL147 compound was well tolerated and induced prolonged stable disease in several cases (Shapiro et al. 2009). Also, preliminary results of a trial evaluating the combination of XL147 and erlotinib resulted in clinical activity and simultaneous inhibition of PI3K and EGFR signaling (Moldovan et al. 2010).

NVP-BEZ235 (Novartis) is an imidazo-quinoline derivative, which exhibits dual pan-PI3 K/mTOR inhibition. Preclinical data show that NVP- BEZ235 has strong anti-proliferative activity in cell lines and tumor xenografts with abnormal PI3K signalling. This therapeutic agent has entered Phase I and II clinical trials in patients with advanced breast, prostate, and brain cancers (Maira et al. 2008). Other PI3K inhibitors that have entered phase I clinical trials include: NVP-BGT226 (a dual class I PI3K and mTOR inhibitor) and NVP-BKM120 (a selective pan-class I PI3K inhibitor) (Brachmann et al. 2009).

Several other phase I studies investigating PI3K inhibitors are ongoing. Two examples of the study drugs are GSK1059615 (GlaxoSmithKline) (Brachmann et al. 2009) and CAL-101 (Calistoga Pharmaceuticals). CAL-101 is a selective agent targeting p110δ. Interim results from a phase I trial with CAL-101 demonstrated favourable clinical results in patients with haematological malignancies such as non-Hodgkin's lymphoma (NHL), mantle cell lymphoma, and chronic lymphocytic leukemia (CLL) (Lannutti 2010)

B. PDK inhibitors Phosphorylation of the threonine residue in the activation loop of the three AKT isoforms and PKC (protein kinase C) is modulated by PDK1. This process stimulates cell growth, proliferation and survival, as well as promoting angiogenesis. Several anti-PDK 1 inhibitors such as UCN-01 were tested in phase I and II clinical trials, however they did not have significant antitumor activity (Welch et al. 2007). Further development of an indoline-based series of PDK1 inhibitors such as BX-517, demonstrated a potent inhibitory effect through binding to the ATP pocket of PDK1 (Islam et al. 2007a, b).

C. AKT inhibitors AKT amplification and activation occurs in a variety of tumors such as melanoma, breast, ovarian and pancreatic cancers. It is critical for phosphorylation of many downstream substrates involved in tumor survival as well as organization of the actin cytoskeleton and invasion (Liu et al. 2009; Carpten et al. 2007). Over expression of AKT2 was reported in late-stage colorectal cancer and metastases suggesting that AKT2 promotes metastatic disease (Rychahou et al. 2008). The involvement of AKT in these processes supports a role for selective targeting of the PI3K/AKT pathway as a strategy for metastasis (Table 27.8) (Vivanco and Sawyers 2002).

Perifosine (Keryx) is a lipid-based phosphatidylinositol analogue that inhibits AKT by targeting the pleckstrin homology (PH) domain of AKT thus blocking AKT membrane translocation. This drug has the end result of reduction of proliferation while also inhibiting AKT. This effect has been shown in a variety of tumors cells such as melanoma, lung, prostate, colon, and breast cancer (Crul et al. 2002). Results from a phase I clinical trial in patients with advanced solid tumors showed that the drug was well tolerated (Unger et al. 2010) with evidence of stable disease in sarcoma (Bailey

Table 27.8 AKT inhibitors that are currently under investigation for various malignancies

Inhibitor	Specificity	Selected tumor types
Perifosine (Keryx)	AKT	Phase I and II in advanced solid tumors
GSK690693	AKT, GSK3 beta, PRAS40, Forkhead	Preclinical studies in ovarian, breast, prostate carcinoma
API-2	AKT	Phase I in advanced solid tumors NSCLC, leukemia
XL418 (Exelixis)	AKT	Phase I in advanced solid tumors
MK2206 (Merck)	AKT	Phase I in advanced solid tumors
Tanespimycin (KOS-953, Kosan)	Hsp90 inhibitor AKT	Phase II metastatic breast cancer Multiple myeloma

et al. 2006) and renal cell carcinoma. However, these results were not clinically validated in phase II clinical studies in breast, pancreas, prostate, head and neck, and lung cancer (Kondapaka et al. 2003; Ummersen et al. 2004; Gills and Dennis 2009).

Other AKT inhibitors that are phosphatidylinositol ether lipid analogues (PIA) which interfere with the PH domain of AKT inhibit the translocation of AKT to the plasma membrane (Hu et al. 2000). Lipid analogues and PH domain-targeting inhibitors were shown to have AKT inhibitory effects (Gills et al. 2007) in addition to reducing tumor cell growth in preclinical studies (Powis et al. 1992).

Inositol polyphosphates such as InsP5, a novel inhibitor of the PI3K/AKT pathway, can compete with PtdIns(3,4,5)P_3 by binding to AKT- PH domain. $InsP_5$ has anti-AKT and antiangiogenic effects resulting in xenograft tumor growth inhibition (Maffucci et al. 2005). A derivative of $InsP_5$, 2-*O*-Bn-$InsP_5$, resulted in enhanced pro-apoptotic and anti-tumor activity through inhibition of PDK1 and mTOR (Falasca et al. 2010). The recent development of the aminofurazan AKT series of inhibitors has led to the identification of GSK690693, a compound that causes dephosphorylation of targets downstream of AKT, including GSK3 beta, PRAS40, and Forkhead (Heerding et al. 2008). Xenograft studies resulted in antitumor activity in ovarian, prostate, and breast carcinoma (Rhodes et al. 2008).

Several AKT antagonists have been identified using high throughput screening. API-1 inhibits AKT by binding to the PH domain and blocking AKT membrane translocation (Kim et al. 2010). API-2 (triciribine phosphate), a water-soluble tricyclic nucleotide selectively induces apoptosis and inhibits cell growth in tumors with PTEN mutations and AKT amplification. This drug is currently being tested in Phase I clinical trials in patients with both solid and haematological malignancies. (Yang et al. 2004)

MK2206 (Merck), an orally active allosteric AKT inhibitor is under evaluation for the treatment of patients with locally advanced or metastatic solid tumors (Tolcher et al. 2009b). Preclinical data showed enhanced anticancer activity for MK-2206 in combination with several anticancer agents (erlotinib, lapatinib) (Hirai et al. 2010) as well as in combination with MEK inhibitor, AZD6244.

XL418 (Exelixis), a small molecule that inhibits the activity of AKT and S6 Kinase (S6K). It has shown inhibitory effects on tumor growth in preclinical studies, including breast and lung adenocarcinomas and has currently entered Phase I clinical trials.

Table 27.9 Summary of mTORC1 and mTORC2 inhibitors currently in clinical trials

Inhibitor	Specificity	Selected tumor types
Rapamycin (Wyeth)	mTOR	Approved advanced RCC Phase I and II in advanced solid tumors
Temsirolimus (Torisel; Wyeth)	mTORC1	Approved advanced RCC and mantle cell lymphoma Phase I-III in advanced solid tumors, ovarian, endometrial carcinoma, NSCLC, melanoma
Everolimus (Afinitor; Novartis)	mTORC1	Approved advanced RCC Phase I-II in advanced breast cancer, lung cancer, pancreatic carcinoma, melanoma or glioma
Ridaforolimus (Merck/Ariad)	mTORC1	Approved soft-tisse and bone sarcomas Phase I clinical trial in patients with advanced malignancies
WYE-132 (Wyeth)	Dual mTORC1 and mTORC2	Preclinical studies in breast, glioma, lung, renal tumors

Hsp90 inhibitors: Both AKT and its activating kinase 3-phosphoinositide-dependent kinase-1 rely on Hsp90 for stability. Hsp90 and its co-chaperones modulate tumor cell apoptosis through formation of AKT-Hsp90 complexes, thus stabilizing the AKT kinase activity and phospho-AKT dephosphorylation (Sato et al. 2000). Several studies indicated that targeting the PI3K-AKT pathway with 17-AAG caused inhibition of AKT phosphorylation, induction of apoptosis and downregulation of multiple AKT and RAF dependent pathways (Workmann et al. 2007; Basso et al. 2002; Georgakis et al. 2006; Hostein et al. 2001; Solit et al. 2002).

D. mTOR inhibitors mTOR has a critical effect through regulation of several intracellular functions including cell growth, cell cycle progression, actin cytoskeleton organization, angiogenesis and apoptotic cell death. Several downstream compounds targeting mTOR have been designed (Faivre et al. 2006) (Table 27.9).

Rapamycin (sirolimus, Wyeth) is a macrolide antibiotic which binds to mTORC1 via FKBP12-rapamycin binding domain adjacent to the catalytic site of mTORC1. It suppresses mTOR-mediated phosphorylation. Analogues of rapamycin, such as temsirolimus (Torisel; Wyeth), everolimus (RAD001/Afinitor) and ridaforolimus (Ariad Pharamceuticals/Merck) have demonstrated antiproliferative activity against a diverse range of malignancies in preclinical studies, and have also been evaluated in multiple clinical trials. Results from phase III clinical trials showed improved clinical outcomes for everolimus in patients with RCC that had progressed after sunitinib or sorafenib therapy. Also, temsirolimus improved overall survival when compared with interferon in patients with metastatic RCC leading to FDA approval (Motzer et al. 2008; Hudes et al. 2007; Motzer et al. 2010). Temsirolimus is also approved for the treatment of mantle-cell lymphoma following results from a phase III clinical trial which reported improved progression free survival (PFS) and objective responses (Hess et al. 2009). Partial response rates were reported in patients with soft-tissue sarcoma, neuroendocrine tumors and endometrial carcinoma and led to phase III trials evaluating everolimus and ridaforolimus in neuroendocrine and soft-tissue sarcoma. However, low response rates have been seen in trials of patients with advanced breast, lung, and pancreatic cancer as well as melanoma and glioma (Dancey 2010).

In addition to inhibiting tumor growth, mTOR inhibitors also act as anti-angiogenic agents, interfering with HIF-1α (hypoxia inducible factor), VEGF and PDGF signalling cascades (Faivre et al. 2006; Thomas et al. 2006). These agents can therefore be effective when used in combination with anti-angiogenic drugs. Evidence of this was seen in a phase II clinical trial investigating the efficacy of the combination of bevacizumab and everolimus which revealed biological activity and good tolerability in the treatment of advanced clear cell renal cancer. This combination had moderate activity in patients with metastatic melanoma (Hainsworth et al. 2010a, b).

Ridaforolimus is an analog of rapamycin that has been shown to inhibit mTOR activity, as evidenced by reduced phosphorylation of 4E-BP1 and S6. This drug inhibits the proliferation of multiple tumor cell lines including breast, colon, lung, prostate, glial, and those of pancreatic origin. This drug was well tolerated with favorable antitumor activity in a phase I clinical trial in patients with advanced malignancies including NSCLC, RCC, and Ewing sarcoma (Mita et al. 2008). Ridaforolimus is currently being evaluated in a phase III clinical trial in patients with advanced sarcoma[4].

Dual ATP-competitive inhibitors of both mTORC1 and mTORC2 are emerging. They have been reported to reduce cancer cell proliferation in vitro and tumor xenograft formation in vivo. In preclinical studies, oral administration of WYE-132 inhibited mTORC1 and mTORC2 and resulted in antitumor activity against breast, glioma, lung, and several renal tumor cell lines (Yu et al. 2010).

References

Abdel-Rahman MH et al (2006) High frequency of submicroscopic hemizygous deletion is a major mechanism of loss of expression of PTEN in uveal melanoma. J Clin Oncol 24:288–295

Adjei AA, Davis JN, Erlichman C, Svingen PA, Kaufmann SH (2000) Comparison of potential markers of farnesyltransferase inhibition. Clin Cancer Res 6:2318–2325

Alberts DS et al (2007) Phase II trial of imatinib mesylate in recurrent, biomarker positive, ovarian cancer (Southwest Oncology Group Protocol S0211). Int J Gynecol Cancer 17:784–788

All-Ericsson C et al (2002) Insulin-like growth factor-1 receptor in uveal melanoma: a predictor for metastatic disease and a potential therapeutic target. Invest Ophthalmol Vis Sci 43:1–8

Appels NMGM, Beijnen JH, Schellens JHM (2005) Development of farnesyl transferase inhibitors: a review. Oncologist 10:565–578

Arcaro A, Wymann M (1993) Wortmannin is a potent phosphatidylinositol 3-kinase inhibitor: the role of phosphatidylinositol 3,4,5-trisphosphate in neutrophil responses. Biochem J 296(Pt2):297–301

[4] NIH's ClinicalTrials.gov. Available from (http://www.clinicaltrials.gov/) and ClinicalTrials-Feeds.org (http://www.clinicaltrialsfeeds.org/) web sites.

Atzori F, Traina TA, Ionta MT, Massidda B (2009) Targeting insulin-like growth factor type 1 receptor in cancer therapy. Target Oncol 4:255–266

Bahr C, Groner B (2005) The IGF-1 receptor and its contributions to metastatic tumor growth-novel approaches to the inhibition of IGF-1R function. Growth Factors 23:1–14

Bailey HH et al (2006) Phase II study of daily oral perifosine in patients with advanced soft tissue sarcoma. Cancer 107:2462–2467

Bakalian S et al (2007) Expression of nm23-H1 in uveal melanoma. Melanoma Res 17:284–290

Barrett SD et al (2008) The discovery of the benzhydroxamate MEK inhibitors CI-1040 and PD 0325901. Bioorg Med Chem Lett 18:6501–6504

Basso AD et al (2002) Akt forms an intracellular complex with heat shock protein 90 (Hsp90) and Cdc37 and is destabilized by inhibitors of Hsp90 function. J Biol Chem 277:39858–39866

Bedikian AY et al (2006) Bcl-2 antisense (oblimersen sodium) plus dacarbazine in patients with advanced melanoma: the oblimersen melanoma study group. J Clin Oncol 24:4738–4745

Beltran PJ et al (2009) AMG 479, a fully human anti–insulin-like growth factor receptor type I monoclonal antibody, inhibits the growth and survival of pancreatic carcinoma cells. Mol Cancer Ther 8:1095–1105

Bennouna J et al (2010) A phase II, open-label, randomised study to assess the efficacy and safety of the MEK1/2 inhibitor AZD6244 (ARRY-142886) versus capecitabine monotherapy in patients with colorectal cancer who have failed one or two prior chemotherapeutic regimens. Investigational New Drugs

Berg T et al (2002) Small-molecule antagonists of Myc/Max dimerization inhibit Myc-induced transformation of chicken embryo fibroblasts. Proc Natl Acad Sci U S A 99:3830–3835

Bernards R, Weinberg RA (2002) A progression puzzle. Nature 418:823

Bianco R, Gelardi T, Damiano V, Ciardiello F, Tortora G (2007) Rational bases for the development of EGFR inhibitors for cancer treatment. Int J Biochem Cell Biol 39:1416–1431

Blackburn EH, Greider CW, Szostak JW (2006) Telomeres and telomerase: the path from maize, Tetrahymena and yeast to human cancer and aging. Nat Med 12:1133–1138

Blagosklonny MV, Toretsky J, Neckers L (1995) Geldanamycin selectively destabilizes and conformationally alters mutated p53. Oncogene 11:933–939

Blanco-Aparicio C, Renner O, Leal JFM, Carnero A (2007) PTEN, more than the AKT pathway. Carcinogenesis 28:1379–1386

Blume-Jensen P, Hunter T (2001) Oncogenic kinase signalling. Nature 411:355–365

Board RE et al (2009) Detection of BRAF mutations in the tumour and serum of patients enrolled in the AZD6244 (ARRY-142886) advanced melanoma phase II study. Br J Cancer 101:1724–1730

Bokemeyer C et al (2009) Fluorouracil, leucovorin, and oxaliplatin with and without cetuximab in the first-line treatment of metastatic colorectal cancer. J Clin Oncol 27:663–671

Bos JL (1989) Ras oncogenes in human cancer—a review. Cancer Res 49:4682–4689

Brachmann S, Fritsch C, Maira S-M, García-Echeverría C (2009) PI3K and mTOR inhibitors–a new generation of targeted anticancer agents. Curr Opin Cell Biol 21:194–198

Brana IPL, Baselga J, Heath EI, Patnaik A, Gendreau S, Laird A, Papadopoulos K (2010) Vall d'Hebron A phase I dose-escalation study of the safety, pharmacokinetics (PK), and pharmacodynamics of XL765 (SAR245409), a PI3K/TORC1/TORC2 inhibitor administered orally to patients (pts) with advanced malignancies. J Clin Oncol 28:15s (suppl; abstr 3030)

Brunner TB et al (2003) Farnesyltransferase inhibitors: an overview of the results of preclinical and clinical investigations. Cancer Res 63:5656–5668

Buettner R, Mesa T, Vultur A, Lee F, Jove R (2008) Inhibition of Src family kinases with dasatinib blocks migration and invasion of human melanoma cells. Mol Cancer Res 6:1766–1774

Burger AM (2007) Highlights in experimental therapeutics. Cancer Lett 245:11–21

Burstein HJ et al (2003) Trastuzumab and vinorelbine as first-line therapy for HER2-overexpressing metastatic breast cancer: multicenter phase II trial with clinical outcomes, analysis of serum tumor markers as predictive factors, and cardiac surveillance algorithm. J Clin Oncol 21:2889–2895

Cantley LC (2002) The phosphoinositide 3-kinase pathway. Science 296:1655–1657

Carpten JD et al (2007) A transforming mutation in the pleckstrin homology domain of AKT1 in cancer. Nature 448:439–444

Chambers AF, Tuck AB (1993) Ras-responsive genes and tumor metastasis. Crit Rev Oncog 4:95–114

Cheng AL et al (2009) Efficacy and safety of sorafenib in patients in the Asia-Pacific region with advanced hepatocellular carcinoma: a phase III randomised, double-blind, placebo-controlled trial. Lancet Oncol 10:25–34

Chernicky CL, Yi L, Tan H, Gan SU, Ilan J (2000) Treatment of human breast cancer cells with antisense RNA to the type I insulin-like growth factor receptor inhibits cell growth, suppresses tumorigenesis, alters the metastatic potential, and prolongs survival in vivo. Cancer Gene Ther 7:384–395

Chiappori A et al (2009) A phase Ib trial of Bcl-2 inhibitor obatoclax in combination with carboplatin and etoposide for previously untreated patients with extensive-stage small cell lung cancer (ES-SCLC). J Clin Oncol (Meeting Abstracts) 27:3576

Chitnis MM, Yuen JSP, Protheroe AS, Pollak M, Macaulay VM (2008) The type 1 insulin-like growth factor receptor pathway. Clin Cancer Res 14:6364–6370

Cimmino A et al (2005) miR-15 and miR-16 induce apoptosis by targeting BCL2. Proc Natl Acad Sci U S A 102:13944–13949

Clayman GL, Frank DK, Bruso PA, Goepfert H (1999) Adenovirus-mediated Wild-Type p53 Gene Transfer as a Surgical Adjuvant in Advanced Head and Neck Cancers. Clinical Cancer Research 5:1715–1722

Cobleigh MA et al (1999) Multinational study of the efficacy and safety of humanized anti-HER2 monoclonal antibody in women who have HER2-overexpressing metastatic breast cancer that has progressed after chemotherapy for metastatic disease. J Clin Oncol 17:2639

Cohen BD et al (2005) Combination therapy enhances the inhibition of tumor growth with the fully human anti–type 1 insulin-like growth factor receptor monoclonal antibody CP-751,871. Clin Cancer Res 11:2063–2073

Coluccia AML et al (2006) SKI-606 decreases growth and motility of colorectal cancer cells by preventing pp60(c-Src)–dependent tyrosine phosphorylation of β-catenin and its nuclear signaling. Cancer Res 66:2279–2286

Cory S, Adams JM (2002) The Bcl2 family: regulators of the cellular life-or-death switch. Nat Rev Cancer 2:647–656

Cotter TG (2009) Apoptosis and cancer: the genesis of a research field. Nat Rev Cancer 9:501–507

Cox AD, Der CJ (2003) The dark side of Ras: regulation of apoptosis. Oncogene 22:8999–9006

Craig C et al (1998) Effects of adenovirus-mediated p16INK4A expression on cell cycle arrest are determined by endogenous p16 and Rb status in human cancer cells. Oncogene 16:265–272

Cripps C, Winquist E, Devries MC, Stys-Norman D, Gilbert R (2010) Epidermal growth factor receptor targeted therapy in stages III and IV head and neck cancer. Curr Oncol 17:37–48

Crul M et al (2002) Phase I and pharmacological study of daily oral administration of perifosine (D-21266) in patients with advanced solid tumours. Eur J Cancer 38:1615–1621

Dancey J (2010) mTOR signaling and drug development in cancer. Nat Rev Clin Oncol 7:209–219

Davies H et al (2002) Mutations of the BRAF gene in human cancer. Nature 417:949–954

Demetri GD et al (2002) Efficacy and safety of imatinib mesylate in advanced gastrointestinal stromal tumors. N Engl J Med 347:472–480

Deng WG et al (2008) Enhancement of antitumor activity of cisplatin in human lung cancer cells by tumor suppressor FUS1. Cancer Gene Ther 15:29–39

Devi GR et al (2005) In vivo bioavailability and pharmacokinetics of a c-MYC antisense phosphorodiamidate morpholino oligomer, AVI-4126, in solid tumors. Clin Cancer Res 11:3930–3938

Dikmen ZG et al (2005) In vivo inhibition of lung cancer by GRN163L: a novel human telomerase inhibitor. Cancer Res 65:7866–7873

Dikmen ZG, Ozgurtas T, Gryaznov SM, Herbert B-S (2009) Targeting critical steps of cancer metastasis and recurrence using telomerase template antagonists. Biochimica et Biophysica Acta (BBA)—Mol Basis Disease 1792:240–247

Douillard J-Y et al (2010) Molecular predictors of outcome with gefitinib and docetaxel in previously treated non-small-cell lung cancer: data from the randomized phase III interest trial. J Clin Oncol 28:744–752
Downward J (2003) Targeting RAS signalling pathways in cancer therapy. Nat Rev Cancer 3:11–22
Druker BJ (2008) Translation of the Philadelphia chromosome into therapy for CML. Blood 112:4808–4817
Eccles SA (2005) Targeting key steps in metastatic tumour progression. Curr Opin Genet Dev 15:77–86
Eccles SA, Welch DR (2007) Metastasis: recent discoveries and novel treatment strategies. Lancet 369:1742–1757
Economou MA et al (2008) Receptors for the liver synthesized growth factors IGF-1 and HGF/SF in uveal melanoma: intercorrelation and prognostic implications. Acta Ophthalmol 86 Thesis 4:20–25
Egger G, Aparicio AM, Escobar SG, Jones PA (2007) Inhibition of Histone Deacetylation Does Not Block Resilencing of p16 after 5-Aza-2'-Deoxycytidine Treatment. Cancer Res 67:346–353
Escudier B et al (2007) Sorafenib in advanced clear-cell renal-cell carcinoma. N Engl J Med 356:125–134
Faivre S, Kroemer G, Raymond E (2006) Current development of mTOR inhibitors as anticancer agents. Nat Rev Drug Discov 5:671–688
Faivre S, Demetri G, Sargent W, Raymond E (2007) Molecular basis for sunitinib efficacy and future clinical development. Nat Rev Drug Discov 6:734–745
Falasca M et al (2010) A novel inhibitor of the PI3K/Akt pathway based on the structure of inositol 1,3,4,5,6-pentakisphosphate. Br J Cancer 102:104–114
Fan Q-W et al (2006) A dual PI3 kinase/mTOR inhibitor reveals emergent efficacy in glioma. Cancer Cell 9:341–349
Flaherty KPI, Sosman J, Kim K, Ribas A, McArthur G, Lee RJ, Grippo JF, Nolop K, Chapman P (2009) Phase I study of PLX4032: proof of concept for V600E BRAF mutation as a therapeutic target in human cancer. in ASCO. J Clin Oncol 27:15s (abstr 9000)
Folkes AJ et al (2008) The identification of 2-(1H-Indazol-4-yl)-6-(4-methanesulfonyl-piperazin-1-ylmethyl)-4-morpholin-4-yl-thieno[3,2-d]pyrimidine (GDC-0941) as a potent, selective, orally bioavailable inhibitor of class I PI3 Kinase for the Treatment of Cancer. J Med Chem 51:5522–5532
Freyer G et al (2003) Phase II Study of Oral Vinorelbine in First-Line Advanced Breast Cancer Chemotherapy. J Clin Oncol 21:35–40
Fry DW et al (2004) Specific inhibition of cyclin-dependent kinase 4/6 by PD 0332991 and associated antitumor activity in human tumor xenografts. Mol Cancer Ther 3:1427–1438
Garcia-Echeverria C et al (2004) In vivo antitumor activity of NVP-AEW541-A novel, potent, and selective inhibitor of the IGF-IR kinase. Cancer Cell 5:231–239
Garlich JR et al (2008) A vascular targeted pan phosphoinositide 3-kinase inhibitor prodrug, SF1126, with antitumor and antiangiogenic activity. Cancer Res 68:206–215
Generali D et al (2007) EGFR mutations in exons 18–21 in sporadic breast cancer. Ann Oncol 18:203–205
Georgakis GV et al (2006) Inhibition of heat shock protein 90 function by 17-allylamino-17-demethoxy-geldanamycin in Hodgkin's lymphoma cells down-regulates Akt kinase, dephosphorylates extracellular signal-regulated kinase, and induces cell cycle arrest and cell death. Clin Cancer Res 12:584–590
Gills J, Dennis P (2009) Perifosine: update on a novel Akt inhibitor. Curr Oncol Rep 11:102–110
Gills JJ et al (2007) Phosphatidylinositol ether lipid analogues that inhibit AKT also independently activate the stress kinase, p38α, through MKK3/6-independent and -dependent mechanisms. J Biol Chem 282:27020–27029
Girnita A et al (2004) Cyclolignans as inhibitors of the insulin-like growth factor-1 receptor and malignant cell growth. Cancer Res 64:236–242

González L et al (2006) Role of c-Src in human MCF7 breast cancer cell tumorigenesis. J Biol Chem 281:20851–20864
Gradilone A et al (2003) Survivin, bcl-2, bax, and bcl-X gene expression in sentinel lymph nodes from melanoma patients. J Clin Oncol 21:306–312
Grand CL et al (2002) The cationic porphyrin TMPyP4 down-regulates c-MYC and human telomerase reverse transcriptase expression and inhibits tumor growth in vivo. Mol Cancer Ther 1:565–573
Gridelli C et al (2007) Erlotinib in non-small cell lung cancer treatment: current status and future development. Oncologist 12:840–849
Gril B et al (2008) Effect of lapatinib on the outgrowth of metastatic breast cancer cells to the brain. J Natl Cancer Inst 100:1092–1103
Gualberto A, Pollak M (2009) Emerging role of insulin-like growth factor receptor inhibitors in oncology: early clinical trial results and future directions. Oncogene 28:3009–3021
Guo LJ, Wu ZY, Zhang S, Zheng JL, Zheng HL (2003) Effect of bcl-2 antisense oligonucleotides on multidrug resistance of cultured uveal melanoma cells. Zhonghua Yan Ke Za Zhi 39:73–76
Hahn O, Stadler W (2006) Sorafenib. Curr Opin Oncol 18:615–621
Hainsworth JD et al (2010a) Bevacizumab and everolimus in the treatment of patients with metastatic melanoma. Cancer 9999:NA
Hainsworth JD et al (2010b) Phase II trial of bevacizumab and everolimus in patients with advanced renal cell carcinoma. J Clin Oncol 28:2131–2136
Haluska P et al (2006) In vitro and in vivo antitumor effects of the dual insulin-like growth factor-I/insulin receptor inhibitor, BMS-554417. Cancer Res 66:362–371
Hanada M, Delia D, Aiello A, Stadtmauer E, Reed JC (1993) Bcl-2 gene hypomethylation and high-level expression in B-cell chronic lymphocytic-leukemia. Blood 82:1820–1828
Harzstark AL RC, Diamond M et al (2007) A phase I trial of nordihydroguareacetic acid (NDGA) in patients with non-metastatic prostate cancer and rising PSA. in ASCO. Clin Oncol 25(18S:15500)
Hashizume R, Gupta N (2010) Telomerase inhibitors for the treatment of brain tumors and the potential of intranasal delivery. Curr Opin Mol Ther 12:168–175
Haupt S, Haupt Y (2004) Manipulation of the tumor suppressor p53 for potentiating cancer therapy. Semin Cancer Biol 14:244–252
Hauschild A et al (2009) Results of a phase III, randomized, placebo-controlled study of sorafenib in combination with carboplatin and paclitaxel as second-line treatment in patients with unresectable stage III or stage IV melanoma. J Clin Oncol 27:2823–2830
Hecht JR et al (2003) A phase I/II trial of intratumoral endoscopic ultrasound injection of ONYX-015 with intravenous gemcitabine in unresectable pancreatic carcinoma. Clin Cancer Res 9:555–561
Heerding DA et al (2008) Identification of 4-(2-(4-Amino-1,2,5-oxadiazol-3-yl)-1-ethyl-7-{[(3S)-3-piperidinylmethyl]oxy}-1H-imidazo[4,5-c]pyridin-4-yl)-2-methyl-3-butyn-2-ol (GSK690693), a Novel Inhibitor of AKT Kinase. J Med Chem 51:5663–5679
Herbst RS et al (2005) TRIBUTE: a phase III trial of erlotinib hydrochloride (OSI-774) combined with carboplatin and paclitaxel chemotherapy in advanced non-small-cell lung cancer. J Clin Oncol 23:5892–5899
Hess G et al (2009) Phase III study to evaluate temsirolimus compared with investigator's choice therapy for the treatment of relapsed or refractory mantle cell lymphoma. J Clin Oncol 27:3822–3829
Hewish M, Chau I, Cunningham D (2009) Insulin-like growth factor 1 receptor targeted therapeutics: novel compounds and novel treatment strategies for cancer medicine. Recent Pat Anticancer Drug Discov 4:54–72
Hidalgo M, Tirado Gomez M, Lewis N, Vuky JL, Taylor G, Hayburn JL, Hsu K, Kosh M, Picozzi VJ (2008) A phase I study of MK-0646, a humanized monoclonal antibody against the insulin-like growth factor receptor type 1 (IGF1R) in advanced solid tumor patients in a q2 wk schedule. in ASCO J Clin Oncol 26: 2008 (May 20 suppl; abstr 3520)

Higa GM, Abraham J (2007) Lapatinib in the treatment of breast cancer. Expert Rev Anticancer Ther 7:1183–1192

Higano CS, Yu Y, Whiting SH, Gordon MS, Lorusso P, Fox F, Katz TL, Roecker JM, Rowinsky EK, Schwartz JD (2007) A phase I, first in man study of weekly IMC-A12, a fully human insulin like growth factor-I receptor IgG1 monoclonal antibody, in patients with advanced solid tumors. J Clinic Oncol 25(18 suppl):139, abstract 3505

Hirai H et al (2010) MK-2206, an allosteric Akt inhibitor, enhances antitumor efficacy by standard chemotherapeutic agents or molecular targeted drugs in vitro and in vivo. Mol Cancer Ther 9:1956–1967

Hoeflich KP et al (2009) In vivo antitumor activity of MEK and Phosphatidylinositol 3-kinase inhibitors in basal-like breast cancer models. Clin Cancer Res 15:4649–4664

Hostein I, Robertson D, DiStefano F, Workman P, Clarke PA (2001) Inhibition of signal transduction by the Hsp90 inhibitor 17-allylamino-17-demethoxygeldanamycin results in cytostasis and apoptosis. Cancer Res 61:4003–4009

Hu Y et al (2000) 3-(Hydroxymethyl)-bearing phosphatidylinositol ether lipid analogues and carbonate surrogates block PI3-K, Akt, and cancer cell growth. J Med Chem 43:3045–3051

Hudes G et al (2007) Temsirolimus, interferon alfa, or both for advanced renal-cell carcinoma. N Engl J Med 356:2271–2281

Huh WK et al (2010) Efficacy and safety of imatinib mesylate (Gleevec→) and immunohistochemical expression of c-Kit and PDGFR-[beta] in a gynecologic oncology group phase II trial in women with recurrent or persistent carcinosarcomas of the uterus. Gynecologic Oncology 117:248–254

Ihle NT et al (2004) Molecular pharmacology and antitumor activity of PX-866, a novel inhibitor of phosphoinositide-3-kinase signaling. Mol Cancer Ther 3:763–772

Invitrogen (2007) INGN 201: Ad-p53, Ad5CMV-p53, adenoviral p53, p53 gene therapy–introgen, RPR/INGN 201. Drugs R D 8, 176–187

Isobe T, Herbst RS, Onn A (2005) Current management of advanced non-small cell lung cancer: targeted therapy. Semin Oncol 32:315–328

Iversen PL, Arora V, Acker A, Mason DH, Devi GR (2003) Efficacy of antisense morpholino oligomer targeted to c-myc in prostate cancer xenograft murine model and a phase I safety study in humans. Clin Cancer Res 9:2510–2519

Jackisch C (2006) HER-2-positive metastatic breast cancer: optimizing trastuzumab-based therapy. Oncologist 11:34–41

Jansen B et al (1988) bcl-2 antisense therapy chemosensitizes human melanoma in SCID mice. Nat Med 4:232–234

Jassem JL, Karp CJ, Mok DDT, Benner RJ, Green SJ, Park K, Novello S, Strausz J, Gualberto A (2010) Randomized, open label, phase III trial of figitumumab in combination with paclitaxel and carboplatin versus paclitaxel and carboplatin in patients with non-small cell lung cancer (NSCLC). in ASCO. J Clin Oncol 28:15s (suppl; abstr 7500)

Jatoi A et al (2010) A phase II study of cetuximab and radiation in elderly and/or poor performance status patients with locally advanced non-small-cell lung cancer (N0422). Ann Oncol 21(10):2040–2044

Javle MM et al (2010) Phase I/II study of MK-0646, the humanized monoclonal IGF-1R antibody in combination with gemcitabine or gemcitabine plus erlotinib (E) for advanced pancreatic cancer. J Clin Oncol (Meeting Abstracts) 28:4039

Ji L, Roth JA (2008) Tumor suppressor FUS1 signaling pathway. J Thorac Oncol 3:327–330

Ji L et al (1999) Induction of apoptosis and inhibition of tumorigenicity and tumor growth by adenovirus vector-mediated fragile histidine triad (FHIT) gene overexpression. Cancer Res 59:3333–3339

Ji Q-s et al (2007) A novel, potent, and selective insulin-like growth factor-I receptor kinase inhibitor blocks insulin-like growth factor-I receptor signaling in vitro and inhibits insulin-like growth factor-I receptor–dependent tumor growth in vivo. Mol Cancer Ther 6:2158–2167

Jiang H (2009) Overview of gefitinib in non-small cell lung cancer: an asian perspective. Jpn J Clin Oncol 39:137–150

Jimeno A, Hong DS, Hecker S, Clement R, Kurzrock R, Pestano LA, Hiscox A, Leos RA, Kirkpatrick DL, Eckhardt SG, Herbst RS (2009) Phase I trial of PX-866, a novel phosphoinositide-3-kinase (PI-3K) inhibitor. in ASCO J Clin Oncol 27:15s (suppl; abstr 3542)

Joannes A et al (2009) Fhit regulates invasion of lung tumor cells. Oncogene 29:1203–1213

Johnston SRD (2001) Farnesyl transferase inhibitors: a novel targeted therapy for cancer. Lancet Oncol 2:18–26

Kang MH, Reynolds CP (2009) Bcl-2 inhibitors: targeting mitochondrial apoptotic pathways in cancer therapy. Clin Cancer Res 15:1126–1132

Kang S, Denley A, Vanhaesebroeck B, Vogt PK (2006) Oncogenic transformation induced by the p110β, -γ, and -δ isoforms of class I phosphoinositide 3-kinase. Proc Natl Acad Sci U S A 103:1289–1294

Karp DD, Paz-Ares LG, Novello S, Haluska P, Garland L, Cardenal F, Blakely LJ, Eisenberg PD, Gualberto A, Langer CJ (2008) high activity of the anti-IGF-IR antibody CP-751,871 in combination with paclitaxel and carboplatin in squamous NSCLC. in ASCO. J Clin Oncol 26:2008 (May 20 suppl; abstr 8015)

Karp DD et al (2009) Phase II study of the anti-insulin-like growth factor type 1 receptor antibody CP-751,871 in combination with paclitaxel and carboplatin in previously untreated, locally advanced, or metastatic non-small-cell lung cancer. J Clin Oncol 27:2516–2522

Keating GM (2010) Panitumumab: a review of its use in metastatic colorectal cancer. Drugs 70:1059–1078. doi:1010.2165/11205090-000000000-000000000

Keating GM, Santoro A (2009) Sorafenib: a review of its use in advanced hepatocellular carcinoma. Drugs 69:223–240 doi:210.2165/00003495–200969020-200900006

Khuri FR et al (2000) A controlled trial of intratumoral ONYX-015, a selectively-replicating adenovirus, in combination with cisplatin and 5-fluorouracil in patients with recurrent head and neck cancer. Nat Med 6:879–885

Kim JK, Diehl JA (2009) Nuclear cyclin D1: An oncogenic driver in human cancer. J Cell Physiol 220:292–296

Kim NW et al (1994) Specific association of human telomerase activity with immortal cells and cancer. Science 266:2011–2015

Kim ES et al (2008) Gefitinib versus docetaxel in previously treated non-small-cell lung cancer (INTEREST): a randomised phase III trial. The Lancet 372:1809–1818

Kim D et al (2010) A small molecule inhibits Akt through direct binding to Akt and preventing Akt membrane translocation. J Biol Chem 285:8383–8394

Kindler HL et al (2010) A placebo-controlled, randomized phase II study of conatumumab (C) or AMG 479 (A) or placebo (P) plus gemcitabine (G) in patients (pts) with metastatic pancreatic cancer (mPC). J Clin Oncol (Meeting Abstracts) 28:4035

Kitagawa M, Aonuma M, Lee SH, Fukutake S, McCormick F (2008) E2F-1 transcriptional activity is a critical determinant of Mdm2 antagonist-induced apoptosis in human tumor cell lines. Oncogene 27:5303–5314

Knudsen ES, Wang JYJ (2010) Targeting the RB-pathway in Cancer Therapy. Clinical Cancer Research 16:1094–1099

Koga F, Kihara K, Neckers L (2009) Inhibition of cancer invasion and metastasis by targeting the molecular chaperone heat-shock protein 90. Anticancer Res 29:797–807

Kolb EA et al (2008) Initial testing (stage 1) of a monoclonal antibody (SCH 717454) against the IGF-1 receptor by the pediatric preclinical testing program. Pediatr Blood Cancer 50:1190–1197

Kolb EA et al (2010) R1507, a fully human monoclonal antibody targeting IGF-1R, is effective alone and in combination with rapamycin in inhibiting growth of osteosarcoma xenografts. Pediatr Blood Cancer 55:67–75

Kondapaka SB, Singh SS, Dasmahapatra GP, Sausville EA, Roy KK (2003) Perifosine, a novel alkylphospholipid, inhibits protein kinase B activation. Mol Cancer Ther 2:1093–1103

Kong D, Yamori T (2008) Phosphatidylinositol 3-kinase inhibitors: promising drug candidates for cancer therapy. Cancer Sci 99:1734–1740

Kulik G, Klippel A, Weber M (1997) Antiapoptotic signalling by the insulin-like growth factor I receptor, phosphatidylinositol 3-kinase, and Akt. Mol Cell Biol 17:1595–1606

Kurzrock R et al (2010) A phase I study of weekly R1507, a human monoclonal antibody insulin-like growth factor-I receptor antagonist, in patients with advanced solid tumors. Clin Cancer Res 16:2458–2465

Lannutti Bea (2010) Demonstration of pharmacodynamic target inhibition and chemokine modulation in patients with cll following treatment with cal-101, a selective inhibitor of the p110 delta isoform of PI3K. in European hematology Association Congress. Barcelona, Spain

Lassus H et al (2006) Gene amplification, mutation, and protein expression of EGFR and mutations of ERBB2 in serous ovarian carcinoma. J Mol Med 84:671–681

Li R, Pourpak A, Morris SW (2009) Inhibition of the insulin-like growth factor-1 receptor (IGF1R) tyrosine kinase as a novel cancer therapy approach. J Med Chem 52:4981–5004

Lim MJ et al (2006) Targeted therapy of DNA tumor virus-associated cancers using virus-activated transcription factors. Mol Ther 13:899–909

Litzenburger BC et al (2009) BMS-536924 reverses IGF-IR-induced transformation of mammary epithelial cells and causes growth inhibition and polarization of MCF7 cells. Clin Cancer Res 15:226–237

Liu P, Cheng H, Roberts TM, Zhao JJ (2009) Targeting the phosphoinositide 3-kinase pathway in cancer. Nat Rev Drug Discov 8:627–644

Llovet JM et al (2008) Sorafenib in advanced hepatocellular carcinoma. N Engl J Med 359:378–390

Loesch D et al (2008) Phase II trial of gemcitabine/carboplatin (plus trastuzumab in HER2-positive disease) in patients with metastatic breast cancer. Clin Breast Cancer 8:178–186

Lombardi G et al An update on targeted therapy in metastatic renal cell carcinoma. Urologic oncology: seminars and original investigations In Press, Corrected Proof

Lopez T, Hanahan D (2002) Elevated levels of IGF-1 receptor convey invasive and metastatic capability in a mouse model of pancreatic islet tumorigenesis. Cancer Cell 1:339–353

LoRusso PM et al (2010) Phase I pharmacokinetic and pharmacodynamic study of the oral MAPK/ERK kinase inhibitor PD-0325901 in patients with advanced cancers. Clin Cancer Res 16:1924–1937

Lowy DR, Willumsen BM (1993) Function and regulation of ras. Annu Rev Biochem 62:851–891

Lu C et al (2009) A phase I trial of intravenous therapy with tumor suppressor FUS1-nanoparticles for recurrent/metastatic lung cancer. J Clin Oncol (Meeting Abstracts) 27:e19065

Macaulay VM, Middleton MR, Eckhardt SG, Juergens RA, Stephens AW, Poondru S, McCarthy SP, Gadgeel SM (2010) Phase I study of OSI-906, dual tyrosine kinase inhibitor of insulin-like growth factor-1 receptor (IGF-1R) and insulin receptor (IR) in combination with erlotinib (E) in patients with advanced solid tumors. J Clin Oncol 28(suppl; abstr 3016):15s, 2010

MacVicar GR et al (2008) An open-label, multicenter, phase I/II study of AT-101 in combination with docetaxel (D) and prednisone (P) in men with hormone refractory prostate cancer (HRPC). J Clin Oncol (Meeting Abstracts) 26:16043

Maffucci T et al (2005) Inhibition of the Phosphatidylinositol 3-Kinase/Akt pathway by inositol pentakisphosphate results in antiangiogenic and antitumor effects. Cancer Res 65:8339–8349

Maira S-M et al (2008) Identification and characterization of NVP-BEZ235, a new orally available dual phosphatidylinositol 3-kinase/mammalian target of rapamycin inhibitor with potent in vivo antitumor activity. Mol Cancer Ther 7:1851–1863

Marshall J-C, Lee J, Steeg P (2009) Clinical-translational strategies for the elevation of Nm23-H1 metastasis suppressor gene expression. Mol Cell Biochem 329:115–120

Martins AS et al (2006) Insulin-like growth factor I receptor pathway inhibition by ADW742, alone or in combination with imatinib, doxorubicin, or vincristine, is a novel therapeutic approach in ewing tumor. Clin Cancer Res 12:3532–3540

Martins CM et al (2008) Expression of the metastasis suppressor gene KISS1 in uveal melanoma. Eye 22:707–711

Maurer CA et al (1998) Apoptosis inhibiting factor Bcl-xL might be the crucial member of the Bcl-2 gene family in colorectal cancer. Dig Dis Sci 43:2641–2648

Mayo MW, Baldwin AS (2000) The transcription factor NF-kappa B: control of oncogenesis and cancer therapy resistance. Biochimica Et Biophysica Acta-Reviews on Cancer 1470:M55–M62

Mita MM et al (2006) A phase I, pharmacokinetic and biologic correlative study of oblimersen sodium (Genasense™, G3139) and irinotecan in patients with metastatic colorectal cancer. Ann Oncol 17:313–321

Mita MM et al (2008) Phase I trial of the novel mammalian target of rapamycin inhibitor deforolimus (AP23573; MK-8669) administered intravenously daily for 5 days every 2 weeks to patients with advanced malignancies. J Clin Oncol 26:361–367

Mitsiades CS et al (2004) Inhibition of the insulin-like growth factor receptor-1 tyrosine kinase activity as a therapeutic strategy for multiple myeloma, other hematologic malignancies, and solid tumors. Cancer Cell 5:221–230

Miyashita T, Reed JC (1995) Tumor-suppressor P53 is a direct transcriptional activator of the human bax gene. Cell 80:293–299

Modi S et al (2007) Combination of trastuzumab and tanespimycin (17-AAG, KOS-953) is safe and active in trastuzumab-refractory HER-2 overexpressing breast cancer: a phase I dose-escalation study. J Clin Oncol 25:5410–5417

Moldovan C, Soria J, LoRusso P, Guthrie T, Song C, Nguyen LT, Martini J, Infante JR, Burris HA III (2010) Institut Gustave Roussy, Villejuif, France. A phase I safety and pharmacokinetic (PK) study of the PI3K inhibitor XL147 (SAR245408) in combination with erlotinib in patients (pts) with advanced solid tumors. in ASCO. J Clin Oncol 28:15s (suppl; abstr 3070)

Molife LR et al (2010) The insulin-like growth factor-I receptor inhibitor figitumumab (CP-751,871) in combination with docetaxel in patients with advanced solid tumours: results of a phase Ib dose-escalation, open-label study. Br J Cancer 103:332–339

Moore MJ et al (2007) Erlotinib plus gemcitabine compared with gemcitabine alone in patients with advanced pancreatic cancer: a phase III trial of the National Cancer Institute of Canada Clinical Trials Group. J Clin Oncol 25:1960–1966

Morali OG et al (2001) IGF-II induces rapid beta-catenin relocation to the nucleus during epithelium to mesenchyme transition. Oncogene 20:4942–4950

Motzer RJ et al (2008) Efficacy of everolimus in advanced renal cell carcinoma: a double-blind, randomised, placebo-controlled phase III trial. Lancet 372:449–456

Motzer RJ et al (2010) Phase 3 trial of everolimus for metastatic renal cell carcinoma. Cancer 9999:NA

Moulder SL et al (2008) Phase I/II study of G3139 (Bcl-2 antisense oligonucleotide) in combination with doxorubicin and docetaxel in breast cancer. Clin Cancer Res 14:7909–7916

Nahta R, Iglehart JD, Kempkes B, Schmidt EV (2002) Rate-limiting Effects of Cyclin D1 in Transformation by ErbB2 Predicts Synergy between Herceptin and Flavopiridol. Cancer Res 62:2267–2271

Naing A et al (2009) Phase I study combining an IGFR inhibitor (IMC-A12) and an mTOR inhibitor (temsirolimus) in patients with solid tumors or lymphoma. J Clin Oncol (Meeting Abstracts) 27:e14535

Nakano K, Vousden KH (2001) PUMA, a novel proapoptotic gene, is induced by p53. Mol Cell 7:683–694

Neidle S (2010) Human telomeric G-quadruplex: the current status of telomeric G-quadruplexes as therapeutic targets in human cancer. FEBS J 277:1118–1125

Nemunaitis J et al (2000) Adenovirus-Mediated p53 Gene Transfer in Sequence With Cisplatin to Tumors of Patients With Non-Small-Cell Lung Cancer. J Clin Oncol 18:609

Nesbit CE, Tersak JM, Prochownik EV (1999) MYC oncogenes and human neoplastic disease. Oncogene 18:3004–3016

Nghiemphu PLAMO, Cloughesy T, Mellinghoff IK, Norden AD, Nguyen LT, Rajangam K, Wen PY (2010) A phase I safety and pharmacokinetic study of XL765 (SAR245409), a novel PI3K/TORC1/TORC2 inhibitor, in combination with temozolomide (TMZ) in patients (pts) with newly diagnosed malignant glioma. in ASCO. J Clin Oncol 28:15s (suppl; abstr 3085)

Nguyen DX, Massague J (2007) Genetic determinants of cancer metastasis. Nat Rev Genet 8:341–352

Nicholson DW (2000) From bench to clinic with apoptosis-based therapeutic agents. Nature 407:810–816

O'Brien S et al (2007) Randomized phase III trial of fludarabine plus cyclophosphamide with or without oblimersen sodium (Bcl-2 antisense) in patients with relapsed or refractory chronic lymphocytic leukemia. J Clin Oncol 25:1114–1120

O'Brien S et al (2009) 5-year survival in patients with relapsed or refractory chronic lymphocytic leukemia in a randomized, phase III trial of fludarabine plus cyclophosphamide with or without oblimersen. J Clin Oncol 27:5208–5212

Olayioye MA, Neve RM, Lane HA, Hynes NE (2000) The ErbB signaling network: receptor heterodimerization in development and cancer. EMBO J 19:3159–3167

Oltersdorf T et al (2005) An inhibitor of Bcl-2 family proteins induces regression of solid tumours. Nature 435:677–681

Ortega S, Malumbres M, Barbacid M (2002) Cyclin D-dependent kinases, INK4 inhibitors and cancer. Biochimica et Biophysica Acta (BBA)—Rev Cancer 1602:73–87

Paez JG et al (2004) EGFR mutations in lung cancer: correlation with clinical response to gefitinib therapy. Science 304:1497–1500

Papadopoulos KP, Markman B, Tabernero J, Patnaik A, Heath EI, DeCillis A, Laird D, Aggarwal SK, Nguyen L, LoRusso PM (2008) A phase I dose-escalation study of the safety, pharmacokinetics (PK), and pharmacodynamics (PD) of a novel PI3K inhibitor, XL765, administered orally to patients (pts) with advanced solid tumors. in ASCO. J Clin Oncol 26: 2008 (May 20 suppl; abstr 3510)

Patel MPa, Masood Ab, Patel PSa, Chanan-Khan AAac (2009) Targeting the Bcl-2. Curr Opin Oncol 21:516–523

Pelengaris S, Khan M, Evan G (2002) c-MYC: more than just a matter of life and death. Nat Rev Cancer 2:764–776

Perez EA, Rodeheffer R (2004) Clinical cardiac tolerability of trastuzumab. J Clin Oncol 22:322–329

Pession A et al (2004) Targeted inhibition of NMYC by peptide nucleic acid in N-myc amplified human neuroblastoma cells: cell-cycle inhibition with induction of neuronal cell differentiation and apoptosis. Int J Oncol 24:265–272

Playford MP, Bicknell D, Bodmer WF, Macaulay VM (2000) Insulin-like growth factor 1 regulates the location, stability, and transcriptional activity of β-catenin. Proc Natl Acad Sci U S A 97:12103–12108

Polager S, Ginsberg D (2009) p53 and E2f: partners in life and death. Nat Rev Cancer 9:738–748

Pollak MN, Schernhammer ES, Hankinson SE (2004) Insulin-like growth factors and neoplasia. Nat Rev Cancer 4:505–518

Ponzielli R, Katz S, Barsyte-Lovejoy D, Penn LZ (2005) Cancer therapeutics: targeting the dark side of Myc. Eur J Cancer 41:2485–2501

Poulikakos PI, Zhang C, Bollag G, Shokat KM, Rosen N (2010) RAF inhibitors transactivate RAF dimers and ERK signalling in cells with wild-type BRAF. Nature 464:427–430

Powis G et al (1992) Selective inhibition of phosphatidylinositol phospholipase C by cytotoxic ether lipid analogues. Cancer Res 52:2835–2840

Pratilas CA, Solit DB (2010) Targeting the mitogen-activated protein kinase pathway: physiological feedback and drug response. Clin Cancer Res 16:3329–3334

Puzanov I et al (2010) Safety and pharmacokinetics (PK) of AMG 479 in combination with erlotinib (E) or sorafenib (S) in patients (pts) with advanced solid tumors. J Clin Oncol (Meeting Abstracts) 28:3018

Ravandi F et al (2001) Expression of apoptosis proteins in chronic myelogenous leukemia. Cancer 91:1964–1972

Raynaud FI et al (2007) Pharmacologic characterization of a potent inhibitor of class I Phosphatidylinositide 3-kinases. Cancer Res 67:5840–5850

Reeves DJ, Liu CY (2009) Treatment of metastatic renal cell carcinoma. Cancer Chemother Pharmacol 64:11–25

Rhodes N et al (2008) Characterization of an Akt Kinase inhibitor with potent pharmacodynamic and antitumor activity. Cancer Res 68:2366–2374

Riedemann J, Macaulay VM (2006) IGF1R signalling and its inhibition. Endocr Relat Cancer 13:S33–43

Rinker-Schaeffer CW, O'Keefe JP, Welch DR, Theodorescu D (2006) Metastasis suppressor proteins: discovery, molecular mechanisms, and clinical application. Clin Cancer Res 12:3882–3889

Rodon J, DeSantos V, Ferry RJ, Kurzrock R (2008) Early drug development of inhibitors of the insulin-like growth factor-I receptor pathway: lessons from the first clinical trials. Mol Cancer Ther 7:2575–2588

Roig JM et al (2004) Adenovirus-Mediated Retinoblastoma 94 Gene Transfer Induces Human Pancreatic Tumor Regression in a Mouse Xenograft Model. Clinical Cancer Research 10:1454–1462

Rose AA, Siegel PM (2010) Emerging therapeutic targets in breast cancer bone metastasis. Future Oncol 6:55–74

Roth JA et al (1996) Retrovirus-mediated wild-type P53 gene transfer to tumors of patients with lung cancer. Nat Med 2:985–991

Rothenberg ML PE, Sandler AB et al (2007) Phase I dose-escalation study of the anti-IGF-IR recombinant human IgG1 monoclonal antibody (Mab) IMC-A12, administered every other week to patients with advanced solid tumors. in AACR-NCI-EORTC International Conference on Molecular Targets and Cancer Therapeutics. Abstr C84. San Francisco

Rowinsky EK (2004) The erbB family: targets for therapeutic development against cancer and therapeutic strategies using monoclonal antibodies and tyrosine kinase inhibitors. Annu Rev Med 55:433–457

Rowinsky EK et al (2007) IMC-A12, a human IgG1 monoclonal antibody to the insulin-like growth factor I receptor. Clin Cancer Res 13:5549s–5555s

Roy V, Perez EA (2009) Beyond trastuzumab: small molecule tyrosine kinase inhibitors in HER-2-positive breast cancer. Oncologist 14:1061–1069

Rudin CM et al (2008) Randomized phase II study of carboplatin and etoposide with or without the bcl-2 antisense oligonucleotide oblimersen for extensive-stage small-cell lung cancer: CALGB 30103. J Clin Oncol 26:870–876

Rusnak DW et al (2007) Assessment of epidermal growth factor receptor (EGFR, ErbB1) and HER2 (ErbB2) protein expression levels and response to lapatinib (Tykerb→, GW572016) in an expanded panel of human normal and tumour cell lines. Cell Prolif 40:580–594

Rychahou PG et al (2008) Akt2 overexpression plays a critical role in the establishment of colorectal cancer metastasis. Proc Natl Acad Sci 105:20315–20320

Sabatini DM (2006) mTOR and cancer: insights into a complex relationship. Nat Rev Cancer 6:729–734

Saleh MN, Pitot H, Maleski J, Leopold L, Forero A (2009) Extended phase I trial of the oral pan-Bcl-2 inhibitor AT-101 by multiple dosing schedules in patients with advanced cancers. J Clin Oncol (Meeting Abstracts) 27:e14537

Samuels Y et al (2004) High frequency of mutations of the PIK3CA gene in human cancers. Science 304:554

Sarantopoulos J, Mita AC, Mulay M, Romero O, Lu J, Capilla F, Chen L, Hwang Y, Friberg G, Rosen LS (2008) A phase IB study of AMG 479, a type 1 insulin-like growth factor receptor (IGF1R) antibody, in combination with panitumumab (P) or gemcitabine (G). J Clinical Oncol 26(suppl):173s, abstract 3583

Sarbassov DD, Guertin DA, Ali SM, Sabatini DM (2005) Phosphorylation and regulation of Akt/PKB by the rictor-mTOR complex. Science 307:1098–1101

Sartorius UA, Krammer PH (2002) Upregulation of Bcl-2 is involved in the mediation of chemotherapy resistance in human small cell lung cancer cell lines. Int J Cancer 97:584–592

Sato S, Fujita N, Tsuruo T (2000) Modulation of Akt kinase activity by binding to Hsp90. Proc Natl Acad Sci U S A 97:10832–10837

Sato M, Shames DS, Gazdar AF, Minna JD (2007) A translational view of the molecular pathogenesis of lung cancer. J Thorac Oncol 2:327–343

Schilder RJ et al (2008) Phase II evaluation of imatinib mesylate in the treatment of recurrent or persistent epithelial ovarian or primary peritoneal carcinoma: a gynecologic oncology group study. J Clin Oncol 26:3418–3425

Segditsas S, Tomlinson I (2006) Colorectal cancer and genetic alterations in the Wnt pathway. Oncogene 25:7531–7537

Shabnam MS et al (2004) Expression of p53 protein and the apoptotic regulatory molecules Bcl-2, Bcl-XL, and Bax in locally advanced squamous cell carcinoma of the lung. Lung Cancer 45:181–188

Shapiro G, Kwak E, Baselga J, Rodon J, Scheffold C, Laird AD, Bedell C, Edelman G (2009) Phase I dose-escalation study of XL147, a PI3K inhibitor administered orally to patients with solid tumors. in ASCO. J Clin Oncol 27:15s (suppl; abstr 3500)

Sharma H, Sen S, Mathur M, Bahadur S, Singh N (2004) Combined evaluation of expression of telomerase, survivin, and anti-apoptotic bcl-2 family members in relation to loss of differentiation and apoptosis in human head and neck cancers. Head Neck 26:733–740

Sharma J et al (2005) Bcl-XL protein levels determine apoptotic index in pancreatic carcinoma. Pancreas 30:337–342

Shen L, Zhang C, Ambrus Jr JL, Wang JH (2005) Silencing of human c-myc oncogene expression by poly-DNP-RNA. Oligonucleotides 15:23–35

Shen M-R et al (2006) Insulin-like growth factor 1 is a potent stimulator of cervical cancer cell invasiveness and proliferation that is modulated by alphavbeta3 integrin signaling. Carcinogenesis 27:962–971

Shepherd FA et al (2005) Erlotinib in previously treated non-small-cell lung cancer. N Engl J Med 353:123–132

Sherr CJ, McCormick F (2002) The RB and p53 pathways in cancer. Cancer Cell 2:103–112

Shields JM, Pruitt K, McFall A, Shaub A, Der CJ (2000) Understanding ras: 'it ain't over 'til it's over'. Trends Cell Biol 10:147–154

Slamon D et al (1989) Studies of the HER-2/neu proto-oncogene in human breast and ovarian cancer. Science 244:707–712

Slamon DJ et al (2001) Use of chemotherapy plus a monoclonal antibody against HER2 for metastatic breast cancer that overexpresses HER2. N Engl J Med 344:783–792

Sobol H et al (1996) Truncation at conserved terminal regions of BRCA1 protein is associated with highly proliferating hereditary breast cancers. Cancer Res 56:3216–3219

Solit DB et al (2002) 17-Allylamino-17-demethoxygeldanamycin induces the degradation of androgen receptor and HER-2/neu and inhibits the growth of prostate cancer xenografts. Clin Cancer Res 8:986–993

Solit DB et al (2008) Phase II trial of 17-allylamino-17-demethoxygeldanamycin in patients with metastatic melanoma. Clin Cancer Res 14:8302–8307

Steeg PS (2004) Perspectives on classic articles: metastasis suppressor genes. J Natl Cancer Inst 96:E4

Steeg PS, Horak CE, Miller KD (2008) Clinical-translational approaches to the Nm23-H1 metastasis suppressor. Clin Cancer Res 14:5006–5012

Strumberg D et al (2007) Safety, pharmacokinetics, and preliminary antitumor activity of sorafenib: a review of four phase i trials in patients with advanced refractory solid tumors. Oncologist 12:426–437

Sugawara Ma, Geffner DLb, Martinez Db, Hershman JMa (2009) Novel treatment of medullary thyroid cancer. [Miscellaneous Article]. Curr Opin Endocrinol, Diabetes Obes 16:367–372

Tait DL, Obermiller PS, Hatmaker AR, Redlin-Frazier S, Holt JT (1999) Ovarian cancer BRCA1 gene therapy: phase I and II trial differences in immune response and vector stability. Clin Cancer Res 5:1708–1714

Tevaarwerk AJ, Kolesar JM (2009) Lapatinib: a small-molecule inhibitor of epidermal growth factor receptor and human epidermal growth factor receptor–2 tyrosine kinases used in the treatment of breast cancer. Clin Ther 31:2332–2348

Thomas GV et al (2006) Hypoxia-inducible factor determines sensitivity to inhibitors of mTOR in kidney cancer. Nat Med 12:122–127

Tol J, Punt CJA (2010) Monoclonal antibodies in the treatment of metastatic colorectal cancer: a review. Clin Ther 32:437–453

Tolcher AW et al (2005) A phase II, pharmacokinetic, and biological correlative study of oblimersen sodium and docetaxel in patients with hormone-refractory prostate cancer. Clin Cancer Res 11:3854–3861

Tolcher AW, Patnaik A, Till ECH, Takimoto KP, Papadopoulos C, Massard D, Mery-Mignard A, Deslandes M, Ozoux J (2008) Soria A phase I study of AVE1642, a humanized monoclonal antibody IGF-1R (insulin like growth factor1 receptor) antagonist, in patients(pts) with advanced solid tumor(ST). J Clin Oncol 26(Suppl173s) Abstract 3582

Tolcher AW et al (2009a) Phase I, pharmacokinetic, and pharmacodynamic study of AMG 479, a fully human monoclonal antibody to insulin-like growth factor receptor 1. J Clin Oncol 27:5800–5807

Tolcher AW, Yap TA, Fearen I, Taylor A, Carpenter C, Brunetto AT, Beeram M, Papadopoulos K, Yan L, de Bono J (2009b) A phase I study of MK-2206, an oral potent allosteric Akt inhibitor (Akti), in patients (pts) with advanced solid tumor (ST). in ASCO. J Clin Oncol 27:15s (suppl; abstr 3503)

Tse C et al (2008) ABT-263: a potent and orally bioavailable Bcl-2 family inhibitor. Cancer Res 68:3421–3428

Unger C et al (2010) First-time-in-man and pharmacokinetic study of weekly oral perifosine in patients with solid tumours. Eur J Cancer 46:920–925

Vaishampayan UN et al (2010) Safety, efficacy, pharmacokinetics, and pharmacodynamics of the combination of sorafenib and tanespimycin. Clin Cancer Res 16(14):3795-3804

Van Cutsem E et al (2009) Cetuximab and chemotherapy as initial treatment for metastatic colorectal cancer. N Engl J Med 360:1408–1417

Van Ummersen L et al (2004) A phase I trial of perifosine (NSC 639966) on a loading dose/maintenance dose schedule in patients with advanced cancer. Clin Cancer Res 10:7450–7456

Vassilev LT et al (2004) In vivo activation of the p53 pathway by small-molecule antagonists of MDM2. Science 303:844–848

Vaux DL, Cory S, Adams JM (1988) BCL-2 gene promotes hematopoietic-cell survival and cooperates with c-MYC to immortalize pre-B-cells. Nature 335:440–442

Vecil GG, Lang FF (2003) Clinical trials of adenoviruses in brain tumors: a review of Ad-p53 and oncolytic adenoviruses. J Neurooncol 65:237–246

Vita M, Henriksson M (2006) The Myc oncoprotein as a therapeutic target for human cancer. Semin Cancer Biol 16:318–330

Vivanco I, Sawyers CL (2002) The phosphatidylinositol 3-Kinase AKT pathway in human cancer. Nat Rev Cancer 2:489–501

Vlahos CJ, Matter WF, Hui KY, Brown RF (1994) A specific inhibitor of phosphatidylinositol 3-kinase, 2-(4-morpholinyl)-8-phenyl-4H-1-benzopyran-4-one (LY294002). J Biol Chem 269:5241–5248

Vogel CL et al (2002) Efficacy and safety of trastuzumab as a single agent in first-line treatment of HER2-overexpressing metastatic breast cancer. J Clin Oncol 20:719–726

Von Hoff DD, LoRusso P, Tibes R, Shapiro G, Weiss GJ, Ware JA, Fredrickson J, Mazina KE, Levy GG, Wagner AJ, Virginia G (2010) Piper cancer center and TGen, scottsdale, AZ; karmanos a first-in-human phase I study to evaluate the pan-PI3K inhibitor GDC-0941 administered QD or BID in patients with advanced solid tumors. in ASCO. J Clin Oncol 28:15s (suppl; abstr 2541)

Wang H, Oliver P, Zhang Z, Agrawal S, Zhang R (2003) Chemosensitization and radiosensitization of human cancer by antisense anti-MDM2 oligonucleotides. Ann N Y Acad Sci 1002:217–235

Wang MY et al (2006) Mammalian target of rapamycin inhibition promotes response to epidermal growth factor receptor kinase inhibitors in PTEN-deficient and PTEN-intact glioblastoma cells. Cancer Res 66:7864–7869

Wang Y et al (2010) A fully human insulin-like growth factor-I receptor antibody SCH 717454 (Robatumumab) has antitumor activity as a single agent and in combination with cytotoxics in pediatric tumor xenografts. Mol Cancer Ther 9:410–418

Ward Y et al (2001) Signal pathways which promote invasion and metastasis: critical and distinct contributions of extracellular signal-regulated kinase and ral-specific guanine exchange factor pathways. Mol Cell Biol 21:5958–5969

Watkins DJ et al (2009) A phase II study of the anti-IGFR antibody MK-0646 in combination with cetuximab and irinotecan in the treatment of chemorefractory metastatic colorectal cancer. J Clin Oncol (Meeting Abstracts) 27:4127

Watters JW, Huang PS (2009) Can phenotypic pathway signatures improve the prediction of response to PI3K pathway inhibitors? Drug Discov Today: Therapeutic Strategies 6:57–62

Wedén S et al (2010) Long-term follow-up of patients with resected pancreatic cancer following vaccination against mutant K-ras. Int J Cancer 9999

Welch Set al (2007) UCN-01 in combination with topotecan in patients with advanced recurrent ovarian cancer: a study of the Princess Margaret Hospital phase II consortium. Gynecol Oncol 106:305–310

Welcsh PL, King M-C (2001) BRCA1 and BRCA2 and the genetics of breast and ovarian cancer. Hum Mol Genet 10:705–713

Wellbrock C, Hurlstone A (2010) BRAF as therapeutic target in melanoma. Biochemical Pharmacology 80:561–567

Wen PY, Prados M, Schiff D, Reardon DA, Cloughesy T, Mikkelsen T, Batchelor T, Drappatz J, Chamberlain MC, De Groot JF (2010) Phase II study of XL184 (BMS 907351), an inhibitor of MET, VEGFR2, and RET, in patients (pts) with progressive glioblastoma (GB). in American Society of Clinical Oncology. J Clin Oncol 28:15s (suppl; abstr 2006)

Werner H, Roberts CT (2003) The IGFI receptor gene: a molecular target for disrupted transcription factors. Genes Chromosomes and Cancer 36:113–120

Westhoff MA et al (2009) The pyridinylfuranopyrimidine inhibitor, PI-103, chemosensitizes glioblastoma cells for apoptosis by inhibiting DNA repair. Oncogene 28:3586–3596

Wiman KG (2007) Restoration of wild-type p53 function in human tumors: strategies for efficient cancer therapy. Adv Cancer Res 97:321–338

Wooster R et al (1995) Identification of the breast cancer susceptibility gene BRCA2. Nature 378:789–792

Workman P, Clarke PA, Raynaud FI, van Montfort RL (2010) Drugging the PI3 kinome: from chemical tools to drugs in the clinic. Cancer Res 70:2146–2157

Workmann P, Burrows F, Neckers L, Rosen N (2007) Drugging the cancer chaperone HSP90. Ann N Y Acad Sci 1113:202–216

Wullschleger S, Loewith R, Hall MN (2006) TOR signaling in growth and metabolism. Cell 124:471–484

Wyman K et al (2006) Multicenter phase II trial of high-dose imatinib mesylate in metastatic melanoma. Cancer 106:2005–2011

Yaguchi S-i et al (2006) Antitumor activity of ZSTK474, a new Phosphatidylinositol 3-kinase inhibitor. J Natl Cancer Inst 98:545–556

Yang L et al (2004) Akt/protein kinase B signaling inhibitor-2, a selective small molecule inhibitor of Akt signaling with antitumor activity in cancer cells overexpressing Akt. Cancer Res 64:4394–4399

Yao E et al (2009) Suppression of HER2/HER3-mediated growth of breast cancer cells with combinations of GDC-0941 PI3K inhibitor, trastuzumab, and pertuzumab. Clin Cancer Res 15:4147–4156

Yarden Y, Sliwkowski MX (2001) Untangling the ErbB signalling network. Nat Rev Mol Cell Biol 2:127–137

Yu EY et al (2009) Phase II study of dasatinib in patients with metastatic castration-resistant prostate cancer. Clin Cancer Res 15:7421–7428

Yu J, Zhang L, Hwang PM, Kinzler KW, Vogelstein B (2001) PUMA induces the rapid apoptosis of colorectal cancer cells. Mol Cell 7:673–682

Yu K et al (2010) Beyond rapalog therapy: preclinical pharmacology and antitumor activity of WYE-125132, an ATP-competitive and specific inhibitor of mTORC1 and mTORC2. Cancer Res 70:621–631

Yuan TL, Cantley LC (2008) PI3K pathway alterations in cancer: variations on a theme. Oncogene 27:5497–5510

Zangemeister-Wittke U et al (2000) A novel bispecific antisense oligonucleotide inhibiting both bcl-2 and bcl-xL expression efficiently induces apoptosis in tumor cells. Clin Cancer Res 6:2547–2555

Zeimet AG, Marth C (2003) Why did p53 gene therapy fail in ovarian cancer? Lancet Oncol 4:415–422

Zeng X, Buck E, Yee D (2009) A Type I insulin-like growth factor receptor kinase inhibitor (PQIP) enhances the cytotoxicity of doxorubicin in human cancer cell lines. In thirty-second annual CTRC-AACR San Antonio breast cancer symposium (Cancer Research 69 (Meeting Abstract Supplement), 6110, San Antonio, TX, 2009)

Zhang S, Yu D (2010) PI(3)King Apart PTEN's Role in Cancer. Clin Cancer Res 16(17):4325–4330

Chapter 28
Metastasis Initiation

Dana Faingold, Dawn Russell-Hermanns and Silvin Bakalian

Metastasis initiation genes are involved in tumor cell motility, invasion and angiogenesis contributing to the dissemination of tumor cells in the circulation. The initiation and progression of tumors depend on oncogene activation and loss or inactivation of tumor suppressor genes at both the primary and metastatic sites. Processes associated with the initiation of metastasis challenge tumor cells during local invasion, angiogenesis, circulation and metastatic niche formation. Most functions for the initiation of both the tumor and metastasis remain essential for cancer cells to continue their metastatic development (Chiang and Massagué 2008).

28.1 Angiogenesis

Angiogenesis supports the primary tumor blood supply, vasculogenic mimicry and provides an escape route by which cells can intravasate into the body's circulatory blood system. After survival into circulation the cells extravasate and initiate formation of the pre-angiogenic micrometastases followed by the development of new blood vessels (Eccles 2004). New vessel formation arises in the hypoxic environment of the tumor which stimulates the synthesis of HIF in the endothelial cells resulting in the production of VEGF that promotes endothelial cell proliferation, migration, survival, expression of adhesion molecules, and increased vascular permeability (Liao and Johnson 2007; Bergers and Benjamin 2003; Carmeliet and Jain 2000). Tumor cells modulate angiogenesis by producing VEGF-A which binds to VEGFR 1 and 2 as well as other angiogenic factors such as placenta growth factor

D. Faingold (✉) · S. Bakalian
Department of Pathology, Henry C. Witelson Ocular Pathology Laboratory, McGill University, Montreal, QC, Canada
e-mail: faingolddana@yahoo.com

S. Bakalian
e-mail: sbakalian@hotmail.com

D. Russell-Hermanns
Henry C.Witelson Ocular Pathology Laboratory, McGill University, Montreal, QC, Canada

J. V. Burnier, M. N. Burnier, Jr. (eds.), *Experimental and Clinical Metastasis*,
DOI 10.1007/978-1-4614-3685-0_28, © Springer Science+Business Media New York 2013

Table 28.1 Anti-VEGF treatment with monoclonal antibodies

Inhibitor	Specificity	Selected tumor types
Bevacizumab antibody	VEGF-A	Approved for colon, breast, NSCLC, GBM
Aflibercept Fusion molecule	VEGF	Prostate cancer, NSCLC, colorectal, and pancreatic cancer
HuMV833 antibody	VEGF-A	Phase I clinical trials
IMCL-1121b (ramucirumab) antibody	VEGFR-2	Breast, colorectal, NSCLC, ovary, prostate, RCC, HCC, melanoma

(PlGF) and VEGFB. These bind to VEGFR1, VEGFC and VEGFD which primarily interact with VEGFR3 stimulating lymphangiogenesis (Ferrara 2004). Hypoxia also promotes neoangiogenesis via HIF-1α which signals through PI3K and MAPK pathways. Hypoxia induces transcriptional activation of uPA, and CXCR4 and influences adhesion, matrix degradation and invasion (Kerbel 2008).

Malignant, stromal or inflammatory cells produce angiogenic factors that stimulate the endothelial cells to proliferate and promote new-vessel formation in tumors. The VEGF pathway contributes to the migratory potential of endothelial cells through induction of proteolytic enzymes such as MMP-2, MMP-9, and uPA (Ferrara and Kerbel 2005).

Anti-VEGF therapy induces cytostatic effects and transient normalization of the tumor vasculature, rendering it more vulnerable to therapy (Table 28.1, Jain 2005).

Antiangiogenic agents: monoclonal antibodies Monoclonal antibodies prevent receptor activation by binding directly to the ligand and were demonstrated to suppress tumor growth and angiogenesis in several studies (Chung et al. 2010; Kim et al. 1993; Gerber and Ferrara 2005). In a large, randomized, double-blind, phase III study the combination between bevacizumab (Avastin®), (a humanized variant of a VEGF-A monoclonal antibody) with irinotecan, 5FU and leucovorin (IFL), showed statistically significant improvement in terms of PFS and overall survival. The study was conducted in patients with metastatic colorectal cancer and clearly established the efficacy of this anti-VEGF antibody in first-line therapy (Hurwitz et al. 2004). The Eastern Cooperative Oncology Group (ECOG) trial evaluated the addition of bevacizumab to FOLFOX (5-FU, LV, oxaliplatin) in colorectal cancer patients and showed increased PFS, overall suvival, and response rates leading to the approval of bevacizumab in combination with chemotherapy in the second-line setting (Giantonio 2007).

The ECOG phase III trial E4599 in patients with NSCLC, randomized 878 stage IIIB/IV patients comparing bevacizumab and chemotherapy with chemotherapy alone. The results showed evidence of improvement in median overall sruvival of more than 12 months in the bevacizumab arm. Hence, bevacizumab in combination with carboplatin and paclitaxel chemotherapy was approved for patients with NSCLC (Sandler 2006). In a phase III clinical trial of patients with metastatic breast cancer, whereby the participants were randomized to receive paclitaxel with or without bevacizumab, the results showed that bevacizumab in combination with paclitaxel improved survival in women with previously untreated metastatic breast cancer (Miller 2007). Several other clinical trials are currently under way studying the use of bevacizumab in the treatment of RCC. The study demonstrated the favourable effects of bevacizumab in a randomized phase II trial in these patients (Yang 2003). Encouraging results are also emerging for other cancers, indicating that the antiangiogenic approach with bevacizumab may have wider applicability, such as in ovarian cancer (Cannistra 2007; Burger et al. 2007) and glioblastoma multiforme (Vredenburgh 2007).

HuMV833, a recombinant humanized IgG4 anti- VEGF monoclonal antibody, demonstrated tolerability, safety and some clinical activity in patients with advanced cancer in phase I studies (Jayson 2005). Several other antibodies targeting VEGF receptors are being clinically pursued. Specifically, fusion soluble receptors such as VEGF-trap (aflibercept), a decoy receptor protein is currently being investigated. This agent is the product of the fusion of the Ig extracellular domains of both VEGFR-1 and VEGFR-2 with the Fc fragment of an antibody that has a high affinity for VEGF-A. The results have been favourable in phase I studies in solid tumors (Tew 2008; Rixe 2006) and is currently being evaluated in phase III trials in prostate cancer, NSCLC, colorectal, and pancreatic cancer (Chung et al. 2010; Grothey and Galanis 2009).

IMC-1121b (ramucirumab) is a fully human monoclonal IgG1 antibody which blocks ligand binding of VEGF-R2. Ramucirumab exhibited good tolerability and safety in phase I clinical trials (Camidge 2006) and therefore phase II clinical studies are now underway for advanced liver, kidney, prostate, ovarian, colorectal, NSCLC and malignant melanoma. This agent has also been evaluated in a phase III clinical trial of docetaxel with or without IMC-1121b as first-line therapy in advanced breast cancer (Ferrara and Kerbel 2005; Grothey and Galanis 2009).

Tyrosine kinase inhibitors Tyrosine kinase inhibitors (TKIs) target the ligand-dependent receptor and inhibit kinase activity by competing with ATP in the tyrosine kinase catalytic domain. Several tyrosine kinase receptors are targets for antiangiogenic therapy for example VEGFR, FGFR, PDGFR and Tie-2 (Morin 2000). The use of anti-VEGF receptor TKIs yielded encouraging results in various advanced cancers such as metastatic colorectal cancer, metastatic NSCLC, metastatic breast cancer, RCC, HCC and recurrent glioblastoma (Table 28.2, Jain 2009).

Sunitinib (SU11248/Sutent; Pfizer), is a multi-targeted TKI having anti-angiogenic and anti growth tumor activities. This is achieved through the selective inhibition of VEGFR2, PDGFR, Kit, Flt3, and REarranged during Transfection (RET) tyrosine kinases. Studies have demonstrated its definitive efficacy in metastatic RCC and in a randomized phase III study assessing sunitinib in the treatment of imatinib-resistant GIST. Currently a phase III clinical study investigates the effect of sunitinib in combination with erlotinib in advanced, platinum-refractory NSCLC (Scagliotti and Govindan 2010).

Another FDA-approved anti-angiogenic agent for cancer treatment is sorafenib (BAY 43-9006, Nexavar®), a TKI that inhibits RAF serine/threonine kinases and receptor tyrosine kinases involved in tumor growth and angiogenesis. This agent acts on the intracellular domain of VEGFR1, VEGFR2, VEGFR3, PDGF receptor

Table 28.2 Examples of anti-VEGF receptor tyrosine kinase inhibitors

Inhibitor	Specificity	Selected tumor types
Sunitinib (SU11248/Sutent; Pfizer)	VEGFR2, PDGFR, Kit, Flt3, RET	RCC, phase III GIST and NSCLC
Sorafenib (BAY 43-9006, Nexavar®)	VEGFR1, VEGFR2, VEGFR3, PDGF receptor β, FLT3, RAF, and c-KIT	Advanced RCC, Approved for HCC
Vatalanib (PTK787; Novartis/Schering AG)	VEGFR1, VEGFR2, VEGFR3, PDGFR- and c-KIT	Phase II/III trials in metastatic colorectal cancer and NSCLC
Vandetanib (Zactima®, ZD6474; AstraZeneca Pharmaceuticals)	VEGFR-2, EGFR, and RET	Phase III clinical trials in NSCLC
Axitinib (AG-013736; Pfizer Inc.)	VEGFR2, PDGF receptor and c-KIT	NSCLC, RCC
Motesanib diphosphonate (Amgen)	VEGFR-1, VEGFR-2, VEGFR -3, RET and c-KIT	Progressive medullary thyroid carcinoma, GIST
Pazopanib (Votrient, GW786034)	VEGFR-1, VEGFR-2 VEGFR-3, PDGF-α, PDGF-β, and c-KIT	Phase III clinical trial in metastatic RCC

β, FMS-like tyrosine kinase 3 (FLT3), RAF, and c-KIT. Phase III data indicate that sorafenib monotherapy results in an increase in median overall survival and a significant increase in PFS in patients with advanced RCC. Sorafenib was also approved for use in HCC after results of an international phase III clinical trial in HCC patients receiving sorafenib had extended survival (Lang 2008).

Vatalanib (PTK787; Novartis/Schering AG) targets VEGFR1, VEGFR2, VEGFR3, PDGFR- and c-KIT. It is currently being studied in phase II/III trials in metastatic colorectal cancer and NSCLC. Encouraging data from a phase II trial examining vatalanib monotherapy administered once or twice daily in previously treated patients with NSCLC have been reported (Scagliotti and Govindan 2010). Vatalanib was investigated in the treatment of metastatic colorectal cancer in double-blind, placebo-controlled, phase III studies: Colorectal Oral Novel Therapy for the Inhibition of Angiogenesis and Retarding of Metastases in First-line (CONFIRM-1 and 2) trials. These trials investigated the effect of 5-FU, leucovorin, and oxaliplatin, (FOLFOX-4) chemotherapy with or without vatalanib as second-line therapy of patients with metastatic colorectal cancer. Although the primary objectives were not achieved in these trials, the PFS time was significantly longer in the vatalanib arm in patients with high LDH levels (Los et al. 2007; Scott et al. 2007).

Another therapeutic approach involves Vandetanib (Zactima®, ZD6474; AstraZeneca Pharmaceuticals) which is an orally available, ATP-mimetic small molecule that inhibits VEGFR-2, EGFR, and RET-tyrosine kinases. Four randomized phase III clinical trials in NSCLC were exploring the efficacy of vandetanib as monotherapy or in combination with chemotherapeutic agents such as docetaxel or emetrexed in NSCLC (Morabito et al. 2009). Preliminary data reported an acceptable safety profile and a modest improvement in the primary endpoint (PFS), however, this agent didn't significantly improve overall survival (Scagliotti and Govindan 2010; Herbst et al. 2010).

Axitinib (AG-013736; Pfizer Inc.) is an anti-VEGFR- TKI, which also acts on PDGFRs and KIT. It has shown dose-dependent antitumor efficacy associated with the blockage of VEGFR-2 phosphorylation in multiple solid tumor settings (Hu-Lowe et al. 2008). Results from a phase II clinical trial with axitinib in patients with advanced NSCLC showed that it was well tolerated (Schiller 2009). There are currently other studies evaluating axitinib in combination with chemotherapy such as those involving nonsquamous NSCLC patients (Scagliotti and Govindan 2010) and others in patients with metastatic RCC with favorable results so far (Rixe et al. 2007).

Motesanib diphosphonate is yet another multi-kinase inhibitor of VEGFR-1, VEGFR-2, VEGFR -3, RET and c-KIT. In patients with progressive medullary thyroid carcinoma, this drug has shown moderate potential with respect to overall disease stability and response rates. (Sherman 2009).

Pazopanib (Votrient, GW786034) is a multi-targeted TKI against VEGFR-1, VEGFR-2 and VEGFR-3, PDGF-α, PDGF-β, and c-KIT. It demonstrated antitumor activity in multiple tumor settings (Sonpavde and Hutson 2007; Bukowski et al. 2010). Pazopanib therapy was well tolerated in a phase II clinical trial in patients with RCC and results from a Phase III clinical trial in metastatic RCC showed clinical activity (Limvorasak and Posadas 2009; Sternberg et al. 2010).

Other multitargeted broad-spectrum TKIs that target the proliferation of metastasis were shown to have indirect antiangiogenic effects (Jain et al. 2006). These agents include lapatinib, (Moy et al. 2007), trastuzumab (Izumi et al. 2002) imatinib (Jain 2005; Stegmeier et al. 2010) and canertinib (CI-1033). Canertinib is a pan-ERB TKI which demonstrated clinically activity in NSCLC (Janne et al. 2007).

Combination therapy with these agents has gained interest and is currently under investigation in certain clinical trials. There have been promising reports of its activity in a randomized phase II trial in patients with previously treated NSCLC using the combination of bevacizumab and erlotinib (Herbst and Sandler 2008). Additionally, cetuximab has shown evidence of antitumor activity in NSCLC and was studied in combination with bevacizumab in a phase II Southwest Oncology Group (SWOG) trial (Scagliotti and Govindan 2010). However, in phase II-III clinical trials in metastatic colorectal cancer, the combined use of cetuximab, panitumumab and bevacizumab had a negative effect on the primary end point (PFS) compared with the arm without the addition of an anti-EGFR antibody (Tol et al. 2009).

Angiogenesis inhibitors have proven themselves with regard to improvement in progression-free or overall survival in a number of malignancies (Table 28.2). However it is unfortunate that with these agents there always remains the threat of eventual drug tolerance and potential side effects. The reported adverse effects of angiogenesis inhibitors are hypertension, fatigue, arterial thromboembolic events, gastrointestinal perforations, impaired wound healing and life-threatening or fatal hemorrhage (Jain et al. 2006). The mechanisms by which these drugs mediate their antitumor effect are not well understood and predictive markers for the efficacy of anti-VEGF therapy have yet to be identified, attesting to the complexity of inhibiting the tumor angiogenic cascade.

28.2 Epithelial Mesenchymal Transition

28.2.1 EMT and Cancer Stem Cells

Motility, intravasation and progression towards metastasis are facilitated by epithelial-to-mesenchymal transition (EMT). This is a process enabled by the loss of E-cadherin (Thiery et al. 2002; Iwatsuki et al. 2010). EMT can be controlled by different signaling pathways such as TGF-β, PI3-AKT and RAS-MAP kinase pathways. Other factors that control this pathway include IGF1R, FGFR, MET and SRC family kinases (Huber et al. 2005).

Transcriptional repressors of the E-cadherin gene (***CDH1***), such as zinc finger proteins (ZEB1, ZEB2), bHLH protein (Twist), and the snail family of zinc finger proteins (Snail, Slug) are inducers of EMT. They are involved in several processes that result in loss of E-cadherin as well as cell–cell junctions resulting in early invasion and metastasis (Thiery 2002; Huber et al. 2005; Tse and Kalluri 2007). Their activity is regulated by cellular pathways known to be involved in EMT such as TGFβ, β-catenin, Wnt signaling pathways, Notch and NF-kappaB-dependent pathways (Voulgari and Pintzas 2009). EMT was linked to the migration of cells from a primary tumor into the circulation and also to the later stages of metastasis (Huber et al. 2005).

Cancer stem cells represent a small population of undifferentiated cells with self-renewal properties that were identified in a variety of solid tumors (Al-Hajj et al. 2003; O/'Brien et al. 2007). This population of cells displays embryonic EMT characteristics and they are signaling through pathways that are found in normal stem cells, such as Wnt, Notch, and Hedgehog. It has been suggested that EMT in tumors could induce the formation of an invasive undifferentiated population of cells, stem cells, which are resistant to anoikis (Mani et al. 2008; Onder et al. 2008). Stem cells were demonstrated to generate different types of tumors including metastases in xenograft immune-deficient mice. Therapeutic targeting of cancer stem cells and development of agents that target critical steps in the Wnt, Notch, and Hedgehog pathways have been proven to inhibit metastasis (Takebe et al. 2011).

The acquisition of a migratory and invasive phenotype during the EMT program may lead to metastatic progression. Therefore, targeting this pathway is representative of yet another viable strategy in the overall management of metastatic disease. EMT-related pathways provide targets such as β-catenin and the transcription factors—Slug, Snail and Twist.

There are various techniques of targeting EMT. One example is the use of antisense oligonucleotides complementary to a specific miRNA (antagomirs) (Krutzfeldt et al. 2005). Other strategies aim to reverse the EMT phenotype utilizing short hairpin RNA (shRNA) delivered to the cancer cells in order to target Snail. In one study, blockage of Snail function induced a mesenchymal-to-epithelial transition (MET) phenotype and also resulted in the up-regulation of E-cadherin (Olmeda et al. 2006).

The blockade of oncogenic cascades with trastuzumab, gefitinib and/or erlotinib also contributes to the inhibition of EMT. Additional pathways that could be targeted include TGF-β, SRC, Wnt/β-catenin, Notch, Hedgehog and NF-kappaB, which all show great potential that their inhibition may actually prevent tumor cells from gaining an invasive phenotype.

Stem cells are representing another way of targeting EMT. Two techniques that have been employed for this purpose include the activation of monoclonal antibodies directed towards CD44 positive cells (Jin et al. 2006) by using promoter-controlled oncolytic viruses. These viruses were shown to have significant antitumor activity in CD44+CD24−/low–derived tumors (Bauerschmitz et al. 2008). Current evidence indicates that systemically administered stem/progenitor cells migrate to and infiltrate primary and metastatic solid tumors. This modality can be used to deliver therapeutic genes selectively to tumor foci. (Aboody et al. 2008)

28.2.2 Transforming Growth Factor Beta Signaling

Transforming growth factor beta (TGF-β) is a cytokine that participates in a number of functions including cell proliferation, survival and immune-surveillance. Early in the development of tumors, TGF-β acts as a tumor suppressor, inhibiting cell proliferation and inducing pro-apoptotic effects. It achieves this by down-regulation of genes encoding c-Myc and up-regulation of CDK- inhibitors (Derynck et al. 2001). In the later stages of tumorigenesis TGF-β is involved in metastatic invasion and colonization of secondary organs promoting angiogenesis, EMT, motility, migration, and homing (Iwatsuki et al. 2010; Padua and Massague 2009).

Therapeutic strategies involving TGF-β include ligand trap monoclonal TGF-β-neutralising antibodies, which were proven effective in reducing the biological activity of TGF-β. A human IgG4 pan-specific monoclonal antibody, GC-1008 (CAT/Genzyme), was shown to neutralize TGF-β. A Phase I/II study of GC-1008 in patients with advanced malignant melanoma or RCC was well tolerated and this agent is currently being evaluated in Phase II studies for patients with metastatic melanoma (Morris et al. 2008).

Antisense technology is being applied with the use of AP12009 (trabedersen), a drug which mediates inhibition of TGF-β2 gene expression. It has been shown to be effective in anaplastic astrocytoma and showed signs of early clinical activity when delivered locally to the tumor in patients with high-grade gliomas (Hau et al. 2009). This therapeutic agent is currently under assessment in a Phase III clinical trial in patients with recurrent or refractory anaplastic astrocytoma following standard radio- and chemotherapy (Hau et al. 2009). It has also been evaluated in phase I and II clinical trials for patients with recurrent or refractory high-grade gliomas, advanced pancreatic carcinoma, metastatic melanoma and metastatic colorectal carcinoma (Schlingensiepen et al. 2006, 2008).

Other therapeutic modalities include small molecule inhibitors of TGF-β receptors (TGF-β RI/II). The novel inhibitor LY2109761, a TGF-βRI kinase inhibitor, was shown to inhibit metastases in xenograft models of pancreatic (Melisi et al. 2008) and breast cancer (Ganapathy et al. 2010). LY2157299 dose escalation studies were safe and well tolerated in a Phase I clinical trial in patients with advanced metastatic malignancies (Calvo-Aller et al. 2008).

28.2.3 Src Signaling Pathways

Src is a non-receptor cytoplasmic tyrosine kinase critical in regulating cell survival and reorganization of the cytoskeleton. It is considered an integral part of metastatic colonization and the invasion pathway (Guarino 2010). Drugs targeting the inhibition of Src and its network effectively prevent the growth of cells undergoing EMT. An example of such an agent is the small molecule inhibitor Dasatinib, which acts by reducing adhesion, proliferation and migration of tumor cells in colorectal cancer, breast cancer and melanoma cells. This drug is currently being investigated in clinical trials in patients with metastatic breast cancer. Encouraging results of dasatinib activity have emerged from a phase II study in patients with metastatic prostate cancer. Moreover, the ability of this agent to also inhibit BCR-ABL has led to its approval for the treatment of imatinib-resistant CML and ALL (Giles et al. 2009).

Another agent, SKI-606 (bosutinib), which is a Src/ABL kinase inhibitor, was proven to have anti-migratory and anti-invasive effects in prostate cancer cells (Rabbani et al. 2010). This drug is currently enrolled in clinical trials for breast cancer and CML. Preclinical studies with AZD0530 (saracatinib), a dual-specific inhibitor of Src showed that this drug resulted in reduced motility and invasion of tumor cells (Vries et al. 2009). Furthermore this compound was well tolerated in phase I clinical trials at doses that resulted in significant inhibition of Src activity (Tabernero et al. 2007) and is currently under evaluation in Phase II clinical trials in patients with advanced metastatic stomach, gastroesophageal junction and ovarian cancer[1].

Other compounds such as KX2–391, a small molecule that targets the protein substrate-binding site on Src has been shown to have preliminary evidence of biological activity in patients with advanced malignancies (Adjei et al. 2009). It is currently under evaluation in a phase II clinical trial in patients with metastatic prostate cancer.

28.2.4 NF-KappaB

The nuclear factor-κB, (NFκB) promotes the oncogenic phenotype through aberrant regulation of BCL-2, BCL-xl, cIAP (integrin associated protein), survivin, TRAF

[1] NIH's ClinicalTrials.gov. Available from (http://www.clinicaltrials.gov/) and ClinicalTrialsFeeds.org (http://www.clinicaltrialsfeeds.org/) web sites.

(TNF receptor associated factor) and COX-2 (Shen and Tergaonkar 2009; Basseres and Baldwin 2006; Mantovani 2010). Also, the NFκB-dependent pathway is required for the induction and maintenance of EMT through regulation of the vascular cell adhesion molecules -MMPs, CXCR4, and uPA. Therefore, this pathway has a key role in promoting angiogenesis, invasion and metastatic colonization (Basseres and Baldwin 2006; Huber et al. 2004).

Preclinical studies have shown that blockage of NFκB activity in highly metastatic human prostate cancer cells affects proliferation, angiogenesis and also causes inhibition of metastasis in a nude mouse model (Huang et al. 2001). Also, re-expression of NFκB inhibitors (microRNA-146a and microRNA-146b), was shown to reduce the metastatic potential in a human breast cancer cell line (Bhaumik et al. 2008).

The NFκB pathway is an important target in clinical studies. A large number of compounds including steroids, non-steroidal anti-inflammatory drugs (NSAIDs), antioxidants and cell permeable peptides have been shown to contribute to the blockade of NFκB activation (Shen and Tergaonkar 2009; Basseres and Baldwin 2006; Baldwin 2001; Gilmore and Herscovitch 2006). Preclinical studies have shown that natural small molecule NFκB pathway inhibitors such as curcumin (Aggarwal et al. 2005), genistein (Li et al. 2005) resveratrol (Bhardwaj et al. 2007) and parthenolide (Sweeney et al. 2005) enhance the apoptotic effects and overall therapeutic activity when combined with chemotherapy and radiotherapy.

Alternative options that target IκB have shown apoptotic activity and antitumor effects in hematological malignancies, prostate cancer cells (Yemelyanov et al. 2005) and in melanoma xenograft models (Yang et al. 2006b).

The NKκB inhibitors discussed so far in this section have only been investigated in pre-clinical trials. Newer agents that specifically target the proteasome, IκB (inhibitor-κB kinase) as well as activation of NF-κB are now under investigation in humans. The synthetic small molecule proteasome inhibitor, Bortezomib (Velcade, Millennium Pharmaceuticals) inhibits NFκB activation in a dose-dependent manner by blocking proteasome-mediated degradation of the NFκB inhibitor, IκB. Bortezomib is currently approved for the treatment of multiple myeloma (MM) (Richardson et al. 2004). Unfortunately, Bortezomib failed to exhibit sufficient clinical activity in patients with metastatic melanoma (Markovic et al. 2005), colon (Mackay et al. 2005) and breast carcinomas (Yang et al. 2006a). It generated modest results in patients with prostate cancer (Papandreou et al. 2004) and RCC (Davis et al. 2004). A number of phase I and II clinical trials demonstrated superior results of the combination of Bortezomib with radiotherapy in patients with HNSCC (Carter et al. 2005). Phase I clinical trials in recurrent ovarian cancer confirmed the safety of the combination of bortezomib with carboplatin (Aghajanian et al. 2005) and similar results were observed in patients with advanced solid tumors (Voortman et al. 2007). In a phase II clinical trial in patients with advanced NSCLC, bortezomib in combination with gemcitabine and carboplatin resulted in improved survival (Davies et al. 2009). Additionally, results from a trial investigating the combination of tanespimycin with bortezomib in patients with MM reported that the drug was well tolerated and demonstrated clinical activity (Taldone et al. 2008; Richardson et al. 2010).

28.2.5 Hedgehog Signaling Pathways

The Hedgehog signaling pathway is one of the key regulators of the stem-cell during embryonic development. Mutation, deregulation and aberrant activation of this pathway has been linked to malignancy in multiple types of human cancer including brain tumors, BCC, pancreatic adenocarcinoma, SCLC, breast and prostate cancer (Magliano and Hebrok 2003). Members of the Hedgehog family bind to Patched1 and Patched2 transmembrane receptors. This inhibits the repression of another transmembrane protein, Smoothened (Smo) by Patched complex.The release of Smo initiates a signalling cascade and transcriptional activation of target genes occurs through the GLI family of proteins (Ruiz i Altaba et al. 2002).

Activation of the Hedgehog pathway in tumors leads to an increase in Snail protein expression and a decrease in E-cadherin. These events contribute to acquisition of a migratory and invasive phenotype and metastatic progression. Moreover, the Hedgehog pathway has been implicated in the regulation of angiogenesis and survival and self-renewal of cancer stem cells (Dai 2009). Therefore, targeting this pathway is representative of yet another viable strategy in the overall management of metastatic disease. Different therapeutic targets including Smoothened (Smo), sonic hedgehog protein (Shh), and Gli are currently under investigation.

Hedgehog signaling inhibitor cyclopamine, is a small-molecule inhibitor acting by direct binding to the transmembrane Smo receptor. This compound was shown to inhibit EMT and metastases in pancreatic cancer cell lines (Cooper et al. 1998). A cyclopamine derived inhibitor IPI-926 (Infinity Pharmaceuticals), entered phase I clinical trials for trials for advanced and metastatic cancer (NCT00761696)[2].

Several other small-molecule Smo inhibitors are currently in clinical trials. The administration of GDC-0449 (Genentech) was well tolerated in patients with advanced solid tumors. In a cohort of 33 patients with locally advanced or metastatic BCC, treated with GDC-0449 the response rate for was 55 % (Hoff et al. 2009). Phase I- II trials are evaluating the efficacy of GDC-0449 alone or in different therapeutic combinations in patients with ovarian cancer, advanced colorectal cancer, advanced BCC recurrent medulloblastoma, advanced pancreatic carcinoma, gastric carcinoma, prostate carcinoma and SCLC (Peukert and Miller-Moslin 2010; Low and Sauvage 2010).

BMS-833923 (Bristol–Myers Squibb, Exelixis) an oral hedgehog pathway antagonist was evaluated BMS-833923 (XL139), in patients with advanced or metastatic solid tumors. This agent is currently tested in multiple myeloma small-cell lung cancer and in metastatic gastric and esophageal adenocarcinoma (Low and Sauvage 2010).

In preclinical studies, blockade of aberrant Hedgehog signalling was achieved with the orally bio-available small-molecule Hedgehog inhibitor, IPI-269609, which induced Snail down-regulation and up-regulation of E-cadherin. Additionally, this

---

[2] NIH's ClinicalTrials.gov. Available from (http://www.clinicaltrials.gov/) and ClinicalTrials-Feeds.org (http://www.clinicaltrialsfeeds.org/) web sites.

drug inhibited systemic metastases in orthotopic xenografts established from human pancreatic cancer cell lines (Feldmann et al. 2008).

Several drugs such as RO4929097 (Roche) and MK0752 (Merck) which are targeting Notch cleavage or DLL4 ligand–receptor interaction are currently evaluated in phase I clinical trials (Takebe et al. 2011).

28.2.6 Wnt Pathway

Wnt (Wingless and Int-1 genes) signals through the β-catenin/T-cell factor-mediated pathway and has an important role in modulating cancer stem cell differentiation and EMT (Reya and Clevers 2005; Fodde and Brabletz 2007). The Wnt ligands, Frizzleds (Fzd) and low-density lipoprotein receptor–related proteins (LRP5 and LRP6), signal through the scaffold protein Axin and the tumor suppressor gene adenomatous polyposis coli (APC). In cancers, deregulation of this pathway results in axin destabilization and nuclear translocation of β-catenin and transcription of several oncogenes involved in proliferation and migration. Examples include c-MYC, cyclin D1, uPAR, MMPs, and EMT-associated target genes (Brabletz et al. 2005). β-catenin was shown to be mutated in approximately 50 % of colorectal cancers. It has been shown that colorectal cancer results from the inactivation of APC or axin (Fodde and Brabletz 2007).

The Wnt pathway is involved in the development of a broad range of human malignancies like melanoma (Alonso and Fuchs 2003), NSCLC (Giles et al. 2003), colorectal carcinoma (Fodde and Brabletz 2007) and breast cancer (Li et al. 2003).

Current strategies targeting Wnt signaling involve compounds that disrupt key components such as β-catenin and axin. These compounds include anti-sense, RNA-interference and protein knockdown strategies (Barker and Clevers 2006; Luo et al. 2007).

In preclinical models, the development of inhibitors of the Wnt pathway is underway. Targeting Wnt with recombinant adenoviral vectors carrying fusion proteins (WIF1-Fc and sFRP1-F) caused down-regulation of *E2F1*, *cyclin D1*, and *c-MYC*. It also promoted cell apoptosis in hepatocellular carcinoma cells and resulted in significant inhibition of xenograft tumors (Hu et al. 2009). At the extracellular level, the Wnt ligands can be targeted by a soluble Wnt receptor comprising the Frizzled8 cysteine-rich domain (CRD) fused to the human Fc domain (F8CRDhFc). This compound exhibited potent antitumor efficacy in teratoma cell lines and retarded the growth of tumor xenografts (Almeida et al. 2007)

High-throughput screening programs identified compounds that have the ability to induce degradation of β-catenin (Ewan et al. 2010; Chen et al. 2009). For example, ICG-001, a small molecule that down-regulates the β-catenin/T cell factor, induced apoptosis and tumor formation in xenograft models of colon cancer (Emami et al. 2004). The recently discovered small molecule, XAV939, stimulates β-catenin degradation by blocking tankyrase activity, which is required for degradation of axin. In preclinical studies XAV939 was shown to inhibit proliferation of APC-deficient

CRC cells (Huang et al. 2009a). A different compound, PKF115–584, was shown to disrupt the interaction of the β-catenin/TCF protein complex. In MM cells, this compound induced cytotoxicity and also reduced tumor growth in xenograft models (Sukhdeo et al. 2007).

NSAIDs were reported to target the Wnt pathway by inhibiting the Wnt target enzyme cyclooxygenase 2 (COX2) or by activating E-cadherin, possibly affecting the level of β-catenin. This supports the use of NSAIDS and selective COX inhibitors for reducing COX-induced prostaglandin levels in Wnt-driven cancers (Castellone et al. 2005).

28.3 Cell Motility and Invasion

28.3.1 MET

The *MET* proto-oncogene and its ligand hepatocyte growth factor (HGF) regulate genetic programs leading to cell proliferation, survival, motility, invasion and protection from apoptosis (Birchmeier et al. 2003). MET gene amplification and mutation, leading to receptor over-expression are associated with tumorigenesis and progression to metastatic disease in several human cancers (breast, lung, hepatocellular carcinoma, multiple myelomas and gliomas) (Migliore and Giordano 2008). Aberrant activation of the c-Met receptor and autocrine stimulation by its ligand, HGF, are involved in regulation of tumor angiogenesis. They also function through enhancement of the invasive growth program by interacting with plexins, integrin, FAK and Src signalling (Eder et al. 2009). Several methods to target the HGF/c-Met signalling pathway are under development including tyrosine kinase-ligand binding inhibitors and monoclonal antibodies (Table 28.3).

AMG102 an anti-HGF/SF-neutralizing antibody that has good pharmacokinetic and safety profiles resulting in antitumor activity when administered in combination with bevacizumab in patients with advanced solid tumors (Jun et al. 2007; Rosen et al. 2010). AMG 102 is currently in Phase II clinical trials against glioblastomas and advanced metastatic RCC.

PF-2341066 (crizotinib) (Pfizer) is a small molecule kinase inhibitor that targets the c-Met kinase catalytic domain and is also an anaplastic lymphoma kinase (Alk) selective inhibitor. Its overall effects are on tumor cell growth and anti-angiogenesis (Zou et al. 2007). This orally available c-Met inhibitor, demonstrated efficacy in reducing tumor burden and increasing survival in a preclinical model of metastatic ovarian cancer (Zillhardt et al. 2010) and is currently undergoing Phase I/II clinical trials in NSCLC.

EXEL-880 (Exelixis,) is a small-molecule kinase inhibitor that targets Met and members of the VEGF receptor tyrosine kinase family by inhibiting phosphorylation. In vivo, these effects were demonstrated in xenograft models of lung metastasis through inhibition of tumor cell proliferation, invasion and angiogenesis mediated by HGF and VEGF receptors. Phase I data indicate that EXEL-880 was well tolerated

Table 28.3 Inhibitors of HGF/c-Met signalling pathway

Inhibitor	Specificity	Selected tumor types
AMG102(Amgen)	HGF/SF	Phase II clinical trials in glioblastomas and renal cancer
PF-2341066 (crizotinib) (Pfizer)	c-Met and ALK inhibitor	Phase I Phase II-III in NSCLC
EXEL-880(Exelixis) Small molecule inhibitor	Met, VEGFR2	Phase I Phase II in papillary renal cancer, gastric and head and neck cancer
ARQ197(ArQule)	Met	Phase I advanced solid tumors Phase II in NSCLC and hepatocellular carcinoma

in patients with a range of solid tumors and partial responses of disease stabilization were reported. The drug is now in Phase II trials in papillary RCC, gastric cancer, and HNSLC (Qian et al. 2009). A different small molecule inhibitor, XL184 (Exelixis) has also been confirmed to exhibit clinical activity and inhibitory effects on both Met and VEGFR2 in patients with progressive glioblastoma (Wen et al. 2010).

ARQ 197(ArQule) is a highly selective small molecule inhibitor that binds to the Met receptor in a non-ATP competitive fashion. Data from phase I clinical trials in a variety of solid tumors have revealed early partial responses and signs of disease stabilization (Eder et al. 2009; Garcia et al. 2007). In a phase II clinical trial the combination between ARQ 197 and erlotinib has demonstrated a 66 % improvement in median progression-free survival (PFS) in patients with advanced, refractory NSCLC (Schiller et al. 2010).This compound is currently being evaluated in clinical trials as a single agent or in combination with other anti-cancer therapies in HCC (Borbath et al. 2010), pancreatic adenocarcinoma, breast cancer, germ cell tumors and CRC[3].

Another small molecule Met inhibitor that is currently under investigation in clinical trials is SGX523 (SGX Pharmaceuticals) which is an ATP-competitive inhibitor that demonstrated potent anti-tumor activity when administered orally in human tumor xenograft models (Buchanan et al. 2009). Unfortunately, the results of a phase II trial showed that patients treated with SGX523 exhibited compromised renal function (Diamond et al. 2010). Another example of these agents is MP470 (SuperGen) which is an oral multi-targeted tyrosine kinase inhibitor that demonstrated inhibitory activity against tyrosine kinase targets, including c-Met, c-Kit, PDGFRα, and mutant Flt-3 (Mita et al. 2009).

28.3.2 CXCR4

Chemokines are signaling molecules that induce the migration of cells toward a gradient. They have recently been implicated in tumor progression and metastasis

[3] NIH's ClinicalTrials.gov. Available from (http://www.clinicaltrials.gov/) and ClinicalTrialsFeeds.org (http://www.clinicaltrialsfeeds.org/) web sites.

(Payne and Cornelius 2002). The chemokine receptor, CXC chemokine receptor 4 (CXCR4) and its ligand CXCL12 (which is expressed in the lungs, liver and bone marrow) may play an important role in guiding disseminating cells to specific locations (Zlotnik and Yoshie 2000). Activation of CXCR4 by CXCL12 leads to the stimulation of a variety of intracellular signal transduction pathways and regulation of cellular survival. Examples include the phosphorylation of PI3K, FAK and the upregulation of MMP-2 and MMP-9 (Fernandis et al. 2004). Hypoxia induced CXCR4 is also upregulated by MET and EGFR.

CXCR4 and its endogenous ligand CXCL12 represent chemokine signaling systems that modulate important pathophysiological processes involved in metastasis. The interaction between CXCR4(expressed by tumor cells) and its ligand CXCL12 plays an important role in facilitating tumor cell migration towards secondary metastatic sites such as the lung, kidney, and bone (Vicari and Caux 2002). However, in addition to the CXCR4-CXCL12 axis, there are other chemokines involved in tumor cell progression supporting organ selectivity. Examples are the CCR7–CCL21/CCL19 axis involved in lymph node metastasis, CCR6 in liver metastasis, and CCL2 and CXCL8 in bone and skeleton metastasis. One of the most intensively reviewed interactions is the CXCL12–CXCR4 axis which has been proven to promote migration, adhesion and invasion of tumor cells (Balkwill 2004).

Disruption of CXCR4 signaling represents an exciting strategy for therapeutic intervention in cancer. Several CXCR4 inhibitors were developed and preclinical studies revealed that the inhibition of the CXCR4/CXCL12 axis significantly decreased the amount of metastasis seen in xenograft models of breast cancer (Muller et al. 2001), RCC, (Pan et al. 2006), HNSCL and in NSCLC (Belperio et al. 2004).

Antibodies to CXCR4 significantly reduced the total bone metastatic load in prostate cancer metastasis models (Wong and Korz 2008; Sun et al. 2005). Also recent studies indicated the possibility of blocking the expression of CXCR4 on the cell surface, with a novel recombinant chimeric protein, TAT/54R/KDE. This agent has been shown to inhibit metastasis mediated by CXCR4/CXCL12 interaction (Ma et al. 2009).

AMD 3100 is a small molecule antagonist of the CXCR4 receptor which competitively binds and prevents the interaction of the receptor with CXCl12 (Persio et al. 2009). The blockage of CXCR4 with AMD3100 has been shown to reduce peritoneal dissemination of epithelial ovarian carcinoma (Kajiyama et al. 2008). In a xenograft model of breast cancer, AMD3100 was shown to delay metastatic growth of breast cancer cells in the lung. In another model, the inhibition of CXCR4 by small interfering RNAi exhibited a substantial delay of growth in experimental lung metastasis (Smith et al. 2004). Another agent, plerixafor (Mozobil®; Genzyme Corp.), was recently proven to mobilize hematopoietic progenitor cells in combination with granulocyte colony-stimulating factor (GCSF) for patients with NHL or ML (Brave et al. 2010). Plerixafor is currently being investigated in clinical trials for the treatment of lymphoma and acute myelogenous leukemia.

A number of preclinical animal studies have shown the effects of peptide therapy against the CXCR4 –CXCL12 axis. TN14003 blocks the receptor by competing with its ligand CXCL12 and demonstrates efficacy in suppressing primary tumor growth in addition to inhibiting lung metastasis in an experimental head and neck cancer model (Yoon et al. 2007).

Another agent, CTCE-9908, which is a small peptide CXCR4 antagonist was proven to inhibit the CXCR4/CXCL12 pathway and to decrease the metastatic burden in xenograft tumors. This demonstrated the potential for CTCE-9908 as adjuvant therapy for metastatic disease (Wong and Korz 2008; Porvasnik et al. 2009; Richert et al. 2009; Kim et al. 2008; Huang et al. 2009b). CTCE-9908 was well tolerated and revealed preliminary signs of efficacy with no dose-limiting toxicities in a phase I/II clinical trial in patients with advanced solid tumors (Hotte et al. 2008). It is currently under evaluation in HCC in combination with trans-arterial chemo-embolization.

28.4 Metastatic Progression and Colonization

Metastatic progression genes are characterized by specific functions that allow the tumor cells to infiltrate and colonize distant organs. They could be expressed in primary tumors involved in metastatic initiation and be included in gene signatures that correlate a primary tumor with metastatic dissemination at a secondary site. Examples include TGF-β induced expression of angiopoietin-like 4 (*ANGPTL4*) which disrupts endothelial contacts in lung capillaries (Padua et al. 2008), lysyl oxidase roles in establishing a metastatic niche and epiregulin and MMP1and MMP2 roles in tumor remodeling and extravasation (Gupta et al. 2007). Multiple therapeutic strategies targeting IGF-1R, c-Met, TGF-β, Src, stem cells and metastatic suppressor genes will be relevant for metastatic progression.

28.4.1 MMPs

MMPs are a family of zinc-dependent proteinases which mediate growth regulatory signals, apoptosis induction, and angiogenic switch during carcinogenesis (Bergers et al. 2000; Kessenbrock et al. 2010). Over-expression of MMPs in cancer causes EMT and induces genomic instability (Egeblad and Werb 2002). They are implicated in the degradation of the extracellular matrix (ECM) and loss of junctional contact between tumor cells, thus promoting their detachment from the primary tumor site (Egeblad and Werb 2002). Increased evidence links MMP-mediated signal transduction to the migration and invasion of metastatic tumor cells (Baker et al. 2001; Friedl and Wolf 2008). In a variety of malignancies, MMP-1 activates the proteolytic cleavage of proteinase-activated receptors (PARs) resulting in increased metastasis (Kessenbrock et al. 2010). MMP-1 proteolytically engage EGF-like ligands, which in turn promotes osteolysis and metastasis to the bone. MMPs were identified in a set of genes resulting in activation of the RANKL pathway and bone or lung metastasis (Minn et al. 2005).

Due to their critical role in tumor growth, angiogenesis and metastasis, MMPs are considered promising therapeutic targets. In preclinical studies MMP- inhibitors were shown to suppress migration and the invasive potential of tumor cells. However, when evaluated in phase III clinical trials, they were not effective in increasing the survival rate of the patients and resulted in dose limiting toxicity (Coussens et al. 2002; Roy et al. 2009; Miller et al. 2004; Hirte et al. 2006).

Other agents under investigation are the peptide-mimetic derivatives (Dublanchet et al. 2005), the gelatinase inhibitors (Krüger et al. 2005) and the small-molecule inhibitors of ADAM proteases (Fridman et al. 2007). MMPs play an important role in tissue remodeling. MMP-1 and MMP-7 were shown to be implicated in the activation of the RANKL (Receptor Activator for Nuclear Factor κB Ligand) pathway, which mediates osteolysis and metastatic dissemination to the bones (Kang et al. 2003). A better understanding of the structure of MMPs and their mode of action will challenge future research in designing additional potent inhibitors (Roy et al. 2009; Cuniasse et al. 2005).

Key points

- Recent advances in genetics, molecular biology and molecular pharmacology have enabled the development of molecular targeted agents
- These novel therapeutic strategies include agents designed to specifically interfere with molecular mechanisms responsible for the malignant phenotype
- Multiple oncogenic pathways functionally disrupted in primary tumors, could be targeted resulting in antiproliferative, anti-invasive and apoptotic effects
- Targeting molecular pathways involved in processes such as angiogenesis, invasion, EMT program and colonization constitute a promising therapeutic approach for metastatic disease
- Targeted agents can be used in combination therapies and may reduce the secondary effects associated with the use of cytotoxic drugs
- There is a need to identify pharmacodynamic markers of drug response and predictive biological markers that enable selection of patients most likely to benefit from targeted therapy

28.5 Summary

The progression to metastatic disease can be a devastating transition in the course of cancer patients. Despite early diagnosis and management of the primary tumor overall mortality rate remains high with metastasis.

In general, the limited therapeutic options available for metastatic disease have minimal efficacy. Therapeutic options that address localized metastatic disease such as surgical resection, regional chemotherapy and chemo-embolization, have failed to show significant improvement in metastatic disease-associated mortality. Systemic chemotherapy has also failed in providing any major influence on survival. This is due to the high resistance to chemotherapeutic agents in various metastatic diseases. These challenges in the management of metastasis have led to the shift towards more targeted therapy. The basis for targeted therapy originated from investigations into the molecular mechanisms that allow the tumor cells to successfully metastasize. These monumental studies have led to the identification of several therapeutic targets involved in apoptosis, proliferation, angiogenesis, invasion and metastasis.

The detection of over-expression of specific molecular targets could biologically predict the aggressive behavior of tumor cells and may provide beneficial information with regard to tumor sensitivity to targeted therapy. Novel techniques including genomics and proteomics have the potential to define better targets in tumors and improve the ability to predict whether certain tumor types or individual patients are particularly sensitive or more resistant to therapy. These techniques could allow for the simultaneous evaluation of samples from an individual patient for the presence of specific targets and evidence of therapeutic activity after the inhibition of a specific target.

The pathways that have been evaluated for the purposes of targeted therapy include Rb, p53, c-Kit, c-Met, VEGF, E-cadherin, HIF-1α, EGFR, NFKB, MMP2, RAS–MAPK and PI3K–Akt pathways. There are also a host of other molecular pathways mentioned in earlier chapters that could potentially be targeted. There are several ongoing clinical trials investigating the use of targeted therapeutic agents alone or in combination with systemic chemotherapy in an effort to delay tumor progression and to potentially arrest metastatic disease. These drugs have been shown to affect signal transduction, cell-cycle control as well as apoptotic processes and may in actuality result in a reduction of the migratory and invasive capacity of the tumor cells.

In this section we have outlined the various therapeutic options for the treatment of metastatic disease. Targeted therapy may potentially provide more viable management options in this patient population. A better understanding of the role of biological targets in the metastatic cascade is essential to the overall progress towards an improvement in the care of patients with metastatic disease.

References

Aboody KS, Najbauer J, Danks MK (2008) Stem and progenitor cell-mediated tumor selective gene therapy. Gene Ther 15:739–752

Adjei AA, Cohen RB, Kurzrock R, Gordon GS, Hangauer D, Dyster L, Fetterly G, Barrientes S, Hong DS, Naing A (2009) Results of a phase I trial of KX2–391, a novel non-ATP competitive substrate-pocket directed SRC inhibitor, in patients with advanced malignancies. in ASCO J Clin Oncol 27:15s (suppl; abstr 3511)

Aggarwal BB et al (2005) Curcumin suppresses the paclitaxel-induced nuclear factor-κB pathway in breast cancer cells and inhibits lung metastasis of human breast cancer in nude mice. Clin Cancer Res 11:7490–7498

Aghajanian C et al (2005) Phase I trial of bortezomib and carboplatin in recurrent ovarian or primary peritoneal cancer. J Clin Oncol 23:5943–5949

Al-Hajj M, Wicha MS, Benito-Hernandez A, Morrison SJ, Clarke MF (2003) Prospective identification of tumorigenic breast cancer cells. Proc Natl Acad Sci U S A 100:3983–3988

Alonso L, Fuchs E (2003) Stem cells of the skin epithelium. Proc Natl Acad Sci U S A 100(Suppl 1):11830–11835

Baker JK et al (2001) Expression of integrins, degradative enzymes and their inhibitors in uveal melanoma: differences between in vitro and in vivo expression. Melanoma Res 11:265–273

Baldwin AS (2001) Control of oncogenesis and cancer therapy resistance by the transcription factor NF-kappa B. J Clin Invest 107:241–246

Balkwill F (2004) Cancer and the chemokine network. Nat Rev Cancer 4:540–550

Barker N, Clevers H (2006) Mining the Wnt pathway for cancer therapeutics. Nat Rev Drug Discov 5:997–1014

Basseres DS, Baldwin AS (2006) Nuclear factor-[kappa]B and inhibitor of [kappa]B kinase pathways in oncogenic initiation and progression. Oncogene 25:6817–6830

Bauerschmitz GJ et al (2008) Tissue-specific promoters active in CD44+CD24-/low breast cancer cells. Cancer Res 68:5533–5539

Belperio JA et al (2004) The SDF-1/CXCL 12/CXCR4 biological axis in non-small cell lung cancer metastases. Chest 125:156S

Bergers G, Benjamin LE (2003) Tumorigenesis and the angiogenic switch. Nat Rev Cancer 3:401–410

Bergers G et al (2000) Matrix metalloproteinase-9 triggers the angiogenic switch during carcinogenesis. Nat Cell Biol 2:737–744

Bhardwaj A et al (2007) Resveratrol inhibits proliferation, induces apoptosis, and overcomes chemoresistance through down-regulation of STAT3 and nuclear factor-{kappa}B-regulated antiapoptotic and cell survival gene products in human multiple myeloma cells. Blood 109:2293–2302

Bhaumik D et al (2008) Expression of microRNA-146 suppresses NF-kappaB activity with reduction of metastatic potential in breast cancer cells. Oncogene 27:5643–5647

Birchmeier C, Birchmeier W, Gherardi E, Vande Woude GF (2003) Met, metastasis, motility and more. Nat Rev Mol Cell Biol 4:915–925

Borbath I, Santoro A, Van Laethem J, Daniele B, Cicalese L, Zeuzem S, Buggish P, Bolondi L, Strosberg JR, Abbadessa G (2010) ARQ 197–215: a randomized, placebo-controlled phase II clinical trial evaluating the c-Met inhibitor, ARQ 197, in patients (pts) with hepatocellular carcinoma (HCC). J Clin Oncol 28:15s (suppl; abstr TPS215)

Brabletz T, Jung A, Spaderna S, Hlubek F, Kirchner T (2005) Migrating cancer stem cells [mdash] an integrated concept of malignant tumour progression. Nat Rev Cancer 5:744–749

Brave M et al (2010) FDA review summary: mozobil in combination with granulocyte colony-stimulating factor to mobilize hematopoietic stem cells to the peripheral blood for collection and subsequent autologous transplantation. Oncology 78:282–288

Buchanan SG et al (2009) SGX523 is an exquisitely selective, ATP-competitive inhibitor of the MET receptor tyrosine kinase with antitumor activity in vivo. Mol Cancer Ther 8:3181–3190

Bukowski RM, Yasothan U, Kirkpatrick P (2010) Pazopanib. Nat Rev Drug Discov 9:17–18

Burger RA, Sill MW, Monk BJ, Greer BE, Sorosky JI (2007) Phase II trial of bevacizumab in persistent or recurrent epithelial ovarian cancer or primary peritoneal cancer: a gynecologic oncology group study. J Clin Oncol 25:5165–5171

Calvo-Aller E, Baselga J, Glatt S, Cleverly A, Lahn M, Arteaga CL, Rothenberg ML, Carducci MA (2008) First human dose escalation study in patients with metastatic malignancies to determine safety and pharmacokinetics of LY2157299, a small molecule inhibitor of the transforming growth factor-beta receptor I kinase. J Clin Oncol 26:2008 (May 20 suppl; abstr 14554)

Camidge DR (2006) A phase I dose-escalation study of weekly IMC-1121B, a fully human anti-vascular endothelial growth factor receptor 2 (VEGFR2) IgG1 monoclonal antibody (Mab), in patients (pts) with advanced cancer [abstract]. ASCO Meeting Abstracts 24:3032

Cannistra SA (2007) Phase II study of bevacizumab in patients with platinum-resistant ovarian cancer or peritoneal serous cancer. J Clin Oncol 25:5180–5186

Carmeliet P, Jain RK (2000) Angiogenesis in cancer and other diseases. Nature 407:249–257

Carter Van W et al (2005) Inhibition of nuclear factor-κB and target genes during combined therapy with proteasome inhibitor bortezomib and reirradiation in patients with recurrent head-and-neck squamous cell carcinoma. Int J Radiat Oncol Biol Phys 63:1400–1412

Castellone MD, Teramoto H, Williams BO, Druey KM, Gutkind JS (2005) Prostaglandin E-2 promotes colon cancer cell growth through a G(s)-axin-beta-catenin signaling axis. Science 310:1504–1510

Chen B et al (2009) Small molecule-mediated disruption of Wnt-dependent signaling in tissue regeneration and cancer. Nat Chem Biol 5:100–107
Chiang AC, Massagué J (2008) Molecular basis of metastasis. N Engl J Med 359:2814–2823
Chung AS, Lee J, Ferrara N (2010) Targeting the tumour vasculature: insights from physiological angiogenesis. Nat Rev Cancer 10:505–514
Cooper MK, Porter JA, Young KE, Beachy PA (1998) Teratogen-mediated inhibition of target tissue response to Shh signaling. Science 280:1603–1607
Coussens LM, Fingleton B, Matrisian LM (2002) Matrix metalloproteinase inhibitors and cancer–trials and tribulations. Science 295:2387–2392
Cuniasse P et al (2005) Future challenges facing the development of specific active-site-directed synthetic inhibitors of MMPs. Biochimie 87:393–402
Dai T (2009) Notch signaling and cancer Cancer Res 2009:71–79
Davis NB et al (2004) Phase II trial of PS-341 in patients with renal cell cancer: a university of chicago phase II consortium study. J Clin Oncol 22:115–119
Davies AM et al (2009) Bortezomib plus gemcitabine/carboplatin as first-line treatment of advanced non-small cell lung cancer: a phase II southwest oncology group study (S0339). J Thorac Oncol 4:87–92.10.1097/JTO.1090b1013e3181915052
DeAlmeida VI et al (2007) The soluble Wnt receptor Frizzled8CRD-hFc inhibits the growth of teratocarcinomas in vivo. Cancer Res 67:5371–5379
de Vries TJ et al (2009) The Src inhibitor AZD0530 reversibly inhibits the formation and activity of human osteoclasts. Mol Cancer Res 7:476–488
Derynck R, Akhurst RJ, Balmain A (2001) TGF-beta signaling in tumor suppression and cancer progression. Nat Genet 29:117–129
di Magliano MP, Hebrok M (2003) Hedgehog signalling in cancer formation and maintenance. Nat Rev Cancer 3:903–911
Diamond S et al (2010) Species-specific metabolism of SGX523 by aldehyde oxidase and the toxicological implications. Drug Metab Dispos 38:1277–1285
DiPersio JF, Uy GL, Yasothan U, Kirkpatrick P (2009) Plerixafor. Nat Rev Drug Discov 8:105–107
Dublanchet A-C et al (2005) Structure-based design and synthesis of novel non-zinc chelating MMP-12 inhibitors. Bioorg Med Chem Lett 15:3787–3790
Eccles SA (2004) Parallels in invasion and angiogenesis provide pivotal points for therapeutic intervention. Int J Dev Biol 48:583–598
Eder JP, Vande Woude GF, Boerner SA, LoRusso PM (2009) Novel therapeutic inhibitors of the c-met signaling pathway in cancer. Clin Cancer Res 15:2207–2214
Egeblad M, Werb Z (2002) New functions for the matrix metalloproteinases in cancer progression. Nat Rev Cancer 2:161–174
Emami KH et al (2004) A small molecule inhibitor of β-catenin/cyclic AMP response element-binding protein transcription. Proc Natl Acad Sci U S A 101:12682–12687
Ewan K et al (2010) A useful approach to identify novel small-molecule inhibitors of Wnt-dependent transcription. Cancer Res 70:5963–5973
Feldmann G et al (2008) An orally bioavailable small-molecule inhibitor of hedgehog signaling inhibits tumor initiation and metastasis in pancreatic cancer. Mol Cancer Ther 7:2725–2735
Fernandis AZ, Prasad A, Band H, Klosel R, Ganju RK (2004) Regulation of CXCR4-mediated chemotaxis and chemoinvasion of breast cancer cells. Oncogene 23:157–167
Ferrara N (2004) Vascular endothelial growth factor: basic science and clinical progress. Endocr Rev 25:581–611
Ferrara N, Kerbel RS (2005) Angiogenesis as a therapeutic target. Nature 438:967–974
Fodde R, Brabletz T (2007) Wnt/[beta]-catenin signaling in cancer stemness and malignant behavior. Curr Opin Cell Biol 19:150–158
Fridman JS et al (2007) Selective inhibition of ADAM metalloproteases as a novel approach for modulating ErbB pathways in cancer. Clin Cancer Res 13:1892–1902
Friedl P, Wolf K (2008) Tube travel: the role of proteases in individual and collective cancer cell invasion. Cancer Res 68:7247–7249

Ganapathy V et al (2010) Targeting the transforming growth factor-beta pathway inhibits human basal-like breast cancer metastasis. Mol Cancer 9:122

Garcia A, Rosen L, Cunningham CC, Nemunaitis J, Li C, Rulewski N, Dovholuk A, Savage R, Chan T, Bukowksi R, Mekhail T (2007) Phase 1 study of ARQ 197, a selective inhibitor of the c-Met RTK in patients with metastatic solid tumors reaches recommended phase 2 dose. in ASCO 2007 J Clin Oncol ASCO Annual meeting proceedings part I. 25:18S (June 20 Supplement, 2007: 3525, 2007)

Gerber HP, Ferrara N (2005) Pharmacology and pharmacodynamics of bevacizumab as monotherapy or in combination with cytotoxic therapy in preclinical studies. Cancer Res 65:671–680

Giantonio BJ (2007) Bevacizumab in combination with oxaliplatin, fluorouracil, and leucovorin (FOLFOX4) for previously treated metastatic colorectal cancer: results from the eastern cooperative oncology group study E3200. J Clin Oncol 25:1539–1544

Giles RH, van Es JH, Clevers H (2003) Caught up in a Wnt storm: Wnt signaling in cancer. Biochim Biophys Acta 1653:1–24

Giles FJ, O'Dwyer M, Swords R (2009) Class effects of tyrosine kinase inhibitors in the treatment of chronic myeloid leukemia. Leukemia 23:1698–1707

Gilmore TD, Herscovitch M (2006) Inhibitors of NF-kappaB signaling: 785 and counting. Oncogene 25:6887–6899

Grothey A, Galanis E (2009) Targeting angiogenesis: progress with anti-VEGF treatment with large molecules. Nat Rev Clin Oncol 6:507–518

Guarino M (2010) Src signaling in cancer invasion. J Cell Physiol 223:14–26

Gupta GP et al (2007) Mediators of vascular remodelling co-opted for sequential steps in lung metastasis. Nature 446:765–U762

Hau P, Jachimczak P, Bogdahn U (2009) Treatment of malignant gliomas with TGF-β2 antisense oligonucleotides. Expert Rev Anticancer Ther 9:1663–1674

Herbst RS et al (2010) Vandetanib plus docetaxel versus docetaxel as second-line treatment for patients with advanced non-small-cell lung cancer (ZODIAC): a double-blind, randomised, phase 3 trial. Lancet Oncol 11:619–626

Herbst RS, Sandler A (2008) Bevacizumab and erlotinib: a promising new approach to the treatment of advanced NSCLC. Oncologist 13:1166–1176

Hirte H et al (2006) A phase III randomized trial of BAY 12–9566 (tanomastat) as maintenance therapy in patients with advanced ovarian cancer responsive to primary surgery and paclitaxel/platinum containing chemotherapy: a national cancer institute of canada clinical trials group study. Gynecol Oncol 102:300–308

Hotte SJ, Hirte HW, Moretto P (2008) Final results of a phase I/II study of CTCE-9908, a novel anticancer agent that inhibits CXCR4, in patients with advanced solid cancers. in 20th EORTC–NCI–AACR Symposium on molecular targets and cancer therapeutics EUR J Cancer, Geneva, Switzerland, 2008

Hu J et al (2009) Blockade of Wnt signaling inhibits angiogenesis and tumor growth in hepatocellular carcinoma. Cancer Res 69:6951–6959

Huang S, Pettaway CA, Uehara H, Bucana CD, Fidler IJ (2001) Blockade of NF-kappaB activity in human prostate cancer cells is associated with suppression of angiogenesis, invasion, and metastasis. Oncogene 20:4188–4197

Huang S-MA et al (2009a) Tankyrase inhibition stabilizes axin and antagonizes Wnt signalling. Nature 461:614–620

Huang EH et al (2009b) A CXCR4 antagonist CTCE-9908 inhibits primary tumor growth and metastasis of breast cancer. J Surg Res 155:231–236

Huber MA et al (2004) NF-kappa B is essential for epithelial-mesenchymal transition and metastasis in a model of breast cancer progression. J Clin Invest 114:569–581

Huber MA, Kraut N, Beug H (2005) Molecular requirements for epithelial-mesenchymal transition during tumor progression. Curr Opin Cell Biol 17:548–558

Hu-Lowe DD et al (2008) Nonclinical antiangiogenesis and antitumor activities of axitinib (AG-013736), an oral, potent, and selective inhibitor of vascular endothelial growth factor receptor tyrosine kinases 1, 2, 3. Clin Cancer Res 14:7272–7283

Hurwitz H et al (2004) Bevacizumab plus irinotecan, fluorouracil, and leucovorin for metastatic colorectal cancer. N Engl J Med 350:2335–2342

Iwatsuki M et al (2010) Epithelial–mesenchymal transition in cancer development and its clinical significance. Cancer Science 101:293–299

Izumi Y, Xu L, di Tomaso E, Fukumura D, Jain RK (2002) Tumour biology: herceptin acts as an anti-angiogenic cocktail. Nature 416:279–280

Jain RK (2005) Normalization of tumor vasculature: an emerging concept in antiangiogenic therapy. Science 307:58–62

Jain RK (2009) Biomarkers of response and resistance to antiangiogenic therapy. Nat Rev Clin Oncol 6:327–338

Jain RK, Duda DG, Clark JW, Loeffler JS (2006) Lessons from phase III clinical trials on anti-VEGF therapy for cancer. Nat Clin Prac Oncol 3:24–40

Janne PA et al (2007) Multicenter, randomized, phase II trial of CI-1033, an irreversible pan-ERBB inhibitor, for previously treated advanced non small-cell lung cancer. J Clin Oncol 25:3936–3944

Jayson GC (2005) Phase I investigation of recombinant anti-human vascular endothelial growth factor antibody in patients with advanced cancer. Eur J Cancer 41:555–563

Jin L, Hope KJ, Zhai Q, Smadja-Joffe F, Dick JE (2006) Targeting of CD44 eradicates human acute myeloid leukemic stem cells. Nat Med 12:1167–1174

Jun HT et al (2007) AMG 102, A fully human anti-hepatocyte growth factor/scatter factor neutralizing antibody, enhances the efficacy of temozolomide or docetaxel in U-87 MG cells and xenografts. Clin Cancer Res 13:6735–6742

Kajiyama H et al (2008) Involvement of SDF-1alpha/CXCR4 axis in the enhanced peritoneal metastasis of epithelial ovarian carcinoma. Int J Cancer 122:91–99

Kang Y et al (2003) A multigenic program mediating breast cancer metastasis to bone. Cancer Cell 3:537–549

Kerbel RS (2008) Tumor angiogenesis. N Engl J Med 358:2039–2049

Kessenbrock K, Plaks V, Werb Z (2010) Matrix metalloproteinases: regulators of the tumor microenvironment. Cell 141:52–67

Kim KJ et al (1993) Inhibition of vascular endothelial growth factor-induced angiogenesis suppresses tumour growth in vivo. Nature 362:841–844

Kim SY et al (2008) Inhibition of the CXCR4/CXCL12 chemokine pathway reduces the development of murine pulmonary metastases. Clin Exp Metastasis 25:201–211

Krüger A et al (2005) Antimetastatic activity of a novel mechanism-based gelatinase inhibitor. Cancer Res 65:3523–3526

Krutzfeldt J et al (2005) Silencing of microRNAs in vivo with 'antagomirs'. Nature 438:685–689

Lang L (2008) FDA approves sorafenib for patients with inoperable liver cancer. Gastroenterology 134:379

Li Y et al (2003) Evidence that transgenes encoding components of the Wnt signaling pathway preferentially induce mammary cancers from progenitor cells. Proc Natl Acad Sci U S A 100:15853–15858

Li Y et al (2005) Inactivation of nuclear factor κB by soy isoflavone genistein contributes to increased apoptosis induced by chemotherapeutic agents in human cancer cells. Cancer Res 65:6934–6942

Liao D, Johnson R (2007) Hypoxia: a key regulator of angiogenesis in cancer. Cancer Metastasis Rev 26:281–290

Limvorasak S, Posadas EM (2009) Pazopanib: therapeutic developments. Expert Opin Pharmacother 10:3091–3102

Los M, Roodhart JML, Voest EE (2007) Target practice: lessons from phase III trials with bevacizumab and vatalanib in the treatment of advanced colorectal cancer. Oncologist 12:443–450

Low JA, de Sauvage FJ (2010) Clinical experience with hedgehog pathway inhibitors. J Clin Oncol 28:5321–5326

Luo J et al (2007) Wnt signaling and human diseases: what are the therapeutic implications? Lab Invest 87:97–103

Ma W-F et al (2009) Phenotypic knockout of CXCR4 by a novel recombinant protein TAT/54R/KDEL inhibits tumors metastasis. Mol Cancer Res 7:1613–1621

Mackay H et al (2005) A phase II trial with pharmacodynamic endpoints of the proteasome inhibitor bortezomib in patients with metastatic colorectal cancer. Clin Cancer Res 11:5526–5533

Mani SA et al (2008) The epithelial-mesenchymal transition generates cells with properties of stem cells. Cell 133:704–715

Mantovani A (2010) Molecular pathways linking inflammation and cancer. Curr Mol Med 10:369–373

Markovic SN et al (2005) A phase II study of bortezomib in the treatment of metastatic malignant melanoma. Cancer 103:2584–2589

Melisi D et al (2008) LY2109761, a novel transforming growth factor β receptor type I and type II dual inhibitor, as a therapeutic approach to suppressing pancreatic cancer metastasis. Mol Cancer Ther 7:829–840

Migliore C, Giordano S (2008) Molecular cancer therapy: can our expectation be MET? Eur J Cancer 44:641–651

Miller K (2007) Paclitaxel plus bevacizumab versus paclitaxel alone for metastatic breast cancer. N Engl J Med 357:2666–2676

Miller KD et al (2004) A randomized phase II feasibility trial of BMS-275291 in patients with early stage breast cancer. Clin Cancer Res 10:1971–1975

Minn AJ et al (2005) Distinct organ-specific metastatic potential of individual breast cancer cells and primary tumors. J Clin Invest 115:44–55

Mita MM et al (2009) A phase Ib dose-escalation study of orally administered MP-470, a multi-kinase inhibitor and supressor of Rad51, in combination with carboplatin doublet containing regimens shows activity in highly refractory solid tumor patients. J Clin Oncol (Meeting Abstracts) 27:e13511

Morabito A et al (2009) Vandetanib (ZD6474), a dual inhibitor of vascular endothelial growth factor receptor (VEGFR) and epidermal growth factor receptor (EGFR) tyrosine kinases: current status and future directions. Oncologist 14:378–390

Morin MJ (2000) From oncogene to drug: development of small molecule tyrosine kinase inhibitors as anti-tumor and anti-angiogenic agents. Oncogene 19:6574–6583

Morris JC et al (2008) Phase I/II study of GC1008: a human anti-transforming growth factor-beta (TGF{beta}) monoclonal antibody (MAb) in patients with advanced malignant melanoma (MM) or renal cell carcinoma (RCC). J Clin Oncol (Meeting Abstracts) 26:9028

Moy B, Kirkpatrick P, Kar S, Goss P (2007) Lapatinib. Nat Rev Drug Discov 6:431–432

Muller A et al (2001) Involvement of chemokine receptors in breast cancer metastasis. Nature 410:50–56

O/'Brien CA, Pollett A, Gallinger S, Dick JE (2007) A human colon cancer cell capable of initiating tumour growth in immunodeficient mice. Nature 445:106–110

Olmeda D, Jorda M, Peinado H, Fabra A, Cano A (2006) Snail silencing effectively suppresses tumour growth and invasiveness. Oncogene 26:1862–1874

Onder TT et al (2008) Loss of e-cadherin promotes metastasis via multiple downstream transcriptional pathways. Cancer Res 68:3645–3654

Padua D, Massague J (2009) Roles of TGF[beta] in metastasis. Cell Res 19:89–102

Padua D et al (2008) TGF[beta] primes breast tumors for lung metastasis seeding through angiopoietin-like 4. Cell 133:66–77

Pan J et al (2006) Stromal derived factor-1 (SDF-1/CXCL12) and CXCR4 in renal cell carcinoma metastasis. Mol Cancer 5:56

Papandreou CN et al (2004) Phase I trial of the proteasome inhibitor bortezomib in patients with advanced solid tumors with observations in androgen-independent prostate cancer. J Clin Oncol 22:2108–2121

Payne AS, Cornelius LA (2002) The role of chemokines in melanoma tumor growth and metastasis. J Invest Dermatol 118:915–922

Peukert S, Miller-Moslin K (2010) Small-molecule inhibitors of the hedgehog signaling pathway as cancer therapeutics. Chem Med Chem 5:500–512

Porvasnik S et al (2009) Effects of CXCR4 antagonist CTCE-9908 on prostate tumor growth. The Prostate 69:1460–1469

Qian F et al (2009) Inhibition of tumor cell growth, invasion, and metastasis by EXEL-2880 (XL880, GSK1363089), a novel inhibitor of HGF and VEGF receptor tyrosine kinases. Cancer Res 69:8009–8016

Rabbani SA, Valentino M-L, Arakelian A, Ali S, Boschelli F (2010) SKI-606 (Bosutinib) Blocks prostate cancer invasion, growth, and metastasis in vitro and in vivo through regulation of genes involved in cancer growth and skeletal metastasis. Mol Cancer Ther9:1147–1157

Reya T, Clevers H (2005) Wnt signalling in stem cells and cancer. Nature 434:843–850

Richardson PG, Hideshima T, Mitsiades C, Anderson K (2004) Proteasome inhibition in hematologic malignancies. Ann Med 36:304–314

Richardson PG et al (2010) Tanespimycin monotherapy in relapsed multiple myeloma: results of a phase 1 dose-escalation study. Br J Haematol 150:438–445

Richert MM et al (2009) Inhibition of CXCR4 by CTCE-9908 inhibits breast cancer metastasis to lung and bone. Oncol Rep 21:761–767

Rixe O (2006) Safety and pharmacokinetics of intravenous VEGF trap plus irinotecan, 5-fluorouracil, and leucovorin (I-LV5FU2) in a combination phase I clinical trial of patients with advanced solid tumors [abstract]. ASCO Meeting Abstracts 24:13161

Rixe O et al (2007) Axitinib treatment in patients with cytokine-refractory metastatic renal-cell cancer: a phase II study. Lancet Oncol 8:975–984

Rosen PJ et al (2010) A phase Ib study of AMG 102 in combination with bevacizumab or motesanib in patients with advanced solid tumors. Clin Cancer Res 16:2677–2687

Roy R, Yang J, Moses MA (2009) Matrix metalloproteinases as novel biomarker s and potential therapeutic targets in human cancer. J Clin Oncol 27:5287–5297

Ruiz i Altaba A, Sanchez P, Dahmane N (2002) Gli and hedgehog in cancer: tumours, embryos and stem cells. Nat Rev Cancer 2:361–372

Sandler A (2006) Paclitaxel-carboplatin alone or with bevacizumab for non-small-cell lung cancer. N Engl J Med 355:2542–2550

Scagliotti G, Govindan R (2010) Targeting angiogenesis with multitargeted tyrosine kinase inhibitors in the treatment of non-small cell lung cancer. Oncologist 15:436–446

Schiller JH et al (2009) Efficacy and safety of axitinib in patients with advanced non-small-cell lung cancer: results from a phase II study. J Clin Oncol 27:3836–3841

Schiller JH, Akerley WL, Brugger W, Ferrari D, Garmey EG, Gerber DE, Orlov SV, Ramlau R, Von Pawel J, Sequist LV (2010) Results from ARQ 197–209: a global randomized placebo-controlled phase II clinical trial of erlotinib plus ARQ 197 versus erlotinib plus placebo in previously treated EGFR inhibitor-naive patients with locally advanced or metastatic non-small cell lung cancer (NSCLC). J Clin Oncol 28:18s (suppl; abstr LBA7502)

Schlingensiepen KH et al (2006) Targeted tumor therapy with the TGF-[beta]2 antisense compound AP 12009. Cytokine Growth Factor Rev 17:129–139

Schlingensiepen KH, Fischer-Blass B, Schmaus S, Ludwig S (2008) Antisense therapeutics for tumor treatment: the TGF-beta2 inhibitor AP 12009 in clinical development against malignant tumors. Recent Results Cancer Res 177:137–150

Scott EN, Meinhardt G, Jacques C, Laurent D, Thomas AL (2007) Vatalanib: the clinical development of a tyrosine kinase inhibitor of angiogenesis in solid tumours. Expert Opin Investig Drugs 16:367–379

Shen HM, Tergaonkar V (2009) NFκB signaling in carcinogenesis and as a potential molecular target for cancer therapy. Apoptosis 14:348–363

Sherman SI (2009) Advances in chemotherapy of differentiated epithelial and medullary thyroid cancers. J Clin Endocrinol Metab 94:1493–1499

Smith MCP et al (2004) CXCR4 Regulates growth of both primary and metastatic breast cancer. Cancer Res 64:8604–8612
Sonpavde G, Hutson TE (2007) Pazopanib: a novel multitargeted tyrosine kinase inhibitor. Curr Oncol Rep 9:115–119
Stegmeier F, Warmuth M, Sellers WR, Dorsch M (2010) Targeted cancer therapies in the twenty-first century: lessons from imatinib. Clin Pharmacol Ther 87:543–552
Sternberg CN et al (2010) Pazopanib in locally advanced or metastatic renal cell carcinoma: results of a randomized phase III trial. J Clin Oncol 28:1061–1068
Sukhdeo K et al (2007) Targeting the beta-catenin/TCF transcriptional complex in the treatment of multiple myeloma. Proc Natl Acad Sci U S A 104:7516–7521
Sun YX et al (2005) Skeletal localization and neutralization of the SDF-1(CXCL12)/CXCR4 axis blocks prostate cancer metastasis and growth in osseous sites in vivo. J Bone Miner Res 20:318–329
Sweeney CJ et al (2005) The sesquiterpene lactone parthenolide in combination with docetaxel reduces metastasis and improves survival in a xenograft model of breast cancer. Mol Cancer Ther 4:1004–1012
Tabernero J, Cervantes A, Hoekman K, Hurwitz HI, Jodrell DI, Hamberg P, Stuart M, Green TP, Iacona RB, Baselga J (2007) Phase I study of AZD0530, an oral potent inhibitor of Src kinase: first demonstration of inhibition of Src activity in human cancers. in ASCO
Takebe N, Harris PJ, Warren RQ, Ivy SP (2011) Targeting cancer stem cells by inhibiting wnt, notch, and hedgehog pathways. Nat Rev Clin Oncol 8:97–106
Taldone T, Gozman A, Maharaj R, Chiosis G (2008) Targeting Hsp90: small-molecule inhibitors and their clinical development. Curr Opin Pharmacol 8:370–374
Tew WP (2008) VEGF-trap for patients with recurrent platinum-resistant epithelial ovarian cancer (EOC): preliminary results of a randomized, multicenter phase II study [abstract]. ASCO Meeting Abstracts 25:5508
Thiery JP (2002) Epithelial-mesenchymal transitions in tumour progression. Nat Rev Cancer 2:442–454
Tol J et al (2009) Chemotherapy, bevacizumab, and cetuximab in metastatic colorectal cancer. N Engl J Med 360:563–572
Tse JC, Kalluri R (2007) Mechanisms of metastasis: epithelial-to-mesenchymal transition and contribution of tumor microenvironment. J Cell Biochem 101:816–829
Vicari AP, Caux C (2002) Chemokines in cancer. Cytokine Growth Factor Rev 13:143–154
Von Hoff DD et al (2009) Inhibition of the hedgehog pathway in advanced basal-cell carcinoma. N Engl J Med 361:1164–1172
Voortman J et al (2007) A parallel dose-escalation study of weekly and twice-weekly bortezomib in combination with gemcitabine and cisplatin in the first-line treatment of patients with advanced solid tumors. Clin Cancer Res 13:3642–3651
Voulgari A, Pintzas A (2009) Epithelial-mesenchymal transition in cancer metastasis: Mechanisms, markers and strategies to overcome drug resistance in the clinic. Biochimica et Biophysica Acta (BBA) – Reviews on Cancer 1796:75–90
Vredenburgh JJ (2007) Bevacizumab plus irinotecan in recurrent glioblastoma multiforme. J Clin Oncol 25:4722–4729
Wen PY, Prados M, Schiff D, Reardon DA, Cloughesy T, Mikkelsen T, Batchelor T, Drappatz J, Chamberlain MC, De Groot JF (2010) Phase II study of XL184 (BMS 907351), an inhibitor of MET, VEGFR2, and RET, in patients (pts) with progressive glioblastoma (GB). J Clin Oncol 28:15s (suppl; abstr 2006)
Wong D, Korz W (2008) Translating an antagonist of chemokine receptor CXCR4: from bench to bedside. Clin Cancer Res 14:7975–7980
Yang CH et al (2006a) Bortezomib (VELCADE®) in metastatic breast cancer: pharmacodynamics, biological effects, and prediction of clinical benefits. Ann Oncol 17:813–817

Yang J, Amiri KI, Burke JR, Schmid JA, Richmond A (2006b) BMS-345541 targets inhibitor of κB kinase and induces apoptosis in melanoma: involvement of nuclear factor κB and mitochondria pathways. Clin Cancer Res 12:950–960

Yang JC (2003) A randomized trial of bevacizumab, an anti-vascular endothelial growth factor antibody, for metastatic renal cancer. N Engl J Med 349:427–434

Yemelyanov A et al (2005) Effects of IKK inhibitor PS1145 on NF-[kappa]B function, proliferation, apoptosis and invasion activity in prostate carcinoma cells. Oncogene 25:387–398

Yoon Y et al (2007) CXC Chemokine receptor-4 antagonist blocks both growth of primary tumor and metastasis of head and neck cancer in xenograft mouse models. Cancer Res 67:7518–7524

Zillhardt M, Christensen JG, Lengyel E (2010) An orally available small-molecule inhibitor of c-Met, PF-2341066, reduces tumor burden and metastasis in a preclinical model of ovarian cancer metastasis. Neoplasia 12:1–10

Zlotnik A, Yoshie O (2000) Chemokines: a new classification system and their role in immunity. Immunity 12:121–127

Zou HY et al (2007) An orally available small-molecule inhibitor of c-Met, PF-2341066, exhibits cytoreductive antitumor efficacy through antiproliferative and antiangiogenic mechanisms. Cancer Res 67:4408–4417

Index

J. V. Burnier, M. N. Burnier, Jr. (eds.), *Experimental and Clinical Metastasis*,
DOI 10.1007/978-1-4614-3685-0, © Springer Science+Business Media New York 2013

Printed by Printforce, the Netherlands